AF566866

The Multiply Injured Patient with Complex Fractures

The Multiply Injured Patient with Complex Fractures

MARVIN H. MEYERS, M.D.
Professor of Surgery
Division of Orthopaedic Surgery, Southwestern Medical School, Dallas, Texas

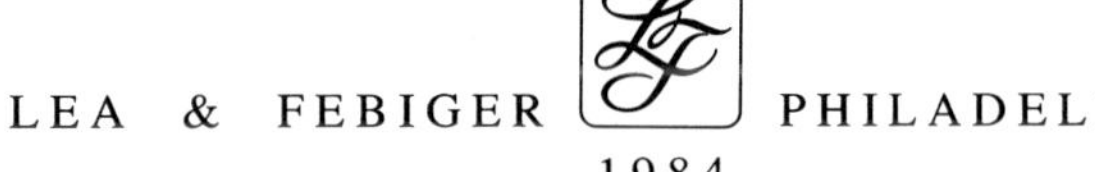

LEA & FEBIGER PHILADELPHIA
1984

LEA & FEBIGER
600 South Washington Square
Philadelphia, Pa. 19106
U.S.A.

Library of Congress Cataloging in Publication Data
Main entry under title:

The multiply injured patient with complex fractures.

Includes bibliographies and index.
1. Wounds and injuries. 2. Fractures. 3. Surgical emergencies. I. Meyers, Marvin H. [DNLM: 1. Fractures. 2. Wounds and injuries. W0 700 M961]
RD93.M84 1983 617'.1026 83-9333
ISBN 0-8121-0882-5

Copyright © 1984 by Lea & Febiger. Copyright under the International Copyright Union. All Rights Reserved. This book is protected by copyright. No part of it may be reproduced in any manner or by any means without written permission of the Publisher.

Printed in the United States of America

Print Number: 5 4 3 2 1

Preface

Management of the multiply injured patient has received increasing interest recently. There are few papers in the orthopaedic literature on this subject. A comprehensive reference book concerned with the treatment of the multiply injured patient with complex fractures is not available. Standard texts on the treatment of fractures contain some information but do not deal in depth with complex injuries of the skeletal system. Few papers have been published in scientific journals that deal with many of the subjects included in this book.

A severely injured patient often has several major body systems traumatized. As a consequence of trauma to the respiratory, vascular, and central nervous systems, the injuries may be life threatening. Therefore, the treating physician must have a plan that enables him to cope with the most serious injuries first to resuscitate the patient. After the patient has been stabilized, the surgeon can evaluate and repair other injuries in the order of their importance.

Management begins with the surgeon who assumes the responsibility for coordinating the efforts of the personnel in the emergency room. The surgeon who has the perspective to treat the patient as a whole is best qualified to take charge. Usually he has a special interest in traumatology. However, the presence of this uniquely qualified surgeon does not absolve other physicians or the orthopaedic surgeon from the obligation to understand the orderly management of the multiply injured patient. The orthopaedic surgeon frequently is the first or only physician available in the emergency room situation. The orthopaedic surgeon also plays a role in the initial assessment of the patient with musculoskeletal injuries and, thereby, contributes to the development of priorities. Frequently the care of other injured systems can be facilitated by temporarily casting or splinting fractures prior to surgical treatment of other systems.

The philosophy in treating some fractures changes from nonoperative to operative when there are multiple injuries. It is generally accepted that recumbency and prolonged bed rest are detrimental to pulmonary physiology, often resulting in death of the multiply injured patient. Early mobilization aids in preventing pulmonary complications and thus, is an urgent preventive measure for the polytrauma patient.

Concomitant ipsilateral extremity fractures are most often best treated by open reduction and internal fixation to mobilize major joints. Stiffness and contracture are common complications of prolonged immobilization in the presence of concomitant ipsilateral fractures, such as of the tibia, femur, and others. Each fracture by itself may be treated by closed methods. However, fractures in the multiply injured patient frequently require open surgery with internal or external fixation.

The need for early mobilization to prevent pulmonary complications and opting for open reduction and internal fixation when multiple bones are fractured are well covered in several chapters of this text. This book includes chapters on shock, the adult respiratory distress syndrome, compartment syndromes, vascular injuries, thoracic injuries, and embolic complications without which it would be incomplete. It was not the intent to cover every conceivable, rare, complex fracture or musculoskeletal injury in adults. The more common complex fractures and fracture combinations have received attention. Specific treatment and management plans discussed in this book may be controversial in some instances. The contributing authors have had considerable experience and frequently have a preferred treatment plan for specific injuries. It is recognized that satisfactory alternative methods may be the choice of other surgeons. Some alternative methods of treatment are discussed in addition to those favored by the authors. Recently, the realization that nutrition is severely impaired in the multiply injured patient has stimulated interest in this subject. Therefore, a chapter on the implications of nutritional deficits on the healing of multiple injuries has been included.

The goals of the text are: (1) To present an approach to the multiply injured patient and complex fractures which time has proved to be satisfactory. (2) To bring the knowledge and recent innovations in the treatment of many complex fractures up to date. (3) To discuss priorities in treating the multiply injured patient as well as orthopaedic priorities. (4) To provide a selected list of references to serve as a source for additional reading. (5) To provide a reference source for the physician and house officers involved in the acute care of the multiply injured patient with complex fractures. (6) To provide a detailed method of treatment for some of the more frequently encountered complex fractures.

In my opinion, this outstanding group of experienced physicians and surgeons have achieved the stated goals.

Dallas, Texas MARVIN H. MEYERS

Contributors

Robert G. Anderson, M. D.

Assistant Professor of Surgery, Division of Otolaryngology, Southwestern Medical School, University of Texas Health Science Center, Dallas, Texas.

Robert W. Bucholz, M. D.

Assistant Professor of Surgery, Division of Orthopedic Surgery, Southwestern Medical School, University of Texas Health Science Center, Dallas, Texas.

Henry M. Carder, M. D.

Clinical Professor of Surgery, Division of Otolaryngology, Southwestern Medical School, University of Texas Health Science Center, Dallas, Texas.

Michael W. Chapman, M. D.

Professor and Chairman, Department of Orthopedic Surgery, University of California School of Medicine at Davis, Davis, California.

Bernd F. Claudi, M. D.

Visiting Associate Professor of Surgery, Division of Orthopedic Surgery, Southwestern Medical School, University of Texas Health Science Center, Dallas, Texas.

McCollister C. Evarts, M. D.

Doris Carlson Hudgins Professor, Chairman, Department of Orthopedic Surgery, University of Rochester School of Medicine, Rochester, New York.

William J. Fry, M. D.

Lee Hudson—Robert R. Penn Professor, Professor and Chairman, Department of Surgery, Southwestern Medical School, University of Texas Health Science Center, Dallas, Texas.

Douglas E. Garland, M. D.

Chief, Head of Trauma and Problem Fracture Services, Rancho Los Amigos Hospital, Downey, California; Clinical Instructor, Department of Orthopedic Surgery, University of Southern California School of Medicine, Los Angeles, California.

Sigvard T. Hansen, M. D.

Professor and Chairman, Department of Orthopedic Surgery, University of Washington, Seattle, Washington.

M. T. Jenkins, M. D.

McDermott Professor, Department of Anaesthesiology, Southwestern Medical School, University of Texas Health Science Center, Dallas, Texas.

Richard E. Jones, M. D.

Associate Professor of Surgery, Division of Orthopedic Surgery, Southwestern Medical School, University of Texas Health Science Center, Dallas, Texas; Chief of Orthopedics, Veterans Administration Medical Center, Dallas, Texas.

MARVIN M. KIRSH, M. D.

Professor of Surgery, Section of Thoracic Surgery, University of Michigan School of Medicine, Ann Arbor, Michigan.

JEFFREY W. MAST, M. D.

Associate Professor of Orthopedics, Department of Surgery, University of Nevada School of Health Sciences, Reno, Nevada.

MARVIN H. MEYERS, M. D.

Professor of Surgery, Division of Orthopedic Surgery, Southwestern Medical School, University of Texas Health Science Center, Dallas, Texas.

BRIAN R. MILNE, M. D.

Visiting Assistant Professor, Department of Anaesthesiology, Southwestern Medical School, University of Texas Health Science Center, Dallas, Texas.

ROBY D. MIZE, M. D.

Clinical Instructor, Department of Surgery, Division of Orthopedic Surgery, Southwestern Medical School, University of Texas Health Science Center, Dallas, Texas.

SCOTT J. MUBARAK, M. D.

Assistant Professor of Surgery, Division of Orthopedic Surgery, University of California at San Diego, San Diego, California.

GEORGE E. OMER, JR., M. D.

Professor and Chairman, Department of Orthopedic Surgery and Rehabilitation, University of New Mexico School of Medicine, Albuquerque, New Mexico.

PAUL C. PETERS, M. D.

Professor of Surgery, Chairman, Division of Urology, Southwestern Medical School, University of Texas Health Science Center, Dallas, Texas.

MELVIN POST, M. D.

Chairman of Orthopedic Surgery, Michael Reese Hospital and Medical Center, Chicago, Illinois. Professor of Orthopedic Surgery, Rush Medical School, Chicago, Illinois.

DANIEL H. RAESS, M. D.

Resident, Department of Surgery, Southwestern Medical School, University of Texas Health Science Center, Dallas, Texas.

SIGURD C. SANDZÉN, M. D.

Clinical Associate Professor of Surgery, Division of Orthopedic Surgery, Southwestern Medical School, University of Texas Health Science Center, Dallas, Texas.

STEVEN D. SCHAEFER, M. D.

Assistant Professor of Surgery, Division of Otolaryngology, Southwestern Medical School, University of Texas Health Science Center, Dallas, Texas.

TAYLOR K. SMITH, M. D.

Professor and Chairman, Department of Orthopedic Surgery, University of Texas Health Science Center, Houston, Texas.

PHILLIP G. SPIEGEL, M. D.

Professor and Chairman, Department of Orthopedic Surgery, University of South Florida Medical Center, Tampa, Florida.

SHANNON E. STAUFFER, M. D.

Professor and Chairman, Department of Orthopedic Surgery and Rehabilitation, Southern Illinois University.

ERWIN THAL, M. D.

Associate Professor of Surgery, Southwestern Medical School, University of Texas Health Science Center, Dallas, Texas.

ROBERT L. WATERS, M. D.

Chief, Surgical Services, Rancho Los Amigos Hospital, Downey, California; Assistant Clinical Professor of Surgery, Department of Orthopedic Surgery, University of Southern California School of Medicine, Los Angeles, California.

JOHN A. WEIGELT, M. D.

Assistant Professor of Surgery, Southwestern Medical School, University of Texas Health Science Center, Dallas, Texas.

ROBERT A. WINQUIST, M. D.

Assistant Professor of Orthopedic Surgery, University of Washington, Seattle, Washington.

Contents

Chapter 1 3

Priorities in the Treatment of the Multiply Injured Patient with Musculoskeletal Injuries
BERND F. CLAUDI *and* MARVIN H. MEYERS

Chapter 2 9

Management of the Upper Airway in the Injured Patient
STEVEN D. SCHAEFER, ROBERT G. ANDERSON, *and* HENRY M. CARDER

Chapter 3 18

Management of NonPenetrating Chest Injuries
MARVIN M. KIRSH

Chapter 4 32

Early Recognition and Treatment of Shock
ERWIN THAL *and* DANIEL H. RAESS

Chapter 5 42

The Adult Respiratory Distress Syndrome
JOHN A. WEIGELT

Chapter 6 55

Urologic Assessment of the Multiply Injured Patient
PAUL C. PETERS

Chapter 7 67

The Fat Embolism Syndrome
C. McCOLLISTER EVARTS

Chapter 8 71

Recognition and Treatment of Compartment Syndromes
SCOTT M. MUBARAK

Chapter 9 90

Major Artery Trauma Associated with Fractures
WILLIAM J. FRY

Chapter 10 96

Anesthetic Considerations in the Multiply Injured Patient
BRIAN R. MILNE *and* M. T. JENKINS

Chapter 11 113

Open Fractures with Major Skin and Bone Defects
RICHARD E. JONES

Chapter 12 128

Recognition and Treatment of Nutritional Deficits in the Multiply Injured Patient
TAYLOR K. SMITH

Chapter 13 134

Extremity Fractures in Head Injured Adults
DOUGLAS E. GARLAND *and* ROBERT L. WATERS

Chapter 14 156

Fractures and Major Nerve Injuries in the Fractured Extremity
GEORGE E. OMER, JR.

Chapter 15 162

Fracture-Dislocations of the Lumbar Spine
E. SHANNON STAUFFER

Chapter 16 179

Fracture-Dislocations of the Cervical Spine
ROBERT W. BUCHOLZ

Chapter 17 196

Complex Fractures of the Pelvis
ROBERT W. BUCHOLZ *and* BERND F. CLAUDI

Chapter 18 210

Concomitant Ipsilateral Fractures of the Hip and Femur
MICHAEL W. CHAPMAN

Chapter 19 218
Segmental Fractures of the Lower Extremity and the Floating Knee
Robert A. Winquist

Chapter 20 249
Major Knee Ligament Injuries and Ipsilateral Fractures
Richard E. Jones, III

Chapter 21 265
Traumatic Dislocation of the Knee
Marvin H. Meyers

Chapter 22 275
Complex Fractures of the Distal End of the Femur
Roby D. Mize

Chapter 23 291
Complex Ankle Fractures
Jeffrey W. Mast *and* Phillip G. Spiegel

Chapter 24 313
Complex Fractures of the Foot
Sigvard T. Hansen, Jr.

Chapter 25 323
Complex Fractures and Dislocations of the Shoulder
Melvin Post

Chapter 26 347
Complex Fractures of the Elbow
Roby D. Mize *and* Bernd F. Claudi

Chapter 27 365
Complex Injuries of the Wrist and Hand
Sigurd C. Sandzén, Jr.

Chapter 28 401
Concomitant Fractures of the Long Bones
Sigvard T. Hansen, Jr.

Index 411

The Multiply Injured Patient with Complex Fractures

Chapter 1 Priorities in the Treatment of the Multiply Injured Patient with Musculoskeletal Injuries

BERND F. CLAUDI
MARVIN H. MEYERS

Management and successful treatment of multiply injured patients are a serious challenge to the general surgeon with special interest in traumatology, to the anesthetist dedicated to the problems of intensive-care medicine, or to the orthopaedic surgeon particularly interested in the needs for early stabilization and restoration of skeletal function. Often other specialists, such as neurosurgeons, maxillofacial surgeons, or urologists, take charge at a certain stage of evaluation and treatment of the polytraumatized patient. The complexity of the most common problems in the field of multiple injuries, however, calls for a team approach,[1-8] characterized by an unselfish readiness of all involved. The team must be highly skilled in giving a prompt and effective evaluation of the extent of the polytrauma, being agreeable to an interdisciplinary discussion of exisiting problems, and, finally, being able to make swift decisions so that no time is lost in performing life-saving procedures.

All this has to be done during the time and at the place where the multiply injured patient is undergoing shock treatment—usually in the emergency department. Under certain circumstances, this can be done as well in an operating room or in a radiology department. In the case of a polytraumatized patient, there is no justification for splitting the evaluation, planning, decision-making, and treatment plans among the different specialists involved. The situation inevitably calls for a team captain whose responsibility must be the permanent care of the patient beginning at the time of admission until the patient is, as a result of all the therapeutic efforts, beyond a life-threatening status. The remaining problems then may be treated best in the facilities of specialty departments. Actually, in most centers, it seems reasonable to accept the general surgeon in the role of team leader. This task can be assumed as well by a neurosurgeon, an anesthetist, or any other specialist. In general, this job should be performed by the best trained and the most skilled physician within a team. In the future, at least in trauma centers, the leader of a trauma team will have to be qualified with special training in the different aspects of polytrauma care, thus enabling that person to be fully aware of all problems involved in the overall management of a multiply injured patient. In actuality, almost all training programs of the different disciplines fall short of preparing the specialist for this outstanding job and its diversified responsibilities.

Although it has been proved that following strict rules in the treatment of polytraumatized patients is difficult and sometimes even impossible, a recommended regimen must be kept in mind. Based on the experience of some major trauma centers,[6,8,9] a multiply staged plan for the treatment of polytraumatized patients is presented. This plan is outlined with reference to the papers by Wolff,[10] Trentz,[6] and Schweiberer[11] and their associates. It consists of five stages:

1. Resuscitation.
2. Phase of immediate operation.
3. Phase of stabilization.
4. Phase of delayed operative procedures.
5. Phase of recovery.

The stages of this plan cannot be described within a clearly defined time frame. Each therapeutic step follows the other and is contingent on the patient's condition before the next procedure can be indicated. These steps should be taken rapidly so that the overall time for the indicated operative procedures is not unnecessarily prolonged. At this point, it already is evident that polytrauma care means a permanent endeavor supported by a team of dedicated nurses and physicians over an unknown period of time. Such an approach is necessary to keep the complication rate low by excluding one of the most common causes of failure: exhaustion of the personnel. Fatigue increases inaccuracy and even negligence during time-consuming and demanding treatment, which may span days or even weeks. The availability of enough properly trained manpower is becoming more and more the key problem for a hospital taking care of polytrauma patients. Available personnel for this purpose is actually limited; therefore, more efforts must be focused at establishing trauma centers throughout the country to which multiply injured patients should be transferred as soon as the patient is stabilized.

The treatment plan previously outlined will be discussed in further detail.

Resuscitation

The resuscitation phase consists of all necessary steps to re-establish vital functions. Thus, it is evident that this important measure should be initiated at all costs beginning at the site of the accident. The personnel in ambulance vehicles must be familiar with basic principles of

1. Maintenance of free airways; if necessary, endotracheal intubation.
2. Intravenous (I.V.) application of volume (Ringer's lactate solution).
3. Appropriate reduction and stabilization of fractures, as well as positioning of the patient.
4. Where to go with a patient with a serious injury pattern.
5. Advance warning to the closest emergency department that is prepared to take care of polytraumatized patients on a routine basis.

(There is an additional advantage in having trauma surgeons permanently on board special ambulances or helicopters.)

The shock treatment initiated at the site of the accident is continued and extended in the emergency department. The treatment of shock and appropriate ventilation will be discussed in greater detail in Chapters 3, 4, and 5. We must stress over and over again that aggressive shock treatment, in combination with early positive end-expiratory pressure ventilation (PEEP), is of utmost importance in the final outcome for a seriously injured patient.[1,12-14]

As long as normal blood pressure in association with adequate volume replacement cannot be achieved, there is no place for further diagnostic procedures that do not exclude life-threatening lesions. This is true to the same extent for re-establishing normal oxygenation. If, however, unstable circulation or insufficient oxygenation obviously is related to major organ system lesions, immediate operative procedures must be performed. In general, at such a point, the polytraumatized patient should already be on a ventilator and provided with central I.V. lines, gastric tube, urinary catheter, and, if indicated, chest tube and peritoneal lavage catheter.

Phase of Immediate Operation

All operations to be performed at this time must be necessary. The life-saving importance of these procedures is, therefore, the only indication. Among these indications are:

1. Persistent life-threatening hemorrhaging due to rupture of great vessels or parenchymatous organs (aorta, liver, spleen, or kidney).

2. Life-threatening hemorrhaging due to crush injuries, such as to the pelvis or extremities.

3. Intracranial hemorrhage, causing symptoms of imminent or complete brain-tissue herniation (closed or open) or open sinus bleeding. Neurosurgical procedures are then indicated.

4. Instances when intubation cannot be carried out (e.g., in case of an associated maxillofacial crush injury). Operations to maintain or restore an airway are then necessary.

All other operations that do not meet the criteria of life-saving procedures can be delayed until the patient is out of shock (to be used here as a common description of a life-threatening status). Thus, even a limb-saving procedure has to be regarded as of a high, but nevertheless secondary, priority. Up to this point, most diagnostic procedures can be performed by relatively simple measures only, such as catheterization of cavities or critical clinical examination and judgment. As long as intracranial bleeding is suspected to be the most serious of all injury patterns, computerized tomography should be performed as the diagnostic procedure of choice to facilitate necessary evacuation of the hemorrhage.[15]

Phase of Stabilization

When all life-saving procedures have been done and/or the appropriate shock treatment proves to be effective, the main objective is to stabilize all other vital functions. For this purpose the patient remains intubated and ventilated, thus meeting the needs for early cardiopulmonary support[1,6,8] and, at the same time, allowing for all further diagnostic procedures. During this phase, which can vary between hours and days, all necessary diagnostic procedures should be performed to evaluate the full extent of the injury. Responsibility for the injured patient cannot be delegated to a physician who takes care of an isolated aspect of polytrauma treatment only, or even worse, to a department, for instance the radiology department. Institutions, as well as specialists, dedicated to single areas only are unqualified to lead the overall treatment and to decide on the sequence of all necessary further procedures. Be it the trauma surgeon, in the function as a team captain, or be it the intensive-care physician, with a profound knowledge and understanding of the particular needs of the multiply injured patient, the same individual must keep the polytrauma patient under strict and permanent control until the patient is either through all necessary diagnostic examinations or is out of life-threatening danger. The patient can then be transferred to an intensive-care unit or an operating room. At this time, the responsibility may be delegated to the nursing (intensive-care) or the operating team, although it seems wise to keep the patient in the hands of the same team until he is through with all operative procedures.

The purpose of the phase of stabilization is to prepare the patient for the treatment of the remaining injuries that need further operations. During this phase, all necessary steps have to be carried out in a prompt and controlled manner to shorten the time until further procedures can be carried out; for example, limb-saving, abdominal, vascular, or thoracic surgery.

Before such procedures can be performed, a few points must be checked. These are:

1. Restoration of stable hemodynamics.
2. Restoration and maintenance of adequate oxygenation/organ perfusion.
3. Restoration of adequate kidney function.
4. Treatment of bleeding disorders.

Restoration of Stable Hemodynamics

The response to shock treatment, with particular reference to volume replacement, has to be controlled continuously. For standard management, central I.V. lines (monitoring of right atrium pressure), intra-arterial catheter (continuous monitoring of blood pressure, repeated blood-gas evaluation), and urinary catheter (precise control of kidney function) serve as supporting measures to the ongoing clinical evaluation of the patient's status. In serious injuries, these techniques remain incomplete and insufficient. As shown by Shoemaker[16] and other authors,[6,10] seriously injured patients have an increased cardiac output, particularly in a shock situation, which thus sometimes calls for aggressive volume replacement. This requires appropriate monitoring of other important hemodynamic criteria, such as pulmonary artery pressure and wedge pressure. A Swan-Ganz catheter should be used to achieve these ends and, at the same time, to measure the actual cardiac output. The application of a Swan-Ganz catheter should be accepted as the method of choice in a patient with multiple-system injury.

Restoration and Maintenance of Adequate Oxygenation (Organ Perfusion)

Although intubation and mechanical volume-controlled ventilation have some risks, there are good reasons for starting aggressive cardiopulmonary care early. Early mechanical, volume-cycled ventilation with PEEP is indicated in many polytraumatized patients to avoid pulmonary insufficiency. As a rule, every polytraumatized patient should be regarded as already in pulmonary insufficiency until the contrary can be proved. This approach occasionally may find a multiply injured patient intubated unnecessarily. However, the benefits of an early volume-cycled ventilation with PEEP are so obvious that this technique of ventilation should be applied despite its existing risks. The earlier the treatment is established, the less severe will be the pulmonary insufficiency, which usually appears as adult respiratory distress syndrome (ARDS) within a few days after injury. Ventilatory support should be maintained throughout the course of treatment until all major operative procedures are completed and the patient's status proves stable. Extubation and spontaneous breathing should be preceded by a systematic weaning period, during which the patient shows he is ready to maintain his respiration without further ventilatory support.

Restoration of Adequate Kidney Function

Restoration of normal kidney function is part of the adequate treatment of shock. Renal failure is almost preceded by reversible oliguria. Hypovolemia represents the most common cause of oliguria, which can be detected early by continuously measuring urine volumes (urinary catheter). As long as the volume replacement remains insufficient, diuretics (mannitol, furosemid) do not help. Diuretics should not be administered until the patient is obviously hypervolemic (hemodynamic parameters). In general, renal failure can be prevented by immediate and appropriate treatment of shock.

Treatment of Bleeding Disorders

Shortly after trauma, bleeding disorders usually start with a hypercoagulation, which is followed by hypocoagulation due to an ongoing waste of coagulation factors by continuous blood loss. The main sources of major blood loss are found in intrathoracic, intra-abdominal, and retroperitoneal lesions, or in combination with compound fractures and associated vascular injuries. As already outlined, part of the immediate operative procedure is to stop this life-threatening hemorrhage. Additional factors participating in post-traumatic bleeding disorders are hemodilution (excessive volume replacement, using crystalloids only) and impaired synthesis of clotting factors (shock-related malfunction of the liver). Continuous blood loss, hemodilution, and lack of clotting factors cannot be treated effectively by application of heparin. Adequate and prompt replacement of blood should be carried out as soon as blood is available. Blood is given not instead of, but in addition to, an ongoing volume replacement with crystalloids. In addition, the application of fresh frozen plasma has been proved effective in the management of post-traumatic bleeding disorders.[17-19] Bleeding disorders can be managed if treatment starts early enough. The disseminated intravascular coagulopathy (DIC) as the final stage of a persisting blood loss, documented by the existence of fibrinogen split products, often has a fatal outcome. Its treatment with heparin in polytrauma remains controversial, since heparin causes an activation of bleeding at any site of severely damaged tissue.

As long as the treatment of an existing coagulopathy has not been effective, further operative procedures are contraindicated, especially in the instance of DIC.

Phase of Delayed Operative Procedures

The time necessary to re-establish the patient's stable condition mainly depends on the injury pattern and the treatment modalities that are applied in a given situation. In general, experienced management of the previously mentioned problems should allow the stabilization phase to be achieved within hours, thus allowing such pending interventions as thoracotomies, laparotomies, procedures in limb-threatening vascular injuries, and stabilization of open fractures to be performed.

All fractures should be handled so that optimal stabilization by means of traction and/or splinting is achieved while waiting to perform operative fixation. Thus, the options for satisfying conservative treatment are initiated. Later, operative procedures for better fracture stabilization and early mobilization of a multiply injured patient, including an upright chest position,[1] can be performed at any time.

Two problems related to associated musculoskeletal injuries in the polytraumatized patient are urgent and will be discussed in more detail. They are both of high priority in the overall treatment plan and should be attacked as soon as the patient's condition permits.

The combined vascular/bone injury as a limb-threatening injury calls for a limb-saving procedure, which can be done only within a short period of time after the injury. Ischemia persisting for longer than 6 to 8 hours inevitably minimizes the chances to restore a full functioning extremity. Every hour of delay in making the diagnosis or carrying out appropriate treatment is an hour closer to amputation. Realizing the specific as well as the general needs of a multiply injured patient, it is obvious that blood flow must be restored as the first priority. Restoration of blood flow might be done, depending on the given circumstances, as a definitive repair by using an interposition venous graft technique or by a temporary shunting. The latter technique seems to be more advisable because it facilitates the internal fixation of the adjacent fracture without increasing the risks of prolonged ischemia.

Next on the priority list is the management of open fractures. Despite the evidence of experimental and clinical studies by the Swiss ASIF group (Association for the Study of Internal Fixation)[20-22] and the clinical findings of other authors,[10,23] the hows and whens of initiating treatment of open fractures still remain controversial. However, all agree that early debridement has to be carried out. With regard to the type of fixation to be applied, some persons oppose and some strongly recommend immediate rigid fixation. As a result of clinical experience, there is no doubt that early internal fixation or the use of external fixators is of extreme benefit. If properly performed, this procedure provides the bone, as well as the soft tissues, with the stability desired to facilitate healing conditions. At the same time, early internal fixation decreases the risk of infection. A critical review of early infections following immediate internal fixation in open fractures reveals that the cause of infection is mainly due to repeated mistakes, including disregard of the basic principles of soft-tissue handling, poor knowledge of appropriate instrumentation, improper application of adequate implants, and, finally, limited technical skills due to lack of significant experience with open fractures.

The treatment of remaining skeletal injuries may be delayed for a few days until the patient's general condition has improved. In general, however, definitive stabilization should be achieved as early as possible, ideally while the patient can profit from continued assisted ventilation. In particular, early stable fixation of long bones, (femur, tibia, forearm, humerus) facilitates nursing care and allows for functional aftercare. The fixation of unstable spine fractures, as well as of articular fractures, is also of high priority during the phase of delayed operative procedures.

Phase of Recovery

All recommendations for treatment modalities in multiply injured patients heretofore outlined aim at the same goals: to optimize the chances of survival, to prevent cardiopulmonary insufficiency, to minimize early complications, such as infection and thromboembolic disorders, and to optimize recovery in a short period of time. The phase of recovery starts after all major surgery is done. Extubation should be performed when the weaning process indicates that the patient is ready. Usually, after another 1 to 2 days, the patient's stable condition allows for a transfer from the intensive-care unit to the ward. Here, all further efforts include continued physiotherapy, psychologic support, and adequate nutrition. Alimentation often remains a neglected aspect in the treatment of polytraumatized patients. Since we know more about the nutritional needs of these patients and how to meet the requirements of hypercaloric alimentation,[24,25] hyperalimentation has to be initiated the first day after injury. Without going into detail, this crucially important aspect stresses once again that the ability for successful management requires a sound understanding of a variety of different pathophysiologic mechanisms of injury. The final outcome depends on cooperation of all specialists, on a well-balanced coordination of necessary surgery, and on a traumatologist who takes the responsibility for the overall treatment of the multiply injured patient.

Summary

Fatal outcome in the multiply injured patient is often related to inappropriate management at the time of resuscitation. Aggressive treatment of shock ideally is initiated at the site of the accident and has to be regarded as the main goal in the initial phase of the overall treatment plan for a polytraumatized patient. The phase of resuscitation, in which vital functions have to be re-established, needs to be controlled by the best trained and most skilled physician on the trauma team. Acting in this particular emergency situation as a team leader, this physician has to have the authority to bring all specialists together at the place and the time they are needed, which is usually the emergency department at the time of admission of a polytraumatized patient. Resuscitation and brief but thorough clinical examination usually run parallel to each other, allowing for swift decision making and outlining in a reasonable sequence the further steps needed to be done (treatment plan). This includes staging of the plan, starting with resuscitation and including a phase of immediate operations, a phase of stabilization, a phase of delayed operative procedures and ending with a phase of recovery. All indicated operations should be carried out at the appropriate time indicated, respecting existing priorities.

Certain priorities must be kept in mind with regard to the management of musculoskeletal injuries. Extremity vascular lesions and open fractures are of the highest priority; however, they should not be treated before all life-threatening problems have been solved. The patient, therefore, needs to be truly stabilized in all vital functions. Remaining skeletal instability can be treated in the phase reserved for delayed operative procedures. The advantages of early rigid fixation of fractures in a multiply injured patient are obvious. Their successive management, however, needs the application of sound basic principles, profound knowledge, and technical skills of the orthopaedic surgeon in charge.

References

1. Border, J. R., LaDuca, J., and Seibel, R.: Priorities in the management of the patient with polytrauma. Prog. Surg., *14*:84, 1975.
2. Border, J. R., et al.: Multiple systems organ failure: muscle fuel deficit with visceral protein malnutrition. Surg. Clin. North Am., *56*:1147, 1976.
3. Claudi, B., Inthorn, D., Hamperl, D., Zumtobel, V.: Operationstaktik bei 150 polytraumatisierten Patienten: eine Zweijahresanalyse. Muenchen, Kongress der Deutschen Gesellschaft fuer Chirurgie, 14-17.5, 1980.
4. Committee on Trauma of the American College of Surgeons: Optimal hospital resources for care of the seriously injured. ACS Bull., *61*:15, 1976.
5. Day, L. J., Hansen, S. T., Jr., and Johnston, R. M.: Instructional Courses on Polytrauma. Las Vegas, American Academy of Orthopaedic Surgeons, 1981.
6. Trentz, O., et al.: Kriterien fuer die Operabilitaet von Polytraumatisierten. Unfallheilkunde, *81*:451, 1978.
7. Walt, A. J.: Initial intrahospital care of the severely injured patient: the early hours. Surg. Clin. North Am., *57*:179, 1977.
8. Chapman, M. W., and Mahoney, M.: The role of early internal fixation in the management of open fractures. Clin. Orthop., *138*:120, 1979.
9. Gustilo, R. B., Chapman, M. W., and Patzakis, M. J.: Management of open fractures and complications. Instructional Course, Las Vegas, American Academy of Orthopaedic Surgeons, 1981.
10. Wolff, G., et al.: Koordination von Chirurgie und Intensivmedizin zur Vermeidung der posttraumatischen respiratorischen Insuffizienz. Unfallheilkunde, *81*:425, 1978.
11. Schweiberer, L., Dambe, L. T., and Klapp, F.: Die Mehrfachverletzung: Schweregrad und therapeutische Richtlinien. Chirurg, *49*:608, 1978.
12. Blaisdell, F. W., and Lewis, F. R., Jr.: Respiratory Distress Syndrome of Shock and Trauma: Post-Traumatic Failure. Philadelphia, W. B. Saunders, 1977.
13. Pontoppidan, H., Wilson, R. S., Rie, M. A., and Schneider, R. C.: Respiratory intensive care. Anaesthesiology, *47*:96, 1977.
14. Wolff, G., et al.: Die akute respiratorische Insuffizienz (ARI) und das Adult Respiratory Distress Syndrom (ARDS). *In* Adult Respiratory Distress Syndrome. Berlin, Springer, 1980.
15. Lanksch, W., Meese, W., and Kazner, E.: Computerized tomography in head injuries. Berlin, Springer, 1979.
16. Shoemaker, W. C.: Pathophysiology of shock as a basis for monitoring and therapy for the critically ill patient. *In* Current Topics in Critical Care Medicine. Vol. 2. Basel, S. Karger, 1976.
17. Hehne, H. J., Nyman, D., Burri, H., and Wolff, G.: Management of bleeding disorders in traumatic-haemorrhagic shock with deep frozen fresh plasma. Eur. J. Intensive Care Med., *2*:157, 1976.
18. Lim, R. C., Olcott, C., Robinson, A., and Blaisdell, F. W.: Platelet response and coagulation changes following massive blood replacement. J. Trauma, *13*:577, 1973.
19. Wilson, R. F., Mammen, E., and Walt, A. J.: Eight years of experience with massive blood transfusions. J. Trauma, *11*:275, 1971.
20. Meyer, S., Weiland, A. J., and Willenegger, H.: The treatment of infected non-union of fractures of long bones. J. Bone Joint Surg. *57A*:6, 836, 1975.
21. Rittmann, W. W., and Perren, S. M.: Cortical Bone Healing After Internal Fixation and Infection. Biomechanics and Biology. Berlin, Springer, 1974.
22. Rittmann, W. W., Schibli, M., Matter, P., and Allgoewer, M.: Open fractures: long term results in 200 consecutive cases. Clin. Orthop., *138*:132, 1979.
23. Gustilo, R. B., and Anderson, J. T.: Prevention of infection in the treatment of one-thousand-and-twenty-five open fractures of long bones. J. Bone Joint Surg., *58A*:453, 1976.
24. Border, J. R.: Metabolic response to short term starvation, sepsis and trauma. *In* Surgery Annual, 1970. Edited by Nyhus and Cooper, New York, Appleton-Century-Crofts, 1970.
25. Dudrick, S. J., and Copeland, E. M.: Parenteral hyperalimentation. *In* Surgery Annual, 1973. Edited by Nyhus. New York, Appleton-Century-Crofts, 1973.

Chapter 2 Management of the Upper Airway in the Injured Patient

STEVEN D. SCHAEFER
ROBERT G. ANDERSON
HENRY M. CARDER

Maintenance of human life depends on adequate respiration. In the chaos often surrounding treatment of the acutely injured patient, this simple fact may be forgotten. Attention may be directed to the more obvious injuries, such as compound extremity fractures or severe facial lacerations. Airway maintenance is of primary importance, and there is no justification for performing complicated life-support maneuvers without first establishing a functional airway.

Confusion in caring for the acutely traumatized patient should be replaced with logical management carried out in an orderly fashion. Because the airway carries the highest priority, individuals concerned with the care of such patients must have expertise in assessing the existing airway and in restoring supportive ventilation as quickly as possible. A knowledge of the anatomy and pathophysiology of this region is essential to rapid assessment and correction of airway problems.

This chapter provides information on airway management based on an understanding of the normal and abnormal upper airway.

Normal Upper Airway

Too often, the vital functions of eating and breathing are lost in the collective phrase, "upper airway." A better phrase to convey the shared responsibilities of the two systems involved with eating and breathing might be the "upper aerodigestive tract." As man evolved beyond his primitive lungfish-like ancestry, a complex system developed to provide for the intake of nutrients and air. Essential to the primitive air breathing animals was a sphincter, the larynx, which could isolate the upper airway from the lower so that ingested matter would not violate the lungs.[1] In man, this system is capable of *slowly* compensating for either intrinsic or extrinsic alterations, but is fragile and easily overwhelmed by sudden changes resulting from acute injuries. Insight into the pathophysiology of the upper aerodigestive tract can be gained by a more careful look at deglutition and respiration.

Deglutition

In the mature individual, eating is voluntarily initiated by the tongue, which propels food posteriorly into the oropharynx through a plunger-like action as it compresses the contents of the oral cavity against the palate.[2] Mediated by cranial nerves, V, IX, and X, the combined action of the soft palate and lateral pharyngeal walls seals off the potential escape of food through the nasopharynx into the nose.[3] Once begun, swallowing progresses involuntarily under the direction of intrinsic innervation and fibers derived from the pons and medulla. Pharyngeal peristalsis becomes a composite wave formed from the actions of the tongue, palate, and pharyngeal constrictors with a velocity of 12 to 25 cm per second.[4] As the food stream passes the larynx, several mechanisms prevent aspiration. First, the larynx is elevated in an anterior direction, bringing it beneath the base of the tongue. Next, sensory fibers from the superior laryngeal branch of the vagus nerve and the glossopharyngeal nerve detect the presence of food in the pharynx and reflexly stop respiration.[5] Concurrently, the laryngeal sphincter closes. The pharyngeal phase of deglutition is completed when the upper esophageal sphincter, the cricopharyngeus muscle, relaxes. The cricopharyngeus muscle is controlled by the pharyngeal plexus (cranial nerves IX and X). This sequence prevents pooling of food in the hypopharynx and subsequent laryngeal and pulmonary insult. Although not essential in the adult, the epiglottis probably plays a minor role in preventing aspiration by diverting some food away from the laryngeal inlet. At the completion of swallowing, coughing clears the larynx of minimal residual food and liquid, which normally collect on the superior surface of the true vocal cords.

Respiration

Respiration is a complex action highly sensitive and responsive to somatic and visceral input. As such, it is incorrect to view the upper respiratory tract as a simple series of static, rigid tubes that connect the mouth and nose to the lungs. As air enters the nose, it is filtered, temperature regulated, and humidified before traversing past the posterior soft palate to reach the oropharynx. At this point, the nasal and oral air mix and share a common pharyngeal passage to the larynx and lungs. The normal flow of air through this region requires constant monitoring by the central nervous system to ensure the functional integrity of the pharyngeal airway. The anatomic integrity of this area is assumed early in fetal development through proper alignment of the mandible, hyoid bone, and larynx.[6] Further stability arises from the appropriate positioning of the cranium, vertebral column, and thorax.[6] At the level of the facial skeleton, upper respiratory function depends on tongue and soft-palate control. The tongue is attached anteriorly to the mandible and hyoid bone. A fracture of the mandible or interruption of the afferent and efferent nerves to this region may compromise the pharyngeal airway, allowing the tongue to fall backward against the posterior pharyngeal wall. The soft palate permits nasal air flow only as long as its tone is maintained via cranial nerves IX and X. In the supine position, the denervated palate obstructs the nasopharynx, a condition known as "palatal valving." In addition to skeletal stability, inferior pharyngeal airway function involves the combined motor input of the pharyngeal constrictors and suspensory muscles of the larynx. Because the larynx evolved primarily as a sphincter of the upper trachea, essential muscular development was directed toward closure of the vocal cords. Only the posterior cricoarytenoid muscle is concerned with dilation and, thus, patency of this segment of the respiratory tract. As the only true abductor of the larynx, bilateral loss of posterior cricoarytenoid muscle function following either neck trauma or central nervous system would lead to laryngeal compromise. The degree of airway restriction is variable, influenced by such factors as the presence of superior laryngeal nerve innervation and the inherent elasticity of the larynx, which favors dilation of this organ.

In viewing the upper aerodigestive tract as a dynamic system that is more than a simple mechanical conduit for food and air, it should be obvious that its proper function depends on several factors. The skeletal anatomy along the entire length of the system must be intact and stable. The nervous system is necessary for both afferent sensory input and maintenance of proper muscular tone. Finally, patency of this region requires a nonedematous and intact soft-tissue lining. For simplicity, the upper aerodigestive tract will be referred to as the "upper airway" in the following discussion.

Abnormal Upper Airway

Because of the complex nature of the upper airway, management may be required for pulmonary insufficiency and toilet, loss of central nervous system control, and obstruction.

Pulmonary Insufficiency and Toilet

Airway management is directed toward providing mechanical ventilation and removing secretions. Successful treatment is directed toward correction of hypoxia or hypercarbia. Such conditions follow venous or fat emboli, shock lung, sepsis, or pulmonary contusion. A healthy young adult often can withstand a significant insult to the lungs without need of an artificial airway. The aged and the very young, however, frequently require direct mechanical conduits to the lower airway for respiratory support following lesser injuries. This support may be provided in the form of an endotracheal tube or a tracheotomy.

Orotracheal or nasotracheal intubation provides immediate airway support. The route of intubation may depend on the skill of the operator, the type of the available tube, patient cooperation, and anticipated duration of maintenance of the artificial airway. The neophyte will probably feel most comfortable using an orotracheal tube. These tubes are manufactured in a variety of sizes and materials. The average adult female and male require a No. 7 (9.5 mm O.D.) and No. 8 (10.9 mm O.D.) tube, respectively (Fig. 2-1). The ideal tube should be made of a disposable plastic with a *low-pressure, high-volume* cuff. This cuff characteristic is particularly important when an endotracheal tube is required for more than 24 hours. Nasal intubation is more difficult, but stabilizes the tube in the nasal cavity and external nares. Compared to orotracheal intubation, this method decreases tracheal trauma due to cuff movement caused by the intermittent positive-pressure action of the mechanical respirator.

Skill at intubation can only be gained by practice. Proper positioning is essential. The supine patient should lie on a flat surface with the head placed on a small headrest or pillow. Two basic types of laryngoscopes are used widely today. The straight laryngoscope blade, such as on a Miller laryngoscope, is placed posterior to the epiglottis and depends on pressure exerted on the laryngeal surface of the epiglottis to expose the larynx. The beginner may find this blade more difficult to use in the conscious patient and may be more likely to dislocate the arytenoid cartilages if the blade is placed posterior to the larynx. The curved laryngoscope blade, on a McIntosh laryngoscope, for example, is inserted anterior to the epiglottis, in the vallecula. The larynx is revealed as the epiglottis is carried forward by the force of the laryngoscope on the base of the tongue. Proper visualization of the larynx by either instrument requires application of an anterio-superior force at the point of laryngoscopic contact, which lifts the offending structures out of the operator's line of vision (Fig. 2-2).

The location of the distal end of the endotracheal tube should be confirmed by a chest roentgenogram immediately after intubation. Routinely inspecting the postintubation roentgenogram and ascultating the chest to listen for bilateral breath sound avoid the inadvertent ventilation of only one lung. The tube cuff is inflated to the point where only a small amount of air escapes during the positive-pressure cycle of the ventilator. Ideal cuff pressure is less than 20 mm Hg and hopefully reduces ischemic necrosis of the tracheal mucosa.

Controversy exists about when a tracheotomy should be performed in the patient who requires prolonged intubation. Most authorities agree that

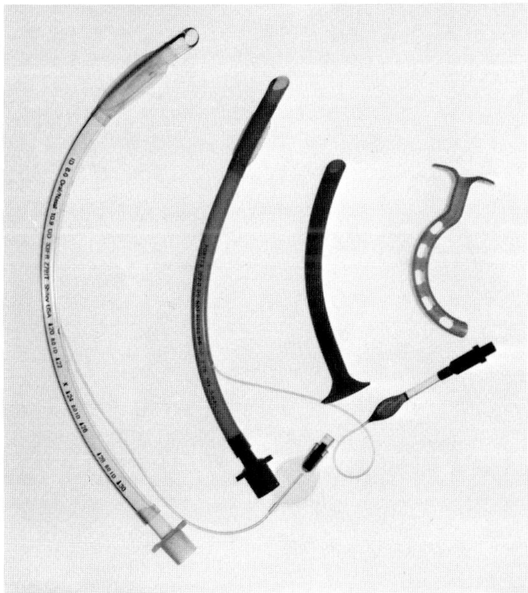

FIG. 2-1. Photograph of various endotracheal tubes and airways (left to right, high-volume, low-pressure endotracheal tube; low-volume, high-pressure endotracheal tube; nasal airway; oral airway).

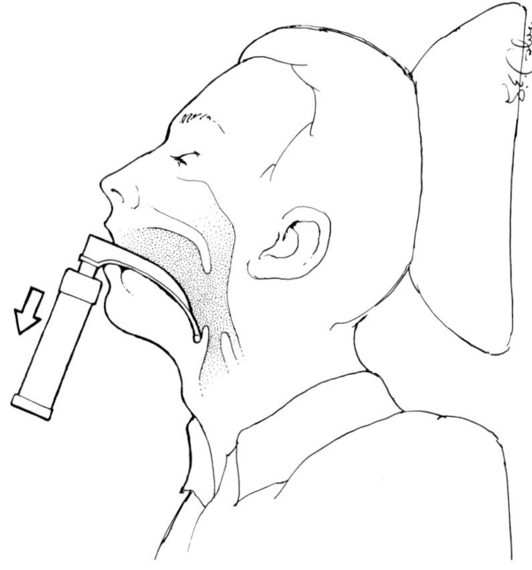

FIG. 2-2. Proper laryngoscopic technique used for orotracheal intubation. Arrow shows direction of force used on left base of tongue.

the likelihood of tracheal and laryngeal damage as a complication of endotracheal intubation increases with: (1) the presence of infection, (2) increased duration of intubation, particularly beyond 1 to 2 weeks in adults, (3) the inexperience of the physician placing the tube, (4) small-volume, high-pressure cuffs, (5) movement of the tube by the mechanical ventilator or by tongue movement on an orotracheal tube in the partially awake patient, and (6) constant inflation of the cuff. Obviously, tracheotomy does not alleviate all these problems. The advantage of tracheotomy is avoidance of further *laryngeal* trauma, ready access for pulmonary suctioning, and decreased airway dead space. The potential for tracheal trauma, however, still exists. Also, long-term tracheotomy has been implicated as a cause of loss of regulation of protective laryngeal closure,[7] and probably accounts for the aspiration problems seen when one attempts to decanulate rapidly the chronic tracheotomy patient. Despite these potential difficulties, tracheotomy is probably the best method of managing the patient requiring long-term airway support.

Loss of Central Control

The airway frequently is jeopardized by loss of central nervous system control as a result of head injury, drug or chemical intoxication, or metabolic coma. Without constant neurogenic input, the parapharyngeal muscles, soft palate, and tongue relax, and breathing is compromised by the collective collapse of these structures. Initial treatment may consist of manipulation of the head to elevate the tongue free from the posterior pharyngeal wall (Fig. 2-3,*A*). After the oropharynx is manually cleared of secretions, two positions are useful. Hyperextension of the head rotates the mandible anteriorly and increases the distance separating the jaw, tongue, and pharynx (Fig. 2-3,*B*). Alternatively, the head may be raised above the thorax by placing it on a pillow and flexing it on the chest. This position carries the tongue anterior to the larynx and away from the posterior pharynx; it is referred to as the "sniffing position" (Fig. 2-3,*C*). In some patients, manual traction at both mandibular angles is required to elevate the tongue. This maneuver can close the mouth and lips, especially in the edentulous patient. Placement of a large, soft, nasal trumpet holds the soft palate away from the posterior nasopharynx and restores the airway by providing a route for breathing through the nose.

The oropharyngeal and nasopharyngeal airways are simple mechanical devices designed to establish a patent pharyngeal passage by either reducing obstruction from the tongue or bypassing the soft palate, respectively. The oropharyngeal mechanical airway is simple to use, but may be insufficient without manual traction on the mandible. The nasopharyngeal mechanical airway requires a minor degree of skill to insert through the nose and has the advantage of avoiding the mouth, which may be inaccessible in some patients with maxillofacial trauma. The next step in airway control is either intubation or tracheotomy, depending on the expected duration of the preciptating central disease process. Whatever the method of management, control of the

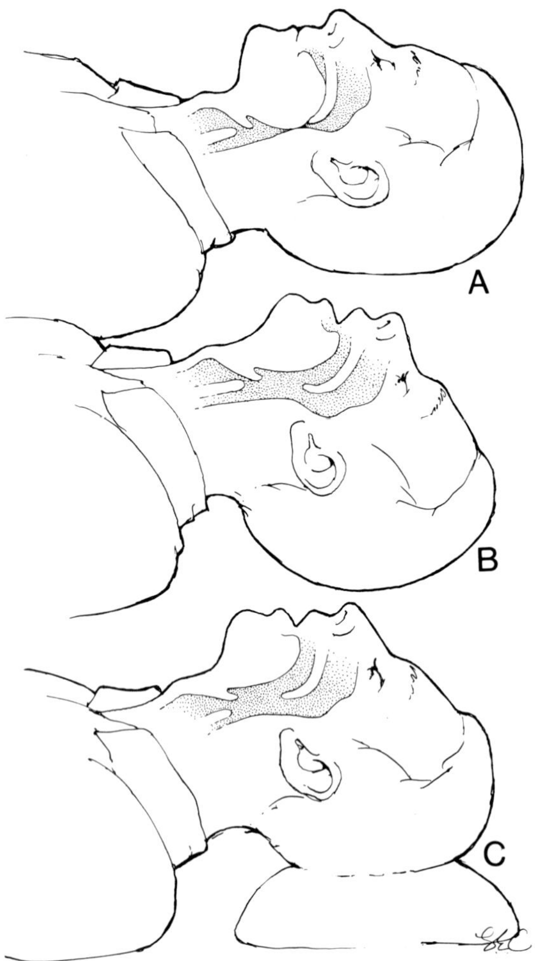

Fig. 2-3. Tongue is shown obstructing pharynx (*A*). Obstruction is corrected by either hyperextension of the head (*B*) or lifting of the head above the thorax (*C*).

airway in the patient with a central nervous system impairment is simplified when one understands the unique anatomy and physiology of this region.

Obstructed Breathing

The obstructed upper airway is both a diagnostic and treatment challenge in the acutely injured patient. A thorough history and physical examination are vital. Unfortunately, some patients may present only moments away from total airway obstruction.

When possible, the history should include the mechanism and site of injury and the clinical course followed since the time of injury. The mechanism of injury may be further divided into blunt and penetrating trauma. Automobile accidents constitute the major source of blunt trauma to the multiply injured patient. The unrestrained occupants frequently suffer severe facial and cranial injuries as their head leads the body in its trajectory through the windshield. A blow to the lower dental arch on the dashboard or windshield can lead to bilateral mandibular or angle fractures, allowing the tongue to fall against the posterior pharynx. The edentulous, atrophic mandible is particularly prone to fracture. If the neck is hyperextended at the time of injury, vital structures in the anterior neck become vulnerable to trauma. A force delivered to the middle cervical region may result in a variable degree of fracture or dislocation of the thyroid cartilage. The extent of fracture depends on the patient's age, the amplitude of the force, and the striking surface. Generally, given the same force and elasticity of the impact surface, older patients are more likely to suffer comminuted airway fractures because of ossification of their laryngeal cartilages and, therefore, less resiliency and elasticity of these structures.

The apparent location or *site of injury* should alert the physician to airway problems, especially in that particular region. An assault victim with trauma to the mouth, for example, might have several missing teeth or dentures with resultant difficulty in breathing. This recent loss of dentition should alert the examiner to the possibility of an obstructing foreign body in the airway. A blow to the lower one third of the neck, such as would be inflicted in motor vehicle or sporting accidents, in an individual who presents with impaired respiration suggests separation of the trachea from the laryngeal cartilages. The astute physician can proceed immediately to appropriate treatment through an understanding of what to expect following trauma to a particular region of the airway (Table 2-1).

Early assessment of penetrating trauma to the upper airway can be hindered by the more obvious and profuse hemorrhage accompanying vascular injuries. An innocent-looking skin wound may be seen with a potentially fatal respiratory tract injury. The physician should mentally try to reconstruct the path of the missile or knife for the purpose of identifying the potentially injured region. Then, an appropriate plan can be formulated to determine the existence of the injury.

The patient's clinical course is included in the history to judge the stability of the airway. For example, an accident victim with multiple system injuries is seen with a history of trauma to the anterior neck. An intravenous line is inserted and the patient's cervical spine is properly immobilized in transit. The paramedics report that the patient had initial hoarseness and hemoptysis. Upon arrival at the emergency room, slight stridor was noted, which increased while the physicians were evaluating a possible cervical spine

Table 2-1. *Upper Airway Compromise Following Trauma.*

Site of Injury		*Airway Problem*
Oral Cavity		—loose teeth or dentures in airway —fractured mandible with tongue obstructing pharynx —swollen or lacerated tongue obstructing pharynx
Anterior Neck	Upper 1/3	—fractured hyoid bone —avulsion of epiglottis —supraglottic lacerations or hematomas —superior laryngeal nerve paralysis
	Middle 1/3	—hematoma, laceration, or thyroid-cricoid cartilage fracture —recurrent or superior laryngeal nerve paralysis —esophageal-hypopharynx laceration
	Lower 1/3	—recurrent laryngeal nerve paralysis —cricoid fracture —laryngotracheal separation —esophageal-hypopharynx laceration

TABLE 2-2. *Signs and Symptoms of Laryngotracheal Trauma.*

Trauma
Ecchymosis
Hoarseness
Dysphagia
Pain and tenderness
Hemoptysis
Crepitus (local)
Loss of thryoid prominence
Drooling
Massive subcutaneous and mediastinal emphysema
Stridor
Cyanosis
Apnea

injury. The patient suddenly experienced a respiratory arrest and died in the emergency room while several physicians attempted orotracheal intubation. This rapid evolution of seemingly innocent airway symptoms should be a "red flag" to impending airway deterioration and the need for prompt treatment. This case also demonstrates the necessity for physicians who care for patients with cervical spine trauma to be particularly aware of the likelihood of coexistent laryngeal injuries. The signs and symptoms of laryngeal trauma are summarized in Table 2-2 and should lead one to prompt recognition and treatment of suspected airway deterioration before it occurs.

When examining the patient with a partial airway obstruction, noisy breathing or *stridor* may be evident. An alteration of, or a foreign body in, the immediate region of the vocal folds (glottis) typically yields stridor on both inspiration and expiration. A supraglottic obstruction, above the vocal cords, is characterized by inspiratory stridor. Such an airway insult might include a lacerated epiglottis falling onto the laryngeal inlet, a fractured mandible with posterior displacement of the tongue, or an aspirated denture resting above the larynx. A further clue to airway obstruction is retraction of the sternum and intercostal spaces on inspiration. Anything that alters airflow through the region between the cricoid cartilage to the segmental bronchi produces expiratory stridor and is analogous to the expiratory wheeze of asthma (Fig. 2-4). Often the stridor cannot be clearly separated into one type or another because the injury traverses two or more regions of the upper airway. Such a problem might arise following a mandible fracture with posterior displacement of the tongue in conjunction with a fractured larynx and a partially avulsed epiglottis. Whatever the presentation, the presence of stridor implies an airway problem.

The adoption of a systematic approach to examining the upper airway is recommended. In the patient with maxillofacial trauma, the mouth and oropharynx are particularly appropriate areas with which to begin the examination. The physician should look for missing dentition, fractures of the jaws, and lacerations of and obstruction by the tongue. Immediate treatment might simply consist of clearing this area of secretions, blood, and loose dentures or applying manual pressure to the bleeding vessel. In the cooperative patient, teeth or foreign bodies lying in the pharynx may be removed under direct vision using the McGill intubation forceps. Distal to the pharynx, bronchoscopy or esophagoscopy under general anesthetic is required for examination of these areas. If cervical spine injury is not present, as

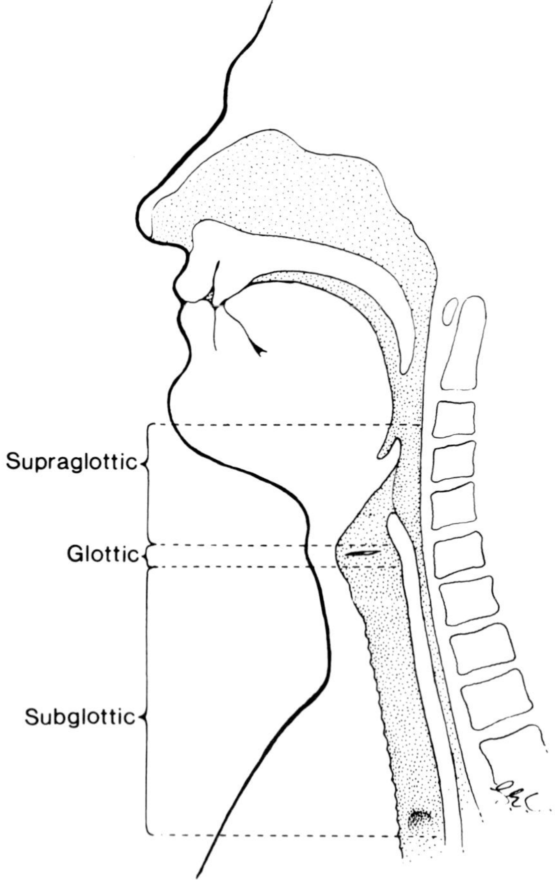

FIG. 2-4. Sagittal diagram of airway indicating level of obstruction that produces stridor.

determined by a cervical spine roentgenogram, obstruction by the tongue can be handled by hyperextension of the neck. When this maneuver is inadequate or contraindicated, pulling the tongue forward should restore breathing. A gauze sponge in the conscious patient or a towel clip in the unconscious individual facilitates grasping a wet or bloody tongue.

Next, inspect the neck for evidence of trauma (Tables 2-1 and 2-2). With clear evidence of a laryngotracheal injury and a patient who is hypoxic or severely stridorous, an *immediate tracheotomy* rather than endotracheal intubation is indicated.[8] Tracheotomy is preferred for these injuries to avoid further damage by the endotracheal tube to the already traumatized larynx. Intubation through a lacerated or fractured larynx can create a false passage adjacent to the airway lumen and avulse the laryngeal mucosa from its cartilage.[8] Such a case is shown in Figure 2-5, *A*

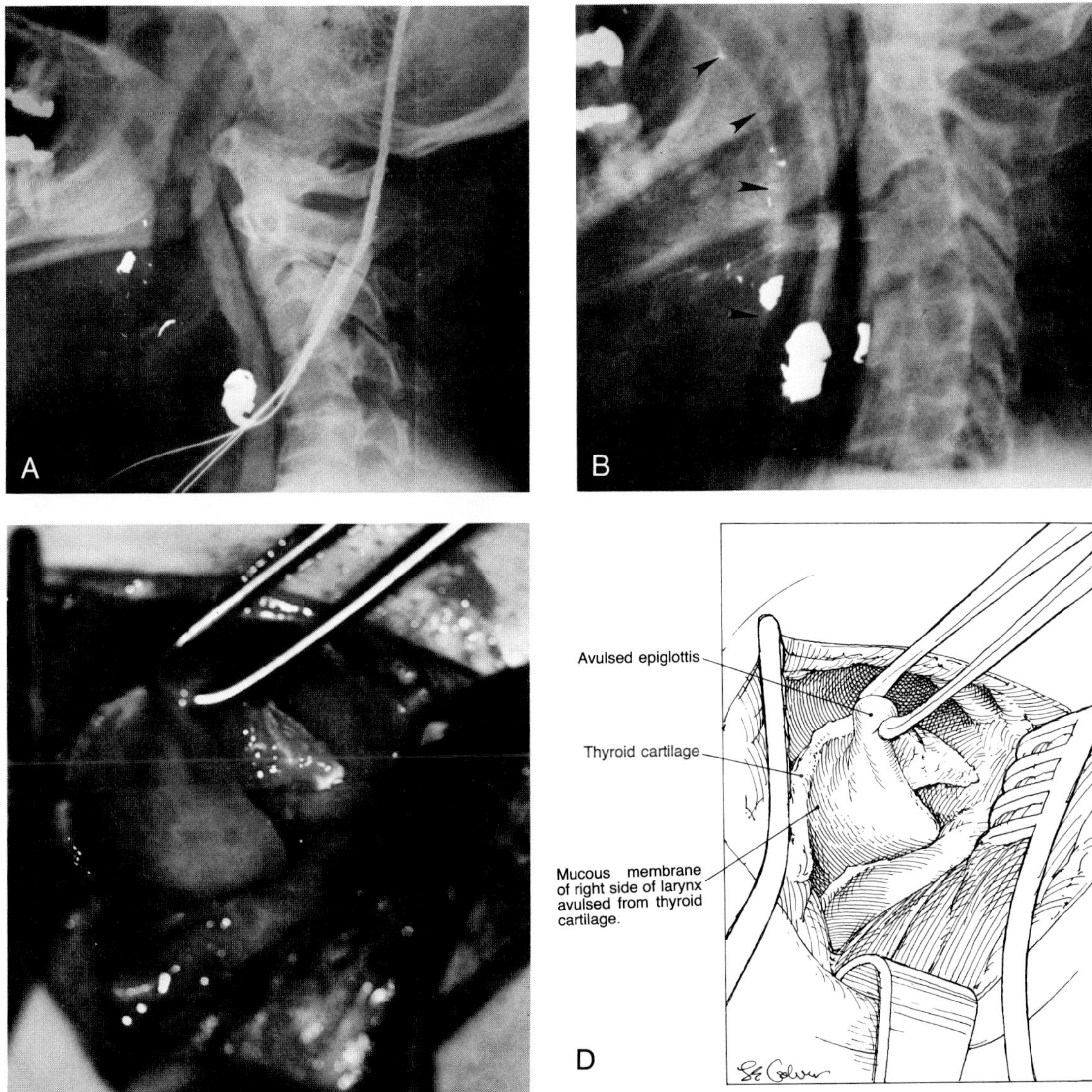

FIG. 2-5. Soft-tissue lateral radiographs of neck in patient with gunshot wound before (*A*) and after (*B*) intubation. Operative photograph of laryngeal injury caused by intubation (*C*) and diagram illustrating injury (*D*).

through *D*. This patient presented with a gunshot wound traversing the tongue and superior larynx. Placement of an orotracheal tube followed the path of the bullet through the epiglottis and disrupted the laryngeal mucosa along the entire length of the thyroid and cricoid cartilages. A second reason for not intubating patients with suspected laryngeal injury is that the entire airway may be dependent on a mucosal bridge that joins the larynx to the trachea. The curved endotracheal tube can sever the mucosa, leaving the patient without an airway. Hence, if the physician suspects a serious laryngotracheal injury, a tracheotomy is the safest way to manage these patients. Unfortunately, not all physicians are trained to perform a tracheotomy. A less desirable method for establishing an airway is the cricothyrotomy. This procedure obviously is dangerous in a laryngotracheal separation, in which the cricothyrotomy has the same effect as an endotracheal tube in potentially disrupting the unstable continuity between the larynx and trachea.

Cricothyrotomy is a means by which an airway is established through a puncture of the fascial membrane between the cricoid and thyroid cartilages. When performed correctly, the puncture or incision includes only the membrane and not the laryngeal cartilages. A small endotracheal tube or catheter is then placed through the operative site into the trachea. Once breathing is restored, an orderly controlled tracheotomy should be performed.

Controversy has recently arisen regarding the advocation of cricothyrotomy as an alternative to tracheotomy in *long-term airway management*. Such a policy neglects the all-too-frequent occurrence of subglottic stenosis at the level of the cricoid cartilage. Stenosis is seen at this region because the cricoid is the only complete cartilaginous ring in the entire airway. The fixed internal diameter of this cartilage restricts airway expansion, and the cricoid mucous membrane is impinged between the endotracheal tube and the cricoid cartilage. A long-term airway through the cricothyroid membrane presents the same laryngeal insult as does endotracheal intubation with the added risk of infection and perichondritis at the wound site. Hence, the incidence of long-term complications may be potentially as great with this form of management as with endotracheal intubation. Further, the injured region in laryngeal trauma may include or lie below the cricoid ring, making this procedure difficult and hazardous. Tracheotomy is preferred in these patients because the artificial airway is placed below the site of injury.

Fortunately, many patients with airway trauma are stable and able to undergo further diagnostic evaluation. A soft-tissue lateral radiograph of the neck provides considerable information (Fig. 2-6). The physician should note the position of the tongue and epiglottis and the continuity of the larynx and trachea. One should also exclude fractures or mass effects due to swelling or hemato-

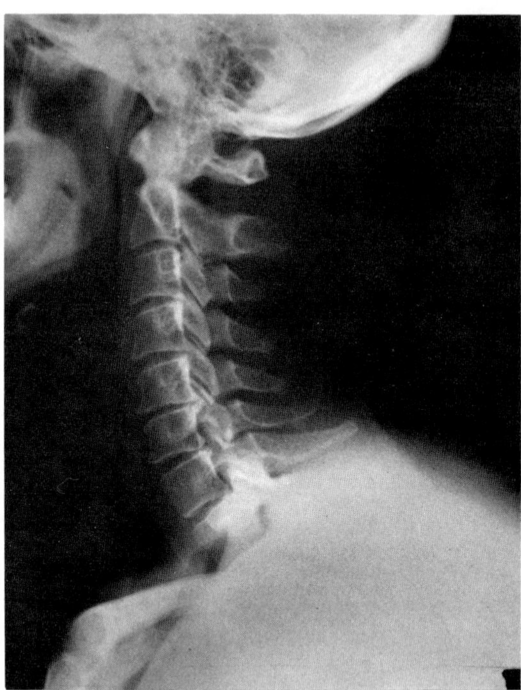

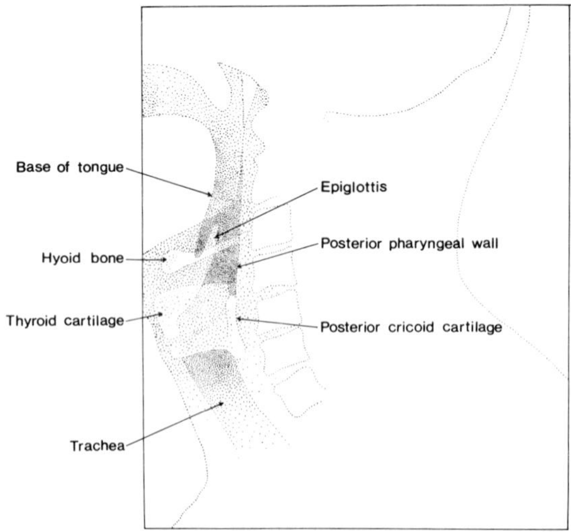

Fig. 2-6. Normal soft-tissue lateral radiograph of neck (*A*) and diagram of same (*B*).

mas, as well as evaluate the *entire cervical spine* for fractures, dislocations, or foreign bodies. In maxillofacial trauma, a facial bone and mandible roentgenogram series complements the physical examination. On these particular radiographs, alterations in the mandible, maxilla, soft palate, floor of mouth, and tongue may be recognized as contributing to airway obstruction. Radiography should never delay performing the appropriate treatment in the patient with a compromised airway. The cervical lateral roentgenogram alone is required prior to any manipulation of the neck. Additional roentgenograms are obtained if indicated *only* when the airway is stable, and only with constant observation by a physician skilled in performing intubation or tracheotomy in patients with suspected airway injury.

Even when the patient has minimal difficulty in breathing, a consultation is frequently required soon after the injury victim arrives in the emergency room. The goal of the consultant initially is to confirm the presence or absence of a significant airway problem. If re-establishing an intact dental arch restores normal breathing, intubation or tracheotomy may be avoided in the lesser injuries. In the patient with an apparently stable airway, but with a change in voice or the occurrence of hemoptysis or dysphagia, carefully performed indirect laryngoscopy may be attempted. The physician must be prepared to perform a tracheotomy immediately should the airway be lost while sitting and positioning the patient for the indirect laryngoscopic examination. Following penetrating trauma to the neck involving the upper aerodigestive tract, there is obvious need for extensive evaluation after establishing a secure airway. We recommend aggressive and early treatment in laryngotracheal injuries (Table 2-3).

In this chapter, we have attempted to develop a rational plan for upper airway management based on the particular needs of the patient and an understanding of the pathophysiology of the region. This approach individualizes patient management while recognizing inherent difficulties when recommending one form of treatment for all upper airway problems.

TABLE 2-3. *Management of Laryngotracheal Trauma.*

Type I

Signs and Symptoms: hoarseness, hemoptysis, no airway compromise, minor laryngeal hematoma, no fractures.

Treatment: indirect laryngoscopy, bed rest, elevation of head of bed, cool mist, tracheotomy tray at bedside.

Type II

Signs and Symptoms: airway compromise, hematoma.

Treatment: tracheotomy, direct laryngoscopy and esophagoscopy. In the absence of lacerations or displaced fracture, the larynx is not opened.

Type III

Signs and Symptoms: airway compromise, large lacerations.

Treatment: tracheotomy, direct laryngoscopy, and esophagoscopy. Midline or paramedian thyrotomy through fracture site. Primary mucosal closure. Stenting ±.

Type IV

Signs and Symptoms: airway compromise, detectable fractures and dislocations.

Treatment: tracheotomy, direct laryngoscopy and esophagoscopy. Midline or paramedian thyrotomy through fracture site. Primary mucosal closure. Open reduction and internal fixation of cartilage. Stenting mandatory.

References

1. Negus, V. E.: The Comparative Anatomy and Physiology of the Larynx. London, William Heinemann, 1949.
2. Scatliff, J. H., and Sabette, M. P.: Pharyngeal cinefluorography in clinical practice. A. J. R., *90*:823, 1963.
3. Argamaso, R. V., et al.: The role of the lateral pharyngeal wall movement in pharyngeal flap surgery. Plast. Reconstr. Surg., *66*:214, 1980.
4. Atkinson, M., Kramer, P., Wyman, S. M., and Ingelfinger, F. J.: The dynamics of swallowing; 1. Normal pharyngeal mechanisms. J. Clin. Invest., *36*:581, 1957.
5. Pressman, J. J., and Keleman, G.: Physiology of the larynx. Physiol. Rev., *35*:506, 1955.
6. Shelton, R. J., Jr., and Bosma, J. F.: Maintenance of the pharyngeal airway. J. Appl. Physiol., *17*:209, 1962.
7. Sasaki, C. T., Suzuki, M., Horuchi, M., and Kirchner, J. A.: The effect of tracheostomy on the laryngeal closure reflex. Laryngoscope, *87*:1428, 1977.
8. Trone, T. H., Schaefer, S. D., and Carder, H. M.: Blunt and penetrating laryngeal trauma: A 13-year review. Otolaryngol. Head Neck Surg. *88*:257, 1980.

Chapter 3 Management of Nonpenetrating Chest Injuries

MARVIN M. KIRSH

Traffic fatalities generally are characterized by multiple injuries of which between 35 and 40% include chest injuries. Statistics from the University of Michigan show that 12% of 235 traffic fatalities were entirely due to thoracic injuries, whereas injury of the thorax was a major contributing factor in another 56.4%.

Initial Management and General Considerations

On arrival in the emergency room, the condition of the person who has sustained severe blunt trauma to the chest varies greatly. The majority of patients are first seen in critical condition and require immediate treatment. On the other hand, there are patients who sustain a life-threatening injury but do not initially appear to be dangerously ill. If the injury is not recognized quickly, death frequently results. The physician caring for patients suffering from blunt chest trauma must not be deceived by an initially good condition and must always be alert for the likelihood of later clinical deterioration. Careful and frequent observation of any patient with a blunt chest injury is as important as the initial evaluation. The physician's attention must not be diverted from thoracic injuries by obvious extrathoracic injuries. After any immediate life-threatening emergencies have been treated, the physician should undertake a careful history, if possible, and methodically examine all systems in the injured patient. Knowledge of the patient's past medical history, allergies, and medications may influence subsequent therapy. Guidelines to the likely injuries may be gained from the knowledge of the circumstances under which the injury occurred. The intrathoracic injuries sutained in a vehicular collision, for example, are different for the driver and for the passenger and are also different from those of a victim who has fallen from a great height.

The major objective in the initial management of patients with blunt chest trauma is the restoration and maintenance of normal cardiopulmonary function. This objective is accomplished by the creation of an adequate airway, establishment of satisfactory ventilation, and correction of hypovolemia or low cardiac output. Although discussed separately, the resuscitative efforts are often carried out simultaneously and are individualized according to the patient's needs.

Airway and Ventilation

The institution and maintenance of an adequate airway and proper ventilation take precedence over all other treatment. The presence of upper airway obstruction is likely if the patient is making efforts to breathe but has little or no movement of air into the lungs, as determined by auscultation. Such a patient also has inspiratory stridor. At times, an adequate airway can be achieved by aspiration of blood, mucus, vomitus, and loose foreign bodies from the oropharynx, forward retraction of the tongue, or insertion of an oral airway. Dentures should always be removed from the patient's mouth. Insertion of a cuffed endotracheal tube is the most satisfactory method of controlling the patient's airway. Before this is done, the patient should be hyperventilated with 100% oxygen by the Ambubag and mask technique. Intubation should be accomplished as quickly as possible, with associated ventilation interposed between attempts.

Laryngeal or cervical tracheal fractures usually prevent endotracheal intubation. These fractures are two of the relatively few indications for emergency tracheostomy. Excessive bleeding into the mouth or pharynx makes endotracheal intubation almost impossible and is another indication for tracheostomy.

Collapse or compression of one or both lungs by accumulation of air or fluid can impair ventilation. Decreased breath sounds, hyperresonance to percussion, and subcutaneous emphysema suggest a pneumothorax, whereas decreased breath sounds and dullness to percussion suggest hemothorax. A tension pneumothorax is suggested by the findings of a pneumothorax plus deviation of the trachea to the contralateral side and apical heart tones. The diagnosis is confirmed by a chest roentgenogram, which should be obtained as soon as possible. If the patient's condition is critical, however, treatment should be instituted without waiting for the chest roentgenogram. Re-expansion of the lung by closed-tube thoracostomy greatly improves ventilation. If possible, an esophagram should be obtained on all patients sustaining blunt chest trauma, especially those with pneumothorax and continued air leak, to rule out associated esophageal injuries, which are often difficult to diagnose.

Other causes of impaired ventilation that require immediate treatment are open pneumothorax (sucking chest wound), flail chest, diaphragmatic hernia, cardiac injuries, pulmonary contusion, pulmonary laceration and aspiration of blood, gastric contents, or foreign body, and acute gastric dilation. Acute gastric dilation causes elevation of the diaphragm and impairs ventilation by reducing the size of the available pleural space. Insertion of a nasogastric tube not only decompresses the stomach, but also lessens the likelihood of aspiration of gastric contents.

The status of a patient's ventilation is best determined by arterial blood-gas studies. If the arterial Po_2 is less than 60 mm Hg while the patient is breathing room air or less than 80 mm Hg while breathing supplemental nasal oxygen, the patient should be placed on a respirator. The severity of the pulmonary dysfunction can be estimated by determining the Pa_{O_2} while the patient is breathing 100% oxygen, either through a rebreathing mask or an endotracheal tube. If the Pa_{O_2} is greater than 300 mm Hg, the patient does not have significant pulmonary dysfunction; however, if the Pa_{O_2} is less than 300 mm Hg, the patient has significant pulmonary dysfunction and should be placed on a mechanical ventilator.

The clinical findings of hypoxia (i.e., agitation, restlessness, apprehension, combativeness, tachypnea, and tachycardia) are too often attributed to other causes, such as alcoholic intoxication, head injury, or pain in general. Patients with these findings should be suspected of suffering from hypoxia until proved otherwise. Narcotics should be administered with caution if the patient is not intubated, since they can depress respiration further. The diagnosis of hypoxia is established by arterial blood-gas studies, and if arterial blood gases cannot be obtained, these patients should be intubated and ventilated with a respirator.

Disturbances of Cardiovascular Function

The circulation may be disturbed in three ways. First, hemorrhage results in reduced venous return to the heart and, consequently, lowers the blood pressure and reduces cardiac output. Second, pericardial blood impedes diastolic filling of the heart, resulting in reduced cardiac output. Finally, the heart itself may be injured, as in myocardial contusion.

Blood loss is the most common cause of reduced cardiovascular function in patients who have sustained blunt trauma to the chest. Hypovolemia in many of these patients is frequently the result of associated extrathoracic injuries. Two to four large-bore No. 15-gauge intravenous catheters should be inserted percutaneously or by cutdown into large veins above and below the diaphragm (subclavian, internal jugular, femoral). One of the catheters should be advanced centrally into the superior vena cava or right atrium for continuous measurement of the central venous pressure (CVP). The constant monitoring of the CVP aids in judging the patient's response to volume administration and in determining the presence or absence of pericardial tamponade. The blood that is initially used for resuscitation is most often bank blood, which has been shown to contain a considerable amount of amorphous debris. The use of fine-screen blood filters in patients receiving multiple transfusions has prevented the debris from entering the pulmonary circulation, plugging the arterioles, and further damaging the lung. All patients with blunt chest trauma requiring transfusion should receive blood passed through a fine-screen filter. Metabolic acidosis should be corrected by the intravenous infusion of sodium bicarbonate (mEq $NaHCO_3 = 0.3 \times$ weight in kilograms $\times$ base deficit). Repeated blood-gas studies should be obtained 30 to 45 minutes after the sodium bicarbonate infusion and additional $NaHCO_3$ given if needed.

The presence of acute pericardial tamponade is difficult to recognize in patients with blunt chest trauma and should be considered in patients whose circulatory collapse is out of proportion to the severity of the wound or blood loss. It should also be suspected in every patient who responds to rapid volume infusion with an elevated central venous pressure rather than with a rise in arterial pressure, regardless of the initial central venous pressure, and in every patient who presents with an elevated central venous pressure or pulsating distended neck veins when he is in the upright position. If the diagnosis of acute pericardial tamponade is suspected, immediate pericardicentesis should be performed with the patient in the upright position (45°), with the use of the subxiphoid approach. As much fluid or blood as possible should be removed. The removal of as little as 15 to 25 ml of blood may be sufficient to decompress the pericardium and temporarily revive the patient. A negative pericardicentesis does not rule out the presence of tamponade. If the diagnosis cannot be established after pericardicentesis and if the likelihood that the patient has cardiac tamponade is great, the pericardium can be explored under local anesthesia with the use of an infraxiphoid retrosternal approach.

An electrocardiogram should be obtained as soon as is feasible to detect the possible occurrence of myocardial contusion. Patients with myocardial contusions should be monitored carefully and any cardiac arrhythmias treated appropriately. Low cardiac output secondary to myocardial contusion is a rare occurrence; if it occurs and an inotropic agent is needed, dopamine or the combination of levarterenol and phentolamine are the preferred agents.

During the initial period of evaluation and resuscitation, and for a period of time afterward, the patient's cardiopulmonary status should be continuously reassessed to determine whether his condition is responding satisfactorily, whether it has deteriorated, or whether a delayed or previously unrecognized complication of blunt chest trauma has developed.

Pulmonary Contusion

Pulmonary contusion is damage to the lung parenchyma resulting in edema and hemorrhage without an accompanying pulmonary laceration; it is a common finding in patients who have sustained blunt trauma to the chest. The incidence of pulmonary contusion reported in patients sustaining major nonpenetrating chest trauma varies between 31.6 and 75.8%. Although often mild and frequently masked by other more dramatic injuries, such as flail chest, pneumothorax, and hemothorax, pulmonary contusion deserves careful consideration in the management of any patient with chest trauma because it has been recognized recently as a distinct lethal entity in itself. The mortality rate from pulmonary contusion alone ranges from 13.7 to 39.0%. Pulmonary contusion plays a major role in one fourth of the deaths due to chest injuries resulting from automobile accidents.

Roentgenographic Findings

The roentgenographic findings depend on the severity of the pulmonary contusion and may vary widely in both distribution and appearance. Pulmonary contusion has an abrupt onset and rapid rate of clearing. The initial chest roentgenogram may show no evidence of intrathoracic injury. This information is valuable because it provides a baseline for later comparison.

Two basic roentgenographic patterns have been described. The more frequent finding is a pulmonary infiltrate characterized by patchy, ill-defined areas of increased parenchymal density. The pathologic basis of these densities is intra-alveolar hemorrhage. The degree of involvement may range from small localized areas to extensive homogeneous opacification. The less frequent pattern is a linear irregular infiltrate with a peribronchial distribution. This appearance is produced by peribroncheolar or perivascular hemorrhage. Signs of resolution usually begin within 48 to 72 hours after injury, but complete clearing may take as long as 14 days to occur. There is usually no evidence of residual pulmonary abnormality after clearing. If resolution does not occur, or if there is progression of the lesion after 48 to 72 hours, a complication should be suspected.

Clinical Features

The clinical picture depends directly on the severity of the injury and can be divided into three categories. It is important to remember that, regardless of the severity of the injury, there may be delay in the onset of symptoms and roentgenographic findings. In addition, the clinical signs of hypoxia may be difficult to recognize, especially in patients with multiple injuries. Arterial blood-gas measurement is the only effective way to evaluate accurately the efficiency of gas exchange. An arterial Po_2 of less than 60 mm Hg with the patient breathing room air or a Pa_{O_2} of less than 300 mm Hg with the patient breathing 100% oxygen is indicative of significant pulmonary dysfunction. The presence of an elevated arterial Pa_{CO_2} (40 mm Hg), in addition to hypoxemia, is an even more ominous finding. Normally, the patient with hypoxemia hyperventilates, and thus any elevation of Pa_{CO_2} is evidence of marked reduction in pulmonary function and indicates the need for support from a respirator. These determinations will help to prevent delays in instituting treatment.

The clinical presentation, management, and prognosis of pulmonary contusion depend on the severity of the injury, and patients can be divided into three groups according to severity of injury.

Group I

Patients in group I may be entirely asymptomatic and may have only roentgenographic evidence of pulmonary contusion. However, these patients usually have symptoms. The patients are usually alert and are able to cough effectively to clear their secretions. Chest pain is present and probably is related to the chest-wall injury rather than to the pulmonary injury. The first evidence of pulmonary contusion if tachypnea, tachycardia, and the presence of rales heard in auscultation. The loose cough produces copious secretions that may be blood tinged. The roentgenographic appearance is usually more severe than the clinical condition of the patient or the degree of change in blood-gas determinations. In most patients, decrease in arterial Pco_2 is minimal.

It should be emphasized that the key to success in management of these patients is good tracheobronchial care that should include intratracheal suction and physical therapy. Bronchoscopy should be performed when secretions cannot be cleared despite these measures. Ultrasonic nebulization by mist or intermittent positive pressure decreases the viscosity of the inspissated secretions. Adequate relief of pain is obtained with narcotics or intercostal nerve block. Because the damaged lung is susceptible to infection, broad-spectrum antibiotics are used. Cultures of the sputum are obtained and antibiotics altered accordingly. Administration of oxygen by mask or nasal cannula may be required in some patients for 24 to 36 hours.

Intravenous fluids should be administered with caution. If large volumes of fluid are needed for resuscitation of the patient, plasma is preferable to Ringer's lactate or saline solution because, as discussed, plasma maintains a normal colloid osmotic pressure. Blood should be administered through a fine-screen filter to remove any platelet or leukocyte aggregates that are present.

The course in these patients is characterized by rapid resolution of the parenchymal abnormality within 72 to 96 hours, disappearance of all signs and symptoms, and return of blood-gas determinations to normal. Survival approaches 100%. The appearance of more extensive lesions after 72 hours in conjunction with clinical deterioration of the patient should raise the suspicion of a superimposed process, such as pneumonia, fat emboli, or pulmonary emboli.

Group II

Patients in group II have sustained a more severe pulmonary injury than those in group I. The contusion occurs frequently without evidence of fracture of the bony thorax, particularly in the younger patient. The seriousness of the underlying pulmonary contusion may be overlooked initially because of the presence of associated extrathoracic injuries that divert attention from the pulmonary problem. If a pneumothorax or hemothorax is present, the extent of the pulmonary contusion may not be fully appreciated until the air or blood is removed, leading to further delay in diagnosis and treatment.

A typical clinical pattern develops in these patients, although it may take 2 to 6 hours for symptoms to develop. Even though minimal symptoms and signs may be present initially, the chest roentgenogram shows the characteristic appearance of severe pulmonary contusion. Alterations in blood-gas values also precede the onset of clinical symptoms and are present at the time of admission, regardless of the clinical status of the patient. The changes occur early and are characterized by a moderate decrease in Po_2 and pH, and an increase in Pco_2.

The first clinical evidence of contusion includes tachypnea, tachycardia, and the presence of scattered "wet" rales heard at auscultation. The essential feature in these patients is the occurrence of copious amounts of mucus, serum, and then frank blood in the tracheobronchial tree. The patient coughs incessantly but is unable to clear the secretions. He becomes restless and apprehensive, and he develops labored respirations. These are early signs of hypoxia, but often are attributed to the associated head injury or to pain. The pattern is one of progressive respiratory insufficiency with increasing dyspnea, tachypnea, and even cyanosis. Coincident with the deterioration in the patient's clinical condition is a progressive fall in arterial Po_2 and pH, widening of alveolar arterial oxygen tension, and rise in Pco_2. There is also roentgenographic evidence of progression. Associated complications, such as hypovolemia, shock, and myocardial contusion, may further complicate management of the patient.

The diagnosis of severe pulmonary contusion must be suspected in any patient who has been subjected to severe thoracic trauma, because survival in these patients depends on early and vigorous therapy. The first 24 hours of treatment are by far the most important. Blood-gas determinations should be performed at the time of admission on all patients sustaining severe thoracic injury. Hypoxia, if present, then will be recognized early, and adequate therapy can be carried out to correct the hypoxia and its lethal sequelae.

The goal of therapy is to restore and maintain oxygenation while avoiding resuscitative measures that might aggravate the pulmonary contusion (Table 3-1).

Endotracheal intubation and control of respiration with a volume-cycled respirator are the best means of achieving adequate oxygenation in patients in group II. Tracheostomy is reserved for patients who require respirator assistance for longer than 31 days. Humidified oxygen helps to raise the Pao_2, endotracheal intubation facilitates removal of secretions, and assisted respiration reduces the work of breathing. Providing adequate humidity in the gas stream is imperative. Although pulmonary ventilation and gas exchange may maintain a normal Pao_2, adequate hemoglobin levels are required to ensure ample delivery of oxygen to tissues.

Table 3-1. *Steps in the Management of Pulmonary Contusion.*

1. Use mechanical ventilation through an endotracheal tube.
2. Use lowest Fi_{O_2} possible to maintain Pa_{O_2} at 60 mm Hg.
3. Use PEEP if unable to maintain Pa_{O_2} of at least 60 mm Hg on an Fi_{O_2} of 0.6.
4. Maintain hematocrit between 40 and 45.
5. Use bronchodilators for bronchospasm.
6. Maintain pH between 7.35 and 7.45.
7. Limit crystalloid solution to 50 ml/hr.
8. Administer furosemide (Lasix), 40 mg intravenously, immediately, and daily thereafter until no longer needed.
9. Administer methylprednisolone, 30 mg/kg of body weight intravenously, immediately, and in divided doses thereafter for 48 hours.
10. Use nasogastric suction.
11. Correct metabolic acidosis with intravenous infusion of sodium bicarbonate.
12. Make frequent cultures of tracheobronchial secretions.

The hematocrit should be maintained at between 40 and 45% by transfusions of whole blood or packed cells. Because bank blood contains a reduced amount of 2,3-diphosphoglycerate and, consequently, the reduced ability of hemoglobin to release oxygen, every effort should be made to keep the patient's pH between 7.35 and 7.45. The tidal volume of the respirator should generally be maintained at 10 to 15 ml/kg of body weight, and the inspiratory inflation pressure should be kept below 40 to 45 cm H_2O. The potential danger of high partial pressures of oxygen in the inspired gas mixture is now well known. This danger can be avoided by using the lowest possible inspired oxygen concentration that will continue to maintain the patient's Pa_{O_2} above 60 mm Hg. Rather than risk the danger of oxygen toxicity by increasing the inspired concentration of oxygen above 60%, it is better to use positive end-expiratory pressure (PEEP).

A nasogastric tube is inserted to avoid gastric distension and aspiration of gastric contents. Intravenous fluids are administered cautiously to avoid pulmonary edema. Large dosages of steroids (30 mg/kg methylprednisolone sodium succinate for injection Solu-Medrol a day) reduce secretions and interstitial edema and should be administered for 48 hours. Diuretics, by decreasing the excess fluid within the lung, and salt-poor albumin, by increasing the serum oncotic pressure, have been shown by Skillman to be of benefit when used together in patients with respiratory failure. Ethacrynic acid (50 mg) or furosemide (40 mg) and 25 g salt-poor albumin are administered immediately after injury and daily until there are no further beneficial results. Despite optimal medical therapy, approximately 15% of these patients die.

Group III

The patients in group III have sustained a severe pulmonary contusion and show signs of early onset of respiratory failure. Even after hypovolemia is corrected, the patients are agitated and restless to the point of being combative. Rapid, labored respirations, tachycardia, and cyanosis are present on admission. Coughing is incessant and produces copious amounts of mucoid, frothy, blood-tinged secretions. Frank hemoptysis is present in many of these patients. Wheezes, rales, and bronchial breathing are scattered throughout both lung fields. Arterial blood-gas determinations show a marked decrease in P_{O_2} and pH, with an increase in PCO_2. The widened alveolar arterial oxygen gradient also reflects the serious degree of involvement.

Despite the early use of respirator support, high concentrations of oxygen in the inspired gas mixture, steroids, and careful regulation of fluid administration, the patient's course is one of rapid, progressive respiratory insufficiency, and death occurs from hypoxia within 72 to 96 hours of injury. Until recently, there was no way to support patients dying from pulmonary insufficiency secondary to pulmonary contusion long enough to allow recovery of pulmonary function. With the development and clinical use of membrane oxygenators, such a means is now available.

Pneumothorax

Pneumothorax is a common complication of blunt chest trauma. The incidence varies between 15 and 50%. When atmospheric air has direct access to the pleural cavity through the wound, the condition is called an open, or communicating, pneumothorax, also often called a sucking chest wound.

When the integrity of the skin and chest wall remains intact and the atmospheric air has no direct access to the pleural cavity, the pneumothorax is termed closed, or noncommunicating. The vast majority of pneumothoraces following blunt chest trauma are of the closed variety. Because the pathogenesis and management of open and closed pneumothoraces are different, the two conditions will be discussed separately.

Closed Pneumothorax

In general, a closed pneumothorax that results from injury to the lung parenchyma tends to be self-limiting because the resultant pulmonary collapse has a sealing effect. Such a closed pneumothorax is termed simple pneumothorax. At times, the pulmonary collapse does not have a sealing effect, however, and the damaged alveoli enlarge during inspiration, thus allowing air to enter the pleural cavity. During expiration, the damaged alveoli close, permitting little or no return during expiration. A flutter valve is thus formed, leading to a buildup of pressure in the pleural cavity. The intrapleural pressures during both inspiration and expiration may rise above atmospheric pressure. This variety of closed pneumothorax is termed tension pneumothorax. Since the pathophysiology, clinical presentation, and management of simple pneumothorax and tension pneumothorax are dissimilar, these conditions too will be discussed separately.

Pneumothorax of the closed variety may also be caused by rupture of the esophagus or fractures of the tracheobronchial tree. The presence of these injuries should always be considered in any patient with either a simple or a tension pneumothorax following blunt chest trauma.

Simple Pneumothorax

Simple pneumothoraces are usually classified according to the volume of the hemithorax occupied by air and the degree of pulmonary collapse. A pneumothorax that occupies 15% or less of the pleural cavity in association with minor degrees of collapse is classified as small; one that occupies between 15 and 60% of the pleural cavity is classified as moderate; and one that occupies more than 60% of the pleural cavity in association with almost complete collapse of the lung is classified as large. As a rule, only patients with moderate or large pneumothoraces are symptomatic. However, in some patients, especially those with pre-existing lung disease, a small pneumothorax may compromise pulmonary function sufficiently to cause symptoms.

The most frequent symptoms in patients with moderate or severe pneumothorax are chest pain and shortness of breath. On physical examination, the breath sounds are distant or entirely absent over the involved hemithorax. At times, this finding may be difficult to interpret because pain and splinting prevent the patient from breathing deeply. Subcutaneous emphysema is present in about 25% of the patients.

The diagnosis of pneumothorax is suggested by the history and clinical findings and is confirmed by a chest roentgenogram, which should be obtained at the earliest possible time to estimate the size of the pneumothorax, but should not take precedence over initiation of emergency treatment. A roentgenographic diagnosis of moderate to large pneumothorax is usually made without much difficulty. The most important sign is separation of the visceral pleura from the parietal pleura by an abnormal collection of air in the pleural cavity.

The treatment of closed pneumothorax depends on the volume of the pneumothorax, the degree of pulmonary collapse, the severity of the respiratory symptoms, the presence or absence of associated injuries, and the likelihood that a nonthoracic operation and general anesthetic may be necessary. Only those otherwise healthy patients whose pneumothorax is small, who are without respiratory symptoms, and in whom the likelihood of an operation is negligible can be treated without the insertion of a chest tube and by careful observation. Another chest roentgenogram should be obtained 6 to 8 hours after the patient's admission and daily thereafter until complete re-expansion of the lung has occurred. If the pneumothorax increases in size, a chest tube should be inserted. Generally, the lungs re-expand fully in 2 to 4 days and remain expanded.

The indications for closed-tube thoracostomy are:

1. Moderate to large pneumothorax.
2. Presence of respiratory symptoms, regardless of size of pneumothorax.
3. Increase in size of pneumothorax that initially was treated conservatively.
4. Recurrence of pneumothorax after initial chest tube was removed.
5. Patient requiring ventilator support.
6. Patient about to undergo general anesthesia.
7. Associated hemothorax.
8. Bilateral pneumothorax.
9. Tension pneumothorax.

If at all possible, the chest tube should be inserted with the patient in the upright or semi-upright position, since the diaphragm may rise as high as the second or third intercostal space when the patient is supine. The second or third anterior intercostal space at the midclavicular line is usually the best site of insertion. The tube can be inserted with the aid of either a trocar or a hemostat. The chest tube is connected to underwater drainage with 15 to 20 cm H_2O suction. For patients with an associated hemothorax, a second chest tube should be inserted in the fifth or sixth intercostal space in the midaxillary line. As soon as the chest tube is secured, a repeat chest roentgenogram should be obtained with the patient in the upright position to verify that the tube is in the correct intrapleural location and is functioning properly to determine the degree of re-expansion of the lung.

Serial chest roentgenograms are a necessity in these patients. The lung usually re-expands fully in 2 to 4 days.

At times, the pneumothorax cannot be completely evacuated, and in addition, it may be associated with a persistent air leak. The most frequent causes of these problems are improper position of chest tube (extrapleural, kinking, not in apex), insufficient number of tubes, inadequate suction, side hole of chest tube mistakenly placed extrapleurally, inadequate seal about site of chest tube, retained bronchial secretions, associated rupture of the tracheobronchial tree, associated ruptured esophagus, and pulmonary laceration. The patient with a persistent pneumothorax and air leak should be systematically evaluated and the cause determined and treated accordingly. When the air leak is secondary to a major intrathoracic injury (e.g., ruptured bronchus, pulmonary laceration), a thoracotomy is necessary.

Tension pneumothorax

Patients with tension pneumothorax are acutely ill and in marked respiratory distress. They are restless, agitated, dyspneic, and even cyanotic. On physical examination, the patients are hypotensive and have tachypnea and tachycardia. There is evidence of nasal flaring and intercostal retraction, in addition to hyperresonance to percussion. Breath sounds are absent over the involved hemithorax; subcutaneous emphysema may or may not be present. The keys to the diagnosis are the presence of displacement of the cervical trachea and cardiac apical impulse toward the uninvolved side.

The diagnosis is confirmed by the chest roentgenogram, which shows collapse of the uninvolved lung, depression of the ipsilateral diaphragm, and shift of the mediastinum toward the unaffected lung.

Tension pneumothorax is life threatening and demands immediate diagnosis and treatment.

Treatment should not be delayed while awaiting roentgenographic confirmation. If no other equipment is available, a large-bore, No. 15- or No. 18-gauge needle can be inserted anteriorly without anesthetic into the involved hemithorax through the second or third intercostal space to achieve partial decompression while the preparations are made for closed-tube thoracostomy. When the needle is inserted into the pleural cavity, a large amount of air escapes under pressure. The preferred method of treatment is closed-tube thoracostomy. Dramatic relief of symptoms is brought about by decompression of the pleural cavity.

Open Pneumothorax

Open pneumothorax (sucking chest wound) that results from blunt chest trauma is associated with large defects in the chest wall. The patients, as a rule, present with the signs and symptoms of respiratory distress. During respiration, a sucking sound is often heard, and the edge of the lung may be seen through the defect. Subcutaneous emphysema is often present and is usually extensive, spreading to involve both hemithoraces, the cervical region, head, and anterior abdominal wall.

Sucking wounds of the chest demand immediate surgical treatment. The patient with an open pneumothorax should be intubated immediately and placed on a respirator, and the wound should be covered with sterile nonocclusive dressings. Endotracheal intubation in these patients may be difficult and should be attempted only by skilled personnel. While the arrival of skilled help is awaited, the wound should be covered with petrolatum gauze extending 3 to 5 inches beyond the wound in all directions. The gauze is supported with 4-by-4-inch pads and held in place with elastic adhesive. An intercostal chest tube should also be inserted in an area removed from the injured area. After the patient has been successfully resuscitated and has undergone all appropriate diagnostic studies, the wound should be explored.

Hemothorax

Like pneumothorax, hemothorax is a common sequel to blunt chest trauma. The incidence of hemothorax reported in patients sustaining nonpenetrating trauma varies between 25 and 75%. The source of bleeding may be the lung, the heart, the great vessels and their branches, an intercostal artery or vein, mediastinal veins, or the vessels of the diaphragm and chest wall. As a rule, bleeding from the lung tends to be self-limiting unless a major laceration has occurred or a large hilar vessel has been injured. Bleeding from an intercostal artery or vein is caused by fracture of the ribs. Because these vessels arise directly from the aorta, bleeding may be brisk and persistent. Hemothorax associated with heart and great-vessel injury will not be discussed.

Diagnosis

If less than 400 ml of blood are lost, there may be little or no change in the patient's appearance and vital signs and fluid may not be present. With large losses (>2000 ml), the findings of internal hemorrhage are present: pallor, restlessness, an anxious expression, tachycardia, and decreased or decreasing blood pressure. The patients may complain of dyspnea and a peculiar tightness in the chest. The pleural fluid is best visualized on a roentgenogram of the chest when the patient is in the upright position. Less than 250 ml of pleural fluid is often not demonstrable on the chest roentgenogram. On the frontal projection, the fluid obscures the costophrenic angle and has the appearance of a homogeneous opacity with a concave upper border, higher laterally than medially. On the lateral chest roentgenogram, the posterior portion of the diaphragmatic silhouette cannot be seen. With massive fluid accumulation, the involved hemithorax appears opaque and the heart and mediastinum are shifted toward the uninvolved side.

The management of patients with hemothorax depends on the severity of the symptoms and the amount of fluid that is demonstrated on the chest roentgenogram. The hemothoraces are arbitrarily classified into three groups: small, moderate, and massive.

Small Hemothorax

Most patients with a small hemothorax (<400 ml blood loss) are asymptomatic and may not even have the physical findings of intrapleural fluid. The chest roentgenogram shows only blunting of the costophrenic angle. No specific therapy other than careful observation is necessary for these patients, since the small amounts of blood in the pleural space are rapidly absorbed within 10 to 14 days. Frequent serial chest roentgenograms are necessary for several days because some of these patients may develop delayed bleeding that, if undetected, may cause difficulty. If removal of the fluid from these patients is deemed necessary, it is preferable to insert a chest tube, since thoracentesis may result in pneumothorax.

Moderate Hemothorax

Patients with moderate hemothorax (500 to 2000 ml blood loss) have the symptoms and physical findings previously outlined. On the chest roentgenogram, the fluid occupies as much as one third of the involved hemithorax. Although hemothoraces can be managed by repeated thoracentesis, they are best managed by insertion of a large-bore (No. 32 or No. 36 Argyle) catheter. Tube thoracostomy allows constant monitoring of continued blood loss, as well as continued drainage for better re-expansion of the lung. The chest tube should be inserted with the patient in the upright or semi-upright position. The chest tube should be inserted through the fifth or sixth intercostal space in the midaxillary line. The chest tube should be connected to underwater seal drainage and high suction (20 to 30 cm H_2O).

Most patients with moderate hemothorax can be treated successfully with volume replacement and closed-tube thoracostomy and do not need a thoracotomy. Bleeding of 200 ml/hr or less usually subsides spontaneously. However, thoracotomy is necessary for control of bleeding in some patients. Immediate thoracotomy is indicated when (1) bleeding through the chest tubes exceeds 300 to 500 ml/hr or is greater than 200 ml/hr for 5 hours, (2) the hemothorax is shown on the chest roentgenogram to be increasing, or (3) the patient remains or becomes hypotensive despite adequate blood replacement.

Massive Hemothorax

Patients with massive hemothorax (>2000 ml blood loss) suffer from the detrimental effects of hypovolemia and hypoxia and are critically ill on admission. They are dyspneic, tachypneic, cyanotic, and hypotensive. The trachea and apical cardiac impulse may be displaced to the contralateral side. The extent of dullness to percussion and absence of breath sounds corresponds to the extent of the hemothorax. On the chest roentgenogram, fluid occupies one half or more of the hemithorax.

A large-bore chest tube should be inserted immediately in the fifth or sixth intercostal space in the midaxillary line. At the same time, vigorous replacement of blood volume should be carried out, and the patient should be intubated and placed on a respirator. In some of these patients, after insertion of the chest tube, the blood drains at a rate that indicates that the patient is about to become exsanguinate. All patients with massive hemothorax should undergo immediate thoracotomy.

Hemopneumothorax

Patients with hemopneumothorax, as identified by air-fluid level on the chest roentgenogram, should have two chest tubes inserted, one through the fifth or sixth intercostal space at the midaxillary line and the other through the second or third intercostal space at the midclavicular line. An alternate technique calls for inserting a multifenestrated chest tube through the fifth or sixth intercostal space and advancing it into the apex of the chest.

Chest-Wall Injuries

Simple Rib Fractures

Approximately 40% of patients sustaining nonpenetrating thoracic trauma sustain fractures of the ribs, the most common of all chest injuries. Fractures of the ribs are more common in adults than in children, because the cartilage in children is more resilient and can absorb the impact without breaking. On the other hand, the ribs of elderly individuals are brittle and can be broken even by minor degrees of trauma. The fifth to ninth ribs are most frequently broken, and fractures on the left side are more common than fractures on the right. If the rib fragment is driven inward, laceration of the pleura, pulmonary parenchyma, and intercostal vessels might occur, resulting in pneumothorax, hemothorax, or both, which may at times be life threatening.

Another delayed complication that is apt to occur in elderly patients or patients with preexisting chronic lung disease is pneumonia and, possibly, respiratory failure. Rib fractures are invariably accompanied by pain. To reduce the pain to tolerable levels, the patient both consciously and unconsciously restricts excursion of the chest wall by shallow breathing. Such shallow breathing results in the ventilation of fewer alveoli. The unaerated alveoli collapse, secretions accumulate, and atelectasis develops. Because coughing causes pain, the patient consciously reduces coughing and thus becomes less efficient in removing secretions. As a result, additional atelectasis develops, thereby setting up a vicious cycle which, if uninterrupted, could lead to death. The pain is most severe and the patient is at the greatest risk from respiratory complications during the first few days after injury. Although this sequence of events is unlikely to occur in young, healthy patients, rib fractures must never be considered insignificant until proved so.

Almost all conscious and alert patients with rib fractures experience a pleuritic type of chest pain that is usually localized to the site of fracture. The pain is localized when one rib is fractured, but it may spread over a wide area when a number of ribs are fractured. The pain is aggravated by coughing, deep breathing, and motion. On physical examination, there is tenderness to palpation, and if displacement is present, bone crepitus may be felt.

The diagnosis is suggested by the history of trauma and the eliciting of pain on palpation; it is confirmed by visualization of the fracture site on chest roentgenogram.

Both an inspiratory and an expiratory chest roentgenogram should be taken of all patients sustaining rib fracture to rule out an unsuspected pneumothorax. Serial chest roentgenograms should be obtained in all patients with rib fractures, since delayed pneumothorax or hemothorax may develop after the initial injury.

When rib fractures are complicated by pneumothorax or hemothorax, these complications must be treated promptly and prior to treatment of the rib fractures. The treatment of the rib fractures depends on the severity of the injury, the age of the patient, the presence of pre-existing lung disease, and the pain threshold of the patient. In young or healthy patients with uncomplicated rib fractures, the relief of pain may be the only therapy that is required. Stronger analgesics or narcotics, such as demerol or codeine, may be needed during the first few days, when the pain is most severe. If pain is not relieved by these analgesics, intercostal nerve block should be used. After the first days, milder analgesics, such as propoxyphene hydrochloride (Darvon) or acetylsalicylic acid (aspirin), usually suffice.

In elderly patients or patients with pre-existing lung disease or a low pain threshold, therapy should be instituted early and aggressively to prevent pulmonary complications. Narcotics should be given immediately to control pain, and they may be repeated as often as necessary. Large doses should be avoided because of respiratory depressant effect. Intercostal nerve block that includes two nerves above and two nerves below the fracture sites relieves pain and permits the patient to ventilate and cough.

First Rib Fractures

Isolated first rib fractures are uncommon, since these ribs usually require an extremely violent force to become fractured. The clinical significance of these fractures is that they may signify either injury to adjacent structures, such as the subclavian artery and vein and brachial plexus, or the other serious intrathoracic injuries, such as rupture of the aorta, rupture of the bronchus, or myocardial contusion. Fracture of the first rib should alert the physician to the possibility of associated serious injuries which should be sought for carefully.

Sternal Fractures

Sternal fracture is an uncommon injury but is increasing in frequency because of trauma caused by steering wheels. Severe trauma is usually necessary to produce a sternal fracture, and this fact accounts for the high incidence of associated serious intrathoracic and extrathoracic injuries listed in Table 3-2. The actual presence of a sternal fracture should alert the physician to the possibility that severe associated injuries might be present and that appropriate investigative studies should be undertaken.

Almost all patients with displaced sternal fractures experience pain at the fracture site, which is aggravated by coughing and deep breathing. The pain is described as sharp and knife-like and, at times, excruciating. On physical examination,

Table 3-2. *Injuries Associated With Sternal Fractures.*

1. Flail chest
2. Pulmonary contusion
3. Ruptured bronchus
4. Hemothorax or pneumothorax
5. Hemopericardium
6. Lacerated pericardium
7. Myocardial contusion
8. Valvular cardiac injuries
9. Cardiac rupture
10. Ruptured thoracic aorta
11. Abdominal visceral injuries
12. Spinal injuries

there is swelling and discoloration overlying the fracture, tenderness to palpation, and, at times, crepitation. The patient with an undisplaced fracture may be asymptomatic, and the fracture may go undetected.

The diagnosis is confirmed by visualization of the fracture site on a lateral or oblique chest roentgenogram. The fracture site cannot be seen on a posterior anterior chest roentgenogram. If the diagnosis is suspected from the history or physical examination, the lateral and oblique views should be obtained to establish the diagnosis.

The treatment of the sternal fracture depends on its severity, and in undisplaced fractures, the treatment should be directed toward the relief of pain. Analgesics usually suffice, but, on occasion, injection of lidocaine or related compounds into and around the fracture site are needed for relief of pain. If pain cannot be relieved by these measures, operative stabilization should be performed. Surgical treatment of the sternal fracture should be delayed until evaluation and possible treatment of the associated injuries have been completed.

Myocardial Contusion

Myocardial contusion is the most common lesion encountered clinically in patients with nonpenetrating cardiac injury. Because cardiac contusion may vary widely in its severity, may occur without external evidence of chest injury, and frequently is associated with other obvious, severe injuries that serve to mask the heart injury, the exact incidence of this disorder is difficult to determine. It is estimated to occur in approximately 25% of nonpenetrating chest injuries. Probably the most frequent cause of contusion is the steering wheel injury resulting from sudden automobile deceleration. It has been reported to occur also after falls from great heights or after blows to the chest.

Symptoms of cardiac contusion may be absent or masked by the other severe injuries. Precordial pain—identical in location, intensity, character, and radiation with those of coronary artery occlusion—is the most frequent symptom. The pain may be immediate or delayed for several hours or days following the injury. This anginal type of chest pain may persist for only 48 to 72 hours. Tachycardia, tachypnea, palpitation, and precordial tenderness may occur, but they are nonspecific.

The diagnosis is suggested by electrocardiography regardless of whether symptoms are present. The most constant findings are elevation in the ST segments and inversion of the T-wave, which result from myocardial or epicardial injury. They may be identical with the changes of coronary artery occlusion. Other electrocardiograms are essential. Frequently, electrical evidence of injury may be delayed for several hours or days. Serum enzyme determinations (SGOT, LDH, CPK) are of no value in establishing the diagnosis because they are usually elevated as the result of the associated musculoskeletal injury.

The treatment is the same as that for acute coronary artery occlusion, with restriction of activity and careful observation until the electrocardiogram has reverted to normal, which may require a period of only 2 to 4 weeks. Mild analgesics relieve the chest pain. Nitroglycerin has been shown to be of no value in such circumstances. Atrial arrhythmias, if they develop, should be treated appropriately. Anticoagulants should not be used during this period of restricted activity because there is danger of extending the hemorrhagic process. Although delayed complications, such as hemopericardium, rupture of the myocardium, or aneurysm formation, have been reported, complete healing of the myocardium and subsequent recovery of the patient generally occur.

The clinical significance of myocardial contusion lies in the fact that the damaged area may serve as a focus of electrical instability that increases the risk of serious arrhythmias, especially ventricular fibrillation, during anesthesia or operation. If contusion of the heart is suspected by the nature of the injury or electrocardiographic findings, procedures that are not urgent should be deferred until stabilization has occurred. Patients undergoing urgent procedures should receive a continuous intravenous infusion of lidocaine (2 mg/kg/hr) during the operation and for 48 to 72 hours postoperatively. If an inotropic agent is needed postoperatively, dopamine is the drug of choice.

Rupture of the Aorta

Only a few emergencies are so sudden in onset and have as high a frequency of catastrophic outcome as does traumatic rupture of the thoracic aorta. At present, it is estimated that 10 to 15% of all persons who die from automobile accidents sustain aortic rupture. There is comparable incidence of traumatic aortic rupture among drivers and passengers, but the occurrence of aortic rupture in persons thrown from the vehicle is more than twice that in persons who are not ejected. The most common site of rupture is at the isthmus of the aorta just distal to the left subclavian artery; 80 to 90% of aortic tears occur in this location. The remainder involve the supravalvular portion of the aortic root, origin of the innominate artery, distal descending aorta, or the left subclavian artery. Multiple sites of rupture have occurred rarely.

The aortic tear is transverse in 80 to 90% of the patients and extends through all layers. Death by exsanguination is instantaneous in these patients. In the remaining 10 to 20%, the aortic tear extends through the intima or media with preservation of the adventitia. The aortic blood is contained by the adventitia, which provides about 60% of the tensile strength of the aorta, pleura, and surrounding tissue. A false aneurysm is formed, and the patient survives at least temporarily. Of the 20% who survive the initial injury, 66% die by 2 weeks, 82% by 3 weeks, and 90% by 10 weeks. Since most of these patients die from secondary hemorrhage within 3 weeks if they are not treated, it is imperative that the diagnosis be established quickly and that repair be carried out.

The most important factor in making the diagnosis of acute traumatic aortic rupture is maintenance of a high index of suspicion and a constant awareness of the likelihood of this lesion in anyone who has sustained an accident characterized by violent and sudden deceleration, regardless of whether there is external evidence of chest injury. More than half of the patients reported in the literature had no external evidence of thoracic injury. The clinical findings are usually meager. An important clinical finding is the sudden onset of hypertension of the upper extremities, especially if it is coupled with evidence of continued blood loss.

Another finding is the presence of a harsh systolic murmur over the precordium or posterior interscapular area. The murmur is thought to be due to the turbulent blood flow across the area of transection. Other findings include diminution in the femoral pulses, dysphagia due to esophageal compression, superior vena obstruction, transient anuria and paraplegia, hoarseness due to recurrent laryngeal palsy, and the presence of blood in the supraclavicular space.

The most common complaint of patients during the immediate post-injury period is retrosternal or interscapular pain. Chest pain is secondary to ''stretching'' or dissection of the adventitia. Recurrence or exacerbation of pain may herald impending rupture of the aneurysm.

Radiographic findings may be invaluable in arousing suspicion of aortic rupture. The importance of careful evaluation of the chest roentgenogram cannot be overemphasized since it is apparent from the literature that too many patients have died because the presence and significance of radiologic abnormalities were not appreciated. The chest roentgenogram may show an increase in the width of the superior mediastinum that could indicate aortic rupture. This sign itself, however, is not diagnostic because there are many causes of mediastinal bleeding. Also, the interpretation of chest roentgenograms obtained from a severely injured patient presents many problems that must be considered when evaluating mediastinal width. Anteroposterior, rather than posteroanterior, examinations often are obtained by portable technique with the patient in the supine or semiapical lordotic projection. Each of these factors tends to magnify the superior mediastinum and to give an abnormal appearance to an entirely normal mediastinum.

Loss of sharpness of the aortic outline, with a loss of aortic knob shadow, almost always is associated with the mediastinal widening of aortic rupture and adds to the importance of this finding. Other roentgenographic findings include deviation of the trachea to the right, inferior displacement of the left main bronchus, pleural effusion, delayed or recurrent hemothorax, widening of the paravertebral strip, first rib fracture, fracture of the sternum, posterior displaced clavicular fracture, obscuration of the medial aspect of the apex of the left lung, and obliteration of the aortopulmonary window.

Although these findings suggest acute traumatic rupture of the aorta, they are not diagnostic, even when associated with upper extremity hypertension or a systolic murmur.

Aortography is the only definitive means for establishing the diagnosis of acute aortic rupture, and it should be performed on any patient who has sustained a high-speed decelerating injury or blunt trauma to the chest whether or not there is external or radiographic evidence of thoracic wall injuries, whether or not there are clinical findings suggesting aortic rupture, and whether or not there are changes in the chest roentgenogram (Table 3-3).

TABLE 3-3. *Indications For Aortography.*

1. History of high-speed decelerating injury
2. Any of the following chest roentgenogram findings:
   a. Superior mediastinal widening
   b. Obscuration of aortic knob shadow
   c. Obliteration of aortic outline
   d. Depression of left main bronchus
   e. Tracheal deviation to the right
   f. Obliteration of aortopulmonary window
   g. Obscuration of medial aspect of left upper lobe
   h. Widening paravertebral stripe
3. Fractured first rib or sternum
4. Unexplained hypotension
5. Massive hemothorax
6. Pulse deficits
7. Upper extremity hypertension
8. Systolic murmur

It is possible with aortography to determine the site or sites of rupture and to estimate the size of the false aneurysm. High-quality aortography can be obtained only by using rapid film changers and by directly injecting the contrast medium into the aorta through a catheter. Retrograde femoral arteriography was used without difficulty in all our patients. We prefer this approach because the examination can be performed easily, even in the severely injured or uncooperative patient. This approach allows angiographic evaluation of other areas of suspected injury, such as lacerations of spleen or liver.

Characteristically, the aortogram in acute aortic rupture demonstrates the presence of a pseudoaneurysm at or near the ligamentum arteriosum without extravasation of contrast medium. When the intimal flap acts as a ball valve, complete interruption of the aorta at the site of transection can be seen without distal filling of the aorta beyond the transection. The internal tears are usually visualized as irregular filling defects within the lumen of the aorta.

Because lethal secondary rupture of the false aneurysm is likely, the treatment of traumatic aortic rupture is immediate surgical repair after the diagnosis is established and the site of rupture localized. Aortography should always precede thoracotomy unless contraindicated by rapid deterioration of the patient's condition.

Innominate Artery Avulsion

Avulsion of the innominate artery from the aortic arch is second in frequency of occurrence only to rupture of the aorta at the aortic isthmus in cases where the patient survives long enough for diagnosis and repair. In two series dealing with the treatment of traumatic aortic rupture, innominate artery avulsion constituted 11 and 33% respectively.

Physical findings of importance include diminution of the radial or brachial pulse and a systolic murmur localized to the aortic area. Chest roentgenogram findings are usually no different from those in aortic isthmus rupture: a widened mediastinum with obscuration of the aortic outline. Aortography establishes the diagnosis. Avulsion of the innominate artery typically shows bulbous dilation of the vessel just distal to its origin associated with a lucent line across the base.

Because of the ever-present danger of sudden, lethal, secondary rupture of the false aneurysm, the treatment is immediate surgical repair.

Subclavian Artery Injury

The diagnosis of subclavian artery injury may be suspected from the physical findings or chest roentgenograms. The cardinal finding of disruption of the subclavian artery is absence of the peripheral pulse with diminution in blood pressure of the involved extremity. Other findings of importance include pallor, coldness, paresthesias or weakness in the involved extremity, a pulsatile mass in the root of the neck, and fracture of the clavicle. The chest roentgenogram shows a widened superior mediastinum with obscuration of the aortic knob shadow. Accurate diagnosis and localization of the injury require aortography. We prefer the retrograde femoral technique. The right posterior oblique position is best for visualization of the origins of the great vessels.

Because of the threat of cataclysmic hemorrhage from secondary rupture of the false aneurysm, the treatment is immediate surgical repair.

References

1. DeMuth, W., and Zinsser, H.: Myocardial contusion. Arch. Intern. Med., *115*:434, 1965.
2. Fulton, R., and Peter, E.: The progressive nature of pulmonary contusion. Surgery, *67*:499, 1970.
3. Fulton, R., and Peter, E.: Physiologic effects of fluid therapy after pulmonary contusion. Am. J. Surg., *126*:773, 1973.
4. Gailbraith, N., Urschel, H., and Wood, R.: Fracture of first rib associated with laceration of subclavian artery. J. Thorac. Cardiovasc. Surg., *65*:649, 1973.

5. Gibson, E., Carter, R., and Hinshaw, D.: Surgical significance of sternal fractures. Surg. Gynecol. Obstet., *14*:443, 1962.
6. Greendyke, R.: Traumatic rupture of the aorta: Special references to automobile accidents. J.A.M.A., *195*:527, 1966.
7. Kirsh, M., et al.: Roentgenographic evaluation of traumatic rupture of the aorta. Surg. Gynecol. Obstet., *131*:900, 1970.
8. Kirsh, M., et al.: The treatment of acute traumatic rupture of the aorta: A 10-year experience. Ann. Surg., *184*:318, 1976.
9. Kirsh, M., and Sloan, H.: Blunt Chest Trauma: General Principles of Management. Boston, Little, Brown and Co., 1977.
10. Kirsh, M., et al.: Management of unusual traumatic ruptures of the aorta. Surgery, *146*:365, 1978.
11. Liedtke, H., and DeMuth, W.: Nonpenetrating cardiac injuries: A collective review. Am. Heart J., *86*:687, 1973.
12. Pontappidan, H., Geffen, G., and Lowenstein, E.: Acute respiratory failure in the adult. N. Engl. J. Med., *287*:690, 1972.
13. Richardson, J., et al.: Pulmonary contusion and hemorrhage crystalloid vs. colloid treatment. J. Surg. Res., *16*:330, 1974.
14. Skillman, J., Parikh, B., and Tannebaum, B.: Pulmonary arteriovenous admixture: Improvement with albumin and diuresis. Am. J. Surg., *119*:440, 1970.
15. Sturm, J., Points, B., and Perryr, J.: Hemopneumothorax following blunt trauma of the thorax. Surg. Gynecol. Obstet., *141*:539, 1975.

Chapter 4 Early Recognition and Treatment of Shock

ERWIN R. THAL
DANIEL H. RAESS

Advanced emergency life support by paramedical personnel, combined with rapid transportation to regional trauma centers, has enabled physicians to care for an increasing number of multiply injured patients. Our highly technologic and sometimes violent society tends to bring a varied group of patients to community hospitals and local trauma centers. Rapid assessment, accompanied by a methodical multidisciplinary approach to patients with multiple injuries, has led to a more efficient means of resuscitation, diagnostic evaluation, definitive treatment, and ultimate decrease in mortality.

Shock continues to be a frequent complication in the multiply injured patient during the early post-injury period. Early recognition, a better understanding of the physiologic, biochemical, and neuroendocrine response to hypovolemia, and a standardized but individualized approach to management have been the cornerstones leading to the successful management of trauma victims. Specialty consultants, who manage complex problems in the critically injured patient, become intimately involved in the overall therapy, which is best coordinated by a trauma or general surgeon. A complete understanding of the significance of shock in the patient with multiple injuries is necessary for the successful management of these patients.

Since Gross defined shock in 1872 as a ''manifestation of the rude unhinging of the machinery of life,'' many modifications have been made. Blalock's classification, made in 1934, is still useful today.[1] The major categories of shock are: (1) hematogenic (hypovolemic), (2) neurogenic, (3) cardiogenic, and (4) vasogenic. Although septic shock may occur later in the course of management in the trauma patient, recognition and understanding of the pathophysiology of neurogenic, cardiogenic, and hemorrhagic shock in the acutely injured patient are essential.

Hemorrhagic Shock

Homeostatic mechanisms, which tend to supplement perfusion of vital organs, assume a primary role in the management of the hemorrhaging patient. Subtleties of regional autoregulation give way to circulatory changes many orders of magnitude greater, causing profound changes in the distribution of circulating blood volume. Hypotension results in increased firing of sympathetic afferents from the carotid sinus and aortic arch baroreceptors. These afferent fibers traversing with cranial nerves IX and X supply the vasomotor center in the medulla, which, in turn, causes increased sympathetic efferent stimuli, thus resulting in arteriolar constriction and increased venomotor tone. As a result, cardiac rate and efficiency increase, peripheral arterial resistance rises, and the effective circulating blood volume increases as a result of decreased venous capacitance. Blood pressure may initially remain normal with minor hemorrhage due to these compensatory mechanisms. A 15 to 25% hemorrhage must be incurred before systolic blood pressure remains below 80 to 90 mm Hg. Catecholamine secretion from the adrenal medulla, as well as from systemic sympathetic nerve ends, also participates in the redistribution of the circulating blood volume. Circulating catecholamines increase vasomotor tone in such areas as the skin, kidney, and viscera, and cause dilation of skeletal muscle arterioles. Vital organs, such as the heart and brain, receive an increased portion of the cardiac output.

The metabolic response to hypovolemia is as complex as the circulatory response. Changes in metabolism may be attributed to the neuroendocrine response to stress and hypoxia at the cellular level. This stress response includes salt and water retention, negative nitrogen balance, and potassium excretion as a result of the pituitary-adrenal response to injury. Catecholamine release results in increased circulating glucagon as well as in the inhibition of production and peripheral utilization of insulin. Antidiuretic hormone is released by the posterior pituitary as a result of baroreceptor firing and reduced left atrial filling pressure. Aldosterone is quickly released during hypovolemia as a result of both decreased renal perfusion pressure and ACTH secretion in the pituitary. As a result of tissue hypoperfusion, glycolysis is abandoned for anaerobic metabolism. Lactic acid accumulation during anaerobic metabolism not only provides less energy per gram of glucose because of its inability to utilize the citric acid cycle, but may also cause significant decreases in blood pH due to severe lactic acidosis.

Clinical and experimental studies have shown that serum lactate is a sensitive and reliable indicator of oxygen debt and a good prognosticator of survival during shock states.[2] Mortality has been found to approach 100% when serum lactate levels reach 8 mM per liter. An important result of the cellular hypoxia in the shock state was demonstrated by Shires and co-workers when they showed sequestration of extravascular extracellular sodium and water into the intracellular space with loss of cellular potassium into the extracellular fluid during hemorrhagic shock in experimental animals.[3,4] Measured transmembrane-potential differences and extracellular fluid potassium accumulation appear to be functions of the magnitude and duration of shock. The exact mechanism for the production of these effects is not known, but appears to represent a reduction in the efficiency of the sodium-potassium ion pump at the cell-membrane level.

If hypotension is prolonged, hypoperfusion of vital organs continues and is manifested by progressive organ failure and decreased mixed venous oxygen concentration. Death results when myocardial and brain oxygen demands cannot be met.

Cardiogenic Shock

Cardiogenic shock is a physiologic state in which hypotension is not the result of a diminished blood volume, but, rather, the result of a primary myocardial failure to maintain an adequate cardiac output. It may result from primary pump failure (myocardial infarction, myocardiopathy, or arrhythmia) or mechanical factors that do not allow the proper pumping of blood in the presence of otherwise normal myocardial function (tension pneumothorax and cardiac tamponade). Partial loss or dysfunction of the myocardium leads to inefficient pumping, decreased ejection fraction, increased left ventricular end-diastolic pressure, and decreased systemic arterial blood pressure. Compensatory mechanisms, such as increased sympathetic tone and the pituitary-adrenal response, are present, as in hemorrhagic shock. Limitation of infarct size and administration of pharmacologic and/or mechanical support are hallmarks of care in ischemic cardiogenic shock.

Chronic congestive heart failure, which decompensates and causes low cardiac output, is easier to recognize because there is usually an antecedent history of heart failure. Chronic signs of ventricular failure, such as dependent edema and other signs of established secondary aldosteronism, may be evident. Filling pressures are elevated in both acute and chronic forms of failure, and the ventricular response to these increased pressures is reflected by the descending limb of the classic Frank-Starling curve. (Fig. 4-1). The rapid infusion of fluids results in a rise in central venous pressure and an increase in pulmonary capillary wedge pressure with no improvement in blood pressure or cardiac output.

Arrhythmias result in inefficient pumping, and if of significant severity, inadequate perfusion may result. Atrial fibrillation or flutter with a rapid ventricular response results in ventricular filling and, hence, failure to generate a peripheral pulse despite relatively normal ventricular contractility. An irregular irregularity in the peripheral pulse or an apical/peripheral pulse ratio greater than 1 is diagnostic of atrial fibrillation.

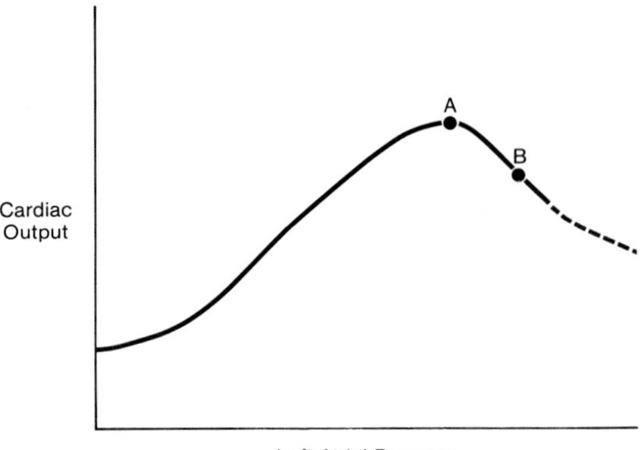

Fig. 4-1. Classic Frank-Starling curve representing cardiac response to increased preload and stretch of myocardial muscle fibers. After maximum cardiac output is achieved with preload augmentation (point A), further increase in volume and left atrial pressure results in decreased cardiac output (point B).

Supraventricular tachycardia with rates greater than 180 may likewise result in hypotension. Ventricular arrhythmias (PVCs and ventricular tachycardia) are potentially life threatening and require emergency therapy. Sinus bradycardia or AV nodal block is usually a manifestation of ischemic heart disease and may result in hypotension if not adequately treated. Certain conditions that prevent diastolic ventricular filling, such as cardiac tamponade or tension pneumothorax, may result in hypotension and should be considered in the diagnosis of the acutely injured hypotensive patient.

Neurogenic Shock

Neurogenic shock refers to a broad spectrum of changes in the effective blood volume due to the increased vascular capacitance, which occurs when the balance between vasoconstrictor and vasodilator impulses to both the arterioles and venules is interrupted. The increase in peripheral vascular capacity, due to less resistance, causes a decreased venous return to the heart and, hence, a reduction in cardiac output. Vasomotor or vasovagal hypotension, such as occurs after an unpleasant event, is usually mild and of short duration. Reflex neurogenic hypotension may be the result of visceral dilation. Spinal shock may be severe and even life threatening with hypoperfusion of vital organs.

In patients with multiple injuries and the potential for both hemorrhagic and neurogenic shock, physical examination usually delineates the source of hypotension. Patients with neurogenic shock (spinal cord injury) have a neurologic deficit, warm, dry, and occasionally flushed skin, and a normal or slow pulse rate. Mentation is generally clear, and urine output is frequently adequate. Hypotension in the injured patient is never assumed to be primarily neurogenic in origin; it is best confirmed by failure to improve blood pressure with volume replacement, lack of evidence for ongoing hemorrhage, and the presence of spinal cord damage.

Patients with closed head injuries rarely become hypotensive unless the event is terminal. The Cushing reflex produces hypertension and either normal or low pulse rates. Diminished blood pressure in the patient with increased intracranial pressure but no spinal cord injury is assumed the result of blood loss until proved otherwise.

Septic Shock

Although septic shock has been most commonly associated with systemic infection caused by gram-negative bacilli, many forms of systemic infection, including gram-positive organisms and fungi, may cause the shock state. Extracellular products of bacteria associated with virulence and invasiveness trigger the hemodynamic sequellae associated with septic shock. These materials have a profound effect on cellular metabolism and cause profound changes in hemodynamics and metabolism at sites far removed from the foci of an infection. Exotoxins, first associated with Pseudomonas aeruginosa infections, are potent inhibitors of protein synthesis.[5] Other proteolytic enzymes and endotoxin appear to emanate from the gram-negative bacilli's cell-wall structure.

Hemodynamic events triggered by endotoxin include changes in the vascular integrity of the endothelium and activation of the kallikrein cascade.[6] Capillary leak results in extravasation of extracellular fluid. Bradykinin, as well as other vasoactive kinins, causes hypotension. The intrinsic clotting cascade is activated as a result of a direct effect of endotoxin and coagulation factor XII, which may set in motion events leading to fibrinolysis and disseminated intravascular coagulation. Complement pathways also appear to be activated and may result in further endothelial damage and vasoactive changes. Hemodynamic changes associated with septic shock differ in various patients and usually depend on the preexisting volume status. A previously normovolemic patient demonstrates a hyperdynamic circulation with increased cardiac output, hypotension, decreased peripheral vascular resistance, and respiratory alkalosis. Patients previously volume depleted, as often seen in the elderly and compromised patient, may demonstrate an early adrenergic type of response, with elevated peripheral vascular resistance, cyanotic cold extremities, hypotension, and a low cardiac output. Metabolic acidosis is not present initially, but will develop if therapy is delayed and is generally considered an ominous but not fatal finding.

Arteriovenous shunting in the peripheral circulation results in lowered peripheral vascular resistance and increased cardiac output. Assuming adequate volume and preload, the heart is a passive partner in this hemodynamic aberration as it attempts to meet the cardiac output required by the systemic circulation. Increased systemic and myocardial catecholamines enable the heart to meet this demand. There is evidence, however, of a humoral myocardial depressant factor in various shock models.[7] These compounds may result in diminished contractility and catecholamine response, and may be important factors in the development of the shock state in man. Pulmonary dysfunction, which is commonly seen in the multiply injured patient, is a result of pulmonary arteriovenous shunting and alveolar collapse with subsequent formation of microatelectasis. Multisystem organ failure is inevitable when appropriate therapy is not instituted prior to the development of a severe metabolic acidosis and circulatory collapse.

Evaluation and Treatment of the Hypotensive Patient

Appraisal and treatment of injuries sustained by an individual begin immediately upon admission to the emergency suite. Hypotension is a symptom of some serious physiologic derangement and not of a disease, per se. As such, it cannot be taken lightly, but, rather, must be recognized as a clinical condition that warrants immediate assessment and management.

The circumstances of injury and patient status prior to admission often can be gleaned from witnesses, family, and paramedical personnel. Thorough physical examination is mandatory in any trauma patient, even if the patient is in extremis and requires emergency life-support measures. Maintenance of the airway, either by simple removal of an oral pharyngeal obstruction, insertion of an oral airway, endotracheal intubation, cricothyroidotomy, or tracheostomy, is of prime importance. Mechanical ventilation, in the event that spontaneous respiration is interrupted, and standard cardiopulmonary resuscitation, in the event of cardiac arrest, take priority over other definitive treatment measures.

In the patient who is not in acute distress, medical history is quickly obtained while vital signs (both in supine and upright positions, if possible) are obtained. Decreased systolic blood pressure, rapid weak pulse, orthostatic hypotension, or increase in pulse denote significant hemorrhage. Skin temperature and color are noted; cyanotic, cold skin denotes severe hemorrhage and profound shock. Good mental status in patients without central nervous system injury is an excellent indication of cerebral perfusion. Apathy to severe injury and pain that progress to coma is an excellent indication of severe shock. As noted in Table 4-1, thirst, often severe, is frequently encountered in the hypotensive patient. Although hemorrhage is the most common cause of hypotension in accident victims, cardiogenic, neurogenic, and vasogenic shock are easily recognized if the physical examination and aberration in hemodynamic measurements are scrutinized. Appropriate early therapy has allowed reduction in morbidity and mortality in each group.

Hemorrhagic Shock

Hypotension in the traumatized patient is assumed to be the result of hemorrhage until proved otherwise. Careful physical examination and routine observation usually delineate the cause of the low blood pressure. External hemorrhage is easily recognized. Amount, duration, and character of the blood loss often may be obtained from companions or emergency medical personnel who have had contact with the patient prior to admission to the hospital. After direct pressure is applied to the bleeding site and blood loss is controlled, a continued, thorough search for other injuries can be made.

Continued internal hemorrhage may result in persistent hypotension, and its recognition and definitive treatment are of the highest priority. Hemothorax is easily demonstrated by physical examination and routine roentgenographic stud-

Table 4-1. *Grading of Shock.*

Degree of Shock	Blood Pressure (Approx.)	Pulse Quality	SKIN: Temperature	SKIN: Color	SKIN: Circulation (Response to Pressure Blanching)	Thirst	Mental State
None	Normal	Normal	Normal	Normal	Normal	Normal	Clear and distressed
Slight	Increased up to 20%	Normal	Cool	Pale	Definite slowing	Normal	Clear and distressed
Moderate	Decreased 20-40%	Definite decrease in volume	Cool	Pale	Definite slowing	Definite	Clear and some apathy unless stimulated
Severe	Decreased 40% to non-recordable	Weak to imperceptible	Cold	Ashen to cyanotic (mottling)	Very sluggish	Severe	Apathetic to comatose, little distress except thirst

From Beecher, H.K., et al.: The internal state of the severely wounded man on entry to the most forward hospital. Surgery, *22*:672, 1947.)

ies. Diagnosis of hemoperitoneum and retroperitoneal bleeding may be more difficult. Blood within the peritoneal cavity may or may not be irritating; hence, physical examination may be deceiving. If central nervous system injury has occurred, equivocal abdominal examination is present, or unexplained hypotension persists, peritoneal lavage is generally performed to rule out intraperitoneal injury.[8,9] Blood loss resulting from fracture sites may not be readily observed. Hematoma from combined tibia/fibula fractures may total 1 to 2 units, and as many as 3 units may be lost from femoral fractures. Humeral fractures may cause blood loss sufficient to produce hypotension. Severe pelvic fractures may produce as much as 6 to 8 units of blood in the retroperitoneal space; consequently, hypogastric artery ligation or selective arterial angiographic embolization may be required for control. Intraoral or pharyngeal blood loss may be swallowed and may not become apparent until nasogastric suction is instituted. Initial determinations of hemoglobin and hematocrit are obtained, but are notoriously inaccurate. Several hours may be required for blood to equilibrate; hence, normal values are common in the presence of acute massive blood loss.

Ability to recover from hemorrhagic shock depends on hemostasis, rapid volume repletion, and return to normal tissue perfusion. Following the work of Shires, which demonstrated intracellular sodium and water sequestration from the extravascular extracellular space, Ringer's lactate solution has been used exclusively for initiation of fluid resuscitation. Shires and Canizaro found that a profound deficit (18 to 26%) of functional extracellular fluid occurred with severe hemorrhagic shock.[10] They concluded that an extracellular fluid mimic, such as Ringer's lactate solution, would replace the lost extracellular fluid that was internally redistributed. Ringer's lactate solution without dextrose is used because rapid infusion of large amounts of sugar may cause an osmotic diuresis. This brisk urine flow robs the patient of needed intravascular volume and creates a false sense of security when good urine volume is taken by the physician to signify adequate volume replacement and renal perfusion. DePalma and associates also demonstrated that hyperosmolar solutions, such as 5% dextrose in Ringer's lactate solution, were less effective than isoosmotic sodium-containing solutions in reversing intracellular damage caused by hemorrhagic shock.[11]

In the hypotensive patient, 2 L of Ringer's lactate solution is given rapidly via a reliable intravenous cannula. Two intravenous routes are recommended in severely injured patients. Care is taken not to begin an infusion in an injured extremity. Although a central line is advantageous and ultimately necessary in patients with hemodynamic instability, the initial concern is rapid volume replacement. These patients are frequently flailing about, uncooperative, and the focus of a lot of activity. For these reasons, subclavian catheters are not recommended for routine use, but, rather, are employed if no other site is available in a rapidly deteriorating patient. Complications of subclavian catheters inserted under duress include venous or arterial perforation, pneumothorax, hydrothorax, contamination leading to sepsis, air embolism, and catheter embolism. Saphenous vein cutdowns are acceptable routes for infusion even with suspected abdominal injuries as long as one upper extremity is also used. All intravenous lines inserted in the field or emergency suite should be removed within 24 hours.

If there is a prompt return of blood pressure to normal and there is no further evidence of ongoing hemorrhage, the infusion is slowed. Blood samples are sent to the blood bank to be typed and crossmatched. If hypotension persists following 2 L of crystalloid infusion or the patient continues to hemorrhage, whole blood is administered as preparations are made to deal definitively with the injury. Available whole blood may be scarce, as many blood banks now have converted to component therapy. Because volume deficiency is the problem, the use of whole blood is most appropriate, but one may need to use packed cells plus volume or fresh frozen plasma. If hypotension does not respond to Ringer's lactate solution and type-specific blood is not available, universal donor blood may be administered. In most blood banks, hepatitis and VDRL screening are omitted in these life-threatening situations.

Patients usually exhibit one of three responses to the administration of 2 L of crystalloid solution over 30 to 45 minutes: (1) when blood loss is minimal (less than 10%), the blood pressure generally returns to normotensive levels, the signs and symptoms of shock are reversed, and the patient remains stable; (2) when blood loss is greater than 10 to 15%, the response may be similar; however, it is generally transient and hypotension reappears in minutes to hours (this may also represent continued bleeding or rebleeding in a previously stabilized patient); (3) if blood loss is massive, the patient rarely responds to the initial fluid infusion and blood replacement becomes urgent. When the patient fails to respond to crystalloid and blood, the prognosis is grave.

The use of albumin in the treatment of hemorrhagic shock is controversial. Although it has been demonstrated that less volume of colloid is required to return the blood pressure to normal in a hypotensive patient, it is also argued that pulmonary edema develops more rapidly with the infusion of these solutions.[12] An alveolocapillary leak allows albumin to pass into the pulmonary interstitium, which draws more water with it and compounds the pulmonary dysfunction. In a series of 978 patients undergoing various operative procedures for severe trauma at Parkland Memorial Hospital in Dallas and in whom Ringer's lactate solution infusion was used exclusively in the treatment of hemorrhagic shock, pulmonary dysfunction developed in only 2.1% and the incidence of the classic adult respiratory distress syndrome was only 1.4%.[13] Pulmonary dysfunction was more closely associated with sepsis irrespective of the presence or absence of shock or the infusion of large amounts of intravenous fluids.

Evidence also shows that resuscitation from hemorrhagic shock with a balanced salt solution in conjunction with red-cell replacement is more effective in restoring renal tubular function than is resuscitation with a colloid fluid.[14] Weaver and associates demonstrated that patients receiving albumin in resuscitation from hypovolemic shock required greater ventilatory assistance and had a higher alveolar arteriolar oxygen gradient than those patients not receiving albumin.[15] Ringer's lactate solution is an excellent, effective, and inexpensive extracellular-fluid mimic, and the use of albumin, Plasmanate, and other volume expanders in the acutely hemorrhaging patient is unnecessary and may result in more pulmonary complications.

Oxygen is given to all patients in shock, generally by nasal cannula or by face mask. Even though hypotensive patients are likely to become acidotic, bicarbonate administration is withheld except in the presence of cardiac arrest. The use of exogenous bicarbonate may lead to a rebound alkalosis, as most of the therapy of the hypotensive patient tends to make the patient alkalotic. Volume replacement is of prime importance. The administration of Ringer's lactate solution does not contribute to the acidosis because the lactate is converted to bicarbonate with one pass through the liver. Nasogastric suction removes acid from the stomach, hyperventilation causes a respiratory alkalosis, and the citrate in blood that is transfused is converted to bicarbonate. Alkalosis causes a shift to the left of the oxygen dissociation curve, which then impairs the unloading of oxygen at the tissue level. It is better for the patients to be slightly acidotic rather than alkalotic.

Another recently developed adjunct in the treatment of hypovolemic shock is the medical antishock trouser (MAST garment). Since the first civilian use of the MAST garment in 1973 by Kaplan and associates,[16] numerous authors have reported effective use of the garment in the treatment of hemorrhagic shock. Early in the use of the MAST garment, inflation and the subsequent squeezing effect on the lower extremities and lower abdomen were assumed to result in an autotransfusion from the lower extremities to the central circulation. A subsequent study by Gaffney and associates revealed little, if any, autotransfusion during MAST garment inflation in supine normovolemic males.[17] Conversely, in the presence of venous pooling in the lower extremities (60° tilt), the MAST garment effectively increased the central intravascular volume. The authors concluded that the increased peripheral vascular resistance and subsequent increase in afterload were the mechanism for increased systemic arterial pressure. Beneficial effects of the MAST garment in hypovolemic hypotensive patients are probably produced by a combination of increased systemic perfusion pressure and redistribution of cardiac output to vital and noncompressed regions.

MAST garments are applied as soon as possible after trauma to receive the maximum benefit; consequently, they are usually applied by the emergency medical technician in the field. External bleeding wounds that can be controlled with simple pressure dressings and are in an area that would be enclosed by the MAST garment do not contraindicate its use. Patients with serious chest injuries, such as flail chest, pneumothorax, or hemothorax, are best treated by delaying inflation of the abdominal compartment until mechanical assistance for ventilation is available.

When a patient wearing a MAST garment arrives in the emergency room, administration of fluid and/or blood should be continued, as appropriate, and vital signs monitored. If the patient remains stable with a systolic blood pressure over 100 mm Hg, gradual deflation with concurrent fluid administration is advised. Blood pressure is monitored before, during, and after separate deflation of each compartment, beginning with the abdominal section. If hypotension recurs, the compartment is reinflated, fluid is administered, and preparations are made for definitive care with the garment still in place.

Patients with lower-extremity fractures and/or pelvic fractures may be easily transported with the garment inflated because it stabilizes both the pelvis and the lower extremities. The urge to look at the injuries under the garment after the patient is admitted to the emergency room must be tempered, and the trousers must not be deflated until preparations can be made to deal with the hypotension that may result.

Myocardial infarction, either suspected or proven, is a contraindication to the use of the MAST garment. Increased afterload results in increased myocardial work and further derangement of the myocardial oxygen supply/demand ratio. Although some authors recommend gradual inflation of the MAST garment in patients with suspected cardiogenic shock, with the premise that rapid decompression results in a reversible transfusion, other authors recommend that the MAST garment not be employed in patients with cardiogenic shock since the rapid increase in afterload may result in further decline in left ventricular function.

Cardiogenic Shock

As stated previously, multiple causes of hypotension occasionally occur in patients sustaining trauma. The heart may be the source of shock as an isolated cause or in conjunction with other factors. History and physical examination with special emphasis placed on the cardiovascular dynamics often lead to the correct diagnosis. Previous symptoms of congestive heart failure in addition to signs of well-established heart failure, such as edema, paroxysmal nocturnal dyspnea, dyspnea on exertion, and hepatomegaly, can be correlated with the findings of decompensated failure, including S_3 gallop, jugular venous distension, hepatojugular reflex, and pulmonary rales, to facilitate the diagnosis.

Central venous pressure is determined by placing a cannula in the superior vena cava. If the patient's condition warrants more careful monitoring, a Swan-Ganz catheter can be inserted to give a better estimate of left-heart filling pressures and central hemodynamics. Although valuable information is obtained from a Swan-Ganz catheter, its use in the emergency room rarely is indicated. Administration of diuretics, only after assurance of adequate volume status, and digitalis preparations usually result in improvement. If hypotension is severe, inotropic support and, occasionally, afterload reduction with vasodilator agents are added. The same principles, with the additional goal of myocardial preservation, apply in patients with acute myocardial infarction and cardiogenic shock. Mechanical assist devices, such as intra-aortic balloon counterpulsation, can be utilized if other modalities fail.

Acute myocardial infarction in the presence of acute trauma is a dangerous problem. Electrocardiograms are routinely obtained on all patients more than 40 years of age, as well as on anyone who complains of chest pain or has a previous history of coronary artery disease.

Myocardial dysfunction is suspected if the rapid infusion of Ringer's lactate solution results not in an increase in blood pressure, but in a rapid increase in central venous pressure. Cardiac rhythm disturbances may result in ineffective pumping by the left ventricle. After electrocardiographic confirmation and determination of serum electrolytes, rapid digitalization or electroconversion can be initiated. Supraventricular tachycardias with a ventricular rate greater than 180 may compromise diastolic filling to such an extent that hypotension results. Carotid massage or Valsalva's maneuver is used only on carefully monitored patients. Hypotension resulting from bradycardia may necessitate temporary transvenous pacemaker placement and subsequent permanent pacemaker placement if indicated by electrophysiologic studies.

Severe hypotension without evident blood loss or reason for extravascular sequestration points to the possibility of a mechanical source for the low blood pressure. Cardiac tamponade is suspected in patients with penetrating trauma who have hypotension, paradoxic pulse, increased venous pressure, and muffled heart sounds. Increased intrapericardial pressure compromises the diastolic filling of the heart and results in such a symptom complex (Beck's triad). A high index of suspicion and early therapy are essential to reverse this process. Needle pericardiocentesis via the subxyphoid route, followed by definitive operative therapy, is the preferred treatment.

Penetrating or blunt thoracic trauma may result in tension pneumothorax, which may cause a mediastinal shift and impaired systemic venous return to the heart. Tension pneumothorax is especially dangerous in the unconscious patient undergoing mechanical ventilation. Physical examination and chest roentgenograms are the key to diagnosis. In the event of severe hypotension and equivocal physical examination, bilateral needle thoracentesis may alleviate this condition, particularly when tension pneumothorax is a possibility and roentgenographic confirmation is not immediately available.

Neurogenic Shock

The patient with neurogenic shock (spinal-cord injury) must be differentiated from the hypotensive patient with a closed head injury. As stated earlier, hypotension associated with an altered state of consciousness is generally due to blood loss. Correction of the volume deficit and restoration of the circulation occasionally reverse the neurologic findings in these patients. On the other hand, patients with a spinal cord injury have an increase in capacitance and are usually normovolemic. Unless there is a concomitant head injury, a change in the level of consciousness is rare.

Patients with closed head injuries and multiple trauma are resuscitated as if there were no head injury. Fluids are not withheld, and blood replacement is provided as indicated previously. When it has been clearly ascertained that there is no blood loss and the volume status is stable, then and only then is fluid restriction considered for the head injury. If a patient has only a head injury and no drop in blood pressure, fluids are administered judiciously.

Mannitol, diuretics, and other drugs used to reduce intracranial pressure are withheld in all hypovolemic patients. Hyperventilation decreases intracranial pressure sufficiently until volume stability can be restored. These drugs are only indicated in normovolemic patients with evidence of increased pressure as shown by either an intracranial pressure manometer or clinical evidence of lateralizing signs. The mere loss of consciousness does not denote an increase in intracranial pressure.

If there is evidence of a spinal-cord injury associated with hypotension, a quick assessment of areas of potential blood loss is made. If there are no fractures, such as in the pelvis and/or long bones, no evidence of bleeding in the chest or abdomen, and no evidence of external blood loss, then and only then is the judicious use of vasoactive drugs considered. The volume status must be stable before using vasopressors. If there is a modest drop in pressure and the patient is cerebrating and maintaining a good urine output, additional support of the pressure may not be necessary. It is equally as important not to overload these patients with fluids and blood when the cause of the hypotension is neurogenic.

Septic Shock

The shock state resulting from systemic bacteremia may be caused by gram-positive organisms, but is more notably caused by gram-negative bacilli. The history of recent genitourinary-tract instrumentation and/or a compromised host, such as seen with the use of chemotherapy, immunosuppressant therapy, or steroids, is common. Differentiation of septic shock from cardiogenic shock or hypovolemia is important, especially when the foci of infection are not readily apparent. Decreased peripheral vascular resistance, increased cardiac output, and low central venous pressure, as well as low pulmonary capillary wedge pressure, are all seen in septic shock states. If septic shock is suspected, volume replacement ensuring adequate preload to the heart, broad-spectrum antibiotic therapy, control of the source of infection, and careful clinical monitoring are essential aspects of treatment. Placement of a pulmonary artery catheter may be helpful, especially in elderly patients with a predilection for congestive heart failure.

Controversy exists concerning the use of corticosteroids in septic shock. Schumer[18] demonstrated decreased mortality after administering 30 milligrams per kilogram of methyl prednisolone for 48 hours. It is emphasized that corticosteroid administration, if used, is not a panacea, and not a substitute for broad-spectrum antimicrobial administration and local control of infection.

Summary

Most cases of hypotension fall into the classification system described by Blalock. If the common sources, such as blood loss, pump failure, and spinal-cord injury, are not readily apparent, the physician must consider less common causes, such as Addisonian states, especially in patients on exogenous steroid therapy, tension pneumothorax, caval obstruction, drug allergies, and tamponade.

Although shock is a symptom complex indicative of some serious underlying pathophysiologic process, its recognition is frequently overlooked. Sole reliance on the blood pressure without regard for other physical findings, such as pulse rate, skin condition, central nervous system response, and urine output, may be misleading. A borderline blood pressure (100 to 110 mm Hg) in the traumatized patient is often an early warning sign of impending disaster and is not to be taken lightly. Most traumatized patients are anxious, apprehensive, and scared, all of which tend to raise the systolic pressure. These patients with marginal pressures must be closely monitored and observed at all times.

Prolonged hypotension may lead to hypoxia, which is manifested by restlessness, combativeness, anxiety, and uncooperativeness. All these signs can be attributed to the drunk and disorderly patient, but, if overlooked, can lead to a fatal outcome.

Although shock in the trauma patient generally is due to hypovolemia, other sources must be considered when resuscitation is unsuccessful. As a general policy, no patient who has had an episode of hypotension, regardless of how transient, should be discharged from a hospital emergency room since the significance and sequelae of that episode in the immediate post-injury period are unpredictable.

References

1. Blalock, A.: Shock, further studies with particular reference to effects of hemorrhage. Arch. Surg. *29*:837, 1937.
2. Weil, M. H., and Afifi, A. A.: Experimental and clinical studies on lactate and pyruvate as indicators of severity of acute circulatory failure. Circulation, *41*:989, 1970.
3. Campion, D. S., et al.: The effect of hemorrhagic shock in transmembrane potential. Surgery, *66*:1051, 1969.
4. Cunningham, J. N., Shires, G. T., and Wagner, Y.: Cellular transport defects in hemorrhagic shock. Surgery, *70*:215, 1971.
5. Young, L. S.: Pathogenesis of septic shock and approaches to management. *In* Aspects of the Management of Shock. K. I. Shine, moderator. Ann. Intern. Med., *93*:723, 1980.
6. Coleman, R. W., Edelman, R., Scott, C. F., and Gilman, R. H.: Plasma kallikrein activation and inhibition during Typhoid fever. J. Clin. Invest., *61*:287, 1978.
7. Lovett, W. L., Wangensteen, S. L., Glenn, T. M., and Lefer, A. M.: Presence of a myocardial depressant factor in patients with circulatory shock. Surgery, *70*:223, 1971.
8. Thal, E. R., and Shires, G. T.: Peritoneal lavage in blunt abdominal trauma. Am. J. Surg., *125*:64, 1973.
9. Thal, E. R.: Peritoneal lavage and local exploration in lower chest and abdominal stab wounds. J. Trauma, *17*:642, 1977.
10. Shires, G. T., and Canizaro, P. C.: Fluid resuscitation in the severely injured. Surg. Clin. North Am., *53*:1341, 1973.
11. DePalma, R. G., Holden, W. D., and Robinson, A. V.: Hemorrhagic shock: ultrastructural effects in liver and muscle. Ann. Surg., *175*:539, 1973.
12. Lowe, R. J., Moss, G. S., Jilek, J., and Levine, H. D.: Crystalloid vs. colloid in etiology of pulmonary failure after trauma: A randomized trial in man. Surgery, *81*: 676, 1977.
13. Horovitz, J. H., Carrico, C. J., and Shires, G. T.: The pulmonary response to major injury. Arch. Surg. *108*:349, 1974.

14. Siegal, D. C., Cochin, A., Geocaris, T., and Moss, G. S.: Effect of saline and colloid resuscitation on renal function. Ann. Surg., *177*:51, 1973.
15. Weaver, D. W., Ledgerwood, A. M., and Lucas, C. E.: Pulmonary effects of albumin resuscitation for severe hypovolemic shock. Arch. Surg., *113*:387, 1978.
16. Kaplan, B. C., et al.: The military anti-shock trouser in civilian prehospital emergency care. J. Trauma, *13*:843, 1973.
17. Gaffney, F. A., et al.: Hemodynamic effects of anti-shock trousers. J. Trauma, *21*:931,
18. Schumer, W.: Steroids in treatment of clinical septic shock. Ann. Surg., *184*:333, 1976.

Chapter 5 The Adult Respiratory Distress Syndrome

JOHN A. WEIGELT

In the United States, trauma is the leading cause of death in the first three decades of life.[1] The initial injuries and subsequent complications are responsible for this high mortality. Pulmonary complications are frequent and impose unwanted morbidity and mortality. The adult respiratory distress syndrome (ARDS) represents the most severe pulmonary insult to the trauma victim.

Definition

ARDS is an acute deterioration of pulmonary function that occurs in specific clinical settings. It is characterized by progressive hypoxemia and its deleterious systemic effects. Unless interrupted by appropriate therapy, the hypoxic cellular dysfunction is incompatible with life. The hypoxemia is due to alterations in alveolocapillary dynamics, which result in an abnormal pulmonary venoarterial shunt. This process is initiated by a yet undefined systemic insult. It has no known relationship to previous disease and is frequently seen in patients with normal cardiopulmonary systems.

The term ARDS has been used to cover a spectrum of pulmonary responses.[2-5] These range from transient episodes of hypoxemia that rapidly correct with therapy to refractory hypoxemia, which is often fatal. We reserve the term ARDS for refractory hypoxemia. Unfortunately, no distinct clinical separation exists between the various degrees of pathologic severity. This lack of uniformity among clinical definitions perpetuates the confusion regarding incidence, morbidity, and mortality figures.

Incidence, Morbidity and Mortality

In the 10-year period from 1966 to 1976, the San Francisco General Hospital averaged 40 cases of severe respiratory failure per year,[6] approximately a 2% incidence among all admitted trauma victims. Fulton reviewed 399 trauma patients and recorded pulmonary insufficiency in 44 (11%).[2] Horovitz and associates studied 49 severely injured patients at Parkland Memorial Hospital of whom only 3 (6%) developed evidence of severe pulmonary failure.[7] A second review of all surgical admissions to the Parkland intensive-care unit revealed a 9% incidence of severe pulmonary failure.[5]

The frequency of ARDS in other reports is much different. Shoemaker and associates studied 152 patients who sustained life-threatening trauma and hemorrhage.[3] Sixty (39%) patients developed ARDS. Gallagher and associates reviewed 421 patients of whom 326 (86%) were believed to have pulmonary failure.[4] Fifty-nine (14%) of these patients were classified as sustaining severe pulmonary failure, based on their need for intensive therapy.

The morbidity of ARDS is greater than that of most pulmonary complications because the severity of insult requires invasive cardiovascular monitoring, prolonged ventilatory support, and continuous intensive care. Each of these manipulations has an inherent complication rate of at least 10%. Mortality is as high as 50 to 70% in overt ARDS.[5,8] A more liberal definition of ARDS results in a higher incidence and a lower mortality (15 to 20%).[3,4] Confusion persists even when ARDS mortality is defined by terminal hypoxemia. One series reports terminal hypoxemia occurring in 11 of 27 (41%) patients with ARDS, while a second reports it among 3 of 59 (5%) patients with ARDS.[4,5] Regardless of differing definitions, ARDS imposes measurable morbidity to the trauma victim.

Pathology and Pathogenesis

Autopsy results reveal that the lungs fill the entire thoracic cavity and show no tendency to collapse. The lungs demonstrate an increased weight and a meaty red appearance with scattered patches of necrosis and abscess formation.[9] The light microscopic picture varies with the stage of disease.[10] Early changes include vascular congestion, alveolar collapse with edema, and inflammatory cell infiltration. As these changes progress, hypertrophy of alveolar lining cells and focal alveolar hemorrhage occur. The final changes include microabscess formation, with or without consolidation, and hyaline membrane deposition in the alveoli.

The exact pathogenesis of the interstitial edema is not known. Although most information suggests that an insult to the pulmonary capillary endothelium results in increased permeability and extravasation of intravascular fluid, the nature of this endothelial insult is not cleary defined.[11] Hypotheses include microembolism, vasoactive substances, immunologic reactions, and direct toxin (endotoxin) effect.[12] Despite the incompletely understood cellular mechanisms, it is fairly clear that a pulmonary vascular insult results in interstitial edema. Subsequent changes include progressive alveolar collapse, decreased compliance, and alterations in pulmonary blood flow. Figure 5-1 represents a general concept of the pathophysiology.

In 1968, Moore and associates published a comprehensive discussion of ARDS, which described four clinical phases and their pathophysiologic features.[13] This description is a succinct outline of the syndrome's natural history.

1. Injury, resuscitation, and alkalosis. A mixed respiratory and metabolic alkalosis results from spontaneous hyperventilation, metabolism of transfused citrate, nasogastric drainage, and antacid therapy.

2. Circulatory stabilization, early respiratory difficulty. This phase may occur within a few hours to five days. It is characterized by a stable cardiovascular system, hyperventilation, a borderline arterial Po_2, and a normal chest roentgenogram.

3. Progressive pulmonary insufficiency. Definite hypoxemia has developed. The resultant hyperventilation produces significant hypocarbia. Intubation is necessary. The chest roentgenogram shows spotty infiltrates bilaterally.

4. Terminal hypoxia and hypercarbia with asystole. Progressive hypoxemia is unresponsive to therapy. Adequate ventilation becomes mechanically impossible, and hypercarbia results. The combined respiratory and metabolic acidosis produces further myocardial compromise. Bradycardia and, finally, asystole or ventricular fibrillation develop.

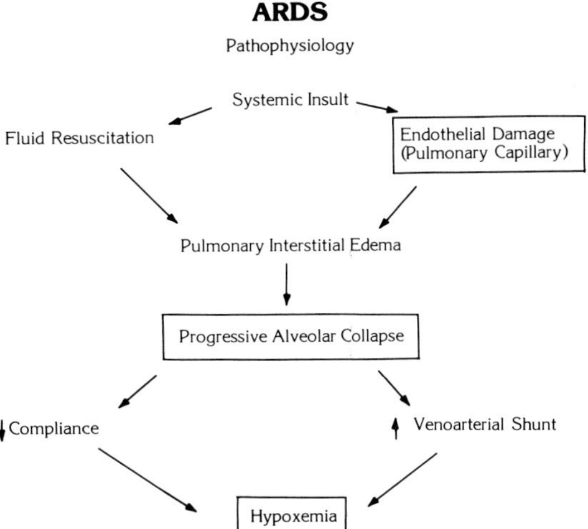

FIG. 5-1. General concept of the pathophysiology of the adult respiratory distress syndrome (ARDS).

Our concepts of the pulmonary response to trauma are presented in Figure 5-2 and Table 5-1. The emphasis is placed on clinically oriented definitions.[5] Pulmonary deterioration includes all

TABLE 5-1. *Diagnostic Criteria of Pulmonary Parenchymal Impairment.*

1. Exclusion of specific causes of respiratory compromise
2. Greater than 96 hours of constant ventilation required
3. Presence of *at least one* of the following.*
   - $P(AaDo_2) > 400$ mm Hg
   - Pulmonary venoarterial shunt > 25%
   - Chest roentgenogram shows diffuse interstitial edema

*Severity classification:
Only one factor present—pulmonary dysfunction
More than one factor present—adult respiratory distress syndrome

TABLE 5-2. *Classification of Adult Respiratory Distress Syndrome.*

I. "NONSEPSIS" RELATED	
Shock	Chest trauma
Fluid overload	Burns
Multiple transfusions	Renal transplantation
Massive trauma	cardiopulmonary bypass
Aspiration	Fat embolism
Pancreatitis (Acute)	Severe cerebral injury
Oxygen toxicity	
II. "SEPSIS" RELATED	
A. Primary Septic Event	
Extrapulmonary	
Pulmonary	
B. Secondary Septic Event ("Nonseptic" ARDS with Septic Complications)	
Extrapulmonary	
Pulmonary	

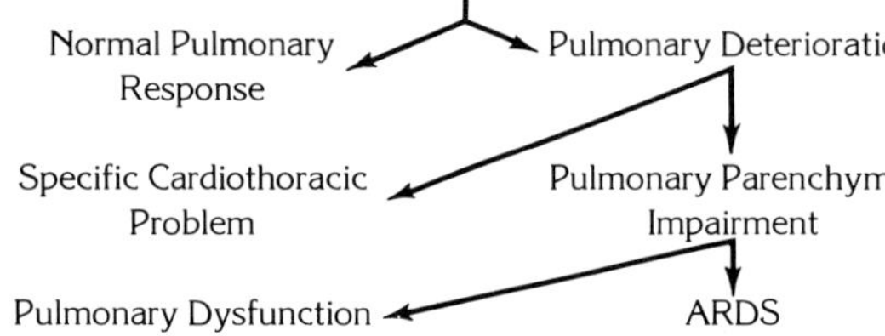

FIG. 5-2. Pulmonary response to trauma.

patients who require ventilation in the post-trauma period. The need for ventilation can be the result of either a specific cardiothoracic or a pulmonary parenchymal problem. Specific cardiothoracic problems include pulmonary contusion, multiple rib fractures, inefficient ventilatory effort (severe head injury), hypoventilation (pain with splinting), cardiac failure, and myocardial contusion. If none of these is present and hypoxemia progresses, the patient has either pulmonary dysfunction or ARDS. If all listed criteria in Table 5-1 are met, ARDS is the diagnosis. If only one of the criteria under number 3 is present, pulmonary dysfunction is the diagnosis.

Diagnosis

Recognition of hypoxemia is the key to diagnosing ARDS. Arterial blood gases confirm hypoxemia, which is defined as an arterial oxygen tension of less than 70 mm Hg while receiving an inspired oxygen concentration of 40% via an endotracheal tube. Changes in the chest roentgenogram aid in the diagnosis of ARDS. Diffuse interstitial infiltrates typify the chest roentgenogram.[14] Unfortunately, hypoxemia and pulmonary radiographic changes are late findings. Patients at risk of ARDS must be accurately identified before hypoxemia develops. Clinical assessment of associated etiologic factors, changes in the chest roentgenogram, pulmonary compliance, venoarterial shunt calculation, and arterial oxygen tensions offer some potential for achieving this early patient identification.

Etiologic Factor Association

Although the exact causes of ARDS are unknown, extensive clinical observation has resulted in a list of clinical conditions known frequently to precede its development. A classification of ARDS is presented in Table 5-2. It emphasizes suspected etiologic contributions and implies a temporal relationship of the insult to ARDS.

Sepsis has a high correlation with ARDS. Fulton reported that sepsis was the only etiologic factor in 42% of patients with ARDS.[2] Eiseman described two groups of patients with ARDS and classified them according to time of onset.[15] The early type related to shock, fluid overload, and massive trauma. This type responded well to therapy with only an 11% mortality rate. The late type, related to sepsis, responded poorly to therapy with a mortality rate of 85%. Clowes and associates found a different mortality rate among patients with early ARDS (12%) and late ARDS (35%).[16] Further, among patients with nonseptic ARDS, 40% subsequently developed septic complications which exacerbated their pulmonary problem. The source of sepsis was extrapulmonary in 90%, and the mortality for these patients was 50%.

Clinical criteria related to this etiologic information may allow accurate early selection of high-risk patients. High-risk criteria include unstable patients with abdominal trauma or intra-abdominal sepsis requiring laparotomy; patients with sufficient thoracic trauma to require continuous ventilation and at least one other serious organ system injury; and unstable patients with long bone fractures and blunt abdominal, thoracic, or central nervous system trauma and documented aspiration requiring ventilatory therapy. Instability is defined as any of the following:

shock (systolic blood pressure < 90 mm Hg) lasting more than 30 minutes or requiring more than 2000 ml of intravenous fluid; deteriorating oxygenation requiring more therapy than supplemental oxygen; and vigorous fluid resuscitation defined as greater than 7% weight gain in 24 hours, more than 6 L of crystalloid, or 6 units of blood in 6 hours. Patients with compromised cardiopulmonary function may also require close scrutiny. Examples of compromised cardiopulmonary function include asthma, chronic obstructive lung disease, heavy cigarette smoking, chest-wall restriction, history of pulmonary emboli, ischemic heart disease, obesity, and ascites.

Unfortunately, the use of etiologic factors with or without high-risk clinical criteria does not result in an improved diagnostic capability. Such criteria predict ARDS in only 50% of evaluated cases.

Chest Roentgenogram Findings

The distinctive changes associated with ARDS that are shown in a chest roentgenogram are produced by fluid accumulation in the lung. Early findings include bilateral interstitial thickening or poorly defined patchy infiltrates without cardiomegaly or pleural effusion. Progression causes these infiltrates to coalesce symmetrically and mimic pulmonary edema. At this point, the changes stabilize and represent advanced disease (Fig. 5-3). Emphasis has been placed on these late changes, and little attention has been given to early radiographic findings.

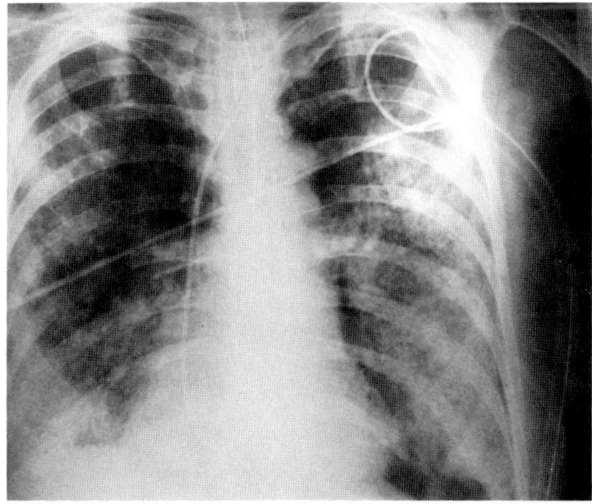

Fig. 5-3. Roentgenogram of chest showing effects of ARDS.

The functional residual capacity (FRC) is the volume of gas present in the lungs following a passive exhalation. It is composed of the expiratory reserve volume and the residual volume. The residual volume is the amount of gas in the lung following forced expiration. FRC is significantly affected by many pulmonary and nonpulmonary factors. Pulmonary factors include rib fractures, flail chest, excess secretions, interstitial edema, and bronchiolar constriction. Nonpulmonary factors include recumbent position, anesthesia, pain, obesity, ascites, muscular weakness, debility, and oversedation. Closure of alveoli and small airways in ARDS substantially reduces FRC.[17] A reduced FRC directly correlates with a decreased compliance and an increased venoarterial shunt.[18]

Direct measurement of FRC requires techniques not easily applied to the clinical situation; however, FRC may be estimated by a routine chest roentgenogram. Figure 5-4 demonstrates the difference between chest roentgenograms before and after a systemic insult resulting in a decrease in FRC. Unfortunately, the nonpulmonary factors influencing FRC cloud the prognostic ability of the chest roentgenogram, and radiographic changes lag behind acute clinical changes.[19]

Pulmonary Compliance

Effective static compliance helps to evaluate pulmonary function during mechanical ventilation. Compliance describes the relationship between inflating pressure and volume. Pulmonary interstitial edema and alveolar collapse result in a loss of lung elasticity. Increased airway pressure is required to overcome this decreased elasticity. If increased airway pressure does not occur, progressively smaller volumes are delivered to the alveoli, thereby promoting further alveolar collapse and decrease in FRC. The compliance decrease in ARDS is proportional to the decrease in total lung capacity and FRC.[11] A positive correlation also exists between compliance and arterial oxygen tension.[20]

The tidal volume and plateau pressure are necessary to calculate effective static compliance in intubated patients. Plateau pressure is obtained by momentarily obstructing expiration and reading the pressure in centimeters of water (cm H_2O) from the pressure gauge on the ventilator. The equation for effective static compliance is listed in the appendix. A normal static compliance is 65

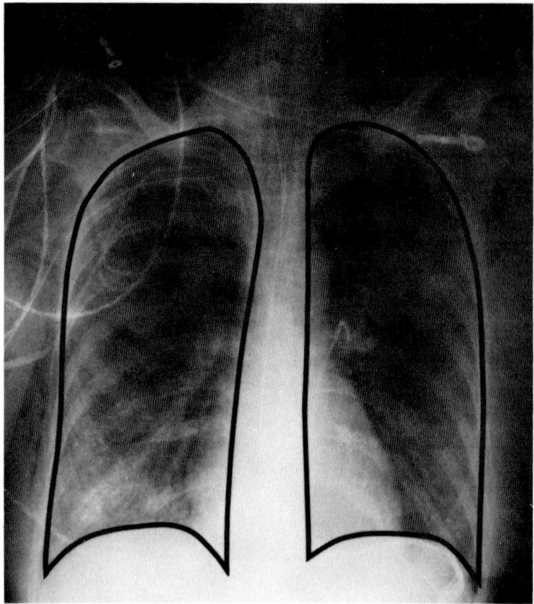

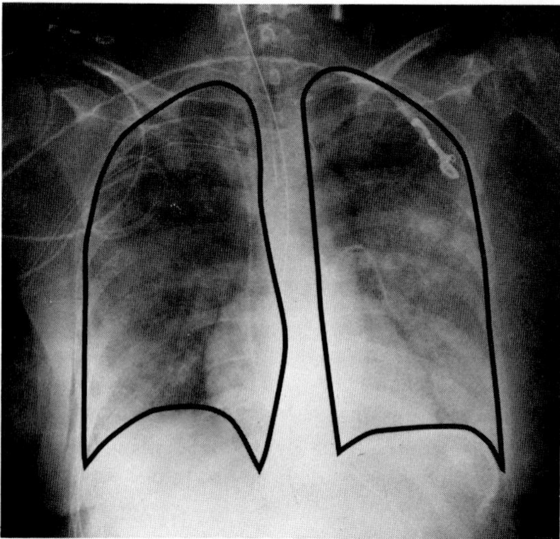

Fig. 5-4. *A,* Functional residual capacity (FRC, outlined) is relatively normal. *B,* Decreases in FRC secondary to systemic insult.

to 75 cm H_2O. A compliance of 50 cm H_2O is acceptable, and a compliance of 25 to 30 cm H_2O is associated with ARDS. Causes of low compliance other than ARDS include conflicting muscular effort and ventilator inspiration, retained tracheobronchial secretions, misplaced endotracheal tube, excessive peak air flow, lobar atelectasis, pneumothorax, fat embolism, pulmonary embolism, and abdominal distension.

The myriad causes of a low compliance and the wide range of acceptable compliance values make compliance a poor early indicator of ARDS. Compliance does help in selecting proper tidal volumes for ventilation and evaluating treatment responses after ARDS has developed.

Venoarterial Shunt

Hypoxemia in ARDS is caused by an increased pulmonary venoarterial shunt. The pulmonary venoarterial shunt is the fraction of blood passing through the lungs without being oxygenated. Shunted blood is divided into anatomic and capillary partitions. In the absence of cardiac abnormalities, the anatomic shunt is constant and normally does not exceed 2 to 3% of the cardiac output. The capillary shunt is variable and is composed of three elements: atelectasis, ventilation-perfusion inequalities, and diffusion hindrances. Increases in any of these three elements are responsible for abnormal shunt fractions. The defect in ARDS is an increase in alveolar units that are perfused but not ventilated.

The finding of an increased pulmonary shunt, which is characteristic of ARDS, may allow selection of high-risk patients. A 15 to 20% venoarterial shunt is claimed to offer diagnostic value, but physiologic shunts of 12 to 15% consistently occur in almost all patients following major trauma and even after uncomplicated upper abdominal surgery.[21] One cannot be sure that a severe parenchymal problem exists until the shunt fraction reaches 25% or greater. Although venoarterial shunt correlates with the severity of insult and eventual outcome, it is not an adequate indicator of early pulmonary parenchymal damage.

Arterial Oxygen Content

Minor alterations in arterial oxygenation, before hypoxemia develops, provide another approach to early identification of pulmonary parenchymal problems. Physical signs of hypoxemia include tachypnea, decreased tidal volume, diffuse rales, and restlessness. These findings are nonspecific, but should prompt an evaluation with arterial blood gases. Most intubated patients receive inspired concentrations of 40% oxygen. It is also common to use brief exposures to 100% oxygen for venarterial shunt calculation.[22]

Arterial blood gases on 40% inspired oxygen (Pa_{O_2} .4) and on 100% inspired oxygen (Pa_{O_2} 1.0) were assessed for their ability to predict pulmonary deterioration prior to hypoxemia. Fifty-nine patients were selected by clinical criteria alone.

All patients were intubated and were not hypoxic when first assessed. Sequential arterial oxygen determinations were performed until a diagnosis of arterial hypoxemia was established or extubation occurred. Accurate prognostic information regarding subsequent pulmonary deterioration was obtained. When the Pa_{O_2} .4 was greater than 100 mm Hg or the Pa_{O_2} 1.0 was greater than 350 mm Hg, the probability of pulmonary deterioration was 10%. When either was below these values, the probability was 60%. When the Pa_{O_2} .4 was below 100 mm Hg and the Pa_{O_2} 1.0 was below 350 mm Hg, the probability of pulmonary deterioration was 95%.

As outlined in Figure 5-2, an ideal situation exists when patients are identified with early evidence of a pulmonary parenchymal problem. We believe the proper monitoring of arterial oxygen tensions allows selection of high-risk patients for whom aggressive monitoring and therapy are indicated (Fig. 5-5).

Therapy

Successful management of ARDS requires careful attention to various pulmonary and cardiovascular aberrations. The intensity of treatment varies with the severity of existing or developing defects. Therapeutic interventions for pulmonary problems include aggressive pulmonary toilet, supplemental oxygen therapy, endotracheal intubation/tracheostomy, positive-pressure ventilation, positive end-expiratory pressure, and a successful weaning method from positive-pressure ventilation.

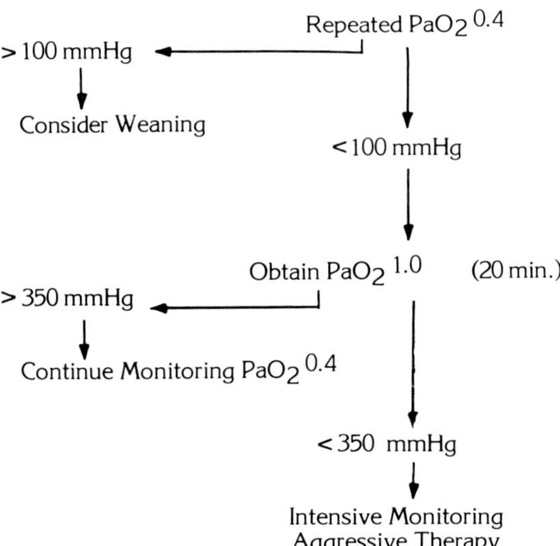

FIG. 5-5. Intensive monitoring includes Swan-Ganz catheterization. Aggressive therapy includes applying 5 cm of positive end-expiratory pressure (PEEP).

Pulmonary Toilet

Mechanical considerations should be directed to the problems of microatelectasis and retained tracheobronchial secretions. Factors that predispose a patient to these problems include low tidal volumes, absence of sigh mechanisms, recumbent position, pain, narcotics, and abnormal fluid balance. Despite the similarities of these pathophysiologic events, distinct differences exist in their therapy.

Therapy for microatelectasis emphasizes the maintenance of normal lung volumes, and the reduction of interstitial pulmonary edema. The treatment techniques include incentive spirometry, frequent position changes, early ambulation, postural drainage, bronchodilators, intermittent positive-pressure ventilation, positive end-expiratory pressure, and avoidance of hypervolemia. Therapy for retained tracheobronchial secretions emphasizes forced expiration, removal of excess secretions, and prevention of inspissated mucus. Treatment techniques include nasotracheal suction, transtracheal irrigation, bronchoscopy, postural drainage, mucolytic agents, tracheostomy, and optimal fluid balance.

Oxygen Therapy

Supplemental oxygen therapy temporarily resolves hypoxemia. Unfortunately, oxygen has no direct beneficial effect on the pulmonary parenchyma and has the potential for causing direct lung toxicity.[23] The toxicity is a vascular insult resulting in perivascular edema and endothelial proliferation. Progression results in pulmonary fibrosis. The incidence is related directly to the inspired oxygen concentration and duration of alveolar exposure.

An inspired oxygen concentration of 50% is considered safe.[24] Higher levels for any prolonged period of time are toxic and should only be used as diagnostic challenges or for a short period following an acute episode of instability.

An inspired oxygen concentration providing a Pa_{O_2} above 60 mm Hg associated with a saturation of 90% or greater is generally adequate to maintain vital functions. If toxic levels of inspired oxygen are being considered, a complete evaluation of the patient should be performed. This evaluation must be directed at cardiac output, oxygen delivery and consumption, and the adequacy of intravascular volume. The Pa_{O_2} alone is not an appropriate guide for increases in oxygen therapy.

Endotracheal Intubation

The purposes of creating an artificial airway in lower respiratory tract disease include decreasing dead-space ventilation, facilitating tracheobronchial suction, and providing a means of positive-pressure ventilation. The indications for intubation can be divided into three broad categories: inadequate ventilation, inadequate oxygenation, and mechanical problems.[25]

Management of the patient with ARDS often requires prolonged periods of endotracheal intubation. Care must be taken to prevent complications associated with the artificial airway. Two main groups of complications exist. The first group is associated with intubation techniques. These complications are similar for all intubated patients and include nasopharyngeal trauma, esophageal intubation, right bronchial intubation, and various tube malfunctions. The second group is associated with long-term intubation and includes sinusitis, hoarseness, vocal cord granulomas, subglottic stenosis, and tracheal stenosis.

All patients intubated for more than 24 hours should have low-pressure endotracheal tubes. The "low-pressure" designation refers to the cuff occlusion pressure. These tubes achieve a tracheal seal without exerting pressures above 25 mm Hg to the tracheal wall, thereby reducing tracheal mucosal ischemia and resulting in a decreased incidence of tracheal stenosis.[26]

We prefer the use of orotracheal tubes for long-term ventilatory support. Prolonged nasotracheal intubation may cause alar and turbinate necrosis. The orotracheal route also allows for a tube with a larger diameter, which decreases airway resistance and gives better access for tracheobronchial suctioning. Intubation with an endotracheal tube no smaller than a No. 8 is preferred.

The decision to perform a tracheostomy for ventilatory support is difficult to make. Recommendations to perform tracheostomy after only 72 hours of intubation are certainly too conservative, but the optimal time for undertaking this procedure is hard to define. Tracheostomy in patients requiring prolonged mechanical support is often performed to decrease dead-space ventilation, improve tracheobronchial toilet, and reduce endotracheal complications. However, the decrease in dead space is minimal and rarely is sufficient to justify a tracheostomy. Improvement of tracheobronchial toilet is often mentioned, but is difficult to substantiate. Endotracheal complications that are avoided are related to the vocal cords; however, the tracheostomy substitutes stomal complications instead. Cuff complications are similar in both approaches because both the endotracheal and tracheostomy tubes have low-pressure cuffs.

Current recommendations for the best time to switch from an endotracheal to tracheostomy tube range from 1 to 4 weeks.[25,27] No prospective study is available to aid in this decision, and we use a maximum time limit of 2 weeks. At this time, the patient is assessed regarding his continued need for ventilatory support. When no immediate hope of extubation is apparent, tracheostomy is performed. A tracheostomy may be performed earlier if deemed necessary for pulmonary care. A common reason for early tracheostomy is deteriorating pulmonary function associated with increased tracheobronchial secretions.

Positive-Pressure Ventilation

Two types of ventilators are available: volume regulated and pressure regulated. Pressure-regulated machines inflate the lungs to a predetermined pressure, regardless of volume. Any change in the patient's position or lung compliance may alter the volume that is administered. A volume-regulated machine delivers a preset volume with each breath, despite changes in pressure. High flow rates and inspiratory pressures are often required for patients with ARDS, and these are more readily obtained with the volume-regulated machines. For these reasons, volume ventilators are preferred.

Most volume ventilators are uncomplicated and require only minimal adjustments for inspired oxygen content, tidal volume, sigh volume, and respiratory rate. The inspired oxygen content that should be used has been discussed. A general practice is to place patients initially on an FI_{O_2} of 40%.

Selection of tidal volume for a patient should

be based on several considerations. A reasonable guide for an initial setting is 12 to 15 ml/kg of body weight. Subsequent adjustments are usually required based on evaluations of inflation adequacy and derived physiologic parameters. Effective static compliance is the most important. The ease with which this relationship is determined makes it a valuable tool in the management of ventilatory therapy. A compliance curve can help to select the optimal tidal volume (Fig. 5-6).

A tidal volume chosen from the steep part of the curve results in the best compliance. This volume results in minimal airway closure and interference with cardiac hemodynamics. A tidal volume may be chosen up to the point at which the curve begins to plateau. Increases above this point are not beneficial to pulmonary or cardiac dynamics. Changes in clinical condition may alter the compliance curve significantly, so it should be replotted at frequent intervals. In practice, the compliance curve is replotted every 24 hours or when ventilatory pressures change acutely.

A sigh volume is important if tidal volumes of 5 to 7 ml/kg are used. Adequate sigh volumes are approximately 40% above normal tidal volumes. The sigh is given intermittently (6/hour) to prevent atelectasis. When a compliance curve is used to select a maximal tidal volume, intermittent sigh is probably unnecessary.[28]

Respiratory rate is usually set at 10/min initially. Adjustments are made to maintain a PCO_2 between 35 and 45 mm Hg. A lower PCO_2 may enhance patient comfort and reduce the tendency to fight the ventilator.

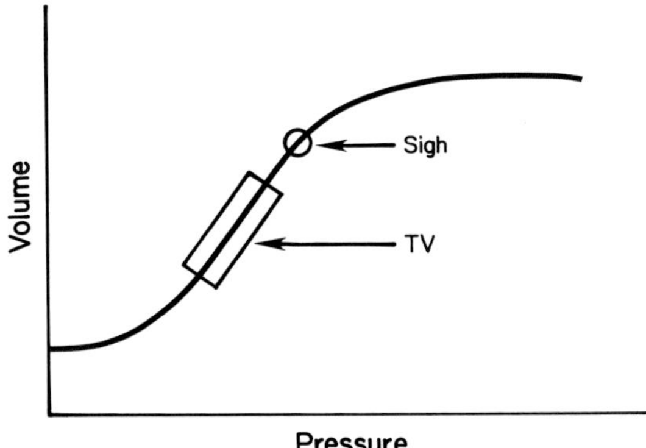

Fig. 5-6. Curve is constructed by inflating lungs with varying tidal volumes and recording pressures.

Fighting the ventilator, or patient ventilator asynchrony, is a common problem in acutely ill patients on controlled ventilation. All causes are not defined, but the result does not represent optimum ventilatory management. Attempts to control this problem should include the following:

1. A brief period of hyperventilation attempting to obliterate ventilatory drive.
2. Tolerable increases in tidal volume and/or rate to obliterate tachypnea. This is limited by the production of significant hypocarbia.
3. Sedation with small, frequent doses of morphine and diazepam (Valium). Doses of 5 to 10 mg/hour of either or both drugs are usually successful in alleviating asynchrony.
4. When sedation is unsuccessful, skeletal muscle paralysis can be used effectively.

Positive End-Expiratory Pressure

Positive-pressure ventilation can be supplemented with positive end-expiratory pressure (PEEP). PEEP is an expiratory retardation that maintains the airway pressure above atmospheric pressure throughout the expiration period. This is accomplished by a valve system incorporated into the ventilator or by placing the exhaust line under water at a depth corresponding to the desired level of PEEP. Positive end-expiratory pressure is measured in centimeters of water. Often, 5 cm H_2O are applied initially. Increases and decreases are made in small increments of 2 to 3 cm H_2O subsequent adjustments of PEEP and tidal volume are selected on the basis of arterial oxygen content, cardiac output, oxygen delivery, oxygen consumption, and compliance.

PEEP is believed to have several therapeutic effects.[4,29,30] It reverses progressive alveolar collapse and reduces interstitial edema, improving alveolar gas exchange and increasing arterial oxygen tensions. Powers and associates demonstrated that PEEP effectively increases the functional residual capacity, increases the Pa_{O_2}, and decreases the magnitude of venoarterial shunt.[29] Sutter and associates demonstrated a relationship between PEEP levels and other cardiopulmonary parameters.[18] Venoarterial shunt and Pa_{O_2} continue to improve with increasing levels of PEEP, but compliance and oxygen transport deteriorate. Compliance and oxygen transport can be used to identify the "best" PEEP level.

These benefits are not without potential side-effects. PEEP may reduce venous return and alter intrathoracic pressure relationships, resulting in a decreased cardiac output.[29,31] The increase in mean airway pressure predisposes the patient to barotrauma, primarily pneumothorax. The detrimental effects of PEEP are most pronounced in hypovolemic patients. Investigation reveals that low levels of PEEP (5 to 10 cm H_2O) are well tolerated.[27] Higher levels of PEEP can be tolerated if the patient is made hypervolemic. This does not imply that all patients who are placed on PEEP should be treated by increasing their intravascular volume.

The appropriate use of positive end-expiratory pressure (PEEP) is still disputed. Certainly, a patient on continuous ventilatory therapy with adequate pulmonary toilet and optimal cardiovascular hemodynamics is a candidate for PEEP when the Pa_{O_2} .4 is less than 65 mm Hg, the alveoloarterial oxygen difference on 100% oxygen is greater than 400 mm Hg, or the venoarterial shunt is greater than 20%.[25,30,32] PEEP is also helpful in improving oxygenation without exposing the patient to toxic levels of inspired oxygen. Evidence also shows that low levels of PEEP applied early to high-risk patients result in significant decreases in the severity of pulmonary parenchymal damage.[5,33,34] A decrease in morbidity and mortality also occurs from this application of PEEP. We routinely apply 5 cm of PEEP to all patients who have arterial gases indicating a high probability of developing ARDS (see Fig. 5-5).

Sedation is frequently required to enhance patient tolerance to high tidal volumes and PEEP. Patient asynchrony with PEEP is more serious than that without PEEP because of the greater potential for barotrauma secondary to the increased ventilator pressures generated. All patients on PEEP do not need musculoskeletal paralysis. Patient assist on PEEP is not harmful if extreme negative pressures and asynchrony do not occur.

Weaning

Various regimens are reported to be successful in weaning the patient from mechanical ventilation.[12,35] The weaning process concerns oxygenation and ventilation adequacy. Inspired oxygen concentration and PEEP are oxygenation factors; respiratory rate, tidal volume, vital capacity, and inspiratory force are ventilatory factors.

A safe FI_{O_2} is necessary before any weaning measures can be attempted. A 40% FI_{O_2} is commonly used, but the FI_{O_2} may be lower if adequate oxygenation is maintained. PEEP is removed as oxygenation improves. PEEP can be decreased safely if the Pa_{O_2} level is 100 mm Hg or greater. PEEP should be decreased only in increments of 2 to 3 cm H_2O per 6 to 12 hours. More rapid removal of PEEP is associated with weaning failures and a worsening of oxygenation.[36]

Ventilation assessment is equally important. A spontaneous respiratory rate of 24 or less is preferred, but a rate of 30 is acceptable. A tidal volume of at least 5 to 7 ml/kg and an ability to increase depth of breathing to at least 15 ml/kg are necessary. The ability to generate a negative inspiratory force of at least 20 cm/H_2O is a final guideline.

The patient who meets these guidelines is a candidate for weaning. Removing mechanical ventilatory support can be accomplished in a number of ways. A popular method is to institute intermittent mandatory ventilation.[35] This form of ventilatory support allows the patient to breathe spontaneously while receiving a controlled minute ventilation. As the patient's ability to maintain adequate oxygenation and ventilation improves, the amount of controlled ventilation is decreased by decreasing the rate of ventilation while the tidal volume remains the same, thereby allowing a gradual weaning process.

Cardiovascular Therapy

The maintenance of adequate intravascular volume and sufficient cardiac function is required when treating patients with ARDS. The major difficulties relate to the inaccuracies in evaluating fluid volumes and the variables imposed by preexistent or concurrent cardiac disease. A further limitation is that the magnitude of relative hypervolemia or increased cardiac function required for each clinical situation has defied quantitation. Monitoring the cardiovascular system allows the best available interpretation. Therapeutic interventions to complement this monitoring include fluid therapy, blood therapy, diuretics, cardiovascular drugs, and nutrition.

Monitoring

Cardiovascular monitoring of patients with ARDS greatly improved following the development of the Swan-Ganz catheter.[37] The Swan-Ganz catheter is a flexible intravascular catheter 120 cm in length. It has an inflatable balloon at its tip, a distal port for measuring pulmonary artery pressure, and a proximal port for measuring central venous pressure. The catheter may also have thermistors, which determine cardiac output by the Fick principle. The catheter comes in different sizes; the most frequently used size is 7F.

The Swan-Ganz catheter is inserted via the venous system and is carried through the right side of the heart into the pulmonary artery. Its passage is monitored by pressure wave forms characteristic of the central circulation (Fig. 5-7). Such monitoring allows the catheter to be placed at the bedside without fluoroscopic control. When properly placed, the catheter is used for measuring pulmonary artery pressures, and pulmonary wedge pressure, obtaining mixed venous blood samples, and determining cardiac output.

Pulmonary artery catheters are placed by various techniques. We favor a percutaneous subclavian vein approach using a modified Seldinger method to cannulate the vein. Fluoroscopy is not employed. Our success rate is 95%. The average time required to place a catheter is 10 minutes. Our complication rate is less than 10% and is primarily related to problems with vein cannulation. Catheters are used for an average of 3.5 days.

The importance of the Swan-Ganz catheter is its ability to measure pulmonary artery pressures, including pulmonary capillary wedge pressure (PCWP). Excellent correlation exists between PCWP, left atrial pressure, and left ventricular end-diastolic pressure.[37] The observed PCWP is the result of a combination of factors including the intravascular volume, ventricular function, transpulmonary pressures, and pulmonary compliance. Some variance that can have clinical importance does occur, but a more valid or feasible measurement is not clinically available. Interpretation of pulmonary artery pressures in patients with PEEP is a common problem. This difficulty arises from the changes in intrapleural and intra-alveolar pressure secondary to continuous positive-pressure ventilation. Elevated values present the primary problem. A low or normal value generally can be accepted as indicating the absence of hypervolemia or ventricular dysfunction. Directional changes with serial measurements are generally valid unless accompanied by PEEP or ventilator changes.

The Swan-Ganz catheter is also useful when aspirating mixed venous blood samples and determining cardiac output. Mixed venous blood samples are analyzed similarly to arterial blood gases. The information can be used to calculate arteriovenous oxygen difference, oxygen consumption, and pulmonary shunt fraction. The equations for these calculations are listed in the Appendix. A normal arteriovenous oxygen difference is 4 to 5 ml of oxygen per 100 ml of blood. This value increases when cardiac output is low and decreases when cardiac output is high. A normal value for oxygen consumption is 250 ml/min. Maintaining this value at a normal or greater than normal value is important to overall management.[3]

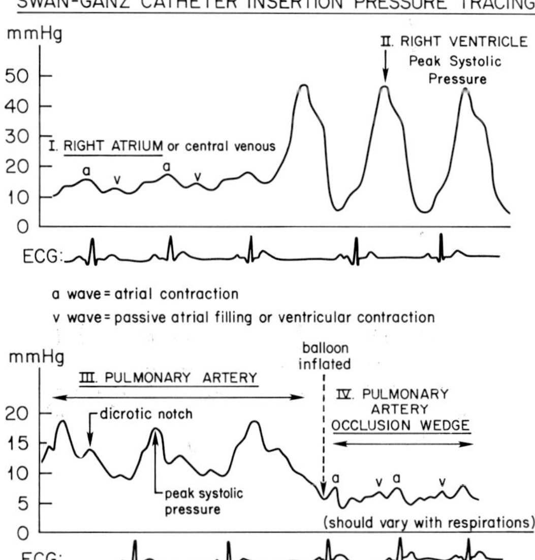

Fig. 5-7. Swan-Ganz catheter insertion pressure tracings.

Fluid Therapy

The type of fluid used for resuscitation and its effect on pulmonary function remain controversial.[38-41] The choice is between crystalloid and colloid.[4] Colloid solutions preserve serum oncotic pressure, which may decrease the amount of fluid lost into the interstitial space. This preservation, however, may have deleterious effects: leakage of colloid into the pulmonary interstitial space increases tissue oncotic pressure, thereby opposing any benefit derived from maintaining serum oncotic pressure. Because a capillary leak is suspected as a major component of ARDS pathophysiology, crystalloid fluid resuscitation is our choice in patients who are candidates for ARDS.

Crystalloid resuscitation often results in a moderate hypervolemia. The exact anatomic site and the exact magnitude of the excess fluid are not entirely clear. However, further fluid overload risks deleterious effects on pulmonary function. Limiting the hypervolemia to what is essential for hemodynamic stability seems prudent. When hemodynamic stability has been accomplished, the basic concepts of postoperative fluid and electrolyte balance must be applied to the patient with ARDS.

Two additional considerations must be remembered when discussing maintenance fluid requirements. Patients who are continuously ventilated have altered intrathoracic pressure relationships and increased ADH secretion.[42] Furthermore, all inspired gases are humidified. Both of these factors promote water retention and may account for as much as 1000 ml of water retained per day. Maintenance fluid is best offered as crystalloid. Some evidence exists that albumin offerred to these patients is detrimental.[41,43]

Blood Replacement

Blood replacement therapy is common in the multiply injured patient. Many investigators have demonstrated adverse effects on pulmonary function secondary to multiple blood transfusions.[41] These adverse effects are believed to result from the aggregation of fibrin, white blood cells, and platelets in the pulmonary capillaries with subsequent endothelial injury. This may be prevented by filtration of blood through a 25- to 40-micron filter. All blood given to multiply injured patients should be filtered, and red blood cells should be replaced to maintain a hemoglobin of 12 g/L. An adequate oxygen-carrying capacity should result for most patients.[44]

Diuretics

Diuretics are used when attempting to mobilize interstitial edema. Skillman and associates demonstrated some improvement in oxygenation by using potent diuretics and albumin.[45] Lucas and associates, however, caution against their routine use.[46] Judicious use of loop diuretics is probably appropriate when monitoring parameters indicate that a hypervolemic state is present. Diuresis should always be induced cautiously and gradually to avoid large fluctuations in intravascular volume and resultant hypoperfusion. Mannitol may be helpful in patients who are unresponsive to loop diuretics, especially when a hypervolemic state is not present. Powers and associates suggest that mannitol might have a beneficial effect on the intrapulmonary shunt associated with ARDS.[47]

Inotropic Support

Cardiotonic drugs are important in patients whose cardiac output is insufficient to meet peripheral demands despite adequate intravascular volume. The presence of isolated myocardial dysfunction is the prerequisite for using these agents. The presence of significant pulmonary insufficiency alone is not an indication for inotropic support or digitalization. When these drugs are used, the monitoring of central filling pressure, pulmonary and systemic vascular resistance, oxygen delivery and consumption, and serial cardiac output is helpful.

Nutrition

Nutrition is a secondary but imperative consideration in major trauma patients with ARDS. Caloric and protein supplementation is required to combat the catabolism that follows the physiologic insult. If such support is not provided, the patient is at increased risk of metabolic and infectious complications.[48] Nutrition is offered by either a parenteral or enteral route, depending on the patient. Patients at our institution are started on nutrition within the first week of admission. All patients with ARDS are supported with at least 40 to 50 calories per kilogram per day and 90 g of protein per day.

Summary

The Adult Respiratory Distress Syndrome is the most severe pulmonary complication that can follow multiple trauma. It is caused by an insult to the pulmonary circulation that results in an increased capillary permeability and subsequent interstitial edema. An increased venoarterial shunt occurs, resulting in arterial hypoxemia. Mortality is at least 50% if treatment is not begun before profound hypoxemia occurs.

Recognition of abnormal cardiopulmonary function before overt hypoxemia develops is important and is best accomplished by attentive monitoring of arterial blood gases. Sequential arterial oxygen tensions obtained on 40% and 100% inspired oxygen concentration are the best guides to selecting patients who have a high probability of pulmonary deterioration. Aggressive cardiovascular monitoring and early treatment with low levels of PEEP offer this group of patients an improved chance of survival.

Appendix

A. Venoarterial Shunt Fraction (Qs/Qt)

$$\frac{Qs}{Qt} = \frac{Cc_{O_2} - Ca_{O_2}}{Cc_{O_2} - Cv_{O_2}}$$

$Cc_{O_2} = Hb \times 1.34 + PA_{O_2} \times .0031$ ml/100 ml blood

$Ca_{O_2} = Hb \times 1.34 \times Sa_{O_2} + (PA_{O_2} \times .0031)$ ml/100 ml blood

$Cv_{O_2} = Hb \times 1.34 \times Sv_{O_2} + (Pv_{O_2} \times .0031)$ ml/100 ml blood

Cc_{O_2} = Oxygen content of pulmonary capillary blood
Ca_{O_2} = Oxygen content of arterial blood
Cv_{O_2} = Oxygen content of mixed venous blood
PA_{O_2} = Alveolar oxygen tension (mm Hg)
Sa_{O_2} = Oxygen saturation of arterial blood (0.00)
Sv_{O_2} = Oxygen saturation of mixed venous blood (0.00)

B. Alveolar − Arterial Oxygen Difference $\{P(A - aD_{O_2})\}$

$P(A - aD_{O_2})$
$= (713 \times FI_{O_2} - 1.25 \times Pa_{CO_2}) - Pa_{O_2}$
Normal = 10 to 44 mm Hg

PA_{O_2} = Alveolar oxygen tension (mm Hg)
Pa_{O_2} = Arterial oxygen tension (mm Hg)

C. Oxygen Delivery

$$O_2del = Ca_{O_2} \times C.O.$$

Normal = 1000 ml/min

C.O. = Cardiac output L/min

D. Oxygen Consumption (V_{O_2})

$$V_{O_2} = C(a - v)D_{O_2} \times C.O.$$

Normal = 250 ml/min

$C(a - v)D_{O_2}$ = arteriovenous content difference

E. Pulmonary Vascular Resistance (PVR)

$$\frac{PVR = PAP - PCWP}{C.O.} \times 80$$

Normal = < 200 dynes − sec cm^{-5}

PAP = Mean pulmonary artery pressure

PCWP = Pulmonary capillary wedge pressure

F. Effective Static Compliance (Ceff)

$$Ceff = \frac{\text{Tidal Volume ml}}{\text{Plateau Inspiratory Pressure cmH}_2\text{O}}$$

Normal = 65 to 75(ml/cmH_2O)

References

1. Baker, C. C., et al.: Epidemiology of trauma deaths. Am. J. Surg., *140*:144, 1980.
2. Fulton, R. L.: Post-traumatic respiratory and pulmonary insufficiency. Contemp. Surg., *8*:41, 1976.
3. Shoemaker, W. C., et al.: Pathogenesis of respiratory failure (ARDS) after hemorrhage and trauma: I. Cardiorespiratory patterns preceding the development of ARDS. Crit. Care Med., *8*:504, 1980.
4. Gallagher, T. J., Civetta, J. M., and Kirby, R. R.: Terminology update: optimal PEEP. Crit. Care Med., *6*:323, 1978.
5. Weigelt, J. A., Mitchell, R. A., and Snyder, W. H.: The effect of early PEEP in the respiratory distress syndrome. Arch. Surg., *114*:497, 1979.
6. Lewis, F. R., Blaisdell, F. W., and Schlobohm, R. M.: Incidence and outcome of post-traumatic respiratory failure. Arch. Surg., *112*:436, 1977.
7. Horovitz, J. H., Carrico, C. J., and Shires, G. T.: Pulmonary response to major injury. Arch. Surg., *108*:349, 1974.
8. Bone, R. C.: Treatment of adult respiratory distress syndrome with diuretics, dialysis, and positive end-expiratory pressure. Crit. Care Med., *6*:136, 1978.
9. Blaisdell, F. W.: Pathophysiology of the respiratory distress syndrome. Arch. Surg., *108*:44, 1974.
10. Teplitz, C.: The core pathobiology and integrated medical science of adult acute respiratory insufficiency. Surg. Clin. North Am., *56*(*5*):1091, 1976.
11. Bowen, J. C., and Miller, W. C.: Pathophysiologic considerations in the diagnosis and treatment of post-traumatic pulmonary insufficiency. Am. J. Surg., *130*:550, 1975.
12. Pontoppidan, H., et al.: Respiratory intensive care. Anesthesiology, *47*:96, 1977.
13. Moore, F. D., et al.: Post-Traumatic Pulmonary Insufficiency. Philadelphia, W. B. Saunders, 1969.
14. Goodman, L. R.: Postoperative chest radiograph: I. Alterations after abdominal surgery. A.J.R., *134*:533, 1980.
15. Eiseman, L. W.: The changing pattern of post-traumatic respiratory distress syndrome. Ann. Surg., *181*:693, 1975.
16. Clowes, G. H. A., et al.: Septic lung and shock lung in man. Ann. Surg., *181*:681, 1975.
17. Pontoppidan, H., Geffin, B., and Lowenstein, E.: Acute respiratory failure in the adult (first of three parts). N. Engl. J. Med., *287*:690, 1972.
18. Sutter, P. M., Fairley, H. B., and Isenberg, M. D.: Optimum end-expiratory airway pressure in patients with acute pulmonary failure. N. Engl. J. Med., *292*:284, 1975.
19. Liebman, P. R., et al.: Limitations of portable roentgenography of the chest in patients with acute respiratory failure. Surg. Gynecol. Obstet., *146*:705, 1978.
20. Fleming, W. H., and Bowen, J. C.: The use of diuretics in the treatment of early wet lung syndrome. Ann. Surg., *175*:505, 1972.
21. Wilson, R. F., et al.: Respiratory failure in clinical shock and trauma. *In* Current Topics in Surgical Research. Vol. I. Edited by G. D. Zuidema, and D. B. Skinner. New York, Academic Press, 1969.
22. Weigelt, J. A., Jackson, G. L., and Mitchell, R. A.: Effects of 100 per cent inspired oxygen on shunt calculation. Curr. Surg., *37*:211, 1980.

23. Deneke, S. M., and Fanburg, B. L.: Normobaric oxygen toxicity of the lung. N. Engl. J. Med., *303*:76, 1980.
24. Blaisdell, F. W., and Lewis, F. R.: Etiologic factors in the respiratory distress syndrome. *In* Respiratory Distress Syndrome of Shock and Trauma, Major Problems in Clinical Surgery. Vol. XXI. Edited by P. A. Ebert. Philadelphia, W. B. Saunders, 1977.
25. Blaisdell, F. W., and Lewis, F. R.: Respiratory management of the respiratory distress syndrome. *In* Respiratory Distress Syndrome of Shock and Trauma, Major Problems in Clinical Surgery. Vol. XXI. Edited by P. A. Ebert. Philadelphia, W. B. Saunders, 1977.
26. Lewis, F. R., Schlobohm, R. M., and Thomas, A. N.: Prevention of complications from prolonged tracheal intubation. Am. J. Surg., *135*:452, 1978.
27. Pontoppidan, H., Geffin, B., and Lowenstein, E.: Acute respiratory failure in the adult (third of three parts). N. Engl. J. Med., *287*:799, 1972.
28. Balsys, A. J., et al.: Effects of sighs of different tidal volumes on compliance, functional residual capacity and arterial oxygen tension in normal and hypoxemic dogs. Crit. Care Med., *8*:641, 1980.
29. Powers, S. R., et al.: Physiologic consequences of positive end-expiratory pressure (PEEP) ventilation. Ann. Surg., *178*:265, 1973.
30. Peters, R. M.: Lifesaving measures in acute respiratory distress syndrome. Am. J. Surg., *178*:368, 1979.
31. Toung, T. J. K., et al.: The beneficial and harmful effects of positive end-expiratory pressure. Surg. Gynecol. Obstet., *147*:518, 1978.
32. Pontoppidan, H., Geffin, B., and Lowenstein, E.: Acute respiratory failure in the adult (second of three parts). N. Engl. J. Med., *287*:743, 1972.
33. Schmidt, G. B., et al.: Continuous positive airway pressure in the prophylaxis of the adult respiratory distress syndrome. Surg. Gynecol. Obstet., *143*:613, 1976.
34. Perel, A., et al.: The variable effect of PEEP in acute respiratory failure associated with multiple trauma. J. Trauma, *8*:218, 1978.
35. Sladen, A.: Weaning from mechanical ventilation. Surg. Rounds, *Sept.*:33, 1979.
36. Luterman, A., et al.: Withdrawal from positive end-expiratory pressure. Surgery, *83*:328, 1978.
37. Swan, H. J. C., and Ganz, W.: Use of balloon flotation catheters in critically ill patients. Surg. Clin. North Am., *55(3)*:501, 1975.
38. Holcroft, J. W., and Trunkey, D. D.: Extravascular lung water following hemorrhagic shock in the baboon: comparison between resuscitation with Ringer's lactate and plasmanate. Ann. Surg., *180*:408, 1974.
39. Nees, J. E., et al.: Comparison of cardiorespiratory effects of crystalline hemoglobin, whole blood, albumin, and Ringer's lactate in the resuscitation of hemorrhagic shock in dogs. Surgery, *83*:639, 1978.
40. Virgilio, R. W., et al.: Crystalloid vs. colloid resuscitation: is one better? Surgery, *85*:129, 1979.
41. Lucas, C. E., Ledgerwood, A. M., and Higgins, R. F.: Impaired salt and water excretion after albumin resuscitation for hypovolemic shock. Surgery, *86*:544, 1979.
42. Sladen, A., Laver, M. B., and Pontoppidan, H.: Pulmonary complications and water retention in prolonged mechanical ventilation. N. Engl. J. Med., *279*:448, 1968.
43. Blaisdell, F. W., Lewis, F. R.: Thromboembolism in the etiology of the respiratory distress syndrome. *In* Respiratory Distress Syndrome of Shock and Trauma, Major Problems in Clinical Surgery. Vol. XXI. Edited by P. A. Ebert. Philadelphia, W. B. Saunders, 1977.
44. Canizaro, P. C., Nelson, J., and Hennessy, J.: Alterations in oxygen transport. *In* Shock, Major Problems in Clinical Surgery. Vol. XIII. Edited by G. T. Shires. Philadelphia, W. B. Saunders. 1973.
45. Skillman, J. J., Parikh, B. M., and Tanenbaum, B. J.: Pulmonary arteriovenous admixture. Am. J. Surg., *119*:440, 1970.
46. Lucas, C. E., et al.: Impaired pulmonary function after albumin resuscitation from shock. J. Trauma, *20*:446, 1980.
47. Powers, S. R., et al.: Hypertonic mannitol in the therapy of the acute respiratory distress syndrome. Ann. Surg., *185*:619, 1977.
48. Meakins, J. L., et al.: Delayed hypersensitivity: indicator of acquired failure of host defenses in sepsis and trauma. Ann. Surg., *186*:241, 1977.

Chapter 6 Urologic Assessment of the Multiply Injured Patient

PAUL C. PETERS

The genitourinary system is often involved in the multiply injured patient. During an average year at Parkland Memorial Hospital, 3200 operations are done on an emergency basis; trauma victims comprise a large percentage of these emergency procedures. Approximately 700 urologic consultations on the trauma patient are rendered each year. A systematic approach to these patients has been developed to give the attending urologist a maximum of information with a minimum of radiation exposure to the injured patient. A concise workup is quickly obtained to exclude major injury or to detect its presence for proper immediate treatment.

Diagnosis

The Trauma Workup

The trauma workup consists of an excretory urogram performed by injecting intravenously 50 ml of an iodine-containing contrast material after a plain film of the abdomen is made. A cystogram and occasionally a urethrogram are performed prior to obtaining the 5-minute film after injection of the contrast material (Fig. 6-1). Routine films are made at 5, 15, and 30 minutes. If possible, a post-voiding film is obtained after the initial cystogram and immediate drainage film are taken. An exception to this general approach is the patient with straddle injury. If a history of straddle injury is obtained, a urethrogram is made prior to passing a soft catheter, which is usually done to obtain a cystogram. The use of isotope studies continues to play a major role in the injured patient. Injections of 99^{m} technetium polyphosphate are being used to measure renal flow, to detect avulsions of renal parenchyma, to determine blood flow to the kidney, and to diagnose the presence of urinary extravasation in selected cases.

Renal and Bladder Injury

Genitourinary injury is usually suspected in patients who have contusions over the eleventh or twelfth ribs posteriorly, hemorrhage or ecchymosis in the flank, and micro or gross hematuria. Only about 80% of patients with severe renal injuries manifest gross hematuria, but the use of the excretory urogram, cystogram, and urethrogram allows prompt detection of the presence of major injuries in nearly all patients. The nonvisualizing kidney by excretory urography represents a major renal artery injury as a rule. Major venous injury, such as severance of the renal vein from the vena cava or segmental arterial injury, results in a nephrogram phase that is apparent after the injection of contrast material. At present, though the nonvisualizing kidney may be recognized, the salvage rate in patients with major arterial intimal tear is still quite poor. By the time the diagnosis is made or the patient reaches the operating room, normothermic ischemia has often destroyed the kidney. Continued suspicion and prompt use of excretory urography and angiography result in earlier diagnosis and greater salvage of these currently disappointing cases.[1]

Intraperitoneal rupture of the bladder has been found to be associated with severe concomitant intra-abdominal injuries. Extraperitoneal rupture of the bladder usually is not associated with major intra-abdominal injuries. In a series of 512 consecutive patients with pelvic fracture seen at Parkland Memorial Hospital, 5% had an extraperitoneal rupture of the bladder. Exploration of the peritoneal cavity is indicated, particularly in the intraperitoneal rupture of the bladder, because of associated concomitant severe injuries. Even if the four-quadrant tap of the abdomen has been done by the trauma surgeon and is negative, the attending surgeon is advised to inspect for injury by opening the peritoneum at the time of repair of an intraperitoneal rupture of the urinary bladder. The overall mortality of patients at Parkland Memorial Hospital with intraperitoneal rupture of the bladder in 1 series of 50 injuries was 20%, not because of the seriousness of the intraperitoneal rupture of the bladder, which may be amenable to simple catheter drainage in some patients, but because of the major associated injuries, such as laceration of the liver, spleen, or crushing chest injury, which often result from the violent force sustained by the patient who has an intraperitoneal rupture of the bladder.

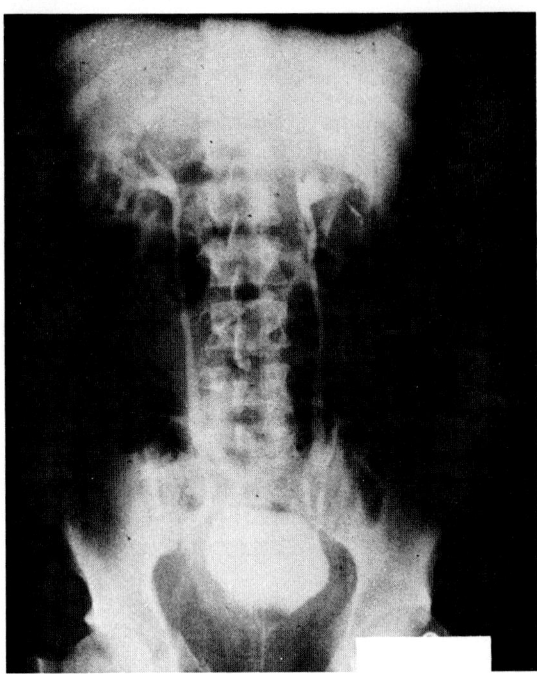

Fig. 6-1. The trauma workup. IVP and cystogram are performed at the same sitting.

Renal Injuries

About 85% of renal injuries are minor and do not require surgery.[2] About 5% of renal injuries result in a shattered, clotted, or severely damaged kidney which must be removed. Therefore, only about 10% of all renal injuries require careful judgmental considerations regarding sequential management.[2] Renal injuries may be divided into major and minor categories. In major renal injuries, lacerations extend completely through the parenchyma and into the collecting system, major pedicle injuries are present, or complete avulsion of the collecting system and interruption of continuity of drainage of urine are present (Fig. 6-2). Minor injuries include intrarenal hematomas, small parenchymal lacerations that do not extend through or into the collecting system, and subcapsular hematomas.

The diagnosis of the presence of a renal injury usually is suspected by the finding of gross or microscopic hematuria or by the presence of a contusion over the flank or over the ribs posteriorly. Fractured ribs are common findings in patients with blunt and penetrating renal trauma. All genitourinary injuries can be triaged conveniently into two general groups—the penetrating or the nonpenetrating injury. The rules of management are thus simplified. All penetrating injuries are explored. Blunt renal injuries are treated by observation, and indications for surgery develop as the diagnostic procedures are performed sequentially or as complications during the hospital course or post-hospital course dictate the need for surgery. The diagnosis can be made in more than 80% of the cases by the excretory urogram.[3] Occasionally, satisfactory information is not achieved. In less than 3% of the cases, a severely contused kidney may fail to visualize at all, and yet no major vascular injury is present. Generally speaking, if even a dense nephrogram is present, the likelihood of the presence of a major reconstructible renal artery lesion is less than 5% (Fig. 6-3). If a delay in function is seen on one side, subsequent films may result in satisfactory visualization. If *no* nephrogram is present, immediate arteriography is indicated, and renal arterial intimal tear must be suspected (Fig. 6-4). Though the current salvage rate of these cases is less than satisfactory, we should not be dissuaded from attempts to make earlier diagnosis so that the patient may be taken to surgery promptly and some kidneys that would otherwise be destroyed by normothermic ischemia can be salvaged.[1]

Injuries caused by sudden deceleration, which are seen in patients involved in auto-pedestrian

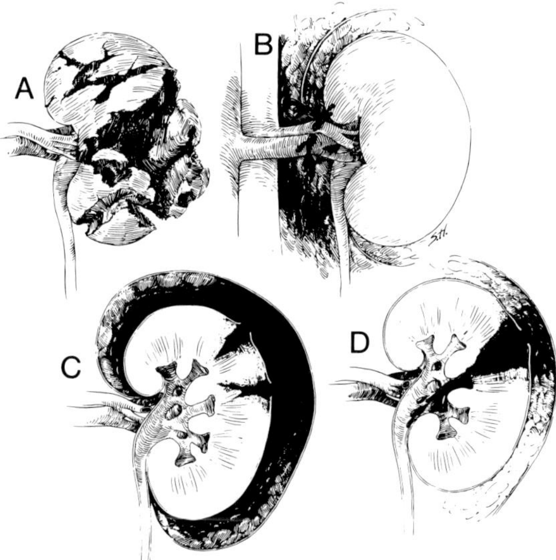

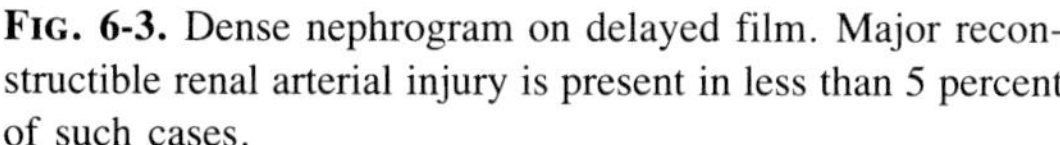

Fig. 6-2. Major renal injuries. *A,* Comminuted kidney; difficult to salvage. *B,* Pedicle tear is nonvisualizing by IVP; difficult to salvage. *C,* Perirenal hematoma with parenchymal tear. Postoperative hypertension a possibility. *D,* Major cortical laceration with gross hematoma; surgical intervention depends on condition of patient.

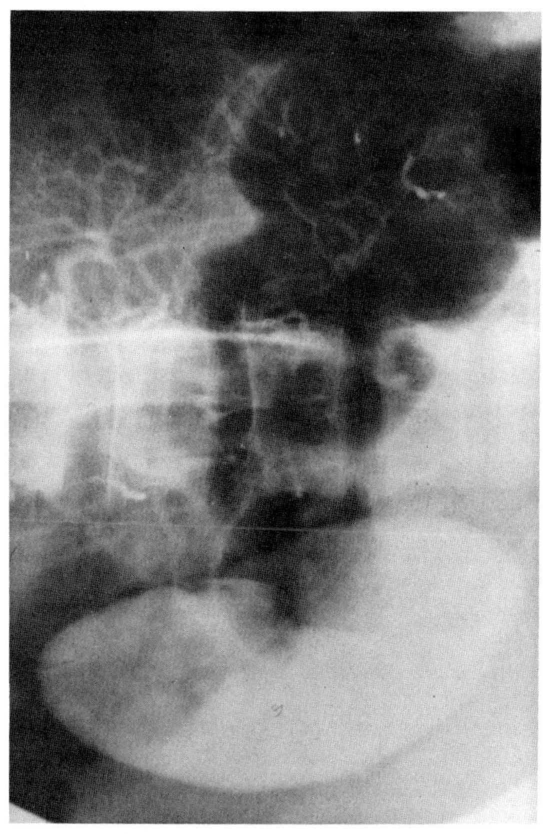

Fig. 6-3. Dense nephrogram on delayed film. Major reconstructible renal arterial injury is present in less than 5 percent of such cases.

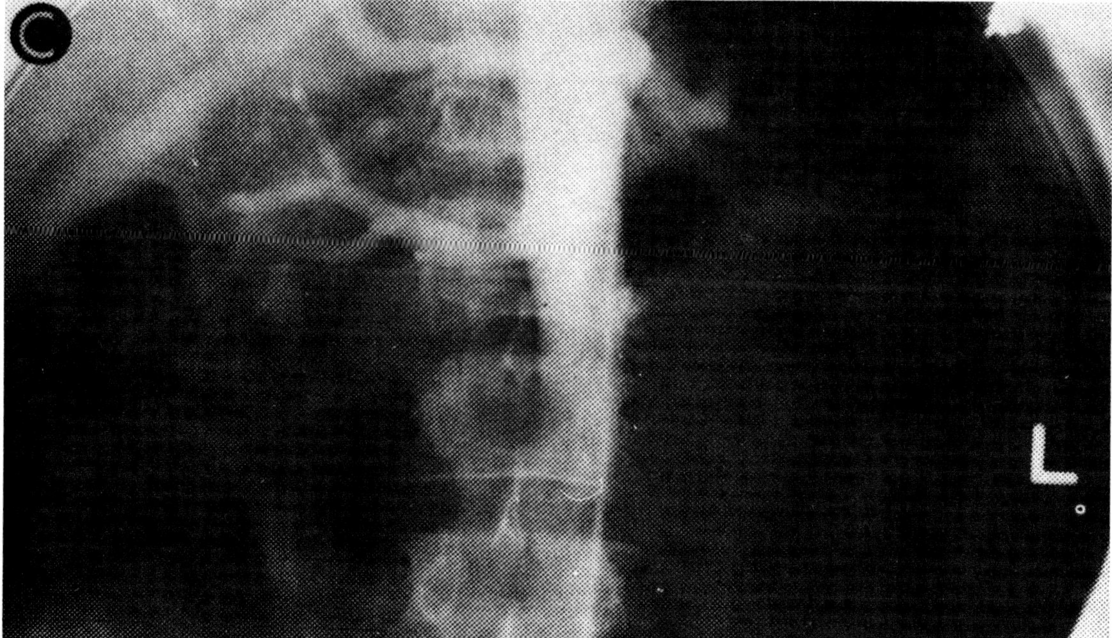

Fig. 6-4. Arteriography showing arterial intimal tear. (Reproduced with permission from Peters, P. C., and Bright, T. C., III: Management of trauma to the urinary tract. *In* Advances in Surgery. Vol. 10. Edited by Longmire, W. P. Jr., et al. Copyright © 1976 by Year Book Medical Publishers, Inc., Chicago.)

accidents or in patients who fell from a height, include arterial intimal tear and, in children particularly, ureteropelvic junction disruption. These injuries may be suspected by delayed function on the excretory urogram and, later, by the presence of extravasation of contrast material in the hilar area of the kidney. Extravasated contrast material appearing early (within 5 minutes) in the renal hilar area is apt to represent a major laceration of the collecting system, whereas a perirenal halo appearing about the convex border of the kidney or diffusely involving the renal fossa usually indicates a minor tear of the collecting system or parenchymal laceration on delayed films. The indication for surgery in such cases must be based on the clinical course of the patient and not on the mere presence of extravasation of urine.

Repair of injuries to the renal collecting system may be accomplished by establishing drainage proximal to the point of injury (nephrostomy or stent) and closing rents in the collecting system with running or interrupted, fine, chromic, gut sutures. Only absorbable sutures are used in repair of the kidney and ureter because of the subsequent danger of stone formation when nonabsorbable sutures are used. Renal injuries secondary to blunt external force that commonly require surgical intervention are complete polar ruptures, renal artery intimal tears, ureteropelvic junction disruptions, major parenchymal lacerations, and, rarely, major renal vein lacerations. Most other renal injuries may be treated by simple observation.

Operative Approach

When exploration of the kidney is indicated after major injury, the lesion is best approached through a transperitoneal midline incision to secure the renal artery first either by performing a medial displacement of the duodenum through the posterior parietal peritoneum on the right side (Kocher's operation) or by incising the parietal peritoneum medial to the inferior mesenteric vein and locating the left renal or right renal arteries at their juncture with the aorta. After the proximal artery is secured on either side with a noncrushing vascular clamp, the colon is reflected and the kidney inspected (Fig. 6-5). The inferior mesenteric vein may have to be divided on the left side to reach more quickly a level directly anterior to the left renal artery. This procedure may be done without concern for infarction of the intestine and allows the operator access to the left renal pedicle in a short period of time.

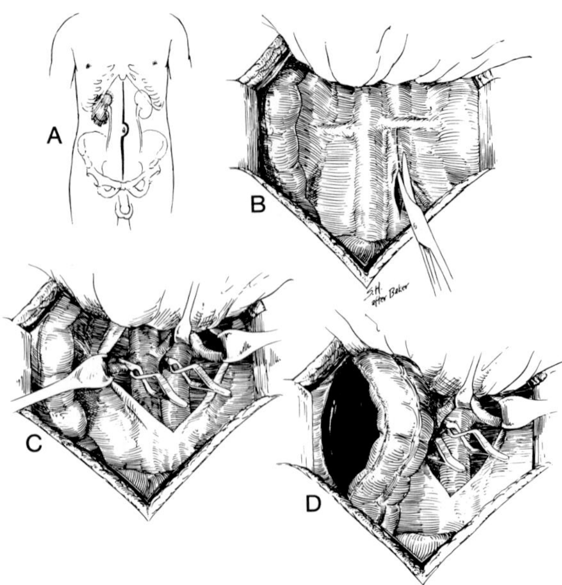

FIG. 6-5. Operative approach to renal pedicle. *A*, Midline xyphoid-to-pubic incision. *B*, Incision of posterior parietal peritoneum over aorta medial-to-inferior mesenteric vein. *C*, Vascular clamps on renal artery and vein. *D*, Reflection of colon to explore Gerota's fascia and enclosed hematoma.

Perirenal and subcapsular hematomas, though historically suspect because of their ability to contract and scar the kidney, thereby resulting in hypertension,[4] have rarely been the cause of subsequent hypertension in my experience. The injured kidney that is most apt to result in renovascular hypertension is the kidney that has sustained a major renal arterial injury (or even a major branch injury), has been repaired at the time of injury, and has subsequently scarred during the follow-up period. In a series of 100 patients reviewed by me, an incidence of hypertension occurred in 5% of the patients. Some incidences of hypertension did not become evident for more than 3 months after the initial injury. I recommend an observation period of 5 years at quarterly intervals following renal arterial trauma and repair. Such a follow-up period is necessary to document renovascular hypertension, though it has been reported as long as 16 years after injury.

The question of management of the patient with multiple organ system injuries is being clarified. Formerly, when simultaneous vascular, colon, and kidney injuries occurred, the urologist was often asked by surgical colleagues to remove the kidney or to assure that no ureteral leak would be present after vascular repair. Consequently, nephrectomy was often performed in borderline cases. Today, the problem is approached by ligation of the ureter and nephrostomy with secondary repair of the ureter at a later date even when associated colon and vascular injuries are present. Ureteral defects of up to 3 cm in size may be compensated for by direct end-to-end anastomosis with mobilization of the kidney above and the ureter and bladder below or by transureteroureterostomy.[5] Defects greater than 3 cm in size may be treated electively after healing of associated injuries by replacing the ureter with a tapered segment of ileum. The segment of ileum may be interposed at any point in the ureter and need not necessarily replace the ureteral defect throughout the length of the ureter.

Ureteral Injuries

Diagnosis

Ureteral injuries are often concomitant with kidney injuries.[2] The diagnosis is often suspected from extravasation on the excretory urogram. Confirmation may be obtained by retrograde pyelography, or if exploration is carried out within a short interval after the patient's admission (as in most cases of penetrating trauma), indigo carmine may be given intravenously and the course of the ureter inspected. The appearance of the blue contrast material outside the lumen of the ureter usually gives the operator a clue to the location of the defect in the collecting system. Patients most suspect of ureteral injuries have a penetrating missile injury in the area of the course of the ureter. Both ureters may need to be inspected if the penetrating missile is lying definitively on the side opposite its point of entry. Only one bilateral ureteral injury caused by a penetrating missile has been seen in 20 years at Parkland Memorial Hospital.

The ureter is seldom injured in blunt trauma patients because it is well protected by the vertebral column and body-wall muscles posteriorly and by the intestines and pelvis anteriorly. However, hyperextension injuries of the spine or deceleration injuries, particularly in children, may cause disruption at the ureteropelvic junction, and the ureter may be disrupted by violent external force to the lumbar spine, particularly when fractures of the transverse processes of multiple lumbar vertebrae are seen.[6]

Management

Ureteral injury, when diagnosed, is treated simply by proximal diversion and stenting. Injuries to the upper third of the ureter may be treated by nephrostomy and internal stent or by ureteropyelostomy and stent if disruptions are complete (Fig. 6-6). Injuries to the middle third are usually treated by direct ureteroureterostomy. An indwelling double-J stent from renal pelvis to bladder may be used, and a drain may be placed near the repair, which should be done with interrupted fine chromic gut sutures.[6] Injuries of the juxtavesical ureter are usually best treated by reimplantation of the ureter into the bladder, usually without stenting unless considerable edema is present. An indwelling stent then may be inserted. When a stent is necessary, I prefer to leave in a double-J stent from pelvis to bladder and to remove it endoscopically 10 days after the repair is made. If more than 6 cm of ureter are lost, an end-to-end ureteroureterostomy or reimplantation into the bladder may not be feasible. In such instances, it is best to ligate the ureter, perform a nephrostomy, and, later, substitute a loop of tapered ileum to replace all or part of the absent ureter. Transureteroureterostomy may be an alternative when sufficient length of proximal ureter remains, usually at least to the pelvic brim (iliac artery level).[5] In cases of major loss of ureteral length, one may simply ligate the ureter, insert a nephrostomy tube, and, after the inflammatory tissue reaction has subsided, substitute a loop of tapered ileum for any length of the ureter desired, thereby salvaging the kidney. Autotransplantation is recommended only in extreme cases

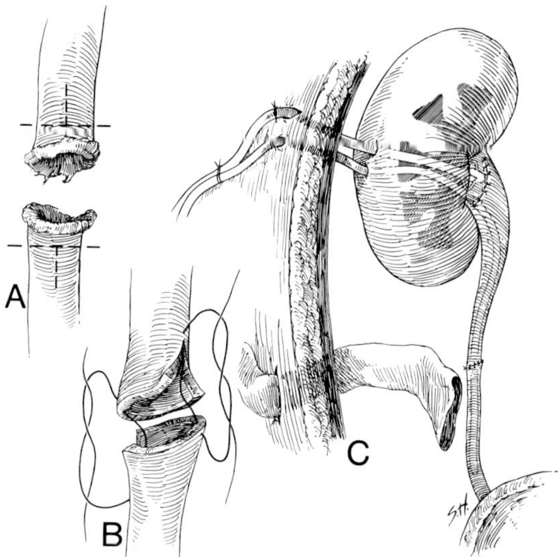

Fig. 6-6. *A* through *C*, Nephrostomy and stenting in ureteral injuries.

in which subsequent use of the ileum is not possible because of disease of the small bowel or because previous loss of an amount of small bowel that makes its further use impossible.

When a penetrating missile has injured the ureter, one must know whether the missile was of high or low velocity. High-velocity missiles are usually military weapons with a muzzle velocity of greater than 2200 ft/sec. Most civilian weapons, such as a .22-caliber or .38-caliber weapon, have a muzzle velocity of 700 to 850 ft/sec and do not cause the "blast" effect on the ureter caused by the high-velocity missiles.[7] The blast effect produces a coagulation necrosis of the ureter, and the extent of the injury is difficult to evaluate at the time of surgery, which is performed a few minutes or hours after the injury. At surgery, the ureter that bleeds freely should be cut back before it is reanastomosed (in the case of complete severance). Ureters that are only partially severed may be treated with indwelling stenting and drainage to the point of injury. Subsequent reconstruction is done only for ureters that fail to heal primarily. Fluorescein dye may be given intravenously, and the cut ureteral edge can be inspected with a Wood's (ultraviolet) filter, which may allow one to determine the viability of tissue (the viable tissue with an intact blood supply fluoresces). This procedure may be of some help in evaluating at the time of operative repair the viability of the ureter that was subject to the blast effect. Currently, there is a certain undeniable failure rate (19 to 54%) because of subsequent fistulization of a poorly vascularized ureter that appeared to be viable at the time of ureteroureterostomy.[6]

Ruptures of the Bladder

Diagnosis and Management

Bladder ruptures are usually classified as intraperitoneal or extraperitoneal. Usually, the patient with an intraperitoneal injury was riding in a motor vehicle, had a full bladder, sustained a violent blow to the lower abdomen, and presented with rather diffuse lower abdominal pain, sometimes well localized in the hypogastrium. A cystogram in patients with intraperitoneal rupture shows contrast material extravasating into the peritoneal cavity and often coming to rest in a subdiaphragmatic position (Fig. 6-7). At least 250 ml of contrast material must be put in the bladder of a patient undergoing cystography following a motor vehicle accident to be certain that the bladder is distended properly to disclose previous ruptures that may have been sealed off temporarily by contraction of the bladder musculature.

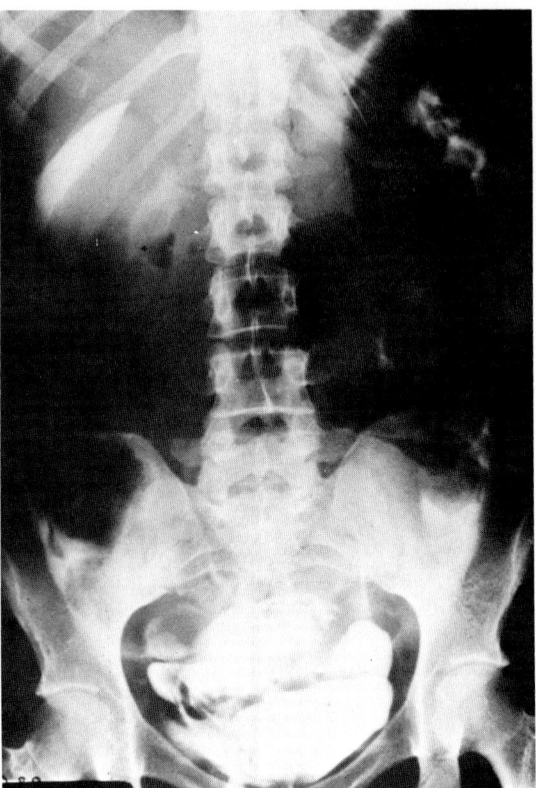

Fig. 6-7. Cystogram of intraperitoneal rupture. Note intrauterine contraceptive device, contrast material around loops of bowel above bladder, and subdiaphragmatic extent of contrast material.

The patient with an intraperitoneal bladder rupture often has sustained severe concomitant injuries. Rupture of the liver or laceration of the spleen is a common accompanying injury often associated with leukocytosis of greater than 20,000 mm^3. I advocate opening the peritoneal cavity for exploration in patients undergoing repair of intraperitoneal rupture of the bladder. The bladder lesion is best repaired by suprapubic drainage via a cystostomy tube brought out from a site separate from the laceration of the bladder, which invariably is found. The laceration should be repaired separately and closed in 3 layers with 5-zero chromic gut suture to the mucosa, 3-zero chromic gut suture to the muscle, and 3-zero chromic gut suture to the adventitia. The cystostomy tube is brought out through a separate stab wound in the bladder and is left in place until cystography shows that healing is complete. If the normal pathway for micturition is open, the fistula created by the placement of the cystostomy tube will close almost without exception in less than 8 hours, even if the tube has been in place for weeks.

Extraperitoneal ruptures of the bladder commonly are associated with pelvic fracture. The urologist is used to looking for the pelvic fracture and bone fragment displacement that have resulted in laceration of the bladder. The characteristic flame-shaped extravasation of the contrast material outside the bladder, which may have a tear-drop configuration because of the pelvic hematoma, is commonly seen (Fig. 6-8). The bladder silhouette nearly always descends to the level of the symphysis in contrast to that of patients who have rupture of the urethra superior to the urogenital diaphragm in whom the bladder may be seen full of contrast material "floating" high above the symphysis (Fig. 6-9). The orthopaedic surgeon, by contrast, finds that only 5 to 6% of patients with a fractured pelvis have a concomitant rupture of the urinary bladder.

Extraperitoneal rupture of the urinary bladder may be treated simply by the insertion of a urethral catheter, and simple catheter drainage is usually all that is necessary. In more severe cases, particularly in male patients, suprapubic cystostomy may be desirable to avoid the lower urinary tract complications (infection, stricture) of prolonged indwelling urethral catheter drainage. A suitable cystostomy in female patients may be done by inserting a perforated male urethral sound, cutting down suprapubically over the sound, tying the catheter to the sound, and pulling the catheter into the bladder. The Lowsley curved prostatic tractor may be used in lieu of the urethral sound, allowing one to do a cystostomy through an 8- or 9-mm suprapubic opening in male or female patients. Once again, the suprapubic tube may be used to instill contrast material for subsequent voiding studies needed to demonstrate the integrity of the urinary tract and voiding mechanisms. The suprapubic fistula closes

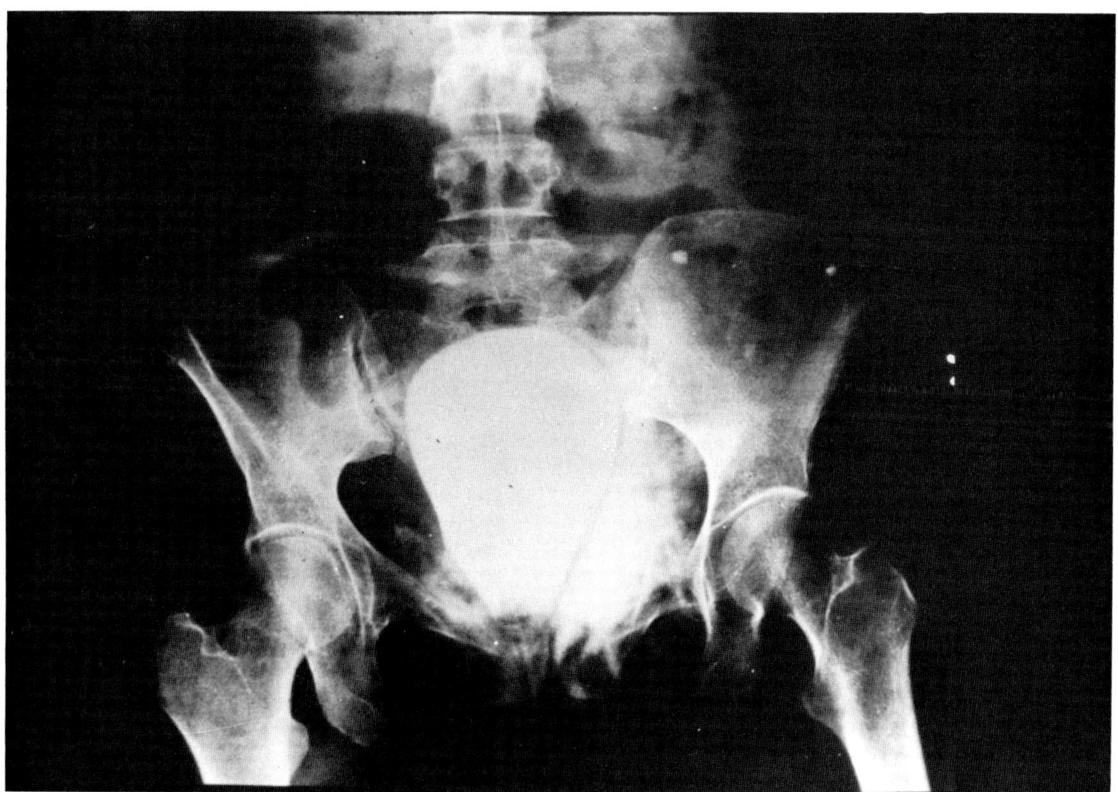

FIG. 6-8. Extraperitoneal rupture of the bladder. Note tear-drop configuration of bladder silhouette. Bladder shadow extends to symphysis.

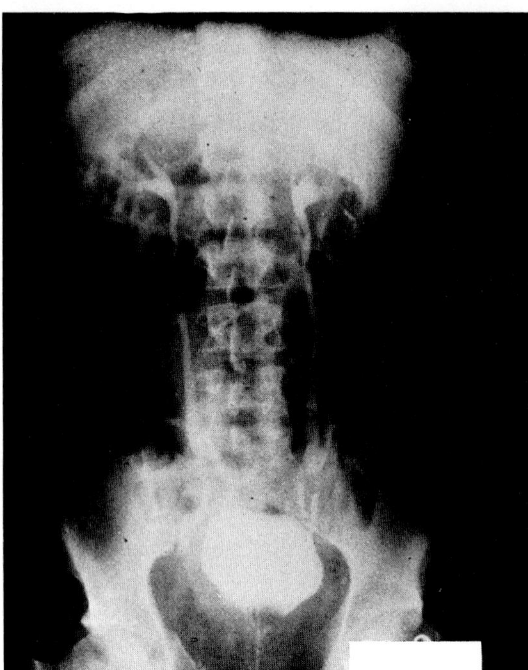

Fig. 6-9. Rupture of urethra superior to urogenital diaphragm.

promptly when the normal urinary tract integrity is re-established and healing is complete (usually within 10 to 14 days after injury). Except in cases of massive injury, extraperitoneal drainage is not necessary, though one may use local infiltrative anesthesia and make a simple stab wound into the extraperitoneal space just above the symphysis to place a Penrose drain in the extraperitoneal space, thereby further ensuring proper drainage. Usually, the suprapubic tube alone suffices, and the extraperitoneal drainage is not necessary. The extravasated urine is resorbed. When the pelvis is comminuted and permanently displaced bone fragments are seen, exploration through a suprapubic incision is indicated. Debridement and removal of bone fragments from the bladder and the establishment of suprapubic drainage through a 28F to 30F cystostomy tube are advocated.

Rupture of the Urethra

Classification and Diagnosis

Urethral ruptures are divided into those superior to and those inferior to the urogenital diaphragm. Urethral ruptures superior to the urogenital diaphragm are associated with severe injury. An enlarged bladder silhouette superior to the symphysis by 3 cm or more is commonly seen (see Fig. 6-9). In male patients, rectal examination discloses that the prostate is difficult to reach or palpate. In these cases, the prostate has been severed with the bladder just superior to the urogenital diaphragm. Often, the puboprostatic ligaments have been torn loose and perhaps 2 or 3 mm of urethra remain above the urogenital diaphragm. The bladder and prostate are displaced high in the pelvis by hematoma, and vesical neck competency prevents drainage of the urinary bladder.

Management of Ruptures Superior to the Urogenital Diaphragm

Unless there is severe comminution of the pelvis with bone fragments mechanically blocking the descent of the prostate, I and others have found that the bladder and prostate invariably descend to the urogenital diaphragm over a period of 2 to 3 months, and reconstruction of the urethra in these cases nearly always is possible with a low incidence of impotence, incontinence, or urethral stricture. Therefore, I advocate only the insertion of a suprapubic cystostomy tube at the time of injury. Unless unusual orthopaedic conditions indicate further exploration of the pelvis,[8] suprapubic cystostomy is the only urinary tract procedure performed at the time of injury.

Reconstruction of the urethra can be done rather simply by a perineal approach or, in selected cases, by a transpubic approach, as advocated by Allen[9] or Waterhouse and associates.[10,11] The incidence of impotence, incontinence, and stricture, the three major complications of this injury, has been markedly reduced in recent years by this initial cystotomy and delayed repair approach,[12] as contrasted with the older and, in my opinion, outmoded efforts to establish continuity at the time of the injury. Attempts to establish continuity over "kissing" sounds or by using indwelling catheters at the time of the injury have the disadvantages of disturbing the pelvic hematoma, converting what may have been a 2- or 3-unit blood loss into a 7- or 8-unit blood loss, taxing the blood-bank facilities of many community hospitals, increasing the risk of hepatitis because of the need for multiple transfusions, and resulting in a much higher incidence of stricture, incontinence, and impotence. The urethral rupture in such cases is usually complete.[13] Many of these injuries, which were, by history, incomplete, were completed by inexperienced operators attempting to manipulate the urethra from below by inserting catheters or sounds. The urethra is best left undisturbed at the time of injury.[13] Simple suprapubic drainage is instituted initially, and subsequent reconstruction is necessary in more than 90% of the cases after a suitable interval for healing, usually not less than 3 months (Fig. 6-10). There are rare exceptions to this approach. Patients with badly comminuted fractures of the pelvis in which bone fragments obviously will impede the descent of the prostate may be treated initially by cystotomy and then by delayed exploration after an interval of 3 to 7 days when the patient's condition is stabilized and facilities for blood fluid replacement are readily available.[8] The best practice to follow at the time of injury is insertion of the suprapubic tube and anticipation of the definitive repair. Rare exceptions do occur, but in 66 injuries handled by Morehouse and MacKinnon, 61 were complete ruptures and reconstruction was necessary after a suitable period of time.[13] Occasionally, in infants with a badly damaged urethra, the injury may be treated simply by sewing the bladder to the abdominal wall, i.e., vesicostomy. This procedure allows for the diversion of the urine in an infant who most likely is still in diapers and allows definitive repair after a suitable interval. In those rare fortunate individuals in whom the lesion is incomplete, the urethra may heal spontaneously, and no surgery other than closure of the vesicostomy is required.[14]

Diagnosis and Management of Ruptures Inferior to the Urogenital Diaphragm

In recent times there has been a marked reversal of the trend for location of ruptures of the urethra. Formerly, 85% were superior to the urogenital diaphragm. In a recent series of 55 ruptures treated at our institution, 40 were found to be inferior to the urogenital diaphragm.[14] Injury to the urethra that occurs inferior to the urogenital diaphragm may be in association with pelvic fracture, but is more commonly associated with straddle injuries. Some are caused by penetrating missiles.

The injury can usually be diagnosed by history of a blow to the perineum or a straddle injury. At times, a drop of blood that has been propelled by a spasm of the bulbocavernosus muscle at the moment of injury may appear at the urethral meatus. Such injuries occur from a kick or blow to the perineum, from a fall while astride a motorcycle or bicycle, or as a result of deviant sexual practices. The diagnosis is confirmed by urethrography with 20 ml of IV contrast material injected through a syringe placed at the urethral meatus.[2] Cystoscopy and inspection of the urethra are indicated in cases subjected to immediate repair.

The rupture of the urethra may be confined by Buck's fascia, in which case it appears essentially as a sleeve of the penis (Fig. 6-11). At other times, when Buck's fascia has been ruptured, the lesion is then contained by Colles' fascia, the at-

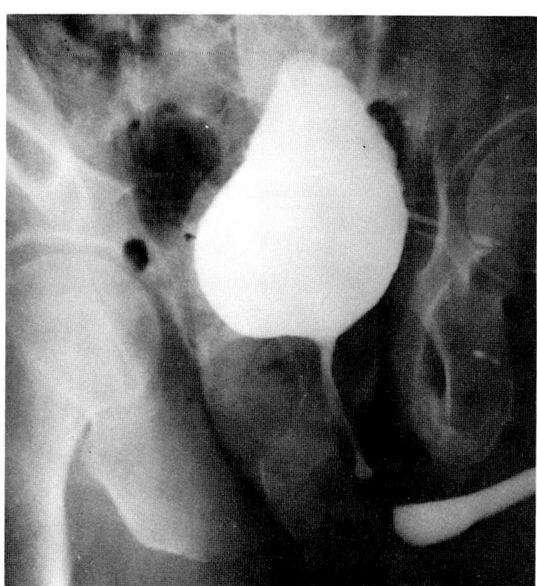

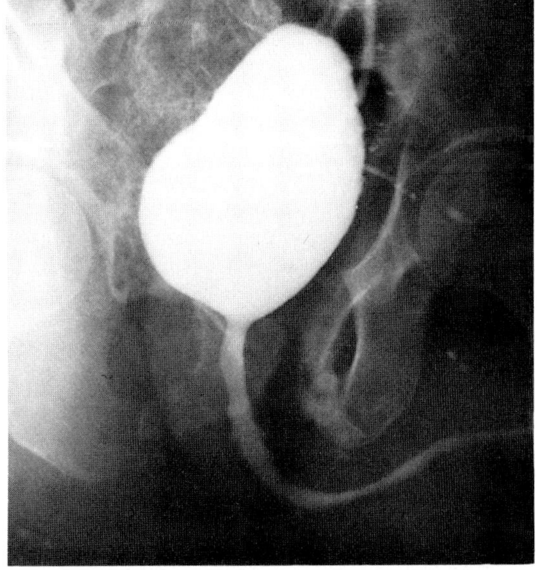

Fig. 6-10. *A,* Combined cystogram and urethrogram of urethra ready for repair at 3 months. *B,* Postoperative result—no stricture, no incontinence, no impotence.

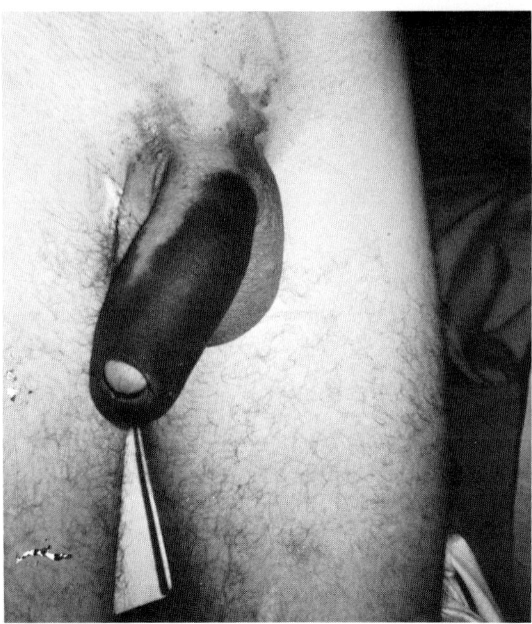

FIG. 6-11. Rupture of urethra confined by Buck's fascia, essentially a sleeve of the penis.

tachments of which are to the fascia lata in the thigh and coracoclavicular fascia in the axillae (Fig. 6-12). By following the fascial planes, extravasations of blood or urine from the urogenital diaphragm may reach the axilla. Posterior extent of these extravasations of blood and urine is confined by the attachment of Colles' fascia to the inferior layer of the urogenital diaphragm.

Immediate repair of the lacerated urethra inferior to the urogenital diaphragm may be accomplished, depending on the extent of the injury. With severe contamination, cystostomy is the treatment of choice, and delayed repair of strictures resulting from healing is carried out after a time interval of 3 months or greater. Penetrating-missile injuries that cause large tissue defects may be treated by producing a preliminary urethrostomy in the area of trauma with secondary repair by one of the methods of reconstruction of the urethra. Currently, staged delayed pedicle flaps and patch grafts are among the most popular methods of repair.[15,16] Initially, the only necessary steps of repair are establishment of drainage of urine and preparation of the tissues for any definitive repair that may be necessary, essentially by producing a urethrostomy in patients in whom primary closure is not possible.

Spatulated, elliptic anastomosis of the urethra using absorbable suture has been advocated by Zinman, et al., who report a favorable experience with this method of repair.[17] Repair may be accomplished at the time of injury without difficulty. An indwelling, stenting, Silastic catheter is usually left in place for 14 to 21 days following the injury to drain the urine satisfactorily. When contaminated wounds are present or maceration of tissues prevents adequate evaluation at the time of injury, cystostomy with subsequent debridement and closure is the preferred method of treatment.

Genital Injuries

Diagnosis and Management

Genital injuries are best classified as penetrating or nonpenetrating. Once again, all penetrating injuries are explored. In injuries to the testis, the testis must be debrided and the tunica albuginea of the testis closed primarily. Drains should not be inserted beneath the tunica albuginea of the testis because they provide an avenue of escape for the seminiferous tubules. Careful debridement of all bits of clothing, gun wadding, and foreign bodies is accomplished. The tunica albuginea then is closed primarily with fine chromic gut suture. A Penrose drain may be placed in the scrotum, but drainage inside the tunica albuginea should not be done.[6] Every attempt should be made to salvage a testis that is demonstrated to have a blood supply, either by bleeding when biopsied at surgery or by the preoperative demonstration of intact blood supply by ^{99m}technetium scanning. ^{99m}Technetium scanning is particularly valuable in the patient with the blunt testis injury. It has been more reliable than the Doppler auscultation in my experience and is recommended for use by the trauma surgeon in assessing the magnitude of injury.

A rupture of the testis may be diagnosed and repaired immediately with anticipation of salvaging at least a portion of the testis. In a series of 30 patients with severe blunt scrotal injury, reported in a personal communication by Waterhouse, 12 patients were found to have a ruptured testis at the time of surgery. Three of these cases could have been diagnosed by the use of the ^{99m}technetium scan. (The gamma camera is finding an increasing use in our emergency room in the evaluation of the trauma patient.)

When managing individuals who have sustained massive injuries with a large amount of tissue loss to the genitalia and perineum, the prin-

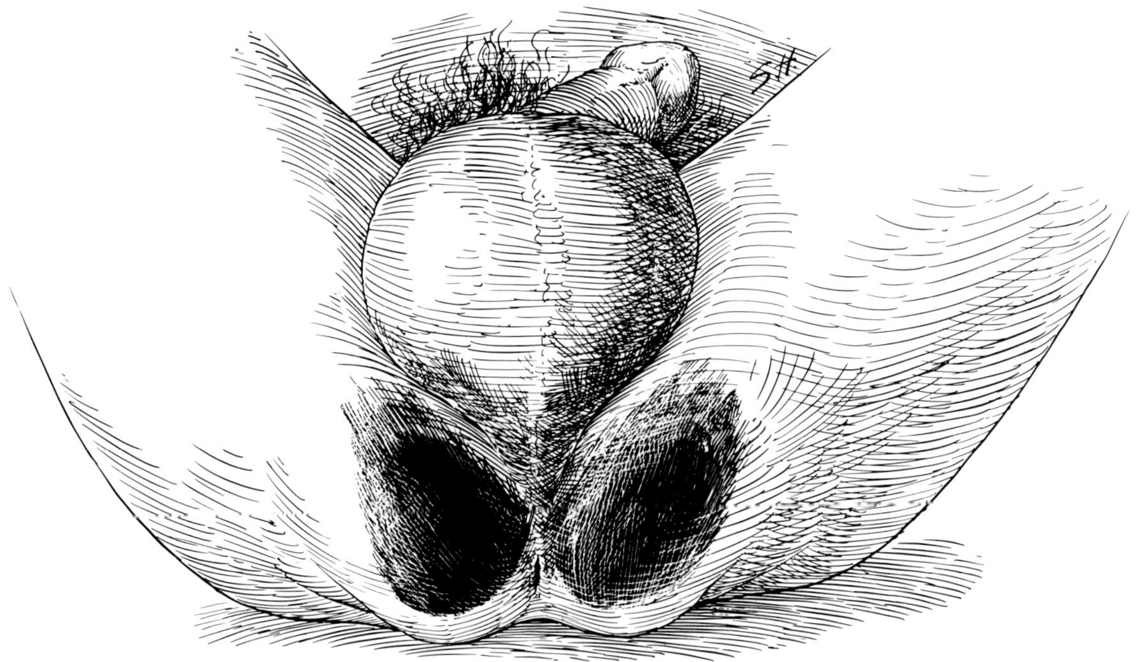

Fig. 6-12. Rupture of urethra confined by Colles' fascia and through Buck's fascia. Note edema and discoloration of scrotum.

ciple once again is to establish proper drainage of the urine. This may be accomplished by cystostomy, or, occasionally, in individuals suffering massive loss of the urethra, a simple perineal urethrostomy can be carried out. The catheter can be inserted directly through the perineal urethra, which has been explosed in such cases into the urinary bladder.

Every attempt should be made to salvage viable-appearing scrotal skin and urethral tissue in such cases. A simple insertion of a Silastic catheter through the perineum into the bladder and the gathering of viable tissues in a "catch as catch can" manner often result in a remarkable cosmetic result.[8] Delayed reconstructive procedures may be carried out at an appropriate time and usually are much less extensive than originally anticipated when the patient was initially seen. Testes that need to be covered when the scrotum has been completely destroyed may be placed in the superficial thigh, where the temperature has been shown by Culp, et al., to be at least 10° less than that of the subcutaneous abdominal wall, a temperature markedly favoring spermatogenesis.[18] Testes may subsequently be placed in the reconstructed scrotum. Even if small bits of scrotum remain, remarkable powers of regeneration of this vascularized tissue have been demonstrated, and the testes may then be inserted back into a regenerated scrotal pouch.

The scrotum is a versatile pedicle flap and can be used for replacing large tissue defects created on the lower anterior abdominal wall and perineum in massive injury cases. One must be careful to remove all tissue to the hair follicles on the undersurface of the scrotum so that the scrotum does not attempt to reconstitute itself when it must lie flat as a pedicle graft for replacement of skin of the anterior abdominal wall or perineum. Scrotal lacerations are best repaired by suture with absorbable material, i.e., chromic catgut, being sure to catch the tunica dartos during closure (whether one or two layers) to minimize chances for postoperative hematoma.

References

1. Bartsch, G., et al.: Successful renal revascularization of unilateral traumatic renal artery thrombosis. J. Urol., *124*:115, 1980.
2. Carlton, C. E., Jr.: Injuries of the kidney and ureter. *In* Campbell's Urology. Vol. 1. Philadelphia, W. B. Saunders, 1978.
3. Peters, P. C., and Bright, T. C.: Management of trauma to the urinary tract. *In* Advances in Surgery. Vol. 10. Edited by W. P. Longmire, Jr. Chicago, Year Book Medical Publishers, 1976.

4. Page, I. H.: The production of persistent arterial hypertension by cellophane perinephritis. J.A.M.A., *113*:2046, 1939.
5. Hodges, C. V., Moore, R. V., Lehman, T. H., and Behnam, A. M.: Clinical experiences with transuretero-ureterostomy. J. Urol., *90*:552, 1963.
6. Bright, T. C., and Peters, P. C.: Ureteral injuries due to external violence: 10 years' experience with 59 cases. J. Trauma, *17*:616, 1977.
7. Demuth, W. E., Jr.: Bullet velocity and design as determinates of wounding capability: an experimental study. J. Trauma, *6*:222, 1966.
8. Turner-Warwick, R.: A personal view of the immediate management of pelvic fracture urethral injuries. Urol. Clin. North Am., *4*:81, 1977.
9. Allen, T. D.: The transpubic approach for strictures of the posterior urethra superior to the urogenital diaphragm. Urol. Clin. North Am., *4*:95, 1977.
10. Waterhouse, K.: Transpubic repair of membranous urethral strictures. Urol. Clin. North Am., *4*:105, 1977.
11. Waterhouse, K., et. al.: The transpubic repair of membranous urethral strictures. J. Urol., *111*:188, 1974.
12. Morehouse, D. D., Belitsky, P., and MacKinnon, K. J.: Rupture of posterior urethra. J. Urol., *107*:255, 1972.
13. Morehouse, D. D., and MacKinnon, K. J.: Posterior urethral injury: etiology, diagnosis, initial management. Urol. Clin. North Am., *4*:69, 1977.
14. Bright, T. C., and Peters, P. C.: Bladder and urethra injuries. *In* Campbell's Urology. Vol. 1. Philadelphia, W. B. Saunders, 1978.
15. Devine, C. J., Jr., Devine, P. C., and Horton, C. E.: Anterior urethral injury: etiology, diagnosis, and initial management. Urol. Clin. North Am., *4*:125, 1977.
16. Devine, C. J , Jr., Devine, P. C., and Horton, C. E.: Secondary reconstruction. Urol. Clin. North Am., *4*:157, 1977.
17. Zinman, L., and Libertino, J.: *In* Reconstructive Urologic Surgery: Pediatric and Adult. Edited by J. Libertino and L. Zinman. Baltimore, Williams & Wilkins, 1977.
18. Culp, D. A., and Huffman, W. C.: Temperature determination in the thigh with regard to burying the traumatically exposed testis. J. Urol., *76*:436, 1956.

Chapter 7 The Fat Embolism Syndrome

C. MCCOLLISTER EVARTS

The occurrence of the fat embolism syndrome as a complication of skeletal and soft-tissue trauma has been of interest for more than a century.[1] With the increase in the incidence of severe musculoskeletal trauma, the multiply injured patient with several fractures may present with an acute respiratory distress syndrome associated with fat embolism. Fat embolism is an important cause of the acute respiratory distress syndrome.[2] Fat embolism produces a clinical syndrome with characteristic findings and pertinent laboratory results. Recent advances in treatment of fat embolism syndrome have contributed to a decrease in morbidity and mortality.[3]

Bagg, et al.,[4] have defined the fat embolism syndrome as "a post-traumatic respiratory distress syndrome occurring within 72 hours of skeletal trauma. The earliest manifestations are an elevation of pulse, temperature of above 100° F, and a falling Pa_{O_2}. The characteristic lung scan confirms the diagnosis."

Historical Aspects

In 1862, Zenker described fat droplets in the lung capillaries of a railroad worker who had sustained a fatal thoracoabdominal injury.[5] In 1865, Wagner described the pathologic features of fat embolism.[6] In 1879, Scriba reviewed and correlated the clinical, pathologic, and experimental observations of fat embolism syndrome.[7] In 1916, Gauss postulated a mechanical origin for embolic fat,[8] and in 1927, Lehman and Moore discussed the physiochemical origin of the fat droplets.[3] In 1964, Sproule and co-authors were the first to report the severe arterial hypoxemia associated with the fat embolism syndrome.[9] In 1966, Ashbaugh and Petty described the use of corticosteroids in the treatment of respiratory failure associated with fat embolism,[10] and in 1973, Beck and Collins published a major review of the theoretic and clinical aspects of the post-traumatic fat embolism syndrome.[11]

Incidence

Clinical signs and symptoms associated with the fat embolism syndrome have been observed in 10 to 15% of patients who sustain long bone fractures. The incidence may be slightly higher in patients with multiple fractures including pelvic injuries. The data necessary to define the exact incidence of this syndrome are difficult to accumulate. The incidence of fat embolism after intramedullary reaming and nailing of long bone fractures is low.[12] Fat embolism also has been reported following fractures of the hip treated with hemiarthroplasty.[13] In a controlled series of 854 patients with fractured hips, the frequency of fat embolism was 4 to 7% among subjects treated without operation.[14] Fat embolism has been reported following total hip and knee replacement.[15] Fuschsig reported a 5.5% mortality directly related to fat embolism syndrome in 5265 deaths among 263,861 trauma patients over a 10-year period.[16] In another study, a mortality rate of 15% occurred in 65 patients with proven fat embolism syndrome.[17] It has been estimated that more than 5000 deaths per year are directly caused by the fat embolism syndrome.

Pathogenesis

The pathogenesis of the fat embolism syndrome continues to be the subject of conjecture and controversy. The source of embolic fat is thought by some to be the bone marrow.[18] Bone marrow fragments have been demonstrated in lung sections, indicating that mechanical fat embolism does, indeed, occur. Also, intravascular fat globules and free fatty acids have been demonstrated following skeletal trauma.[19,20]

However, there is also evidence that the fat embolism syndrome can occur via other mechanisms in the absence of skeletal trauma.[21] The physiochemical theory of fat embolism postulates that changes in the lipid stability occur after trauma that alters the microcirculatory flow patterns, thereby resulting in inadequate tissue perfusion, subsequent tissue hypoxia, and the fat embolism syndrome.[22,23] The exact source of embolic fat is not known; however, more than one possibility exists for the source of the embolic fat, and the causes are not mutually exclusive.

Clinical Manifestations

It is well to distinguish between the clinical entity, the fat embolism syndrome, as the cause of acute respiratory insufficiency and the presence of intravascular fat emboli, which have been described in a variety of conditions including pancreatitis, osteomyelitis, diabetes, burns, and prolonged steroid therapy. Thus, although fat emboli may be manifest in the lungs and other organs at autopsy, this finding does not mean that the patient necessarily had the fat embolism syndrome.

The importance of the early diagnosis of the fat embolism syndrome must be emphasized, especially since prompt respiratory management often can affect the ultimate outcome of acute respiratory distress. The signs and symptoms of the fat embolism syndrome in association with musculoskeletal trauma are predominantly those of the adult respiratory distress syndrome. Therefore, a history of trauma with multiple fractures of long bones, coupled with hypovolemic shock and the early development of respiratory distress, should alert the physician to the possible onset of fat embolism syndrome.

In one prospective study of patients admitted to a trauma unit with fractures of the pelvis, femur, and tibia, the criteria of an elevated pulse and marked elevation in temperature above 100° F provided identification of all cases.[4] By using these criteria, no cases of fat embolism syndrome can be missed. The earliest signs to occur are elevations in pulse and temperature. Tachypnea, with a respiratory rate of 30 or higher, is one of the earlier signs and may often be followed by the onset of dyspnea, which may be marked and accompanied by cyanosis.

Additional clinical signs involve changes in the mental state, including drowsiness, restlessness, confusion, and, occasionally, an obstreperous behavioral pattern. These are not the earliest signs of fat embolism syndrome, but rather reflect the hypoxic nature of the syndrome. In addition, petechiae may occur across the root of the neck, in the axilla, and in the conjunctiva on the second or third day following the onset of the fat embolism syndrome. The petechiae can be noted in the conjunctiva and are sharp, distinct, and observed by looking at the eyelids. Also, retinal lesions can be identified by funduscopic examination and appear as microinfarcts at the ends of retinal arterioles.[24] Approximately 50% of patients with fat embolism syndrome demonstrate petechiae, but they may be transient and fleeting in nature. (Note that the petechiae of fat emboli differ in site from that of the petechiae seen in patients with subacute bacterial endocarditis.) The neurologic examination in the patient with the fat embolism syndrome may show pathologic reflexes that disappear or change rapidly.

The signs and symptoms of fat embolism syndrome are present in 60% of the patients within 24 hours following trauma and in 85% of the patients within 48 hours. The temporal delay is thought to be secondary to the evolving effects of the fat within the lung fields and the onset of hypoxemia with subsequent hypoxia.

The major pathophysiologic feature of the fat embolism syndrome is respiratory failure. The pulmonary involvement that accompanies this syndrome features a loss of lung surfactant; small-vessel perfusion is hindered, endothelial damage occurs within the pulmonary capillary beds, and ventilation perfusion mismatches occur, resulting in vascular congestion, interstitial hemorrhage, severe alveolar wall damage, and airway collapse.[25]

Laboratory Findings

Arterial hypoxemia is the hallmark of the fat embolism syndrome and should be observed immediately following trauma. Measurement of the arterial blood bases (Pa_{O_2}, PCO_2, and PA_{O_2} values) is critical to the diagnosis and management of fat embolism syndrome. Serial determinations of arterial blood gases identify the severity of the emerging acute respiratory distress syndrome. Arterial Pa_{O_2} values of less than 60 mm Hg are regarded as significant and indicate the presence of hypoxemia. In addition, serial chest roentgenograms may reveal the presence of fluffy exudates within the lung fields. A dense pulmonary infiltrate may develop in both lung fields and may be confused with pulmonary edema. The changes in the chest roetgenograms are characteristic but not specific.

Other laboratory findings that aid in the diagnosis of the fat embolism syndrome are serial measurements of the hematocrit levels. A decrease in the hematocrit value has been observed in association with the fat embolism syndrome. Thrombocytopenia may occur with platelet values of less than 150,000 mm.

Electrocardiographic changes may occur with the demonstration of prominent S-waves, arrhythmias, inversion of T-waves, and right bundle branch blocks. These changes are not specific. Measurement of the intravascular fat droplets by a cryostat frozen section is of help in the identification of the fat embolism syndrome.[26] Another specific test is the lung scan, which reveals the presence of widespread embolic phenomena within the lungs.[24]

The diagnosis of fat embolism syndrome is best made after analysis of the history, clinical manifestations, and laboratory findings. An essential asset when making an early diagnosis is a high index of suspicion. The critical laboratory finding is a low Pa_{O_2}, indicating the presence of the arterial hypoxemia.

Treatment

Many different forms of therapy have been suggested for patients with the fat embolism syndrome.[1,27-29] The various modes of therapy are derived from studies that are anecdotal and without controls. The many theories regarding the pathogenesis of the fat embolism syndrome have resulted in a multitude of therapeutic suggestions.

Certain general and specific measures, however, should be utilized in the treatment of the fat embolism syndrome. Initially, the patient who has sustained multiple injury must have an open and functioning airway, blood volume must be restored, and fluid and electrolyte balance maintained. Initial treatment of fractures should consist of splinting, and unnecessary transportation should be avoided.

The specific measures for the management of the fat embolism syndrome involve the early recognition and treatment of the impending respiratory failure. First, the hypoxemia should be decreased by the administration of oxygen by face mask or nasal tubing. If respiratory distress increases, as determined by serial Pa_{O_2} values, one should not hesitate to utilize endotracheal intubation and provide ventilatory assistance. The management of the respiratory complications has improved with the use of volume ventilations and positive end-expiratory pressures. Tracheostomy rarely has to be performed in the patient with fat embolism syndrome. Usually (within 2 to 3 days), the patient starts to improve and can be removed from the volume cycled ventilator.

Although few prospective studies exist, there is strong anecdotal and clinical evidence that the administration of methylprednisolone (30 mg/kg body weight every 6 hours) decreases the respiratory distress.[30] Rokkanen, et al.,[31] suggest the administration of steroids to multiply injured patients (prednisone 10 mg/kg body weight every 8 hours) beginning in the emergency room. Stoltenberg and Gustilo randomized the treatment of 64 patients with isolated lower extremity fractures and showed that the steroid-treated group did not have clinical evidence of the fat embolism syndrome.[32] Arterial oxygenation was improved in the patients with fat embolism in the control group. The steroid-mediated improvement in oxygenation is felt to be due to a decreased inflammatory response in the lungs. Capillary endothelium may be protected and vascular integrity preserved along with the stabilization of the lysosomal membrane granulocytes.

Low-molecular-weight dextran has been given to patients with the fat embolism syndrome primarily because of its role as an improver of microcirculatory flow. In the first 24-hour period following trauma, 500 ml of low-molecular-weight dextran has been given by slow intravenous infusion. Others have suggested the use of low-dose heparin primarily as a chylolytic agent rather than an anticoagulant. The suggested dose has been 1000 IU every 8 hours intravenously.[28]

The fat embolism syndrome as a variant of adult respiratory distress syndrome is a frequent complication in the multiply injured patient. This syndrome has characteristic clinical manifestations and pertinent laboratory findings. Modern techniques in the management of respiratory distress have led to a decrease in mortality and morbidity. Recent clinical research suggests that steroid administration may aid in the treatment of the fat embolism syndrome.[34]

References

1. Sevitt, S.: Fat Embolism. London, Butterworth, 1962.
2. Blaisdell, F. W., and Lewis, F. R.: Respiratory distress syndrome of shock and trauma. *In* Major Problems in Clinical Surgery. Vol. 21. Philadelphia, W. B. Saunders, 1977.
3. Lehman, E. P., and Moore, R. M.: Fat embolism; including experimental production without trauma. Arch. Surg., *14*:621, 1927.
4. Bagg, R. J., Stein, S., Urban, R. T., and McKay, D.: Parameters of the fat emboli syndrome (F.E.S.). Orthopaedic Transactions, *3*(#3):278,1979.
5. Zenker, F. A.: Beitrage zur Anatomie und Physiologie der Lunge. Dresden, J. Braunsdorf, 1861.
6. Wagner, E.: Die Fettembolie der Lungencapillaren. Arch. Heilk., *6*:369, 1865.
7. Scriba, J.: Untersuchungen uber die Fettembolie. Leipzig, J. B. Hirschfeld, 1879.
8. Gauss, H.: Studies in cerebral fat embolism: with reference to the pathology of delirium and coma. Arch. Intern. Med., *18*:76, 1916.
9. Sproule, B. J., Brady, J. L., and Gilbert, J. A. L.: Studies on the syndrome of fat embolization. Can. Med. Assoc. J., *90*:1243, 1964.
10. Ashbaugh, D. G., and Petty, T. L.: The use of corticosteroids in the treatment of respiratory failure associated with massive fat embolism. Surg. Gynecol. Obstet., *123*:493, 1966.
11. Beck, J. P., and Collins, J. A.: Theoretical and Clinical Aspects of Posttraumatic Fat Embolism Syndrome. A.A.O.S. Instructional Course Lectures. Vol. 22. St. Louis, C. V. Mosby, 1973.
12. Weisz, G. M.: Fat Embolism: Current Problems in Surgery. Chicago, Year Book Medical Publishing, 1974.
13. Gresham, G. A., Kuxzynski, A., and Rosborough, D.: Fatal fat embolism following replacement in arthroplasty for transcervical fractures of femur. Br. Med. J., *2*:617, 1971.
14. Sevitt, S.: Fat embolism in patients with fractured hips. Br. Med. J., *2*:257, 1972.
15. Lanchiewicz, P. F., and Ranawat, C. S.: Fat embolism syndrome following bilaterial total knee replacement with total condylar prosthesis: a report of two cases. Clin. Orthop., *160*:106, 1981.
16. Fuschsig, P., Brucke, P., Blumel, G., and Gottlob, R.: A new clinical and experimental concept on fat metabolsim. N. Engl. J. Med., *276*:1192, 1967.
17. Peltier, L. F.: An appraisal of the problem of fat embolism. Inst. Obst. Surg., *104*:313, 1957.
18. Gauss, H.: The pathology of fat embolism. Arch. Surg., *9*:593, 605, 1924.
19. Armin, J., and Grant, R. T.: Observations on gross pulmonary fat embolism in man and the rabbit. Clin. Sci., *10*:441, 1951.
20. Jacobs, R. R., et al.: Fat embolism: a microscopic and ultrastructure evaluation of two animal models. J. Trauma, *13*:980, 1973.
21. Bergentz, S. E.: Studies on the genesis of posttraumatic fat embolism. Acta Chir. Scand. [Suppl.], *282*:1, 1961.
22. LeQuire, V. S., et al.: A study of the pathogenesis of fat embolism based on human necropsy material and animal experiments. Am. J. Pathol., *35*:999, 1959.
23. LeQuire, V. S., Hillman, J. W., Gray, M. E., and Snowden, R. T.: Clinical and pathologic studies of fat embolism. A.A.O.S. Instructional Course Lectures, *19*:12, 1970.
24. Kearns, T. P.: Fat embolism of the retina; demonstrated by flat retinal preparation. Am. J. Ophthalmol., *41*:1, 1956.
25. Greenfield, L. J., Barkett, M., and Coalson, J. J.: The role of surfactant in the pulmonary response to trauma. J. Trauma, *8*:735, 1968.
26. Gurd, A. R.: Fat embolism: An aid to diagnosis. J. Bone Joint Surg., *52B*:732, 1970.
27. Bivins, B. A., Madauss, W. C., and Griffen, W. O., Jr.: Fat embolism syndrome: a clinical study. South. Med. J., *65*:937, 1972.
28. Evarts, C. M.: The fat embolism syndrome: a review. Surg. Clin. North Am., *50*:493, 1970.
29. Peltier, L. F.: The diagnosis and treatment of fat embolism. J. Trauma, *11*:661, 1971.
30. Alho, A., et al.: Corticosteroids in patients with a high risk of fat embolism syndrome. Surg. Gynecol. Obstet., *147*:358, 1978.
31. Rokkanen, P., et al.: The efficacy of corticosteroids in severe trauma. Surg. Gynecol. Obstet., *138*:69, 1974.
32. Stoltenberg, J. J., and Gustilo, R. M.: The use of methylprednisolone and hypertonic glucose in the prophylaxis of fat embolism syndrome. Clin. Orthop., *143*:211, 1979.
33. Evarts, C. M.: Low-molecular-weight dextran. Med. Clin. North Am., *51*:1285, 1967.
34. Gossling, H. R., and Pellegrini, V. D., Jr.: Posttraumatic Fat Embolus: A Conceptual and Clinical Review. (In Publication) 1982.

Chapter 8 Recognition and Treatment of Compartment Syndromes

SCOTT J. MUBARAK

The skeletal muscles of the extremities are grouped into compartments enclosed by a relatively noncompliant osteofascial envelope. A buildup of fluid within the muscle compartment is not easily dissipated, owing to the inelastic nature of the surrounding fascia. A compartment syndrome is a condition in which the high pressure within a closed muscle compartment compromises the circulation to the nerves and muscles within the involved compartment. If the pressure remains sufficiently high for several hours, permanent damage to the indwelling muscles and nerves can result. With severe involvement, a Volkmann's ischemic contracture of the limb may occur. To prevent the myoneural ischemia and injury produced by a compartment syndrome, the physician must make a prompt diagnosis and decompression of the compartments must be performed (Fig. 8-1).

The compartments of the leg and forearm are involved most frequently, but compartment syndromes in the shoulder, arm, hand, buttocks, thigh, and foot also occur. This chapter will deal with the more frequent causes of compartment syndromes in the forearm and leg only.

Diagnosis

To arrive at an early diagnosis and treatment of this entity, the physician must have a sound knowledge of the following subjects as they relate to the compartment syndrome: the most frequent causes, the anatomy of the limbs, the clinical findings, the laboratory investigations that aid the diagnosis, and the differential diagnosis.

Causes

In 1976, Sheridan and Matsen reported on 44 compartment syndromes in which the 3 most common causes were fractures, soft-tissue injury, and post-ischemic injury.[1] The primary causes in our experience are identical (Fig. 8-2).[2]

Fracture. In our prospective study of nearly 100 cases of acute compartment syndromes documented by pressure measurement, the most common cause is fracture (45%).[2] Of this group, fractures of the tibia predominate. The tibial fractures usually involve the diaphysis and, most typically, are closed injuries. However, compartment syndromes may follow open tibial fractures, tibial plateau fractures, and ankle fractures. Elective operations on the tibia, including the Hauser procedure (transplantation of the tibial tubercle),[3] tibial osteotomies, tibial leg lengthening, and use of the tibia for donor bone-graft site, have been associated with compartment syndromes.[4]

Fractures also represent the most common cause of compartment syndrome in children. Recently, Mubarak and Carroll reviewed the causes of Volkmann's contracture in 55 children (Fig. 8-3).[5] Of the contractures, 36% were caused by femur fractures, usually following inappropriate selection of traction techniques. Supracondylar fractures of the humerus, the most

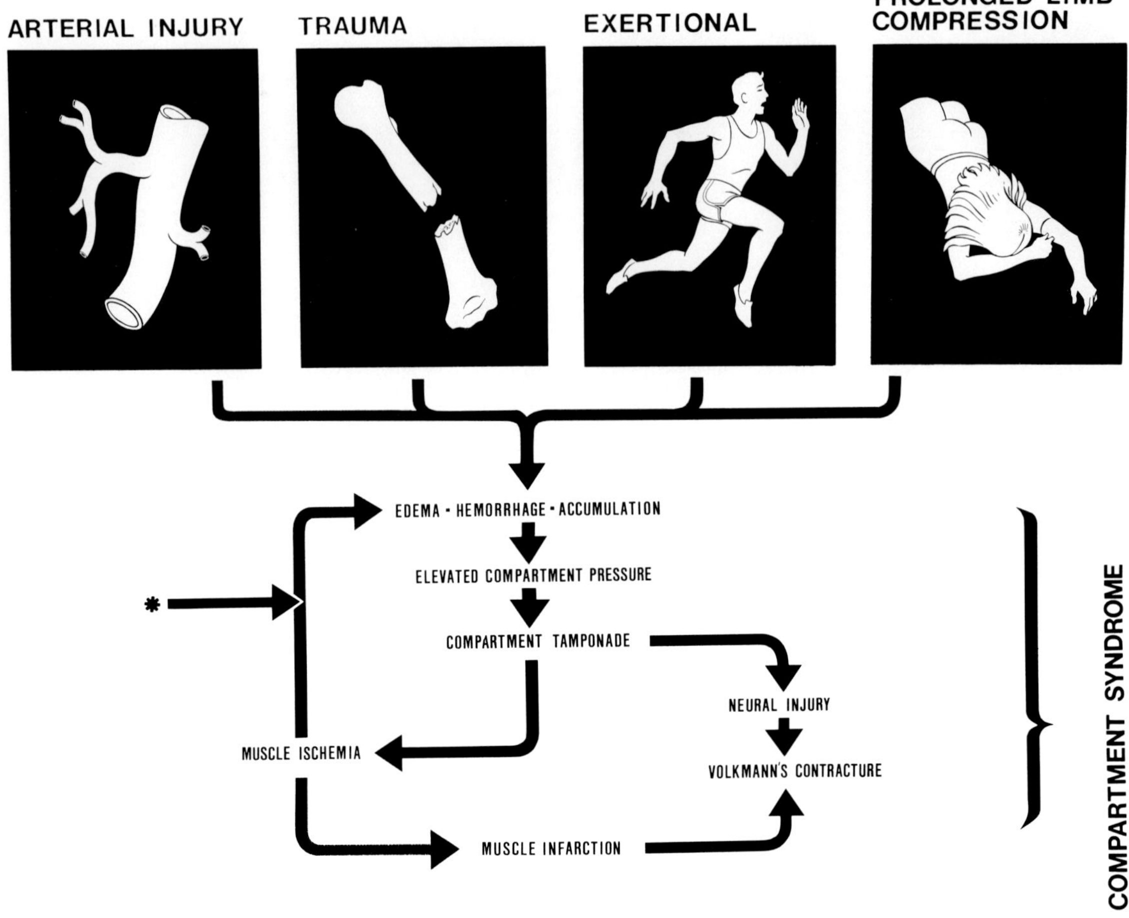

Fig. 8-1. Multiple causes may initiate a compartment syndrome, which, if untreated, may result in a Volkmann's contracture. Immediate surgical decompression is necessary to break this vicious cycle (see asterisk). (With permission from Mubarak, S. J., and Hargens, A. R.: Diagnosis and management of compartment syndromes. *In* AAOS Symposium on Trauma to the Leg and Its Sequellae. St. Louis, C. V. Mosby, 1981).

infamous injury associated with a Volkmann's contracture, still remained a frequent cause (16%). This injury is particularly difficult to evaluate because of its frequent association with arterial and neural injury.

Soft-Tissue Injury. In our experience, soft-tissue injury without fracture is the second leading cause of a compartment syndrome. In many cases, soft-tissue injury may represent severe trauma, but syndromes may follow even after a minor contusion to the anterior compartment of the leg.

Post-Ischemic Swelling. Ischemia to the leg occurs following an acute arterial injury or occlusion. After repair of the artery and/or removal of the clot, the circulation is restored. If the ischemic period is greater than 4 hours, post-ischemic swelling may initiate a compartment syndrome when a prophylactic fasciotomy has not been performed (Fig. 8-4).

Drug Overdose—Limb Compression. Prolonged immobilization in drug overdose victims or after a general anesthetic in the knee-chest position is a common cause of compartment syndromes and the crush syndrome. The pathogenesis of this compartment syndrome is due to the patient's torso compressing the extremity over a prolonged period of time. The intramuscular pressures generated in this situation range from

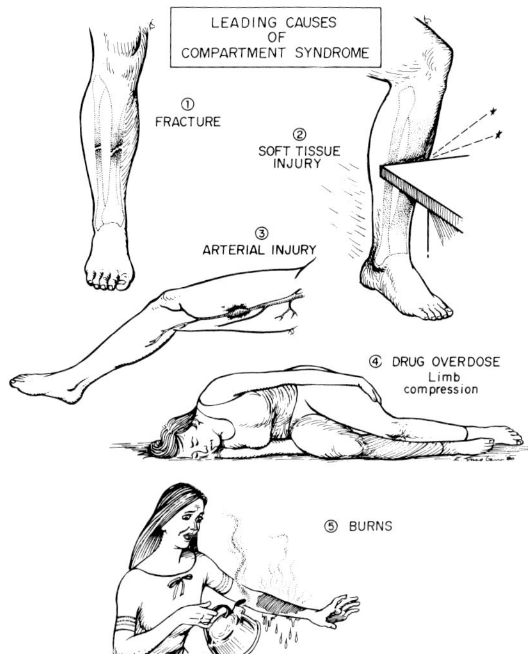

Fig. 8-2. Causes of the compartment syndrome. (With permission from Mubarak, S. J., and Hargens, A. R.: Compartment Syndromes and Volkmann's Contracture. Philadelphia, W. B. Saunders, 1981.)

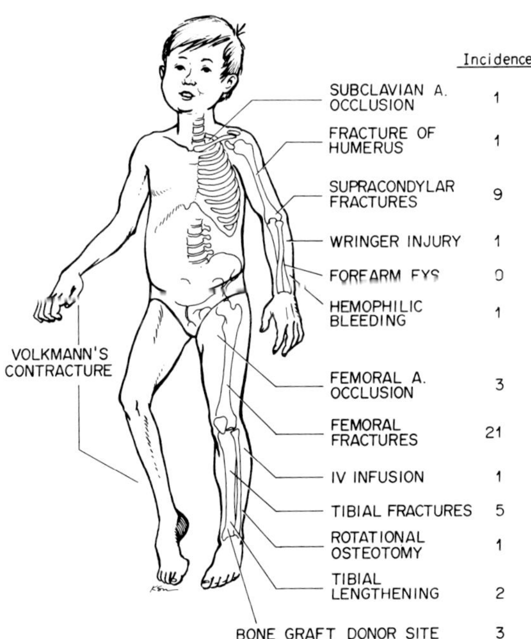

Fig. 8-3. Causes of Volkmann's contracture in 58 limbs (55 children). (With permission from Mubarak, S. J., and Carroll, N. C.: Volkmann's contracture in children: aetiology and prevention. J. Bone Joint Surg., *61-B*:285, 1979.)

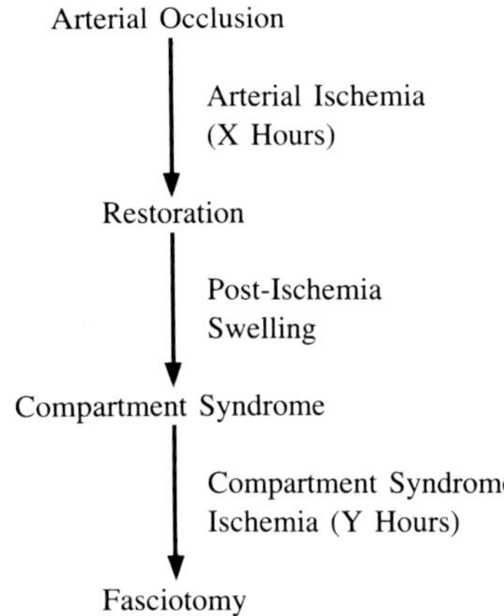

Total Ischemia = X Hours + Y Hours

Fig. 8-4. Pathogenesis of post-ischemia-initiated compartment syndromes. (With permission from Mubarak, S. J., and Hargens, A. R.: Compartment Syndromes and Volkmann's Contracture. Philadelphia, W. B. Saunders, 1981.)

30 mm Hg to over 200 mm Hg (Fig. 8-5).[6] The drug overdose patients seek medical attention late and, when hospitalized, frequently have other overlying problems, such as respiratory depression and renal failure, that delay the diagnosis of their compartment syndromes (Fig. 8-6). For this reason, the incidence of limb functional loss and frequency of Volkmann's contracture are high.[5]

Burns. Severe burns to the limbs cause the skin as well as the fascia to become a rigid envelope that constricts the underlying edematous soft tissues. Escharotomy and fasciotomy are required to decompress the underlying tissues.

Miscellaneous. Bleeding diathesis secondary to such conditions as hemophilia or to the use of anticoagulants may cause compartment syndromes. Venomous snakebites and exercise are rare causes.[2]

Anatomy

The forearm has two basic compartments. The *volar compartment* consists essentially of the flexors and pronators of the forearm and wrist. These may be further divided into superficial and deep areas (Fig. 8-7). The superficial muscles are the flexor carpi ulnaris, palmaris longus, flexor carpi radialis, and pronator teres. The deeper group of muscles consists of the flexor digitorum

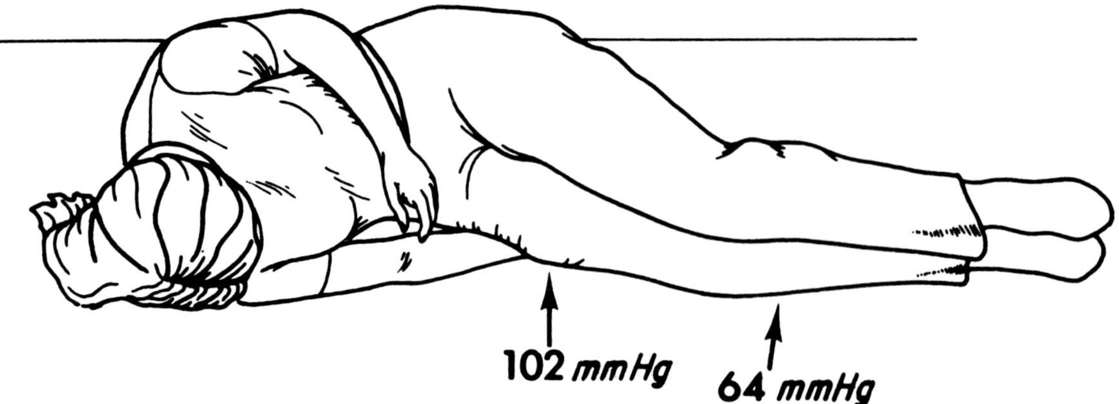

Fig. 8-5. Trunk compression of forearm (pressure range, 30 to 160 mm Hg) and leg (pressure range, 29 to 160 mm Hg). (With permission from Mubarak, S. J., and Hargens, A. R.: Compartment Syndromes and Volkmann's Contracture. Philadelphia, W. B. Saunders, 1981.)

superficialis and profundus, the flexor pollicis longus, and the pronator quadratus. The nerves of the volar compartment are the median and ulnar.

The *dorsal compartment* consists mainly of the wrist and finger extensors. The *mobile wad* (brachioradialis and extensor carpi radialis longus and brevis muscles) is physically and functionally a subcompartment between the dorsal and volar forearm compartments. The major nerve of the dorsal compartment is the posterior interosseous, the continuation of the radial nerve.

The leg consists of four compartments (Fig. 8-8). The *anterior* is the most frequently involved compartment in the body. The other compartments are the *lateral, superficial posterior,* and *deep posterior*. Each of these compartments contains two or more muscles, and a specific nerve courses through each compartment. The lateral compartment contains the common peroneal nerve, which divides into the deep and superficial branches. The deep peroneal nerve, originating in the lateral compartment, courses into the anterior compartment, where it follows the anterior tibial artery to the first toe-web space on the dorsum of the foot. The superficial peroneal nerve remains in the lateral compartment and courses along the anterior intermuscular septum. In the lower one third of the leg, the superficial peroneal nerve pierces the fascia, and its two terminal

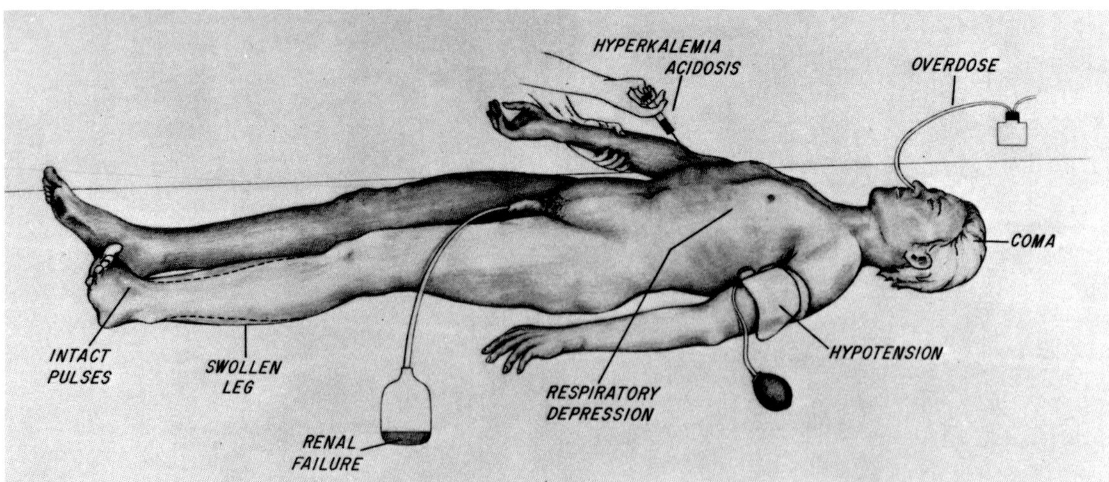

Fig. 8-6. Typical findings soon after hospital admission of a drug overdose patient sustaining limb compression with resulting crush syndrome. (With permission from Mubarak, S. J., and Owen, C. A.: Compartmental syndrome and its relationship to the crush syndrome: a spectrum of disease. Clin Orthop., *113*:81, 1975.)

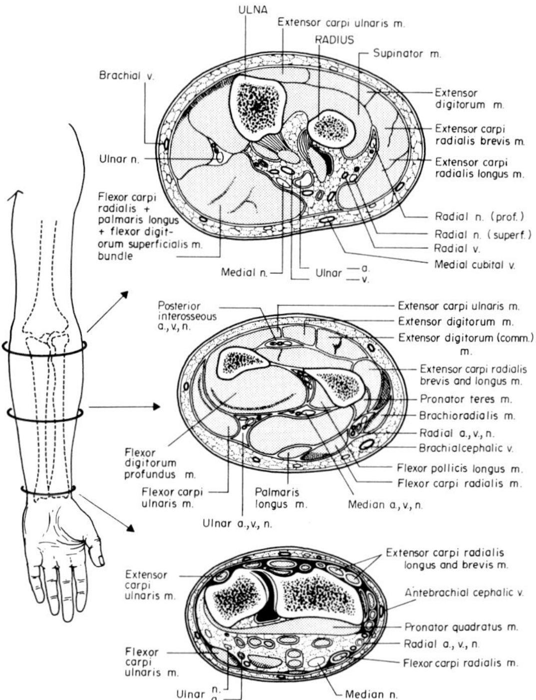

Fig. 8-7. Forearm compartments: transverse sections through left forearm at various levels. (With permission from Mubarak, S. J., and Hargens, A. R.: Compartment Syndromes and Volkmann's Contracture. Philadelphia, W. B. Saunders, 1981.)

branches supply sensation to the dorsum of the foot (Fig. 8-9).

Clinical Findings

Physical findings of a compartment syndrome depend on the compartments involved (Fig. 8-10). The earliest and only truly objective finding is a swollen and tense compartment that is a manifestation of increased pressure. The increased pressure equilibrates rapidly throughout the compartment, and thus, perceptible tenseness should be demonstrated throughout the extent of the compartment. Although even the experienced physician cannot consistently estimate by palpation the degree to which compartment pressures are elevated, the presence of tenseness throughout the compartment suggests that a syndrome may be present. Conversely, if the compartment is soft, the physician may be reassured, for the moment at least, that this entity is not present.

Pain with stretch of the muscles is the next clinical finding noted. Pain is quite subjective and depends on the reliability of the patient and the patient's threshold of pain. Following any injury or fracture, a patient has pain. Differentiating between ischemic muscle pain and pain from the original injury is frequently difficult. Pain out of proportion with that expected for a given injury or pain that progresses certainly should make the treating physician suspicious of an ischemic

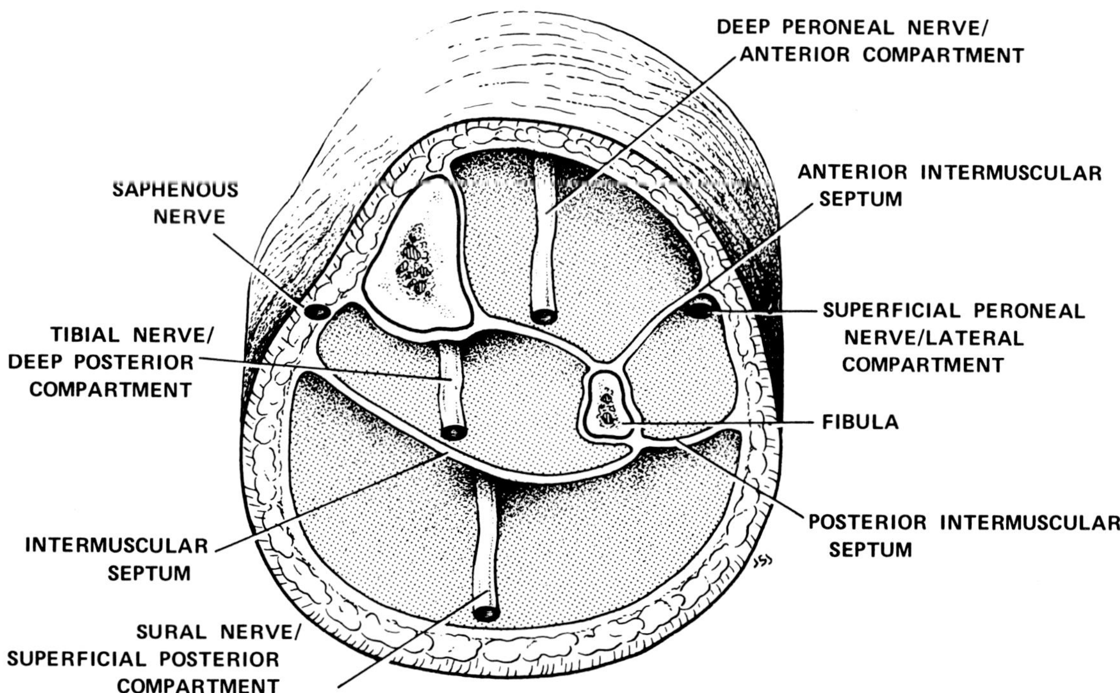

Fig. 8-8. Cross section at junction of middle and distal thirds of the leg illustrating the four compartments and their respective nerves. (With permission from Mubarak, S. J., and Owen, C. A.: Double-incision fasciotomy of the leg for decompression and compartment syndromes. J. Bone Joint Surg., *59-A*:184, 1977.)

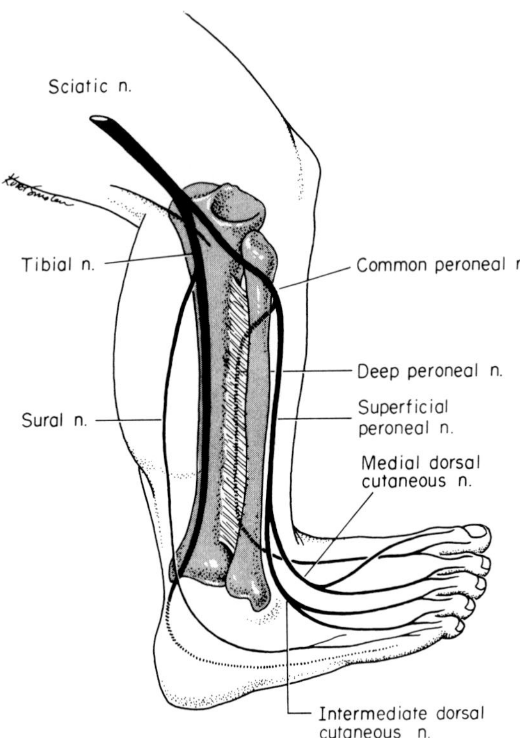

Fig. 8-9. Peripheral nerves of the leg. (With permission from Mubarak, S. J., and Hargens, A. R.: Compartment Syndromes and Volkmann's Contracture. Philadelphia, W. B. Saunders, 1981.)

situation. If the limb is anesthetic secondary to nerve ischemia, the pain with muscle stretch may be decreased markedly or absent. Thus, although pain is an early finding in a compartment syndrome, its evaluation and quantitation are often difficult.

Motor deficit, whether paresis or paralysis, likewise is difficult to interpret. This condition may arise secondary to either nerve ischemia, primary ischemia of the muscle, guarding secondary to pain, or a combination of the above.

The most helpful physical finding is a sensory deficit. Providing the patient is reliable and can cooperate, a careful sensory examination should allow evaluation of the involved compartments. As previously noted, each of the major compartments of the forearm and leg has at least one nerve coursing through it; consequently, careful sensory examination aids in confirming the involved compartment (Figs. 8-7 and 8-8). Two-point discrimination is mandatory for the early detection of any sensory deficit. Initially, nerve ischemia is evident by paresthesia in the distribution of the involved nerve. Later, hypesthesia and possibly anesthesia may result if the syndrome is left untreated.

Peripheral pulses usually are present in a compartment syndrome. The compartment pressures rarely are high enough to occlude the major artery coursing through a compartment (Fig. 8-11). Although palpation of the pulses may be difficult at times because of swelling, a Doppler blood-flow meter confirms their presence. If peripheral pulses are absent, the patient should be evaluated for arterial obstruction, and arteriography may be indicated.

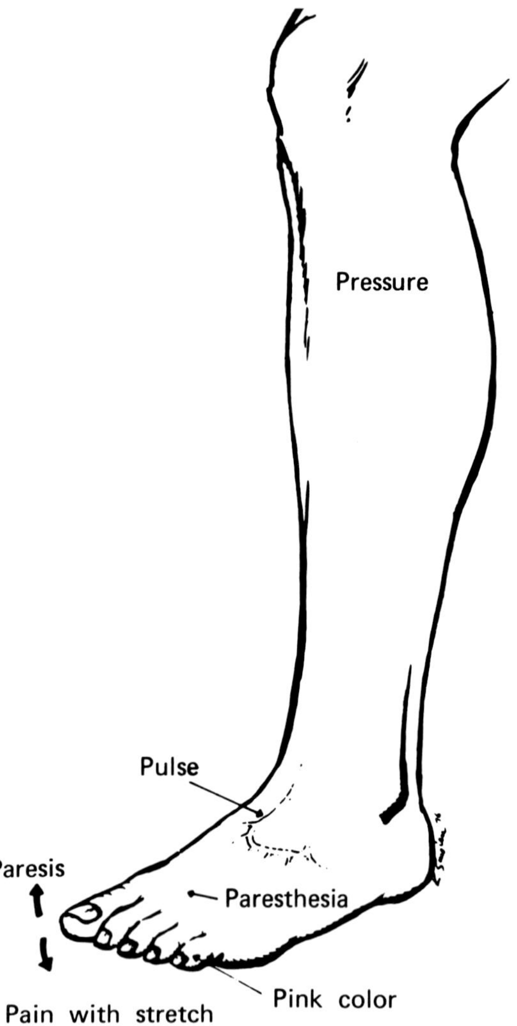

Fig. 8-10. Early findings of a compartment syndrome illustrated in anterior tibial compartment. Of these six "Ps," increased pressure is the earliest finding. (With permission from Mubarak, S. J., et al.: Muscle pressure measurement with the wick catheter. *In* Practice of Surgery. New York, Harper & Row, 1978.)

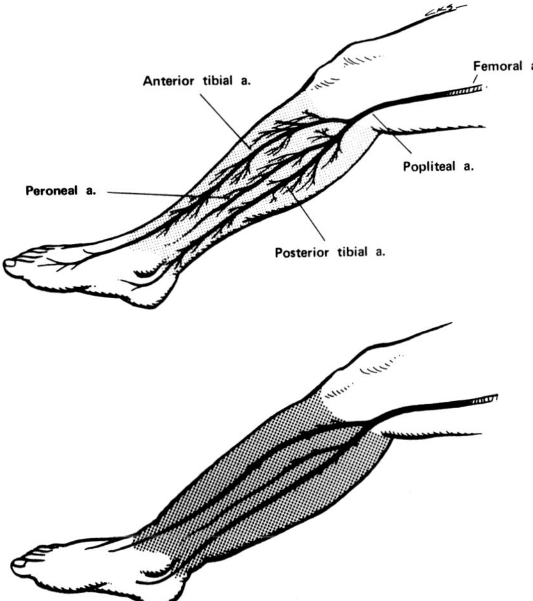

Fig. 8-11. Capillary-blood ischemia associated with compartment syndromes. *A,* At tissue-fluid pressures below 30 mm Hg, blood flows normally from arteries into arterials and capillaries. *B,* When pressure rises above 30 mm Hg, blood-flow through intracompartmental capillaries is impeded while central-artery and collateral circulations remain normal. During capillary ischemia, blood flow is confined to large arteries, veins, and nonnutritional arteriovenous anastomoses. Typically, pulses are present in tissues distal to the region of elevated tissue pressure; this may give the physician a false sense of security, believing that normal circulation is present in the muscle compartments. (With permission from Mubarak, S. J., and Hargens, A. R.: Compartment Syndromes and Volkmann's Contracture. Philadelphia, W. B. Saunders, 1981.)

Laboratory Tests

Intramuscular Pressure Measurement. As previously noted, the earliest finding of a compartment syndrome is increased pressure.[7] The needle technique has been popularized by Reneman[8] and Whitesides, et al.[9] It employs commonly available hospital equipment and does not require a transducer and recorder. Matsen, et al., modified the needle technique with the use of a syringe-infusion pump, pressure transducer, and recorder.[10] This infusion technique is frequently useful for long-term monitoring of a compartment over a number of days.

The wick catheter technique was first described in 1968 and later modified for clinical use (Fig. 8-12).[11] This technique uses a fluid-filled catheter connected to a pressure transducer and recorder. Wick material at the catheter's tip allows measurement of tissue pressure under equilibrium conditions. Recently, Rorabeck and associates developed the slit catheter (Fig. 8-13), which uses the same principles as the wick catheter.[12] The advantage of the slit catheter technique is ease in manufacture with more reliability of construction of the catheter tip. The slit and wick catheter techniques use the same electronic equipment (a pressure transducer and recorder) that anesthesiologists use to record direct arterial blood pressure.

Normal intramuscular pressures range from 0 to 8 mm Hg. Pressures greater than 20 mm Hg are elevated markedly and suggest an impending compartment syndrome. Intracompartmental pressures greater than 30 mm Hg for a time period greater than 8 hours have been demonstrated to produce changes in muscle and nerve function and have been accepted generally as the threshold for decompression in my clinic (see indications that follow).[7]

Electromyography and Nerve Conduction. These tests have been utilized primarily in the laboratory investigation of compartment syndromes. Clinically, Matsen and associates have used a small, battery-powered nerve stimulator to differentiate a direct nerve injury from a compartment syndrome.[13] This technique is performed in patients unable to contract a muscle group voluntarily. It stimulates the motor nerve, which innervates the muscles under consideration at a point just proximal to the muscle compartment. Response to this stimulation is reduced or absent when the myoneural junction is rendered ischemic in an acute compartment syndrome. Conversely, normal muscle contraction is observed if a primary neurapraxia is present proximal to the site of nerve stimulation. However, if the nerve injury is located between the stimulation site and the neuromuscular junction, the finding is ambiguous, and intramuscular pressure measurements are necessary to differentiate a primary neurapraxia from an acute compartment syndrome. This technique is also not helpful in prospective monitoring of patients at risk of developing a compartment syndrome.[13]

Peripheral Circulation Assessment. In the investigation of a patient with a possible major artery injury and/or a compartment syndrome, noninvasive studies, such as Doppler blood-flow and pulse-reappearance time, may be helpful. On

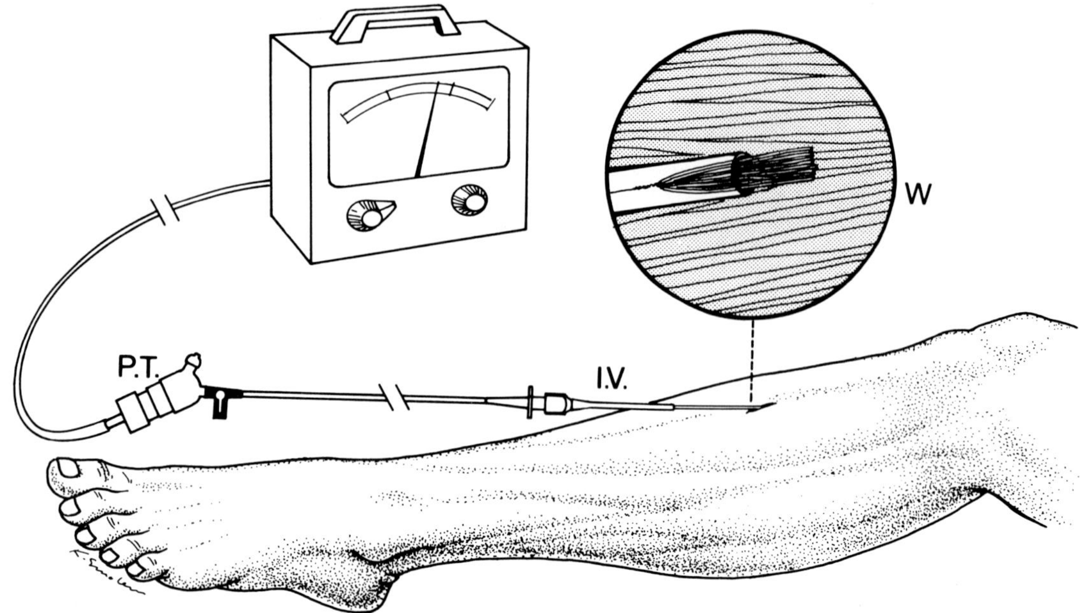

Fig. 8-12. Wick catheter technique for continuous measurement of equilibrium and tissue-fluid pressure in a muscle compartment. An intravenous placement unit (IV) aids insertion of the sterilized saline-filled catheter. Before insertion, the wick catheter is connected to a pressure transducer (P.T.) and recorder and is calibrated. A closeup view of the catheter's tip (W) illustrates how catheter patency and continuous fluid transmission are maintained by the numerous wick fibers. (With permission from Owen, C. A., et al.: N. Engl. J. Med., *300*:1169, 1979.)

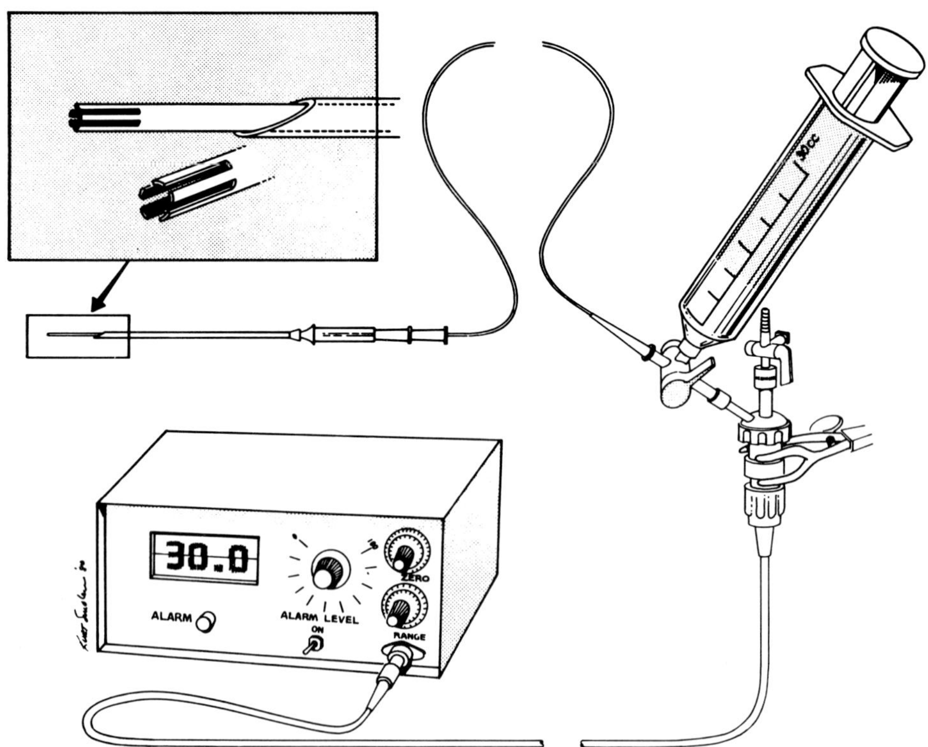

Fig. 8-13. Slit catheter technique for continuous measurements of equilibrium in a compartmental pressure. Prior to insertion into a muscle compartment, the sterile slit catheter is connected to the pressure transducer and digital recorder and then is filled with saline via a 30-ml syringe. The catheter tip protrudes from the insertion needle during filling so that the tip can be checked for air bubbles (see closeup, upper left). Prior to insertion into muscle, the catheter is pulled entirely within the needle. (With permission from Mubarak, S. J., and Hargens, A. R.: Compartment Syndromes and Volkmann's Contracture. Philadelphia, W. B. Saunders, 1981.)

other occasions, arteriograms may be necessary. With a typical acute compartment syndrome without an associated arterial injury, the arteriogram demonstrates patent major arteries with extrinsic compression and closure of the smaller arteries and arterioles.

Although used in the study of model compartment syndromes, such laboratory techniques as radioisotope–blood-flow studies, muscle Po_2, Pco_2, and pH, and technetium pyrophosphate scanning have not as yet become practical in the evaluation of acute compartment syndromes in human beings.[14-16]

Blood and Urine Tests. Blood levels of plasma creatine phosphokinase (CPK) can be used as an index of skeletal muscle ischemia and necrosis. Normal CPK values reach up to 130 IU. Acute compartment syndromes raise plasma CPK to levels of 1000 to 1500 IU, and multiple compartments, as seen in the crush syndrome, have CPK levels of greater than 10,000 IU with levels reaching as high as 150,000 IU. Other enzymes that are elevated include adolase, SGOT, and LDH.[5] Other blood parameters may be elevated with a severe crush syndrome: white blood count, hematocrit, and serum potassium. Creatinine elevated up to 10 mg/100 ml (normal level near 1 mg/100 ml) and blood urea nitrogen (BUN) at levels between 10 to 150 mg/100 ml indicate renal failure.[5]

Urinalysis frequently can detect the presence of myoglobulinuria (positive benzidine test for occult blood with absence of red cells) (Table 8-1).

Differential Diagnosis

The most difficult diagnosis arises in trying to distinguish a compartment syndrome from nerve injury and/or arterial injury (Table 8-2). The nerve injury associated with a fracture or contusion is most commonly a neurapraxia. The typical findings include sensory and motor deficits with little pain due to the nerve injury per se. However, a neurapraxia usually is associated with fractures or soft-tissue injury, which, of course, produce pain. Neurapraxia has intact pulses, and the compartment is soft.

An arterial injury is usually associated with absent peripheral pulses. However, intimal tears, pseudoaneurysms, or adequate collateral circula-

TABLE 8-2. *Typical Clinical Findings of Compartment Syndrome, Arterial Occlusion, and Neurapraxia.*

	Compartment Syndrome	*Arterial Occlusion*	*Neurapraxia*
Pressure increased in compartment	+	−	−
Pain with stretch	+	+	−
Paresthesia or anesthesia	+	+	+
Paresis or paralysis	+	+	+
Pulses intact	+	−	+

With permission from Mubarak, S. J., and Carroll, N.: Volkmann's contracture in children: aetiology and prevention. J. Bone Joint Surg., *61B*:290, 1979.

TABLE 8-1. *Typical Urinalysis in Patient with the Crush Syndrome and Myoglobulinuria (Occult Blood: Positive and RBC = 0).*

Macroscopic			*Microscopic*		
Color	—	Reddish-brown	RBC	—	0
Appearance	—	Clear	WBC	—	Rare
Specific gravity	—	1.008	Renal cells	—	0
pH	—	7.0	Bacteria	—	0
Protein	—	2+	Squamous epithelium	—	Few
Glucose	—	Negative	Mucous threads	—	0
Ketones	—	Negative	Crystals	—	0
Occult Blood	—	Large amount (positive)	Casts	—	0

With permission from Mubarak, S. J., and Hargens, A. R.: Compartment Syndromes and Volkmann's Contracture. Philadelphia, W. B. Saunders, 1981.

tion can sustain a distal pulse. The other associated findings of an arterial injury include ischemic stretch pain, hypesthesia, weakness, and pallor. The compartment clinically is soft.

The compartment syndrome findings have been noted previously. The major differentiating point between this entity, neurapraxia, and arterial injury is the tense compartment with elevated pressure. In this case, measurement of compartment pressure may be important in differentiating compartment syndromes from the other problems, especially when more than one of these problems are present and/or the patient is uncooperative or unresponsive. Other useful techniques include the Doppler blood-flow meter and arteriography to evaluate the arterial status.

Indications/Contraindications

Our indications for decompression are: (1) the clinical findings of a compartment syndrome and (2) intracompartmental pressure ≥ 30 mm Hg in a normotensive individual. Most patients with compartment syndromes can be diagnosed clinically, and documentation of elevated compartment pressure may be only confirmatory. However, pressure measurement is helpful in uncooperative, unreliable, or unresponsive patients, and in those with a nerve deficit.

At present, opinions differ with respect to the threshold pressure at which decompression is required. Whitesides, et al.,[9] and Matsen, et al.,[13] suggest that fasciotomies be performed in patients with intracompartmental pressures of 50 to 70 and 45 mm Hg, respectively. Although the needle injection[9] and infusion techniques[10] measure pressures that are systematically higher than pressures measured by the wick and slit catheter techniques, larger differences of opinion regarding a threshold pressure for fasciotomy are not explained by methodologic peculiarities alone.[17]

Our clinical and animal studies to date support the conclusion that the threshold intracompartmental pressure at which fasciotomy is recommended is 30 mm Hg for an 8-hour pressurization period.[2,14-17] Myoneural necrosis at pressure levels above 30 mm Hg after 8 hours is significantly high based on pyrophosphate uptake, muscle histology, studies of nerve function, and Starling force.[14-16] Since the time parameter is usually unknown in most cases of acute compartment syndromes, we recommend that any intracompartmental pressure greater than 30 mm Hg, combined with the other clinical findings, requires fasciotomy. Undoubtedly, a spectrum of tolerances to elevated intracompartmental pressure exists among human beings, but we believe that it is prudent to use a value close to the capillary blood pressure (20 to 25 mm Hg) before the muscle and nerve are injured by ischemia as a criterion for decompression. However, one must remember that this threshold compartment pressure of 30 mm Hg alone is a relative indication for decompression that must be tempered by the patient's cooperation and reliability, overall condition, blood pressure, peripheral perfusion, trend of symptoms and signs, and trend of intracompartmental pressures.[17]

There are few contraindications for decompression of acute compartment syndromes. Even patients with bleeding disorders, such as hemophilia, with severe burns, or who are extremely ill require decompression. If the patient is too tenuous to undergo anesthesia in the operating room, the decompression can be performed under local anesthesia on the ward or in the intensive-care unit.

When is decompression not indicated? With a delay in diagnosis, it is sometimes more prudent not to open the limb and to risk infection in the presence of necrotic tissue. In these circumstances, the late findings of a compartment syndrome, including anesthesia and paralysis, are present, but the compartment feels "woody" by palpation. If pressure measurement is near normal, decompression is not recommended. However, if the pressures are elevated above 30 mm Hg, decompression should be performed in hopes of reversing some of the muscle and nerve ischemia.

Treatment Options

Early Evaluation and Care

When evaluating a patient with a traumatized limb and a neurocirculatory deficit, the physician should document carefully the time of injury and examination. The examination should be performed carefully and should include motor, sensory, and circulatory evaluation. When a neurologic deficit is observed in a painfully traumatized and swollen limb, the physician must evaluate and treat the patient promptly. Initially, cast splitting and "windowing" over any involved nerve, such as the common peroneal nerve at the fibular head, should be performed. If the neurologic deficit persists without improvement for more than an hour, removal of the cast and all circular dressings is mandatory (Fig. 8-14).

If the compartments clinically are observed to be tense, measurement of pressure is necessary. At this stage, one must differentiate the troublesome problems of compartment syndrome, neurapraxia, and arterial injury. The neurapraxia associated with a fracture or soft-tissue injury usually is treated by observation alone. With time and prompt diagnosis, nearly all function returns. The arterial injury requires immediate restoration of the circulation, whether by repair of the artery or removal of a thrombosis. Similarly, the compartment syndrome must be treated by immediate decompression. Thus, the problems must be sorted in an organized fashion and a diagnosis arrived at promptly.

Forearm Decompression

Eichler and Lipscomb described an approach to the patient with a forearm compartment syndrome.[18] They outlined a stepwise scheme that included a division of forearm skin, subcutaneous tissue, and fascia. In 1972, Eaton and Green described a specific operative technique in which their skin incision began distal to the elbow flexion crease and medial to the biceps tendon, and extended distally in the longitudinal axis of the midforearm to the transverse flexion crease at the wrist.[19] The forearm fascia was incised longitudinally along its full length. The epimysium of all poorly vascularized muscles was sectioned. The fascia was left open, and delayed closure with split-thickness skin grafts and relaxing incisions was performed 48 to 72 hours later.

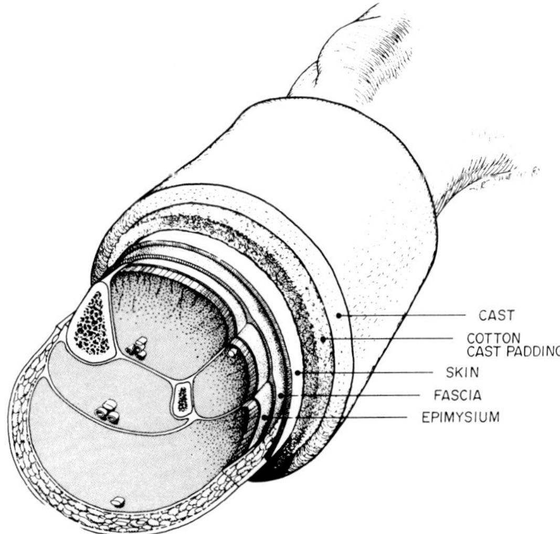

FIG. 8-14. The surrounding envelopes of a muscle compartment. (With permission from Mubarak, S. J., and Hargens, A. R.: Compartment Syndromes and Volkmann's Contracture. Philadelphia, W. B. Saunders, 1981.)

Neumeyer and Kilgore reported their experience with 14 patients who had forearm compartment syndromes.[20] Their incision began adjacent to the medial epicondyle, extended obliquely across the antecubital fossa over the volar mobile wad, and returned to the midline in the distal forearm. It continued in a curvilinear fashion across the carpal canal to the midpalm. This report recommended wide exposure of all three possible areas of involvement—the volar and dorsal compartments of the forearm and the intrinsics of the hand. Closure was accomplished by split-thickness skin grafting after several days.

Whitesides and associates described another operative approach in which their incision began above the elbow laterally and was carried transversely across the antecubital fossa to the proximal-medial forearm.[21] The incision was continued distally along the ulnar border of the forearm to the wrist, where it curved laterally in the flexor crease of the wrist and extended into the palm in the thenar crease. The fascia was opened from above the elbow to the midpalm. The carpal tunnel and all neurovascular and muscular envelopes were opened fully. They noted that subcutaneous fasciotomy should never be performed in the forearm. The fascia was left open and was closed by split-thickness skin grafting 48 to 72 hours later. Similarly, Matsen and associates used the volar-ulnar approach.[13] They frequently performed carpal tunnel releases and epimysiotomy as recommended by Eaton and Green.[19] The advantage of this volar-ulnar approach is that the flexor tendons and median nerve are not left exposed in the distal forearm.

In 1978, Gelberman, et al.,[22] recommended decompression of the forearm with a volar-curvilinear incision and a straight longitudinal dorsal incision, which is my preferred technique (Fig. 8-15).

Leg Decompression

In 1967, Kelly and Whitesides stressed the anatomic importance of the four compartments and suggested that the fibulectomy-fasciotomy through a single lateral incision was an adequate means of decompressing these compartments.[23] The specific details of this procedure were outlined more completely by Ernst and Kaufer[24] and later by Whitesides and associates.[21] Patman and

Thompson favored fibulectomy for: (1) severe cases, (2) cases with obvious myonecrosis or paralysis, and (3) cases in which fibulectomy would aid exposure and repair of a distal popliteal artery.[25]

Willhoite and Moll advocated decompression without fibulectomy through a single lateral incision.[26] Similarly, Matsen and associates have recommended the parafibular approach for decompressing all four compartments.[13]

Patman and Thompson advocated the double-incision method for early compartment syndromes.[25] The double-incision technique for decompression of the leg described in detail in 1977 remains my preferred technique.[27]

Preferred Method

I prefer a volar and dorsal fasciotomy to decompress the forearm and a double-incision fasciotomy to decompress the leg.

Volar and Dorsal Fasciotomy of the Forearm[17]

Since 1974, I have utilized a single, longitudinal curvilinear incision for decompression of the volar forearm. This incision allows an easy approach to antebrachial fascia and transverse carpal ligament, as well as exposure of the arteries and nerves of the forearm and the mobile wad.[22,28] The incision is nearly identical to McConnell's combined exposure of the median and ulnar neurovascular bundles, as described by Henry (1973).[29] I prefer a straight longitudinal incision for the dorsal compartment of the forearm.

The effectiveness of the volar forearm fasciotomy was evaluated initially in a series of cadaver experiments.[22] The major volar incisions made were the volar-ulnar incision described by Whitesides, et al.,[21] and the curvilinear, midline volar incision (Fig. 8-15). Both were effective in lowering pressures in the volar forearm, and both also lowered pressures within the mobile wad and dorsal regions in approximately one half of the limbs. The volar forearm pressure generally fell to normal values when the antebrachial fascia had been divided from the lacertus fibrosus to the junction of the middle and distal thirds of the forearm. When the dorsal pressures remained elevated following volar fasciotomy, a dorsal fasciotomy was performed.

Furthermore, since 1974 the adequacy of forearm decompression using the curvilinear volar incision has been confirmed intraoperatively with the wick catheter in 18 patients.[28]

Double-Incision Fasciotomy of the Leg

I prefer the double-incision technique for decompression of the four compartments of the leg. This technique was compared to fibulectomy-fasciotomy in a series of cadaver experiments. When properly performed, both techniques are effective in obtaining an adequate decompression. However, the double-incision technique offers several advantages over fibulectomy-fasciotomy:

1. It is simpler and requires minimal dissection. The procedure can be performed under local anesthesia if necessary.
2. It is faster and relatively safer. Both procedures require close attention to anatomic detail to avoid damaging important cutaneous nerves. However, the double-incision method involves less risk, primarily because all the fascial incisions are superficial and avoid deep neurovascular structures.
3. The fibula is left intact. Concern by surgeons regarding the sequelae of fibulectomy in a child or an adult may lead to delay of treatment with potentially disastrous results.

The double-incision technique also has advantages over the long, single, lateral skin incision method:

1. Two shorter skin incisions offer better cosmesis, as delayed primary closure usually can be performed at around 1 week. In over 90% of our patients, skin grafting has not been required.
2. Any portion of the double-incision technique may be used for decompression of any specific combination of compartments fewer than four.
3. Two incisions provide an opportunity to perform a double decompressive dermotomy if required. In these rare cases in which the skin is a limiting envelope, a single incision may not be sufficient for complete decompression, and therefore, double decompressive dermotomies are required.
4. Debridement is facilitated through these skin incisions if necrotic muscle is encountered.

In our prospective study of acute compartment syndromes started in 1974,[4] the double-incision fasciotomy has been utilized on more than 40 patients.[2] In most of these patients, we have verified the adequacy of decompression and the technique with intraoperative pressure monitoring.

Operative Technique[17]

Volar and Dorsal Fasciotomy of the Forearm

Volar Approach

A complete, single skin incision, beginning proximal to the antecubital fossa and extending to the midpalm, can be utilized for volar forearm decompression. The incision begins 1 cm proximal and 2 cm lateral to the medial epicondyle and is carried obliquely across the antecubital fossa and over the volar aspect of the mobile wad. It is gently curved medially, reaching the midline at the junction of the middle and distal thirds of the forearm (See Fig. 8-15), and is continued straight distally to the proximal wrist crease, just ulnar to the palmaris longus tendon. The forearm incision is extended across the volar wrist crease in the curvilinear fashion. It is carried no farther radially than the midaxis of the ring finger to avoid injury to the palmar cutaneous branch of the median nerve. The incision is terminated in the midpalm at a level even with the base of the thumb-index web. The carpal tunnel has been released as a standard part of forearm decompression.

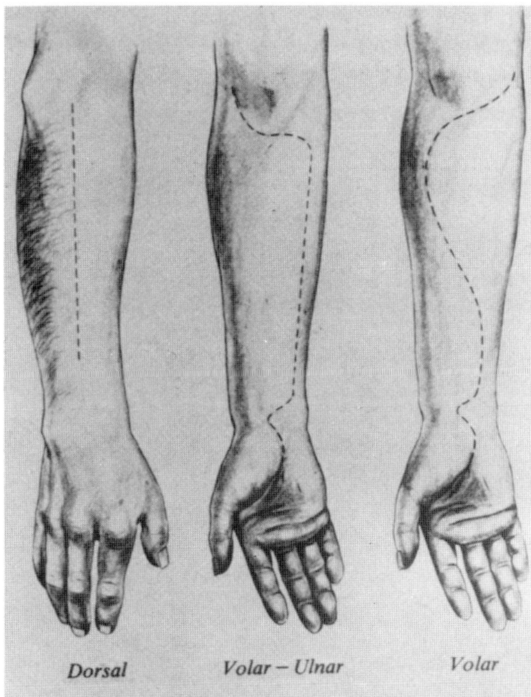

FIG. 8-15. Dorsal, volar-ulnar, and curvilinear volar incisions. The curvilinear volar incision is preferred because of the exposure afforded the major nerves, brachial artery, and mobile wad. (With permission from Gelberman, R. H., et al.: Decompression of forearm compartment syndromes. Clin. Orthop., *134*:225, 1978.)

In patients with median nerve dysfunction in addition to the carpal tunnel release, the median nerve should be explored in the proximal forearm. There are three areas of potential neural compression in the proximal forearm. The most proximal, the lacertus fibrosus, is always released as part of the fasciotomy. The next area of possible compression is the proximal edge of the pronator teres, and the third is the proximal edge of the flexor digitorum superficialis. The surgeon should be certain that the nerve lies freely in all three regions.

An additional incision for the mobile wad has not been necessary, as this area can be exposed easily with the curvilinear volar incision.

It is highly advisable that tissue pressure measurements be available intraoperatively. Volar and dorsal pressures are measured prior to the skin incision. Following the volar fasciotomy, the pressure in the dorsal compartment is remeasured. When the pressure is elevated, a dorsal fasciotomy is performed.

Dorsal Approach

The incision begins 2 cm lateral and 2 cm distal to the lateral epicondyle (see Fig. 8-15). It is extended straight distally toward the midline of the wrist for 7 to 10 cm, depending on the size of the forearm. The skin edges are undermined, and the dorsal fascia of the entire forearm is incised directly in line with the skin incision; thereby completing the decompression of the volar and dorsal regions of the forearm. If intraoperative pressure monitoring has been performed, a final pressure in each compartment is checked. The wounds are packed open, and a bulky, compressive hand dressing extending above the elbow with plaster forearm and elbow splints is applied. Skin incisions are not closed at the time of fasciotomy.

If the diagnosis was delayed and some muscle appears necrotic, a superficial debridement is carried out. More definitive debridements are carried out secondarily when muscle viability can be determined more accurately.

After Care

The extremity is elevated continuously in the bulky dressing. At 3 to 4 days postfasciotomy, the patient is returned to the operating room. The skin of the hand and wrist and the proximal few centimeters of the wound frequently can be closed at this time. The large central portion of the wound may be skin grafted at this time. Skin grafts have been necessary in nearly all our patients.

If some of the forearm musculature is necrotic, further debridement is carried out every 3 to 4 days until the granulating bed is healthy. Quantitative cultures are used to determine the appropriate time for grafting.

Active and active-assisted range of motion of the hand is started on the second day postfasciotomy while the patient is still in the bulky dressing. Exercises are discontinued for 7 days after split-thickness skin grafting is performed, and are then reinstituted. The bulky dressing is discontinued at 2½ to 3 weeks, and the patient is placed in a splint with the thumb in opposition and the wrist neutral. The elbow is left free.

Double-Incision Fasciotomy of the Leg

Skin Incisions

A limited incision approximately 15 cm long (roughly one third of the length of the leg) can be utilized for both the anterolateral and posteromedial incisions. This incision is best utilized if the compartment syndrome is diagnosed and treated promptly. If the limited approach is utilized, intraoperative tissue pressure measurement should be used to documcnt the adequacy of decompression.

The limited-incision technique has advatanges in that less muscle is exposed and delayed closure can be accomplished at 5 to 7 days without skin grafting in nearly all cases. The disadvantages of the limited incision are twofold. First, on rare occasions when swelling is massive, the skin may limit tissue decompression. Second, particularly in the case of a less experienced surgeon, fasciotomy may not be complete if the scissors or fasciotome* slip off the fascia.

Longer skin incisions (20 to 25 cm in length) on both the anterolateral and posteromedial leg are advisable when intraoperative tissue pressure measurement is not undertaken. Also, if the case is delayed and a great deal of swelling is present, longer incisions should be made. The presence of necrotic muscle frequently requires longer incisions for adequate exposure and debridement. Finally, if the surgeon has any doubt regarding the completeness of the fasciotomy, the exposure should be extended for the full length of the compartment. A disadvantage of the more extensive incision is that skin grafting is required in most cases.

Anterolateral Approach (Anterior and Lateral Compartments)

The incision is placed halfway between the fibular shaft and the tibial crest, approximately over the anterior intermuscular septum dividing the anterior and lateral compartments, and allows easy access to both. The skin edges are undermined proximally and distally to allow for wide exposure of the fascia (Fig. 8-16). Following this

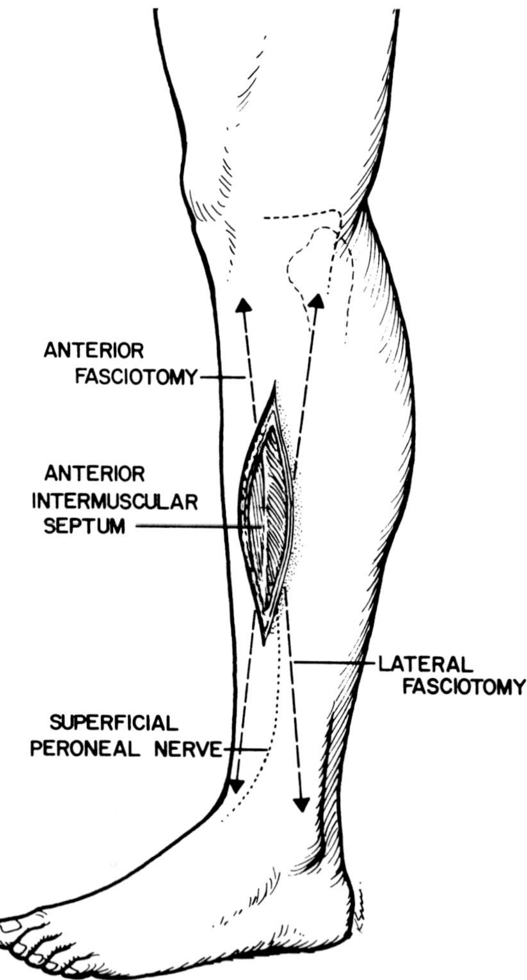

Fig. 8-16. Anterolateral incision. The skin incision utilized to approach the anterior and lateral compartments is placed halfway between the fibular shaft and the tibial crest. (With permission from Mubarak, S. J., and Hargens, A. R.: Diagnosis and management of compartment syndromes. *In* AAOS Symposium on Trauma to the Leg and Its Sequellae. St. Louis, C. V. Mosby, 1981.)

procedure, one should be able to visualize almost the full extent of the compartment fascia. This step is important when using a more limited incision.

A transverse incision is made just through the fascia to identify the anterior intermuscular septum that separates the anterior compartment from the lateral compartment. Identification of this septum is necessary to find the superficial peroneal nerve that lies in the lateral compartment next to the septum. Using a 12-inch Metzenbaum scissors or fasciotome, the anterior compartment fascia is opened. Visualization is aided by retraction with right-angled retractors. The scissors are pushed with the tips opened slightly in the direction of the great toe distally and toward the patella proximally. If the surgeon suspects that the tip of the scissors has strayed from the fascia, the instrument is left in place, and a small incision is made over the tip of the scissors. If the fasciotomy is incomplete, further release can be performed through this accessory incision.

The lateral-compartment fasciotomy is made in line with the fibular shaft. The scissors or fasciotome is directed proximally toward the fibular head and distally toward the lateral malleolus. In this way, the fascial incision is posterior to the superficial peroneal nerve. This procedure completes the decompression of these compartments.

Posteromedial Approach (Superficial and Deep Posterior Compartments)

The medial incision is slightly distal to the previous incision and 2 cm posterior to the posterior tibial margin. By making the incision at this location, one avoids injuring the saphenous nerve and vein, which course along the posterior margin of the tibia in this locale (Fig. 8-17). Once again, the skin edges are undermined. The saphenous nerve and vein are retracted anteriorly. A transverse fascial incision is made to allow identification of the septum between the deep and superficial posterior compartments. The tendon of the flexor digitorum longus in the deep posterior compartment and the Achilles tendon in the superficial posterior compartment are identified. The superficial posterior compartment is usually easiest to decompress first. This fasciotomy is extended proximally as far as possible, and then distally behind the medial malleolus. The deep posterior compartment is released distally and then proximally under the soleus bridge. If the soleus attaches distally to the tibia more than halfway, it should be released. Occasionally we have encountered the soleus muscle or fascia extending to near the ankle, completely covering the deeper-lying fascia of the deep posterior compartment. In this instance, the deep posterior compartment is not visualized until the superficial posterior compartment has been opened and the soleus retracted.

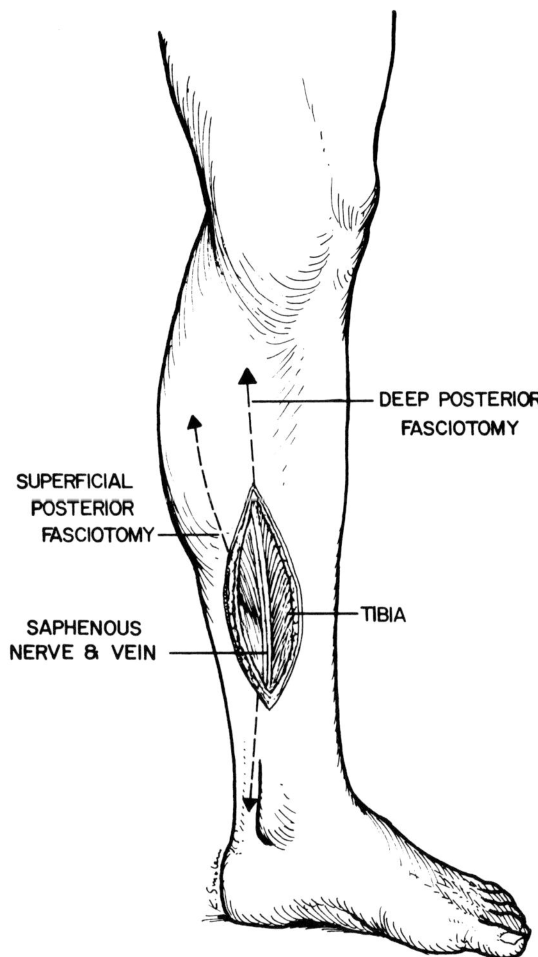

Fig. 8-17. Posteromedial incision. The skin incision used to compress the superficial and deep posterior compartments is placed 2 cm posterior to the posterior tibial margin. (With permission from Mubarak, S. J., and Hargens, A. R.: Diagnosis and management of compartment syndromes. *In* AAOS Symposium on Trauma to the Leg and Its Sequellae. St. Louis, C. V. Mosby, 1981.)

This procedure completes a four-compartment decompression (Fig. 8-18). If intraoperative pressure monitoring has been utilized during this procedure, a final pressure check of each compartment is not performed. The wounds are

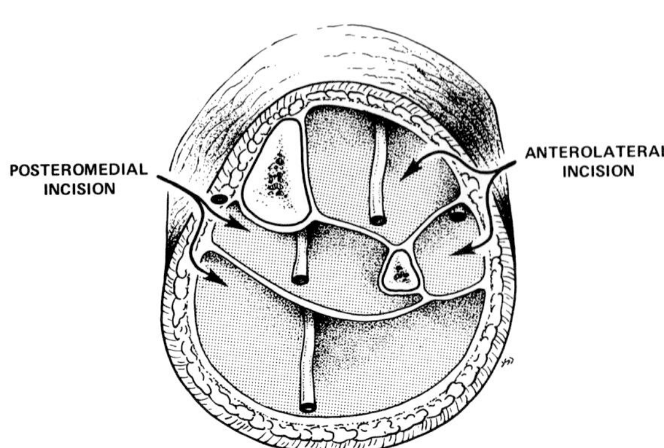

Fig. 8-18. Composite illustrating four-compartment decompression using the double-incision method. (With permission from Mubarak, S. J., and Owens, C. A.: Double-incision fasciotomy of the leg for decompression compartment syndromes. J. Bone Joint Surg., *59-A*:184, 1977.)

packed open and dressings are applied. Usually the leg is immobilized with a posterior splint.

If the procedure is delayed, little muscle should be debrided at the time of initial decompression. Differentiating infarcted muscle from ischemic, but recoverable, muscle is difficult in this situation.

After Care

Approximately 5 to 7 days after fasciotomy, the patient is returned to surgery. After this period, and if a more limited skin incision has been made, closure is almost always possible. We have found that vertical mattress suturing (near-far-far-near technique) is the best technique for skin closure following fasciotomy. Again, tissue pressure measurement helps to verify that pressure has not risen to ischemic levels during the closure.

With large wounds or too much swelling, split-thickness skin grafting is necessary. If there is necrotic muscle, the wounds are debrided repeatedly or twice weekly until a satisfactory granulation bed is present. Quantitative bacteria counts decide when to perform grafting.

Do not overlook the insiduous development of contractures, as even with early diagnosis, contractures may develop in the subacute phase due to splinting secondary to pain, anterior compartment weakness, or posterior compartment muscle involvement. Posterior splinting of the ankle in the neutral position is mandatory.

Special Problems

Several problems associated with compartment syndromes require special considerations.

Fractures of Radius and Ulna and Compartment Syndromes of the Forearm

Acute forearm compartment syndromes are sometimes associated with fractures of the radius and ulna. In most cases, internal fixation of both bones should be undertaken at the time of fasciotomy.

Arterial Injuries and Compartment Syndromes of Forearm

Arterial injuries associated with compartment syndromes most often occur following supracondylar fractures, forearm fractures, or external penetrating injuries. If an arterial injury associated with a compartment syndrome and supracondylar fracture is suspected, the patient should be taken immediately to the operating room (Fig. 8-19). The fracture should be reduced and the pulses and hand circulation reassessed. If reduction of the fracture gives no improvement in the circulation, the physician should consider obtaining a transfemoral-brachial arteriogram instead of immediately exploring the fracture site, depending on the ease in obtaining the arteriogram. Subsequently, exploration and repair of the artery should be performed.

Fasciotomy of the forearm is indicated when the clinical signs of a compartment syndrome are present and the intracompartmental pressure is greater than 30 mm Hg. The fracture is best treated by percutaneous pin fixation or overhead olecranon pin traction. Wound management is identical to that described earlier for forearm fasciotomy.

Tibial Fractures and Compartment Syndromes of the Leg

When a limited incision is employed with a stable tibial fracture, a long leg cast can be used to immobilize the fracture and allow wound care. External pin fixator, or more commonly, internal fixation devices have been used to facilitate wound and fracture management. The major disadvantages of the pins are that mobilization of the skin for delayed primary closure is not as easy, and skin grafting is usually required.

Prophylactic Fasciotomy of the Leg

Prophylactic fasciotomy is considered for any patient with an increased risk of developing a

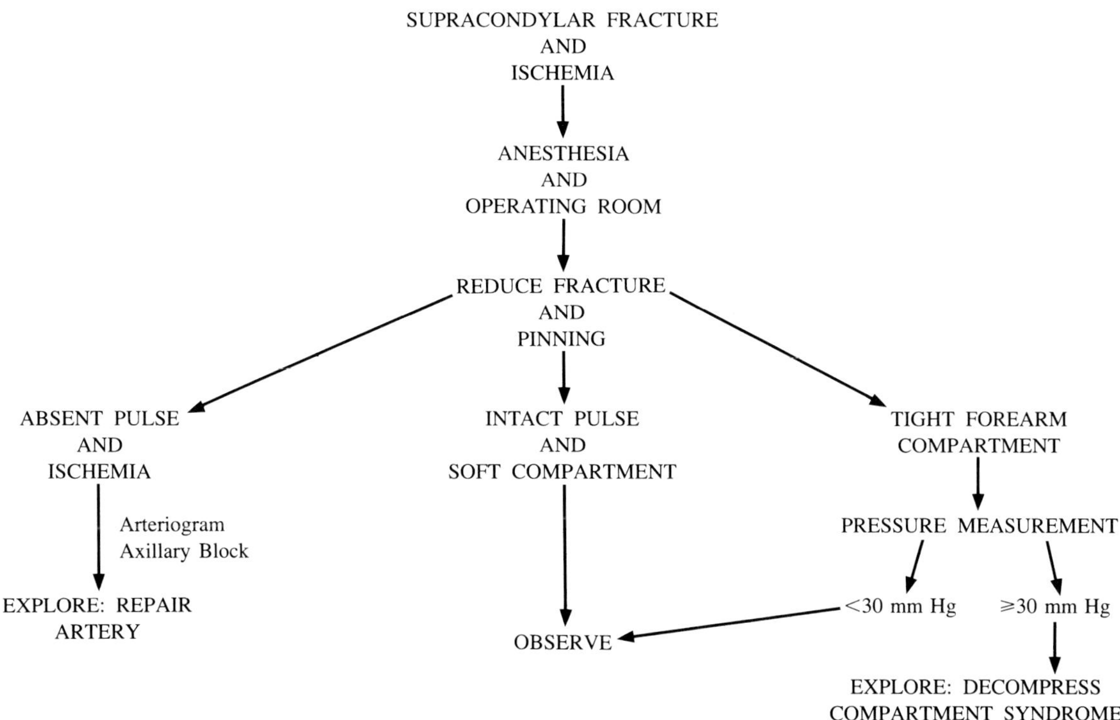

FIG. 8-19. Schema for management of supracondylar fractures associated with upper-extremity ischemia. (With permission from Mubarak, S. J., and Hargens, A. R.: Compartment Syndromes and Volkmann's Contracture. Philadelphia, W. B. Saunders, 1981.)

compartment syndrome. I recommend that prophylactic fasciotomies should be performed on most elective tibial operations, such as leg lengthenings or rotational osteotomies.

Patients who have sustained an arterial injury or thrombosis or who have a femoral artery bypass are especially prone to the development of compartment syndromes after restoration of the arterial circulation. If the arterial ischemia lasts for more than 4 hours, prophylactic, 4-compartment fasciotomy of the leg is warranted at the time of arterial repair.

Complications and Results

The major local complication of an untreated compartment syndrome is a Volkmann's contracture. The contracture and neurologic deficit may result in a severe functional loss to the limb. The subsequent reconstructive surgery for this problem is covered elsewhere.[17] The major systemic complication of multiple compartment syndromes is the crush syndrome with associated renal failure. This problem is almost entirely limited to compartment syndromes initiated by drug overdose with limb compression, which was discussed earlier in this chapter.

In our prospective study of compartment syndromes, approximately 75% of the patients have a normal or near-normal result, and 15% have some functional impairment. The incidence of Volkman's contracture is about 10%. The worst results occurred in patients who developed compartment syndromes following severe burns, drug overdose with limb compression, or postischemic swelling. In these patients, the severity of the original injury and, sometimes, delays in diagnosis and treatment accounted for the poor prognosis.

The result of a compartment syndrome depends on a number of significant variables: the type and severity of the injury, the magnitude of the pressure elevation, and the duration of the compartment syndrome. The magnitude of intracompartmental pressure elevation can be documented, but the duration of the pressure elevation above ischemic levels cannot be determined accurately. The lag phase from the time of injury to the onset of symptoms may vary from 4 hours to 4 days (Fig. 8-20). However, only the duration of

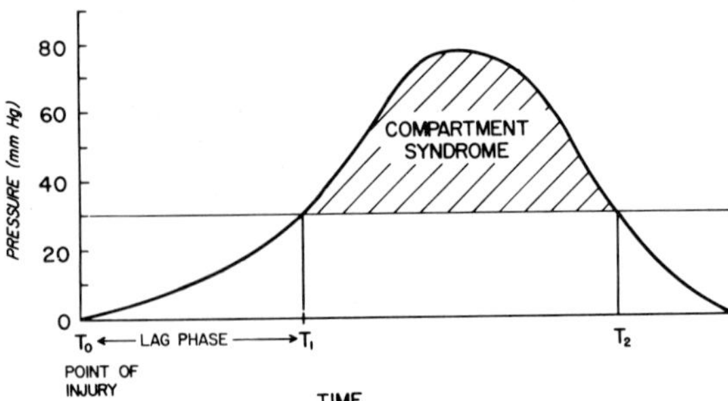

FIG. 8-20. The time between injury and the onset of findings of a compartment syndrome may vary from hours to days (lag phase T_0-T_1). Ischemia of the muscles and nerves of the compartment does not take place until the pressure rise is greater than 30 mm Hg (horizontal line). Thus, the time from injury to diagnosis and treatment is only a relative indicator of the ischemia unless one has monitored the tissue pressure from the point of injury. (With permission from Gelberman, et al.: Compartment syndromes of the forearm: diagnosis and treatment. Clin Orthop. *134*:225, 1978.)

the compartment syndrome can be influenced by the physician promptly treating the patient.

To prevent the complication of a Volkmann's contracture, the physician must have, above all, a high index of suspicion and an awareness of the cardinal signs and symptoms of a compartment syndrome. I recommend displaying a "Prevent Volkmann's" poster in the emergency room and on the wards as a reminder of this problem for house staff, nurses, and physicians (Fig. 8-21).

References

1. Sheridan, G. W., and Matsen, F. A.: Fasciotomy in the treatment of the acute compartment syndrome. J. Bone Joint Surg, *58A*:112, 1976.
2. Mubarak, S. J., and Hargens, A. R.: Unpublished data.
3. Wall, J. J.: Compartment syndrome as a complication of the Hauser procedure. J. Bone Joint Surg., *61A*:185, 1979.
4. Mubarak, S. J., and Carroll, N. C.: Volkmann's contracture in children: aetiology and prevention. J. Bone Joint Surg., *61-B*:285, 1979.
5. Mubarak, S. J., and Owen, C. A.: Compartmental syndrome and its relation to the crush syndrome: a spectrum of disease. Clin. Orthop., *113*:81, 1975.
6. Owen, C. A., et al.: Intramuscular pressures with limb compression: clarification of the pathogenesis of the drug-induced muscle-compartment syndrome. N. Engl. J. Med, *300*:1169, 1979.
7. Mubarak, S. J., et al.: Acute compartment syndromes; diagnosis and treatment with the aid of the wick catheter. J. Bone Joint Surg., *60-A*:1091, 1978.
8. Reneman, R. S.: The anterior and the lateral compartmental syndrome of the leg due to intensive use of muscles. Clin. Orthop., *113*:69, 1975.
9. Whitesides, T. E., Jr., Haney, T. C., Morimoto, K., and Hirada, H.: Tissue pressure measurements as a determinant for the need of fasciotomy. Clin. Orthop., *113*:43, 1975.
10. Matsen, F. A., Mayo, K. A., Sheridan, G. W., and Krugmire, R. B.: Monitoring of intramuscular pressure. Surgery, *79*:702, 1976.
11. Mubarak, S. J., et al.: The wick catheter technique for measurement of intramuscular pressure: a new research and clinical tool. J. Bone Joint Surg., *58-A*:1016, 1976.
12. Rorabeck, C. H., Castle, G. S. P., Hardie, R., and Logan, J.: The slit catheter: a new device for measuring intra-compartment pressure. Proc. Can. Orthop. Res. Soc., 14th Annual Meeting, Calgary, Canada, June 8–9, 1980, p. 12.
13. Matsen, F. A., Winquist, R. A., and Krugmire, R. B.: Diagnosis and management of compartmental syndromes. J. Bone Joint Surg., *62-A*:286, 1980.
14. Hargens, A. R., et al.: Fluid balance within the canine anterolateral compartment and its relationship to compartment syndromes. J. Bone Joint Surg., *60-A*:499, 1978.

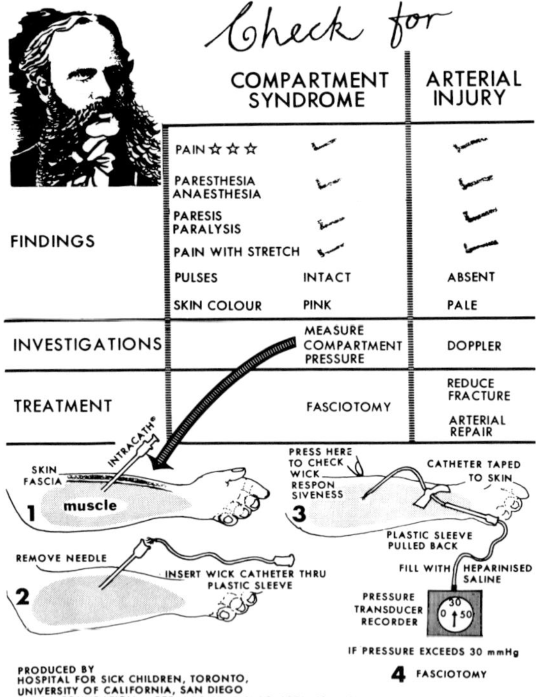

FIG. 8-21. Poster outlining the clinical findings, investigations, and treatment of compartment syndromes and arterial injuries. The poster is used to alert medical and nursing staff to the diagnosis and prevention of Volkmann's contracture. (Poster by Rang, M., Toronto, Ontario, Canada and Mubarak, S. J., San Diego, California.) (With permission from Mubarak, S. J., and Hargens, A. R.: Compartment Syndromes and Volkmann's Contracture. Philadelphia, W. B. Saunders, 1981.)

15. Hargens, A. R., et al.: Peripheral nerve conduction block by high muscle compartment pressure. J. Bone Joint Surg., *61-A*:192, 1979.
16. Hargens, A. R., et al.: Quantitation of skeletal-muscle necrosis in a model compartment syndrome. J. Bone Joint Surg. *63A*:631, 1981.
17. Mubarak, S. J., and Hargen, A. R.: Compartment Syndromes and Volkmann's Contracture. Philadelphia, W. B. Saunders, 1981.
18. Eichler, G. R., and Lipscomb, P. R.: The changing treatment of Volkmann's ischemic contractures from 1955 to 1965 at the Mayo Clinic. Clin. Orthop., *50*:215, 1967.
19. Eaton, R. G., and Green, W. T.: Epimysiotomy and fasciotomy in the treatment of Volkmann's ischemic contracture. Orthop. Clin. North Am., *3*:175, 1972.
20. Neumeyer, W. L., and Kilgore, E. S., Jr.: Volkmann's ischemic contracture due to soft tissue injury alone. J. Hand Surg., *1*:221, 1976.
21. Whitesides, T. E., Jr., Hirada, H., and Morimoto, K.: Compartment syndromes and the role of fasciotomy, its parameters and techniques. A.A.O.S. Instructional Course Lectures, *26*:179, 1977.
22. Gelberman, R. H., et al.: Decompression of forearm compartment syndromes. Clin. Orthop., *134*:225, 1978.
23. Kelly, R. P., and Whitesides, T. E., Jr.: Transfibular route for fasciotomy of the leg. J. Bone Joint Surg., *49A*:1022, 1967.
24. Ernst, C. B., and Kaufer, J.: Fibulectomy-fasciotomy: an important adjunct in the management of lower extremity arterial trauma. J. Trauma, *11*:365, 1971.
25. Patman, R. D., and Thompson, J. E.: Fasciotomy in peripheral vascular surgery. Arch. Surg., *101*:663, 1970.
26. Willhoite, D. R., and Moll, J. H.: Early recognition of impending Volkmann's ischemia in the lower extremity. Arch. Surg., *100*:11, 1970.
27. Mubarak, S. J., and Owen, C. A.: Double-incision fasciotomy of the leg for decompression in compartment syndromes. J. Bone Joint Surg., *59-A*:184, 1977.
28. Gelberman, R. H., et al.: Compartment syndromes of the forearm: diagnosis and treatment. Clin. Orthop., *161*: 252, 1981.
29. Henry, A. K.: Extensile Exposure Applied to Limb Surgery. Edinburgh, E. & S. Livingstone Ltd., 1950.

*Fasciotome—made by Down Surgical Company, Toronto, Ontario, Canada.

Chapter 9 Major Artery Trauma Associated with Fractures

WILLIAM J. FRY

Major trauma to a portion of an extremity with combined injuries to both the skeletal support and arterial supply is commonly encountered in the trauma center. Although we have seen major arterial disruption with fractures in all areas of the body, including the spine and pelvis, two areas are the most common and the most troublesome to the surgeon whose practice involves the trauma victim. Fractures in and about the area of the knee and the elbow consistently place the blood supply at jeopardy because of the close proximity of the vessels in these areas to the bony components. The arterial supply in these two areas is relatively fixed in its position because of multiple branches penetrating dense fascial compartments. Thus, the arterial conduit is disrupted easily by fractures and dislocations of these areas.

Initial Evaluation and Diagnosis

When vascular disruption occurs, time is of the essence. The pressure of time, however, should not deter the surgeon from performing a complete and careful evaluation of the patient. Initial therapy must include careful evaluation and resuscitation of the trauma victim (see previous chapters). In most instances, disruption of major neurovascular structures is obvious because of absence of distal pulses and loss of motor function distal to the injury. Because of the extent of the trauma or marked edema, there may be questionable findings. In this instance, the Doppler blood-flow meter may be helpful. Experience with the pocket Doppler meter gives the examining surgeon the ability to discern a normal signal from one dampened by obstruction, as well as to note the complete absence of any arterial signal. The novice should use the Doppler meter frequently to gain familiarity with the various signals that may be heard with normal and occluded arterial circulation. The triphasic sound characteristic of a normal pulse cannot be heard when a main arterial segment is disrupted or occluded.

Listening with a stethoscope over the area of injury is helpful, but is not highly diagnostic. In a recent review of all traumatic arteriovenous fistulae seen at Parkland Memorial Hospital, Dallas, Texas, only 18% had an audible bruit at the time of initial evaluation.[1]

Physicians treating patients with ischemia of an extremity distal to a fracture or a dislocation should attempt reduction to relieve any arterial entrapment.[2] Return of pulses with reduction of dislocation or with traction of the fracture signals the return of normal circulation. Again, this can be assessed by utilizing the Doppler meter and by careful examination of the distal pulses. The return of distal pulses does not rule out the possibility of arterial damage, and in most instances, the patient should be evaluated further. The greatest pitfall associated with the therapy of these patients is believing that some blood flow exists and that an expectant attitude should be taken. Most catastrophies are associated with the lack of an aggressive attitude toward evaluating the patient with marginal blood supply to the extremity.

In an extensive review conducted at this institution,[3] arteriography was found not only safe but accurate in the delineation of arterial injuries secondary to all types of extremity injuries. We feel that arteriography is mandatory in most instances in the evaluation of patients who have had an ischemic episode or who continue to have questionable circulation to the involved extremity. Although this procedure has been reported by some to be time consuming, the competent arteriographer can accomplish angiography quickly, and the problems facing the surgeon are demonstrated accurately in a way that cannot be accomplished by another technique. Utilization of arteriography allowed us to eliminate unnecessary vessel exploration and made operative procedures more expeditious. Most arteriograms should be done in two planes to outline accurately all aspects of the vessel in question. Arteriography has been exceedingly accurate, particularly in blunt injuries.

When the clear diagnosis of vascular disruption has been made, one should consider venography, particularly in injuries about the knee. Unattended venous obstruction jeopardizes the best arterial repair and, ultimately, the viability of the extremity. Thrombus within the vein is also a common finding. Venography helps to show the site of venous obstruction and, in addition, demonstrates accessory venous channels that may preclude the necessity of concomitant venous repair.[4]

Therapy

After careful evaluation of the patient and delineation of specific vascular disruption, injuries are treated on a priority basis, depending on their severity and life-threatening nature. In the occasional patient with massive multisystem trauma, an extremity may be sacrificed in an effort to save the patient's life. Certainly, long delays may take place for operations on the chest, abdomen, and head. These situations are rare, and the decision to sacrifice an extremity purposely is not a common occurrence. The pursuit of viability of an extremity in the presence of major life-threatening injuries is without value.

The treatment options in arterial injuries associated with fractures have been debated for a long time. Generally, we have taken the attitude that the viability of the extremity takes priority over the treatment and stabilization of the fracture. We make every attempt to re-establish arterial and venous blood flow first. Regardless of the efficiency of the emergency room and the trauma surgeons, hours usually have passed from the time of injury to the start of the operative procedure. The first priority should be dissection, through a medial approach, of the distal end of the disrupted artery (Fig. 9-1). Careful extraction of the thrombus should be carried out with the use of the Fogarty catheter. We then use an infusion of cold (4°C) Ringer's lactated solution, with 1000 units of heparin and 12½ g of mannitol per liter, in the distal arterial bed. This proce-

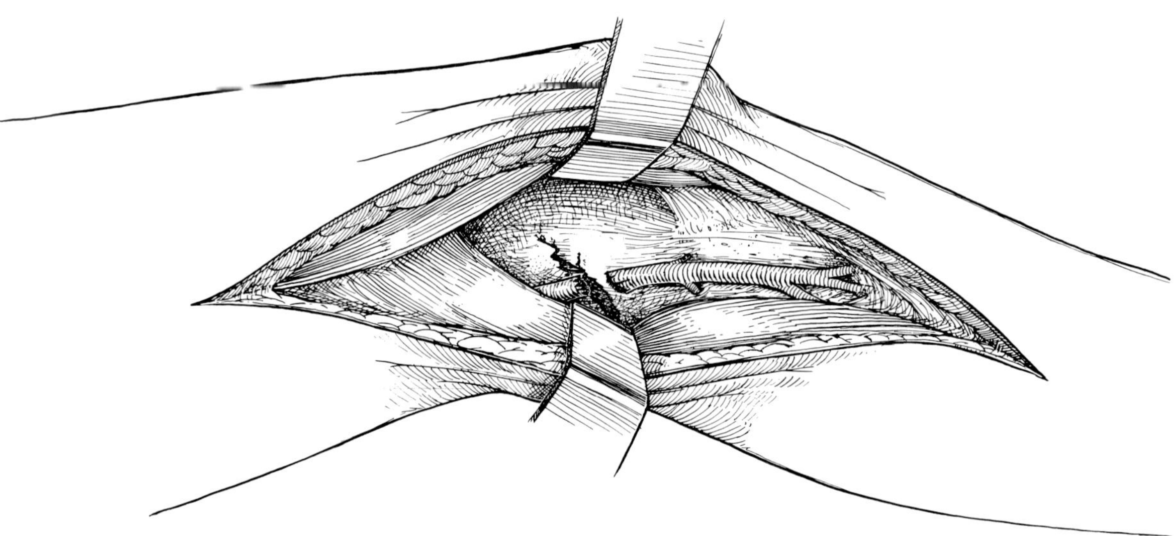

Fig. 9-1. The medial approach to the popliteal artery.

dure cools the extremity and prevents thrombosis of the capillary bed; the mannitol prevents excessive edema during the perfusion. The popliteal vein, if intact, should be vented to prevent infusion of large quantities of fluid into the systemic circulation. In massive injuries where venous disruption also has occurred, the effluent readily extravasates, allowing venous repair to be done prior to arterial reconstruction (Fig. 9-2, *A*, *B*). While the perfusion is being carried out, the proximal end of the disrupted artery can be dissected free and debrided. The decision is then made as to whether an end-to-end anastomosis can be performed or whether a vein graft must be utilized. In most instances of arterial disruption secondary to fracture and dislocations, the artery is damaged in such a way that a vein graft is necessary to bridge the gap between the two ends of the vessel.

Because of the crushing trauma involved in these injuries, the vessel must be debrided back to normal tissue. Once the proximal vessel has

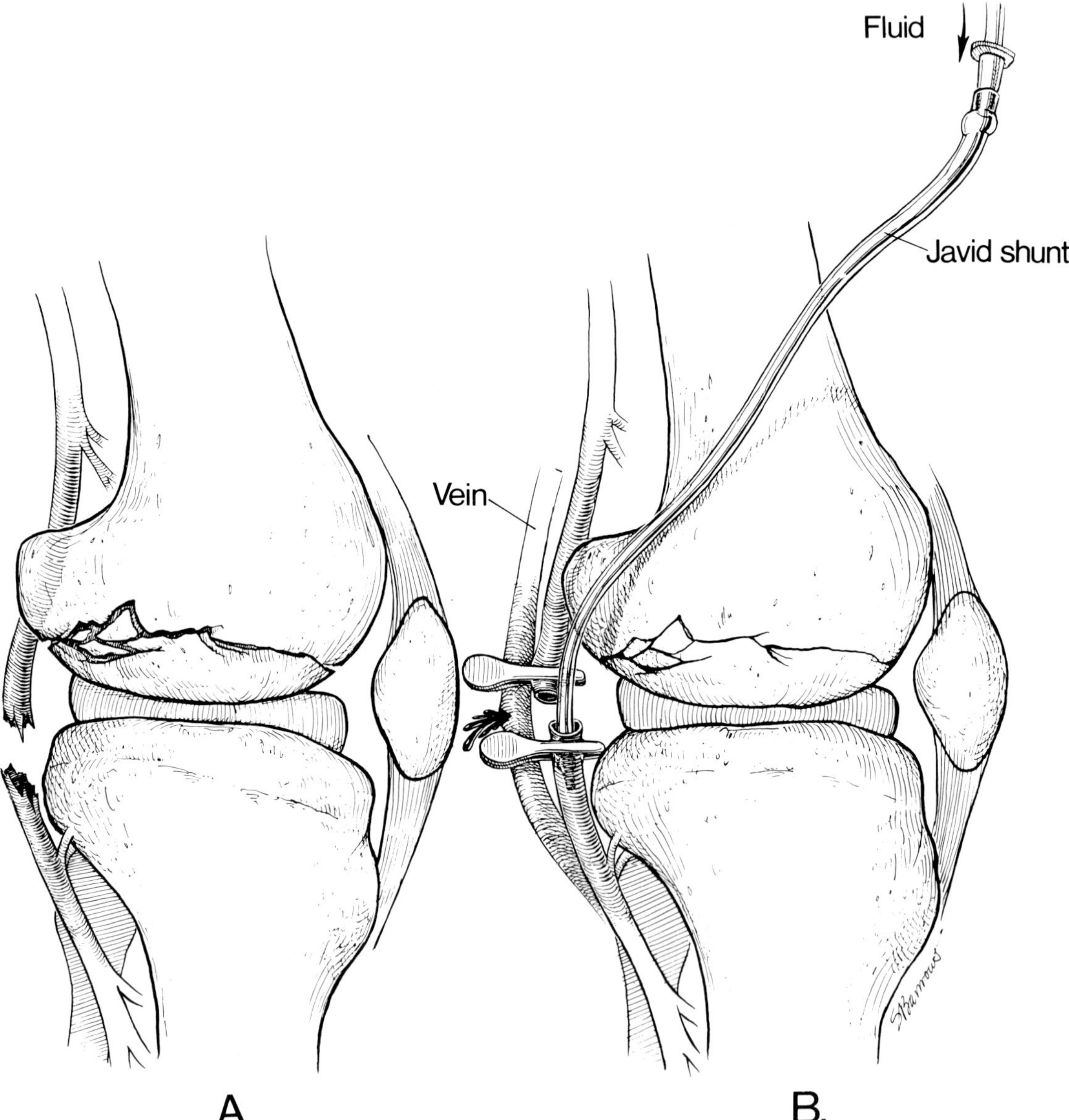

Fig. 9-2. *A* and *B*, Demonstration of perfusion technique utilized in popliteal artery disruption. Note venting of popliteal vein in *B*.

been dissected free, the use of the Fogarty catheter eliminates any thrombus that is present. If the patient cannot be totally anticoagulated with heparin because of multiple injuries, dilute heparin solution should be instilled in the distal end of the vessel and then occluded with a vascular clamp. This approach temporarily prevents thrombosis in this vessel and allows an opportunity to harvest a saphenous vein, if necessary. In crushing injuries of the extremity, a saphenous venous conduit from the other extremity should be used, if possible. This approach allows all possible venous return through normal channels and eliminates, as much as possible, the chance for venous hypertension and potential failure of arterial repair. Following the harvesting of the suitable vein, anastomoses are carried out in a routine fashion; care is taken to spatulate both the artery and the vein so that the anastomosis is approximately three times the circumference of the artery itself (Fig. 9-3 *A*, *B*, and *C*). This technique prevents narrowing at the suture line and subsequent stricture from scarring at the area of anastomosis. I have found this technique helpful in maintaining a patent anastomosis without subsequent stricture.

Long ischemic episodes invariably result in severe distal edema and subsequent compartment syndrome. We have found it useful to administer large doses of mannitol intravenously 10 minutes prior to the release of the arterial clamps and restoration of arterial circulation. Infusion of 20 g of mannitol at this time, with 10 g of mannitol given every hour thereafter for the subsequent 5 hours, virtually has eliminated the occurrence of the compartment syndrome in our patients with prolonged ischemia. An additional benefit from this use of mannitol is the safeguard against renal failure caused by myoglobulinemia.

Following the reinstitution of arterial blood flow and repair of any venous injury, an orderly approach to the fracture may be carried out. Care must be taken to safeguard against undue manipulation and stretching of any vascular anastomosis. With the utilization of vein graft replacement, such manipulation and stretching have not proved to be a problem in our experience. In extremities in which viability is questionable, we have chosen to leave the fracture unattended until the viability of the extremity can be defined clearly. The utilization of a posterior splint for stability of the fracture site has proved to be helpful and, at the same time, has allowed constant observation of the involved extremity. As was pointed out in Chapter 8, constant monitoring of the extremity for the occurrence of the compartment compression syndrome is mandatory, and extensive fasciotomy should be carried out when this problem occurs.

Avulsion and loss of soft tissue in and about the injured portion of the extremity occurs in some injuries. Every effort should be made to cover the vascular graft or anastomosis with viable tissue. This generally is possible, but may be difficult about the elbow and knee. We prefer to use a biologic dressing over the blood vessels to protect them from drying and infection.[5] Autograft skin is the best dressing possible in a wound that is relatively clean. In extremities in which viability of surrounding tissue is still in question because of trauma, we have utilized either homograft skin or pig skin as a dressing to promote healing and production of granulation tissue. These dressings diminish the possibility of local infection.

In some injuries about the elbow, vascular disruption does not occur. Vascular occlusion may occur without blood vessel disruption. Hemorrhage within a closed fascial space causes vessel compression and diminished blood flow. On the arteriogram, compression of the vessel shows tapering and attenuation of the major arterial conduit and has been likened to the appearance of spasm. Simple fasciotomy in the area of the elbow, with incision of the lacertus fibrosus, allows evacuation of thrombus with complete restoration of blood flow.

In rare instances when multiple trauma has caused spasm of a vessel because of direct injury in multiple areas, we have found injections of tolazine hydrochloride to be helpful.[6] A small catheter is inserted into the artery proximal to the area of injury, and 20 mg of tolazine hydrochloride are infused slowly every hour. This technique has been expedient in salvaging the multiply injured extremities by relieving the spasm attendant to direct trauma.

The most dreaded complication of traumatic injuries is the incidence of infection in the postoperative period with erosion of arterial anastomoses and/or vein graft interposition. Although infection cannot be eliminated totally, the utilization of wide debridement at the time of the operative procedure and frequent observation of the wound have cut down remarkably on the incidence of extreme infections. We believe this treatment, in combination with the routine use of a biologic dressing, has eliminated much of the

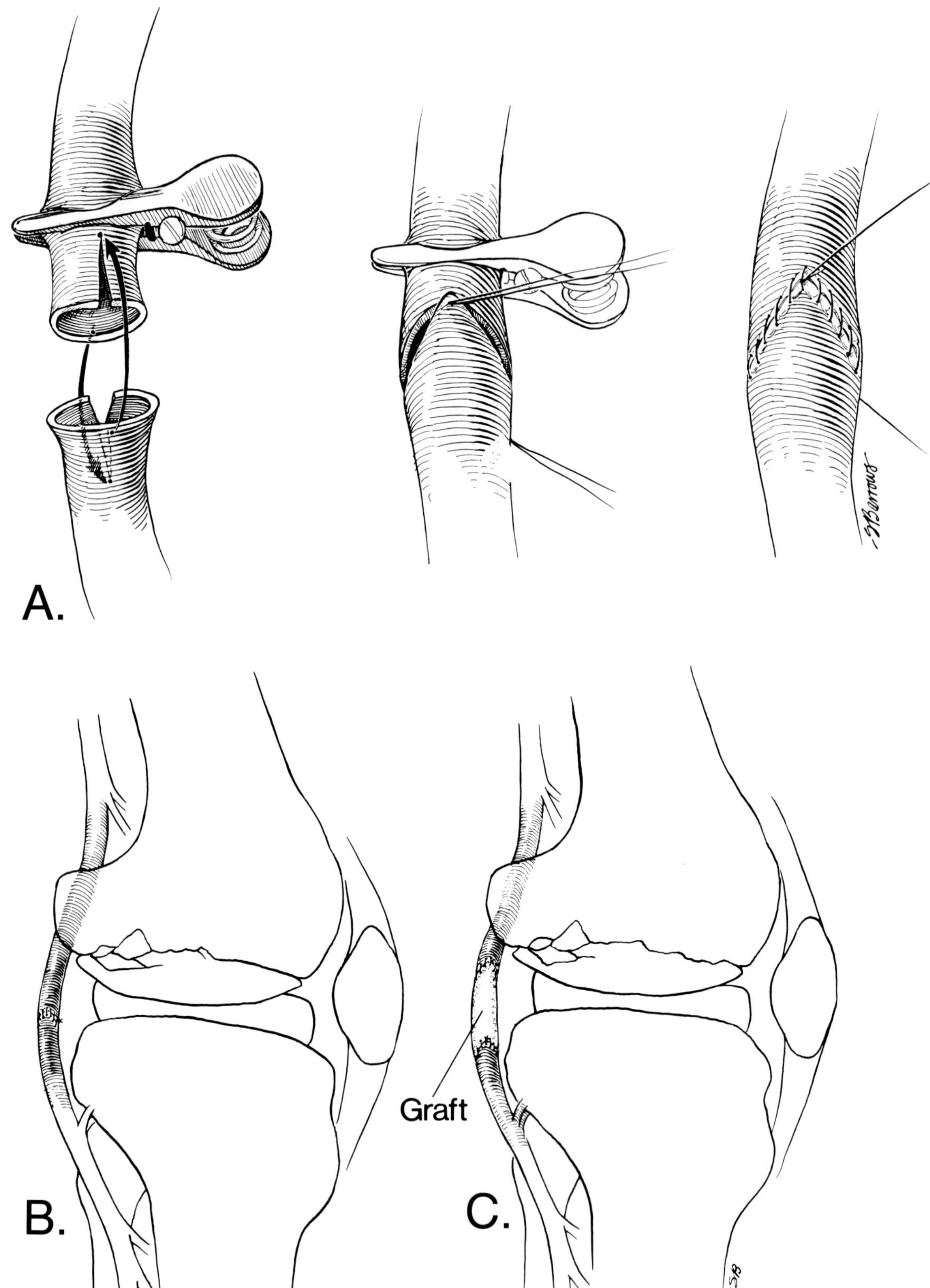

FIG. 9-3. Technique utilized in anastomosing small- and medium-sized arteries. Note the spatulation of the vessels to ensure a large circumference to prevent suture-line stenosis *(A)*. *B* and *C* depict completed anastomosis with an end-to-end repair and with a vein graft interposition.

difficulty encountered in the past with such problems.

The main reasons for thrombosis of an arterial anastomosis are:

1. Technical. With the institution of standard techniques in vascular surgery, this has virtually been eliminated.

2. Venous outflow problems. This thrombosis has been eluded to, and with the recognition of venous obstruction as a major cause of arterial graft failure, this problem should no longer be prominent.

3. Infection. Infection has been discussed. With care, the incidence of marked problems resulting from infection and subsequent necrosis of vascular anastomosis has been reduced. Again, the utilization of a biologic dressing is paramount in extremities with massive tissue loss.

4. Fracture instability. Although a potential cause of vascular disruption, fracture instability has not been a problem when care and cooperation between the vascular surgeon and the orthopaedic surgeon have been practiced. Delay in treatment of the fracture and stabilization of the extremity can be done safely without jeopardy. Care is taken to splint the fracture or dislocation site and to maintain observation of the operative wound.

The results of treatment of major arterial disruption associated with fractures and dislocations have been good, as pointed out by several authors. A recent review of all popliteal injuries at this institution revealed a limb salvage rate of over 85%.[7] The loss of extremities from severe ischemia because of delayed diagnosis and improper transportation has become a rarity.

References

1. Kollmeyer, K. R., Hunt, J. L., Ellman, B. A., and Fry, W. J.: Epidemiology and treatment of acute and chronic civilian traumatic arteriovenous fistulae. Arch. Surg. *116*:697, 1981.
2. Jones, R. E., Smith, E. C., and Bone, G. E.: Vascular and orthopedic complications of knee dislocations. Surg. Gynecol. Obstet., *149*:554, 1979.
3. Snyder, W. H., Thal, E. R., and Bridges, R. A.: The validity of normal arteriography in penetrating trauma. Arch. Surg., *113*:424, 1978.
4. Gerlock, A. J., Thal, E. R., and Snyder, W. H.: Venography in penetrating injuries of the extremity. A. J. R., *126*:1023, 1976.
5. Legerwood, A. M., and Lucas, C. E.: Biological dressings for exposed vascular grafts: a reasonable alternative. J. Trauma, *15*:567, 1975.
6. Dickerman, R. M., Gewertz, B. L., Foley, D. W., and Fry, W. J.: Selective intraarterial tolazoline infusion in peripheral arterial trauma. Surgery, *81*:605, 1977.
7. Snyder, W. H., Watkins, W. L., Whiddon, L. L., and Bone, G. E.: Civilian popliteal artery trauma: an eleven-year experience with 83 injuries. Surgery, *85*:101, 1979.

Chapter 10 Anesthetic Considerations in the Multiply Injured Adult

BRIAN R. MILNE
M. T. JENKINS

The anesthesiologist's most critical and fundamental role is as part of the hospital accident team dealing with the immediate care of critically injured patients.[1] The traumatized patient scheduled for an emergency operation presents many anesthetic or physiologic problems that are not commonly encountered during elective procedures for prepared patients. Airway problems may be compounded by food in the stomach that is not removed readily by a gastric tube. Further, the tracheobronchial tree already may have been transgressed by silent aspiration during a period of unconsciousness, hypotension, or nonresponsiveness. The patient's ability to breathe may be impaired greatly by injuries specifically encroaching on the upper airway, as in maxillofacial trauma. Damages to the chest wall or to the myocardium may not appear significant, and breath sounds may be present bilaterally until a pneumothorax develops during controlled ventilation or until arrhythmias develop during the course of anesthesia.

Unusual diagnostic skill may be needed to assess associated injuries with physiologic effects that are evidenced only after an operation has progressed in other anatomic areas. For example, during an operation involving extremity fractures, hemorrhage from a lacerated spleen or fractured liver may be minimal as the procedure begins, but may impose important diagnostic questions when hypotension ensues.

During assessment of the multiply injured patient, problems may arise in establishing priorities of sites for operative intervention.

When the severely injured patient is admitted to the emergency room for resuscitation and then is brought directly to the operating room, it is difficult, if not impossible, to obtain an adequate history of pre-existing diseases, allergies, or the nature of chronic drug therapy. Many drugs commonly utilized by patients exert effects on basic homeostatic mechanisms. These effects are compensated for in various ways by the noninjured or nonanesthetized individual, but trauma and anesthesia may severely attenuate the patient's compensatory mechanisms for such drug effects.

A percentage of the traumatized patients is in either a hypometabolic or a hypermetabolic state. The effects of trauma and the responses of the patient to anesthesia at either extremity of metabolic balance require precise diagnosis and exacting care to prevent serious intraoperative or postoperative complications.

Often, a question arises about whether to proceed at once with a corrective operation or to delay while assessing and correcting the full extent of the patient's deranged physiology. Immediate surgical intervention is indicated for patients who are actively bleeding, who have unresolved airway obstruction, and who have penetrating abdominal wounds or compound fractures. Anesthetic problems may be minimized, however, when a definitive surgical procedure for most other trauma is delayed (usually not more than 6 hours) until cardiovascular or respiratory dynamics are re-established, adequate diagnostic information is obtained, and treatment of associated conditions is initiated.[2]

In a 1-year study during which anesthesia was administered to 1161 patients with acute trauma, the overall mortality rate was 5.34%. However, the relative contribution of anesthetic factors to this figure cannot be identified accurately.[3] The mortality rate among patients with pre-existing disease was 7.2%. This mortality rate cannot be applied nationally because of many factors that lie outside the actual anesthetic experience. As more communities employ emergency medical technicians who begin resuscitation of victims at the geographic locale of injury, an increasing number of patients will reach the hospital alive to be further resuscitated in emergency rooms staffed by full-time, trained, emergency physicians. For many patients, the subsequent course will be improved, perhaps reducing the mortality rates.

In the present era, trauma is the leading cause of death among Americans of both sexes from ages 1 to 45 years; it ranks fourth as a cause of death in all age groups. Anesthesiologists must recognize and understand the special problems posed by the trauma victim. The orthopaedist must recognize the contribution to patient care made by the anesthetic procedure, as well as the inherent dangers and limitations of anesthesia. The potential contribution of the practicing anesthesiologist to the overall care of the trauma patient has been well summarized by Baskett, who emphasizes the anesthesiologist's participation in the accident and emergency services at all stages.[4]

Assessment

Before selecting an anesthetic agent or technique, a rapid assessment of the patient must be made. A decision must be made either to accept the patient for immediate anesthesia and operation or to delay if there is time for further resuscitation and preparation. Those accepted immediately without further indicated preoperative preparation usually include patients with unchecked hemorrhage, obstructed airway, penetrating wounds of the abdomen, and/or compound fractures.

Lack of Full Preanesthetic Evaluation

In the preparation of a patient for an elective operative procedure, a careful history and physical examination should reveal pre-existing diseases of the respiratory system, cardiovascular system, endocrine system, liver, and kidneys. Special attention can be paid to the detection of such disease entities as diabetes mellitus, hyperthyroidism, emphysema, asthma, coronary artery disease, treated hypertension, cirrhosis, and chronic renal failure. Also, a history of allergies can be elicited, particularly those involving unusual responses to barbiturates, antibiotics, and narcotics. Many patients on the elective schedule cannot identify the drugs they use on a regular basis, but in taking the history, emphasis should be placed on any ongoing patient therapy with antihypertensives, diuretics, drugs to treat cardiac diseases, steroids, and antibiotics.

When an adequate history and physical examination cannot be conducted, a rapid determination of trauma status can be made while applying and inserting devices for extensive monitoring of several physiologic parameters (Table 10-1). The extent of hemorrhage and circulating blood volume may be estimated; ventilation and cardiac status and the presence of a urine output can be determined rapidly by monitors (Table 10-1).[5]

Presence of Multiple Injuries

It has been stated that 20% of all trauma patients have multiple injuries,[6] but in cases resulting from motor vehicle accidents, multiple injuries are found in 65% of patients.[7] Because some injuries may be unrecognized at the time of induction of anesthesia, the anesthesiologist must be aware and suspicious of common patterns of injury and their diagnosis and management. For example, if operative blood loss is minimal during a procedure on a lower extremity, but physical signs are consistent with vascular instability, the team should rule out intra-abdominal blood loss, as from a ruptured spleen or liver, and developing pneumothorax or hemothorax.

Presence of Airway and Ventilation Difficulties

A wide range of injuries can cause respiratory obstruction, hypoventilation, or both. Such injuries include trauma to the face, jaw, or upper airway; aspiration of foreign bodies, such as teeth or food; and injuries to the neck or chest resulting in airway distortion or compression producing a pneumothorax, hemothorax, flail chest, and/or paradoxic respirations. Moreover, a depressed conscious level secondary to head injury, intoxication, or shock may also cause hypoventilation in the trauma victim. Any of these circumstances represents compelling reasons for introducing an

TABLE 10-1. *The Physical Signs and Symptoms Commonly Seen in Previously Healthy Patients with Hemorrhagic Shock, Classified as Trauma Status I, II, and III.*[5]

	Status I	*Status II*	*Status III*
Respiratory system			
Respiratory distress	no distress	mild distress	severe distress
Blood gases	normal	abnormal $Pa_{O_2} \downarrow$ $Pa_{CO_2} \downarrow$	abnormal $Pa_{O_2} \downarrow\downarrow$ $Pa_{CO_2} \downarrow$ or $\uparrow$
Cardiovascular system			
Blood pressure	no change	decreased	not measurable
Central venous pressure	normal or $\uparrow$	decreased	marked decrease
Pulse	normal or $\uparrow$	mild increase	marked increase
Peripheral circulation	slight decrease	moderate decrease	marked decrease
Urinary system			
Urine output	normal	decreased	absent
Central nervous system	normal	disoriented	impaired consciousness $\downarrow$ coma
Blood loss	$<10\%$	$\approx 30\%$	$>50\%$

artificial airway. Either orotracheal or nasotracheal intubation may be used, depending on the reflex responsiveness of the patient, location of the injury, and type of surgical repair indicated. Even when tracheostomy is surgically indicated, the patient's physical status may be improved by assisted or controlled ventilation with oxygen through an endotracheal tube while deliberately and carefully carrying out the surgical maneuver of tracheostomy.

If the maxillofacial damage is of such severity to preclude introduction of an endotracheal tube from above, oxygenation of the patient can be carried out by high-volume flows of oxygen through an 18- or 15-gauge needle introduced into the tracheal lumen through the cricothyroid membrane. An adult patient cannot ventilate for himself through an 18-gauge needle if this is the sole source of airway for spontaneous respiration, but oxygenation of the blood can be restored by insufflation through a transcricothyroid needle if the structure of the lung has not been disrupted by the patient's primary trauma. If the patient does not have complete subglottic obstruction, the chest will not be overinflated by a high flow of oxygen through the cricothyroid needle. Because of the concavity of the structure of the larynx from the subglottic approach, the vocal cords open in response to increasing pressure in the tracheobronchial tree. Performance of a tracheostomy can proceed with care while controlled ventilation is carried out by the transcricothyroid insufflation.

A tracheostomy must be performed at some stage in the operative care of the patient with jaw fractures, a nasal injury or fracture, and intact teeth. Blood clots and edema of nasal passages prevent postoperative nasal breathing. If the patient's jaws are wired together and if he has a full set of teeth, he will be able to breathe only with continued concentrated effort; if several teeth are missing, the patient will be able to maintain his airway only if he learns automatically to keep his lips apart.

If an endotracheal tube can be introduced, the surgical opening of the trachea is usually best deferred until the corrective operation for the pirmary trauma has been accomplished.

Extent of Injury and Hemorrhage

The signs of hypovolemia should be sought and the degree of shock assessed. Table 10-1 describes the physical signs and symptoms commonly exhibited in previously healthy patients with hemorrhagic shock, here classified as trauma status I, II, and III. Note that, in geriatric patients and those with pre-existing disease, the same signs may appear with lesser degrees of blood loss. Furthermore, normovolemic patients may simulate the signs of shock as a result of injury to the spinal cord, pneumothorax, or cardiac tamponade. The interests of the patient are served best by attempting to restore normovolemia and hematocrit prior to the induction of anesthesia, but one must recognize that surgical intervention must take precedence on occasion.

Intoxication

The patient's vital signs, behavior, and subsequent anesthetic management may be modified by intoxication with alcohol or other drugs. More than half of the motor vehicle accidents in the United States directly involve intoxicated drivers.[8,9] Further, one study of drinking drivers revealed that 21% had been simultaneous users of other drugs.[10] Further care of the intoxicated patient is described in the section entitled Special Situations.

Presence of Potential "Full Stomach"

All trauma patients should be considered at risk of regurgitating gastric contents, and appropriate measures should be instituted to prevent contamination of the tracheobronchial tree. Significant morbidity and mortality arise from the dangers of inhalation of gastric contents, immediate obstructive or bronchospastic symptoms, and delayed pneumonitis. The rate of gastric emptying is reduced markedly following injury, and delay of operation for the traditional 6 hours from the time of last oral intake probably has little effect on the volume of gastric contents. Of more importance is the time interval from the last meal to the time of injury, when gastric motility usually ceases.

General Principles of Anesthetic Management

The general principles for the successful management of the multiply injured patient are as follows.

Premedication

It is probably safest to withhold premedication in the patient undergoing an urgent operation or in whom physiologic derangements have not been corrected. In general, oral premedicants are contraindicated in the nonelective patient, since their systemic effects are unpredictable in the presence of delayed gastric emptying. Small doses of intravenous analgesics may be prescribed under strict supervision provided no contraindication exists, such as head injury or respiratory embarrassment. Barbiturates have no real role in the course of treatment as they may lead to disorientation of and combativeness by the patient in the presence of pain.

There are fewer indications now for anticholinergic drugs as part of the premedication schedule. If they are utilized, intravenous administration prior to induction is the preferable method. Atropine, scopolamine, and glycopyrrolate decrease the tone of the lower esophageal sphincter and thus make regurgiation of gastric contents more likely.[11] General anesthetic agents in use today have minimal sialogogic effects; consequently, the need for routine use of a drying agent has decreased.

There is a good indication for the oral administration of preinduction antacids; the one major contraindication is proven or suspected penetrating injury of the gastrointestinal tract. The rationale for their use lies in the observation that the severity of aspiration pneumonitis is reduced markedly when the pH of the inhaled gastric contents is greater than 2.5. Milk of magnesia in an oral dose of 30 ml has been shown to be an effective antacid when given 10 to 80 minutes prior to the induction of anesthesia.[12] Preinduction antacids do not provide the complete answer to the problem of significant aspiration, a condition associated with a mortality rate of 28%.[13]

Technique

In the majority of multiply injured patients requiring operative intervention, general anesthesia is the technique of choice because of the need to control respiration. Spinal anesthesia may be the choice for patients with traumatized lower extremities if the central nervous system is not involved, if the blood volume has been replaced, or if the patient is not intoxicated or otherwise unmanageable. Generally, spinal anesthesia is contraindicated in problems associated with severe hypovolemia.

Regional blocks, such as sciatic-femoral for lower extremity work or brachialplexus for upper extremity operations, can be utilized. Administration of intravenous regional anesthesia (Bier's local antesthesia) is a simple and easily learned technique with a gratifyingly high rate of success. For operating on the forearm of an adult, an intravenous block can be accomplished with 30 ml of 0.5% lidocaine injected below a tourniquet after the extremity has been partially exsanguinated by using an Esmarch's type of bandage.

A larger volume, such as 50 ml of 0.5% lidocaine, may be used similarly for lower extremity blocks.[14]

General anesthesia is preferred when trauma is severe or when the head, neck, or trunk is involved in addition to an extremity. The anesthesiologist should select agents and techniques that tend to facilitate resuscitation or that produce such minimal changes that resuscitation can be carried out more successfully. The first consideration should be to ensure that the combined effects of the preoperative trauma and the anesthesia will have the least depressant effects on the basic mechanisms of respiratory, cardiovascular, and metabolic compensation. The details of individual anesthetic techniques are not discussed in this chapter, but a general anesthetic method should be chosen and altered as indicated by the patient's physical and fluid status, the nature and extent of the proposed operation, and the presence of specific contraindications to a particular technique.

The advantages of local or regional anesthesia include diminished physiologic upset to the patient, lower risk of aspiration of gastric contents, and good pain relief without use of narcotics, thus allowing continuous observation for the presence of suspected head or abdominal injuries.

Monitoring

The anesthesiologist's role in monitoring the condition of the trauma patient is of vital importance, and, indeed, in the massively traumatized, severely hypotensive patient, the anesthesiologist's role may be solely that of monitoring and applying resuscitation while withholding anesthesia. The extent of monitoring depends in large part on the clinical condition of the patient and on the facilities available.

General Condition

In addition to utilizing sophisticated monitoring devices, the experienced anesthesiologist also employs simple measures, such as observation of skin color and turgor, capillary refill time in the nail beds and skin over the forehead, quality of the peripheral pulses, and respiratory efforts.

Blood Pressure

In many cases, measurement of the blood pressure by the traditional sphygmomanometer and stethoscope is adequate. An oscillometer tends to give a greater degree of accuracy at lower levels of blood pressure. The automatic electronic oscillometer is a useful device in the emergency situation because it frees the anesthesiologist for other maneuvers. Direct cannulation of a peripheral artery with electronic display of the blood pressure has become a valuable technique, although it is not without the hazards of temporary radial artery thrombosis and thromboembolism.[15] The radial, ulnar, or dorsalis pedis arteries may be cannulated with a 20- to 22-gauge Teflon cannula, nontapered, "over-the-needle" catheter, which is regarded as the least dangerous technique.[16] Arterial cannulation is useful in rapidly fluctuating clinical conditions and for intermittent sampling of arterial blood gases; it is essential for the management of patients undergoing cardiopulmonary bypass operations.

Respiratory Function

Simple measures, such as observation of skin and blood color, respiratory movements, and ventilator gauges, provide useful information. Heart and breath sounds can be auscultated through precordial or esophageal stethoscopes. Assessment of alveolar ventilation by expired air capnographs or arterial blood-gas analysis is a useful maneuver.

Urine Output

All trauma patients with moderate to severe injuries should have a urinary catheter inserted, and urine output should be measured every 30 to 60 minutes. A urine flow of at least 0.5 to 1 ml/kg of body weight should be achieved through expansion of the extracellular fluid volume.

Electrocardiogram

The ECG should be used in all cases since it provides information on cardiac arrhythmias, myocardial ischemia, electrolyte anomalies, and the effects of drugs.

Temperature

All trauma patients require monitoring of the core temperature, since hypothermia is a frequent complication of trauma surgery. Elevations of temperature are much less common, but may occur secondary to febrile or hemolytic transfusion reactions, sepsis, or the malignant hyperthermia syndrome. These conditions must be detected early for appropriate therapy to have a chance for success. Esophageal temperature reflects the temperature at the heart, and a nasopharyngeal or tympanic probe gives an indication of brain temperature.

Fluid Balance

Estimates of blood loss, both preoperatively and intraoperatively, frequently are erroneous. Recourse often is made to serial measurements of the hematocrit, which may be erroneously high if the balanced salt solution infused is not equal to the translocated extracellular fluid volume. In general, adequacy of fluid replacement can be assessed on the basis of the patient's general condition, blood pressure, and urine output.

When significant blood loss has occurred, or massive fluid infusion is necessary, more sophisticated measurement techniques may be required. Serial measurements of central venous pressure (CVP) may provide a useful index of fluid replacement, but there are limitations to the technique.[17,18] Physiologists suggest that a low CVP indicates that the patient's blood volume is too low for the capacity of his vascular system, particularly that of the venous reservoir, which normally contains at least 50% of the total blood volume. There is also evidence that substantial fluctuations of blood volume sometimes occur without accompanying changes in CVP. Changes in CVP may not occur partly because of the inherently large compliance of the venous reservoir and partly because of the action of cardiovascular reflexes, which adjust venous tone in response to changes of cardiac output and arterial blood pressure. Physiologists further suggest that a high CVP indicates either hypervolemia or failure of the cardiac pump. A high CVP measurement should be interpreted with care and in relation to other monitoring parameters.

Cannulaton of a central vein via the external jugular vein, aided by a J-wire, is used frequently to monitor central venous pressure.[19] Morbidity of this technique is low. Management of the fluid balance of critically ill patients and those with disparity of right and left ventricular function may be assisted by the use of a pulmonary artery flotation catheter (Swan-Ganz). Insertion of a flotation catheter in the opening sequences of massive trauma management usually is not practical.[20]

Miscellaneous

For the patient with major trauma, serial measurements of acid-base status and coagulation studies are indicated, particularly when large volumes of fluid or blood have been administered or when low output states or hypothermia have existed. Other useful monitors in certain contexts include intracranial pressure monitors and peripheral nerve stimulators.

Induction and Intubation

The anesthesiologist should assume that the trauma victim has a full stomach or, at least, a nonemptied stomach and, therefore, is at high risk of regurgitating gastric contents, either actively by vomiting or passively under anesthesia as esophageal sphincters relax. During anesthesia, the tracheobronchial system should be isolated from the gastrointestinal system by the use of a cuffed endotracheal tube. The critical period most often is the induction-intubation time.

Two techniques are widely used for induction and intubation in the emergency patient—either the rapid-sequence induction and intubation method or the awake intubation technique.[21]

The rapid-sequence induction (colloquially and undesirably known as "crash induction") involves a specific series of events undertaken at the induction of general anesthesia and developed to minimize the period from loss of consciousness to protection of the airway. Preoxygenation for at least 5 minutes is desirable to replace pulmonary nitrogen, thereby providing a small reservoir of oxygen during the period of apnea following drug induction. During this interval, nasogastric tubes should be aspirated as thoroughly as possible and may then be withdrawn and not replaced until after successful tracheal intubation. Whether one should remove the nasogastric tube is a debatable question, and indications for or against removal are not absolute.[22]

Two minutes prior to induction, a small dose of a nondepolarizing relaxant (d-tubocurarine or pancuronium) is given to reduce the fasciculations commonly associated with the depolarizing block of succinylcholine. Anesthesia is induced either with an "ultra-short-acting" thiobarbiturate for the patient exhibiting vasomotor stability or with the phencyclidine congener, ketamine, for the patient with less stabilized blood pressure. Muscle relaxation to facilitate endotracheal intubation is provided by succinylcholine given immediately following the induction agent.

As soon as consciousness is lost, an assistant should apply cricoesophageal compression (Sellick maneuver)[23] and should maintain this pressure until the airway is protected by inflation of the cuff of the endotracheal tube. When the airway is secured, anesthesia can be maintained with appropriate agents. Cricoid pressure reduces but does not eliminate the likelihood of regurgitation, particularly if inexpertly applied.[24]

Intubation of awake patients, in contrast, allows the patient to control his airway and maintain intact his protective reflexes. This type of intubation probably is indicated when any difficulty with laryngoscopy and intubation is anticipated, especially in the presence of partial airway obstruction or distorted anatomy. High bowel obstruction is another relative indication. Contraindications to this type of intubation include patients with penetrating wounds of the neck, penetrating eye injuries, or elevated intracranial pressure. The oral or nasal route may be employed. Topical anesthesia is applied to successive parts of the upper airway to allow gentle insertion of the endotracheal tube, with or without the aid of a laryngoscope, while avoiding full depression of the protective laryngeal reflexes. Small amounts of sedative medications, such as diazepam, may be given intravenously to produce a tranquil and sedated yet conscious patient. If the nasal route is chosen, local vasoconstriction is useful to reduce the chance of hemorrhage caused by the tracheal tube. Once the endotracheal tube is in place, general anesthesia can be induced rapidly by the intravenous route.

The massively traumatized, hypotensive patients of trauma status III may be so critically ill that their pain appreciation and basic reflexes are depressed to such an extent that they offer minimal resistance to awake laryngoscopy without adjuvant therapy.

At the conclusion of surgery, the endotracheal tube should be left in place until the patient has recovered consciousness and has competent laryngeal reflexes. If the patient is judged to require postoperative ventilation, the tube should remain in place even longer.

Maintenance of Anesthesia

Many techniques are available for maintenance of general anesthesia in the trauma patient. There are good indications for the nitrous oxide relaxant technique, in which neuromuscular blocking drugs are used to produce an immobile, compliant patient with muscular relaxation in the presence of so-called ''light'' anesthesia. Advantages include excellent muscle relaxation for intra-abdominal surgery and the facilitation of artificial ventilation, which allows the anesthesiologist to control ventilation when hypoventilation could otherwise occur in the traumatized patient. Though artificial ventilation is not without hazard, the nitrous oxide relaxant technique, aptly described as providing minimum physiologic trespass, is suited particularly to the needs of the trauma victim requiring general anesthesia in whom intravenous narcotics can be added for analgesia.

Pharmacologic Considerations

Induction Agents

Sodium pentothal is the standard intravenous induction agent and is well tolerated by the low-risk, well-hydrated patient. All short-acting barbiturates cause direct depression of myocardial contractility; the degree depends on the dose administered and the rate of injection. They do not significantly alter systemic vascular resistance but markedly increase the capacitance of the peripheral venous system. In the normal individual, therefore, induction of anesthesia with thiopental sodium (Pentothal) causes mild arterial hypotension but little change in the cardiac index. However, when hypovolemia, heart disease, or adverse posture exists, normally safe doses of thiopental sodium may prove too depressant to the heart. There is little difference between the two popular barbiturates, thiopental sodium (Pentothal) and methohexital sodium (Brevital), although following equipotent anesthetic doses, the latter may maintain cardiac index to a slightly higher degree.[25]

Ketamine is a so-called dissociative anesthetic agent that can be used intravenously or intramuscularly for the induction of general anesthesia. It is unique among induction agents in that it is reported to stimulate cardiac performance in the absence of other drugs affecting the cardiovascular or central nervous systems.

Typical responses in unpremedicated patients given the usual intravenous induction doses of ketamine are an increased cardiac output of 41%, an increased mean arterial pressure of 23%, and an increased heart rate of 33% occurring within 5 minutes.[26] The increase in cardiac output is secondary to both positive inotropic and chronotropic effects on the heart; left ventricular filling pressure does not change.[27]

Therefore, in the hypovolemic patient or in the inadequately resuscitated patient, induction of anesthesia by ketamine is preferable to induction with a thiobarbiturate drug.

Muscle Relaxants

The depolarizing relaxant, succinylcholine, produces a paralysis of rapid onset and short duration and thus is the relaxant of choice in the "rapid-sequence induction." Following the depolarizing block of succinylcholine in the normal individual, the level of serum potassium rises approximately 0.5 mEq/L. Such an increase is transient and of little consequence. Marked rises of levels of serum potassium, with the possibility of subsequent serious cardiac arrhythmias, can occur after the administration of succinylcholine to patients with severe crush injuries, multiple trauma with muscle drainage, burns, and recent acute spinal-cord transections. The drug probably is safe in the immediate post-injury period.[28] Care must also be exercised when using succinylcholine in the presence of a penetrating eye injury because it increases intraocular as well as intracranial pressure and may cause extrusion of the ocular vitreous.

Of the nondepolarizing, long-acting muscle relaxants used for paralysis in the nitrous oxide relaxant technique, pancuronium is the agent of choice in the trauma victim because of its useful cardiovascular effects. Most studics of thc hemodynamic effects of pancuronium in human beings show moderate stimulation, including a rise in heart rate of 22% and in cardiac output of 8%.[29] Moreover, pancuronium given in sufficiently large doses provides intubating conditions immediately after injection comparable to those of succinylcholine, and it does not increase intraocular or intracranial pressure. Pancuronium, therefore, is a useful alternative agent when even a minor increase in intraocular or intracranial pressure is contraindicated.

Narcotics

These powerful analgesics often are used as adjuvant drugs in general anesthetic techniques. In the main, they have few adverse cardiovascular effects. The synthetic derivative, fentanyl, is a potent, short-acting agent with even less propensity than morphine to cause hypotension in the patient whose extracellular fluid status has not been restored. It can be given to the trauma patient in small increments for analgesia.

Inhalational Anesthetic Agents

The most commonly used vapors, halothane and ethrane, are potent myocardial depressants and, to a lesser extent, exert peripheral vasodilator action. A depressed cardiac output can be anticipated when using these agents in the presence of hypovolemia. The relatively weak gas, nitrous oxide, is also a myocardial depressant. In a study involving healthy volunteers, 40% nitrous oxide in oxygen produced a reduction in cardiac output of 15 to 20% due to decreases in heart rate and contractility. However, systemic vascular resistance in these subjects rose by 20%, and consequently, the overall effect on systemic blood pressure was minimal.[30]

Fluid Therapy

Perioperative fluid administration in the multiply injured patient is one of the more important resuscitative roles of the anesthesiologist. (The literature covering this subject is vast, and for more comprehensive reviews, the reader is referred to recent publications.[31])

Essentially, fluid administration includes balanced salt solutions plus whole blood or blood components as dictacted by the clinical situation. Fluid therapy strives to restore blood pressure to a level deemed normal for that patient, to attain a cardiac output appropriate to the patient's metabolic demands, and to maintain a hematocrit at an acceptable level with normovolemic hemodilution. Oxygen transport capacity reaches its maximum at a hematocrit value of 30% and falls below the baseline value only when the hematocrit falls to 20 to 25%. Improvement in oxygen transport capacity implies also improvement in the tissue oxygen supply as a result of the improved rheologic properties of diluted blood.[32]

The rationale for the use of balanced salt solutions (BSS) has been summarized recently by Giesecke.[33]

1. In response to trauma, obligatory edema occurs in the injured areas of the body; its magnitude depends on the extent of injury, blood loss, and surgical manipulation.
2. The edema is formed at the expense of healthy extravascular extracellular fluid, intracellular fluid, and plasma volume.
3. A deficit occurs in the healthy functional extracellular fluid (ECF) as a result of the contribution to the edema space.
4. Balanced salt solutions are given to correct the deficit of function ECF.
5. After appropriate resuscitation, the patient gains an amount weight approximately equivalent to the volume of the acutely sequestered edema.

6. During the phase of resolution, usually 2 to 4 days post-injury, the edema is mobilized from the injured area and is lost as urine in the stage of diuresis.

Volume therapy with both BBS and blood or components should be administered until a satisfactory cardiovascular status has been attained. To this end, intraoperative monitoring is crucial. An acceptable blood pressure, heart rate, central venous pressure, urine output, and, if available, pulmonary wedge pressure are sought.

For hemorrhagic shock, 1 to 2 L of balanced salt solution given rapidly correct hypotension when blood losses of 20% or less have been sustained by adults. When blood loss is severe or continuing, the beneficial effects of the quantity of BSS are transient and vital signs deteriorate again. By this time, however, type-specific whole blood usually is available for transfusion along with the continued infusion of BSS.

Depending on the extent of surgical manipulation, balanced salt solutions are continued at a rate of 10 ml/kg of body weight/hour, with careful monitoring of the vital signs, urine output, and, if available, central venous pressure.

Packed red blood cells are given when blood loss exceeds 15 to 20% of the estimated blood volume, or earlier if hematocrit is less than 25% or if signs of shock are present. Packed cells are commonly diluted with saline to a volume of approximately 500 ml to facilitate rapid administration.

In addition to their effectiveness in the role of temporary support of the circulation, balanced salt solutions are inexpensive, nontoxic, isotonic, and easily stored.

Resuscitation with massive quantities of BSS leads to transient hyponatremia and dilution of clotting factors and platelets. Replacement with packed cells or less-than-fresh whole blood does not correct these deficiencies. Further therapy should include administration of 2 units of fresh frozen plasma and 2 units of platelets with every 10 units of packed cells, or as dictated by laboratory studies.

Another physiologic advantage of BSS described in the literature includes a low incidence of oliguric renal failure.[34] Moreover, renal failure occurring in the presence of adequate urine flow (high-output renal failure) is associated with a mortality rate of 18%, whereas oliguric renal failure is 50 to 70% fatal.

Postoperative pulmonary function appears relatively unaffected by the use of large volumes of BSS, provided gross overloads are avoided.[35] The adult respiratory distress syndrome occurring postoperatively in the trauma patient appears related more to the presence of sepsis, aspiration, fat embolism, microembolism from blood transfusion, direct pulmonary injury, oxygen toxicity, and/or severe central nervous system damage.[36]

Common Intraoperative Problems

Hypothermia

Hypothermia is a common finding in the trauma patient before, during, and after operations. Loss of heat occurs for a number of reasons, such as infusion of cold solutions intravenously, including blood, cold environment in the operating room, lack of covering of the patient during examinations, loss of heat from an open abdomen or chest, and the intraoperative use of cold irrigation solutions.

The hypothermic patient is affected adversely by a number of problems, including an impaired metabolism of drugs, prolongation of action of nondepolarizing muscle relaxants, shift of oxyhemoglobin dissociation curve to the left, which impairs oxygen delivery to the tissues, cardiac dysfunction and arrhythmias, obligatory shivering in the immediate postoperative period with consequently increased oxygen and cardiac output requirements, marked peripheral vasoconstriction, increased half-life of drugs, thrombocytopenia, and lactacidosis. In addition, there are difficulties in interpretation of blood-gas data.

Hence, all possible attempts should be made to help the patient to retain heat. The use of warming blankets on the patient, a warm environment in the operating room, the use of a low-flow circle system, the warming of all intravenous fluids, and short operating times help to achieve this goal.

Warmed and humidified oxygen (approximately 40% or more, as the situation demands) should be supplied postoperatively to all patients recovering from general anesthesia because of the anticipated post-anesthetic hypoxemia. A compelling argument can be made for not extubating the patient until the core temperature exceeds 35° C.

Hypotension

Probably the most common adverse finding during general anesthesia for multiple trauma is hypotension. The traditional classification of the causes of hypotension fall into three categories—hypovolemic, cardiogenic, and vasogenic. Hypovolemic hypotension usually is caused by blood loss and is the prime indication for volume therapy with crystalloids, colloids, and/or blood as necessary. Reduced venous return to the heart also belongs in this category when due to tension pneumothorax, cardiac tamponade, adverse posture, or physiologic effects of positive-pressure ventilation.

Cardiogenic hypotension indicates central pump failure in the presence of normovolemia and normal peripheral vasculature. Its causes include cardiac arrhythmias, cardiac tamponade, myocardial contusion, relative overdose of anesthetic agent, and myocardial infarction or preexisting heart disease. Cardiac arrhythmias causing hemodynamic upset should be treated promptly with antiarrhythmic drugs while considering the possible roles of hypoxia, hypercardia, hypothermia, and electrolyte or acid-base disturbances in their causation. Similarly, cardiac tamponade from pericardial collections of fluid should be treated by pericardiocentesis. Withdrawal of depressant anesthetic agents always is appropriate. Pharmacologic support of the failing heart may be necessary. Dopamine administered by intravenous infusion at a rate appropriate to the clinical situation is increasingly popular as the first-choice agent.[37] In low dosage (½ μg/kg/min), stimulation of dopaminergic receptors in the kidney occurs and causes renal vasodilation, increase in renal blood flow, and a rise in glomerular filtration rate (GFR) and renal sodium excretion. Doses from 2 to 10 μg/kg/min stimulate β_1-adrenergic receptors, causing increased cardiac output and heart rate. Doses in excess of 10 μg/kg/min produce direct stimulation of α-receptors with resultant increased peripheral vascular resistance at the expense of reduced renal blood flow. Thus, in conditions of severe hypotension, high doses of dopamine may be used to increase blood pressure and thereby increase coronary blood flow. At present, severe hypotension is the main indication for norepinephrine infusion.

Hypotension in the presence of bradyarrhythmias may be an indication for isoproterenol infusion, while hypotension associated with supraventricular tachyarrhythmias is the prime indicator for the use of digitalis glycosides.

Vasogenic hypotension includes hypotension resulting from spinal-cord transections, chemical sympathectomy associated with spinal or epidural anesthesia, inappropriate vasodilator therapy, and septic shock. Septic shock is rarely an early manifestation in the multiply injured patient. Therapy is primarily directed toward volume replacement, and pressor agents are rarely needed.

Acid-Base Disturbances

Acid-base disturbances are common predictable occurrences in the multiply injured patient. A metabolic acidosis may arise secondary to low cardiac output. Metabolic acidosis may result from impaired peripheral circulation consequent to hypothermia, from clamping of major blood vessels, and from infusion of old blood with its high acid content. Whenever possible, attention to the underlying cause is desirable.

Sodium bicarbonate infusion remains the usual alternative treatment for acidosis. Often, sodium bicarbonate is given empirically, but one is best guided by blood-gas analysis, which allows the administration of sodium bicarbonate according to one-half the deficit derived from the traditional equation, and also allows remeasurement before additional administration of sodium bicarbonate.

$$\text{mEq sodium bicarb necessary} = 0.3 \times \text{body weight in kg} \times \text{base deficit}$$

A respiratory acidosis may result from any of the causes of impaired ventilation. Therapy is directed toward improving ventilation. A metabolic alkalosis is sometimes seen following massive transfusion when the circulation is restored effectively. Hepatic conversion of the citrate anticoagulant to sodium bicarbonate increases body buffer base, thereby leading to alkalosis.[38] Similarly, iatrogenic metabolic alkalosis may be a consequence of energetic sodium bicarbonate therapy. Usually, special treatment is not required for this alkalosis. A respiratory alkalosis occurs following hyperventilation, as seen with some head injuries, or secondary to pain or fear. Iatrogenic respiratory alkalosis occurs from deliberate overventilation, as is used in the therapy for some head injuries. Treatment should be directed at the underlying cause. (When a mixed picture of acid-base imbalance is encountered in the multiply injured patient, interpretation may be more complex.)

Coagulopathies

Following a massive transfusion, defined as an acute infusion of blood in an amount equivalent to 1½ to 2 times the patient's estimated blood volume, some degree of coagulopathy often arises.

Exact identification of the cause of nonsurgical bleeding requires complex laboratory tests, but a rapid evaluation can be made by obtaining a prothrombin time and a platelet count while also observing the whole-blood coagulation time. Clot retraction and lysis abnormalities in these tests suggest a multifactoral coagulopathy, known as disseminated intravascular coagulopathy (DIC).[39]

The most common cause of a bleeding disorder in massive transfusion is dilutional thrombocytopenia. Dilution of labile clotting factors V and VIII is less important since, for example, only 30% of normal levels of factor VIII suffice for adequate hemostasis. Therefore, when massive transfusion of blood is likely, platelets and fresh frozen plasma should be available from the blood bank. It is a common practice to administer 2 units of platelets and 2 units of fresh frozen plasma after each 10 units of bank blood. Laboratory studies may dictate further intervention. Each unit of platelets increases the platelet count by 10,000 per mm^3.

Other coagulopathies, such as DIC, require further tests. In an attempt to combat this hypercoagulable state, the fibrinolytic system is activated to lyse the excessive fibrin. A high incidence of DIC occurs in patients with multiple organ injury and hypovolemic shock.[40]

Inappropriate Deterioration in Condition

When the patient's condition deteriorates out of proportion to the operative status and the blood loss and replacement, some other previously undiagnosed major injury may be the cause. Common causes of intraoperative deterioration include intra-abdominal or intrathoracic hemorrhage, pneumothorax, myocardial contusion or cardiac tamponade, and spinal-cord transection. Head injury per se is rarely a cause of shock.

The physician should be aware of common patterns of injury. For example, 7% of motor-vehicle accident victims have neck and cervical spine injuries.[41] In a report on 100 patients sustaining blunt trauma to the chest, 22 had associated neurologic injuries, 38 had fractures in areas other than the chest cage, 28 had abdominal injuries, and 23 of those with abdominal injuries required laparotomy. The overall mortality rate was 11%.[42]

Special Situations

Massive Trauma/Exsanguination

These patients fit into the category of trauma status III (see Table 10-1). A loss of 50% or more of their estimated blood volume results in impaired consciousness or coma. Operative intervention must be immediate in most cases, thus accentuating the anesthetic problems. These patients present challenges since the administration of even severely limited doses of potent anesthetic agents, whether intravenous or inhalational, may precipitate irreversible cardiovascular collapse.

Resuscitation, provision of adequate operating conditions by rendering the patient immobile with curarizing agents, and judicious administration of anesthetic agents as tolerated by the patient are the appropriate responses to this critical state. The severely hypotensive and traumatized patient has a dulled appreciation of pain and rarely resists intubation when awake. Administration of 100% oxygen through the endotracheal tube and provision of muscle relaxation by increments of pancuronium are sufficient at this early stage. As the clinical situation improves, indicated by an elevation in blood pressure and slowing of the pulse, some depression of the patient's sensorium may be indicated. Increasing proportions of nitrous oxide are given as tolerated by the patient, although small doses of ketamine intravenously allow the continued administration of 100% oxygen.

The sequence of endotracheal oxygen with assisted or controlled ventilation associated with intravenous ketamine and pancuronium has become an acceptable technique for the patient in shock who is not exsanguinated.[43,44]

Finally, as the condition of the patient stabilizes at a satisfactory level, the anesthesiologist may resort to the conventional nitrous oxide relaxant narcotic technique. Consideration should be paid to the predictable problems of hypothermia, acid-base disturbances, and coagulopathies.

Head Injury

In a study by Crighton and Giesecke of trauma patients requiring surgery, head injury was present in 28% of the patients.[3] Head injury commonly occurs in association with other injuries, notably of the neck, chest, and abdomen. The presence of disorientation or coma makes evaluation of other injuries more difficult. In addition, disorientation may not be readily distinguishable from intoxication.

Ideally, the patient with a closed head injury without an obviously operable intracranial lesion would be observed and monitored for a period of 6 to 24 hours prior to the administration of general anesthesia. However, the multiply injured patient may require early operative intervention for other injuries. In such instances, factors that may adversely affect intracranial pressure must be avoided.[45] A desirable anesthetic technique features smooth induction and emergence, moderate hyperventilation, absence of hypoxia, control of arterial and venous pressures, and avoidance of drugs known to raise intracranial pressure (halogenated agents, d-tubocurare, succinylcholine).

In patients with head injuries, adjuvant therapies, such as steroids in variable doses, hyperosmotic agents, prolonged artificial ventilation in an intensive-care unit, or deliberate barbiturate coma, have useful functions. Decisions regarding these modalities should be made in conjunction with the surgeon involved.[46]

Injuries of Neck and Cervical Spine

Seven percent of motor-vehicle accident victims have injuries to the neck and cervical spine. Trauma to the soft tissues of the neck, especially following gunshot wounds or bomb blasts, can cause extensive edema leading to airway obstruction.[47] Early control of the airway is necessary. Laceration of the large blood vessels in the neck by car windshields may produce torrential hemorrhage. Blunt trauma to the larynx and trachea is infrequent, but nevertheless represents a real anesthetic hazard because of its subsequent laryngospasm or airway obstruction caused by tissue drainage and distortion.[48]

Fracture dislocations of the cervical spine, especially if previously undetected, may result in spinal-cord injury following manipulation of the head and neck for intubation or positioning for operation. In the conscious patient, spasm of the neck muscles maintains relative stability of the fracture/dislocation. In such cases, therefore, the use of muscle relaxants to facilitate intubation is contraindicated. Intubation either by nasal or oral routes after generous topical anesthesia may be safer for the awake patient. Stabilization of the neck for intubation may be achieved manually or by the use of the VAC-PAK collar.[49] Other possible maneuvers in this situation include the catheter-guided intubation technique[50] or the use of the fiberoptic endoscope.

In patients whose physical status is compatible with spinal-cord transection, the pattern of injury conventionally is divided into two phases. Phase 1, spinal shock, lasts for 1 to 3 weeks and is characterized by loss of sensation, flaccid paralysis, and absent reflexes. Phase 2, autonomic hyperreflexia, is marked by return of reflexes, which may be hyperactive and/or discoordinated. Respiratory problems arise as a result of intercostal and possibly diaphragmatic paralysis, which impairs coughing ability and reduces both tidal volume and vital capacity. Aspiration of gastric contents is a constant hazard, as are atelectasis and pneumonia which may occur later.

Autonomic hyperreflexia may appear as arterial hypertension, cardiac irregularities, headaches, and sweating, especially when lesions are above the midthoracic level. This hyperreflexia is likely to occur during operation and may require control of the elevated blood pressure by the intravenous titration of trimethaphan or by the addition of halothane in the breathing circuit. The reflex can be prevented by subarachnoid block.[51] The use of succinylcholine in the paraplegic patient may result in an immediate though temporary increase in serum potassium levels sufficient to cause cardioplegia.[52]

Maxillofacial Injuries and Airway Obstruction

Upper respiratory obstruction is a frequent consequence of trauma and a likely cause of early death. Any region of the upper respiratory tract from the mouth to the trachea may be involved, and the causes of injury are manifold.[50,53] Attention to the airway before, during, and after anesthesia remains the cornerstone of treatment.

Of special concern to the anesthesiologist is the emergency patient who uses accessory muscles of respiration prior to the beginning of anesthesia. The accessory respiratory muscles are active when there is partial airway obstruction caused by external pressure of a hematoma or by internal pressure from damaged tissue or foreign bodies in any part of the airway. The accessory muscles of respiration may be considered as volitional. When a patient who uses these muscles is heavily sedated or when general anesthesia of any type is started, the patient usually becomes completely apneic. Apnea that occurs at the beginning of anesthesia, when sensory reflexes are not obtunded and airway anatomy is distorted, poses problems to the anesthesiologist who is attempting to establish an airway. If a rapid-sequence induction including a curarizing agent is planned, the patient's safety will be better assured when oxygenation is carried out before beginning the anesthesia.[54]

Maxillofacial trauma presents many problems to the anesthesiologist: airway obstruction is always a real or potential threat, the stomach is probably holding swallowed blood, and, indeed, continuing hemorrhage in the mouth and pharynx is likely. Also, bone or tooth fragments may be free in the mouth and pharynx and consequently represent an aspiration hazard.

No particular difficulty in intubation is expected with isolated mandibular fractures. When more extensive trauma is present, nasotracheal intubation under topical anesthesia in an awake, sedated patient may be the best approach. Visualization aided by the laryngoscope reduces the hazard of pushing bone fragments ahead of the endotracheal tube into the trachea. A suction catheter passed through and protruding beyond the nasal endotracheal tube serves as a leader and prevents mucosal injury, submucosal tunneling, entry into a false passage, and scooping of debris into the lumen of the tube. The suction catheter should be withdrawn when the endotracheal tube reaches the hypopharynx. Nasotracheal intubation should be avoided when severe nasal trauma or a fracture of the floor of the anterior fossa is present or suspected. Preliminary tracheostomy is indicated when there is a combination of nasal injury, jaw fracture, and intact teeth or whenever intubation in the awake patient has failed.[55]

A variety of techniques has evolved for placement of orotracheal or nasotracheal tubes in the obstructed or potentially obstructed airway of the patient, including awake intubation,[55] fiberoptic intubation,[56] catheter-guided intubation,[50] and oxygen by transcricothyroid insufflation.[57]

The endotracheal tube should remain in situ at the end of operation until the patient is awake and the protective reflexes have returned. The patient whose jaws are wired shut must be observed closely following extubation. Because vomiting after extubation could prove fatal, wire cutters and a tracheostomy set should be immediately available at the patient's bedside. The nasotracheal tube should not be removed unless it can be reintroduced easily. Removal of the tube over a small catheter whose distal end remains in the trachea leaves the catheter as a guide for immediate reintroduction of an endotracheal tube if needed.

Chest and Heart Trauma

Cardiac injury after trauma is surprisingly common. Many patients without external evidence of chest injury demonstrate evidence of cardiac contusion after motor-vehicle accidents. When chest trauma is obvious, cardiac injury occurs in a significant percentage of patients. Injury to the heart may appear as electrocardiographic abnormalities (e.g., ST changes, dysrhythmias, heart block), contusion or laceration of myocardium and valves, acute coronary occlusion, or acute right or left ventricular failure. An anesthetic technique that minimizes adverse myocardial effects should be planned, including controlled ventilation with high concentrations of oxygen. Perhaps such patients should be managed as though they had suffered a recent myocardial infarction; however, anticoagulants should not be used.[58]

A particularly hazardous situation arises when a pericardial effusion is present. When the effusion is large enough to cause cardiac tamponade, a fixed low cardiac output results from a combination of reduced filling of the heart and depressed ventricular activity. The hallmarks of this condition are increasing venous pressure, hypotension, muffled heart sounds, and a paradoxic pulse; however, these signs by no means are constant. Further reductions in cardiac output caused by anesthetic maneuvers, e.g., myocardial depressant drugs, vasodilator drugs, and controlled ventilation with constant positive pressure, further endanger the patient. The treatment of choice is pericardiocentesis under local anesthesia prior to induction of general anesthesia.[59]

Traumatic rupture of the thoracic aorta usually results in immediate death, but some patients reach the hospital alive, demonstrating that adventitia and pleura still are intact and preventing free bleeding. This condition is suspected when a widened mediastinum is apparent on the chest roentgenogram.[60] It has been stated that 36% of these patients have minimal evidence of chest trauma.[61] The diagnosis can be confirmed by aortography if the clinical condition permits.

With regard to chest trauma excluding the heart, approximately 37% of motor-vehicle accident victims have thoracic and thoracic spine injuries. These injuries include fractured ribs or sternum, flail chest, pneumo- or hemothorax, pulmonary contusion, bronchial tear, and ruptured diaphragm. When a pneumothorax or hemothorax is present, water-sealed chest drains should be inserted preoperatively. Undiagnosed pneumothorax is likely to be worsened intraoperatively by a combination of positive-pressure ventilation and nitrous oxide diffusion. A developing pneumothorax is a common cause of unexpected deterioration in the patient's condition. A tension pneumothorax is particularly hazardous because it can distort the heart and great vessels to such an extent that cardiac output is diminished significantly.

A persistent air leak through a chest drain suggests a bronchial tear. The affected bronchus can be isolated by the use of a double-lumen endobronchial tube. Hemothorax is associated most commonly with penetrating injuries of the chest but can also occur in closed-chest injuries in the absence of fractured ribs. Hemorrhage may arise from the pulmonary, intercostal, and great vessels, and also from the heart. In addition to loss of blood from the circulation, such a hemorrhage causes mechanical interference with ventilation. Chest drains are mandatory.[58]

Fractured ribs may inhibit adequate spontaneous ventilation and the ability to clear secretions from the chest, particularly if a flail segment has been produced. The extent of compromise of these functions determines the mode of treatment; prolonged controlled ventilation is required for the more severely affected patient. Recently, the use of local anesthetic drugs or narcotics administered epidurally has appeared as a promising innovation when chest splinting and hypoventilation are the result of pain.[62]

Pulmonary contusion has been estimated to occur in 70 to 75% of patients with major chest trauma and is one of the primary causes of posttraumatic respiratory failure.[63] In such cases, the occurrence of infection, fluid overload, hemorrhagic hypotension, and embolic phenomena must be minimized.

Eye Injuries

Injuries to the eye are occasionally seen in patients with multiple trauma. In particular, penetrating injuries of the globe pose an anesthetic problem. Most authorities agree that the use of succinylcholine, the usual relaxant used in the rapid-sequence induction, is contraindicated in this instance since it leads to an increase in intraocular pressure with the resultant possibility of extrusion of intraocular contents. Nasogastric decompression is also contraindicated since any retching or vomiting so induced may result in increased intraocular pressure mediated through raised venous pressure.[64] Induction of anesthesia with thiopental sodium (Pentothal) and use of the nondepolarizing relaxant, pancuronium, in generous doses (50 to 100% higher than normal) allow intubating conditions almost as rapidly as does succinylcholine, but without the increase in intraocular pressure.[65] Thereafter, controlled ventilation to normocapnea and smooth gentle anesthesia provide desirable operating conditions.

Burns

In the acute stage, extensive burns present the potential problems of hypovolemia and thermal injury to the respiratory tract. Many burned patients require multiple operations. Such procedures may be prolonged and extensive; as a result, intraoperative blood loss and heat loss become important considerations. Moreover, such patients are often anemic, septic, hypovolemic, undernourished, and exhibit some degree of respiratory failure.

The anesthetic technique of choice for repeated operations is probably the nitrous oxide-relaxant technique supplemented by narcotics. The depolarizing relaxant, succinylcholine, should be avoided because it has a peculiar effect in the burned patient, of causing a sudden rise in serum potassium sufficient to produce cardiac arrest.[52] The dissociative agent, ketamine, has been advocated for these patients because it provides intense analgesia and relative safety to the airway. The possibility of its intramuscular administration becomes a useful property when veins are difficult to find.

Thermal injury to the respiratory tract appears acutely as carbon monoxide poisoning or upper airway obstruction, and later as the smoke inhalation syndrome.[66]

Intoxication

The emergency trauma victim may be intoxicated with alcohol and other drugs. Although alcohol is a potent respiratory, cardiovascular, and central nervous system depressant, the patient may be combative and/or disoriented. In 169 intoxicated and traumatized patients with blood-alcohol levels of less than 250 ml/dl, Lee, et al., were unable to demonstrate any increase in post-anesthetic morbidity or mortality when compared with 530 sober patients. Allowances may have been made in the anesthetic management of these patients because of their apparent intoxication and may have aided in preventing complications. However, at higher blood-alcohol levels, mortality rates were increased.[67]

A number of useful guidelines have evolved for the anesthetic management of patients intoxicated with alcohol:[68]

1. Because of the decreased ability of intoxicated patients to withstand hemorrhage, blood replacement therapy probably should be instituted earlier in the intoxicated patient than in the sober patient.
2. Because the chronic alcoholic actually may be iso-osmotically overhydrated, fluid therapy must be planned with care.
3. Because of the tendency to hypoglycemia, glucose should be added to the fluid management regimen.
4. Because of the enzyme induction effect resulting from chronic ethanol ingestion, anesthetic agents that are in part metabolized are perhaps best avoided. Increased biotransformation of inhalational anesthetic agents appears to be associated with their toxicity.
5. Because ethanol is a central nervous system depressant and tends to induce a lack of recall, supplementation of the nitrous oxide relaxant technique with narcotics or other depressant drugs should be reduced or eliminated in the acutely intoxicated patient.
6. Because acutely intoxicated individuals are more prone to hypothermia, the core temperature should be monitored intraoperatively. All intravenous fluids should be warmed, and a warming blanket should be employed, if necessary, to maintain body temperature.

Patients may be under the influence of drugs other than ethanol, or may be nonintoxicated chronic abusers of such drugs. Some of these substances cause both physical and psychic dependence. These patients may experience physiologically disturbing withdrawal syndromes, such as tremors, twitchings, delirium, hypotension, vomiting, and convulsions, during the postoperative period. Other characteristics of withdrawal may include prolonged sleepiness, apathy, and mental depression. Such findings may confuse the usual evidences of recovery from anesthesia and operation.[69]

Postoperative Considerations

Anesthetic involvement with the multiply injured patient continues into the postoperative period. The effects of massive trauma may not be apparent at the same time. Following the successful, definitive, operative correction of injuries in one or more areas, the patient must be observed closely for evidences of occult damage in other sites or for progressive neurocardiorespiratory deterioration.

Respiratory function must be monitored carefully, and a composite assessment must be made from clinical impression, spirometry, radiography, and blood-gas analysis. All patients have some temporary impairment of oxygenation after general anesthesia. Such impairment in the multiply injured patient may be due to hypoventilation, impaired gas exchange, or defective oxygen transport. Artificial ventilation may be necessary until adequate spontaneous respiration is demonstrated, hematologic, biochemical, and acid-base values are satisfactory, fluid balance is optimized, and core temperature is restored toward normal. Respiratory support may be necessary for a period of hours or days or longer, necessitating admission to an intensive-care unit.

Delayed recovery from anesthesia also demands anesthetic involvement. In addition to the usual explanations, consideration must be made in the multiply injured patient to such factors as head or spinal-cord injury, cerebral damage from hypotension or hypoxia, persistent narcosis with alcohol or other intoxicants, hypothermia, and hypoglycemia. Rare causes of failure to awaken include sickle-cell crisis, the severe metabolic acidosis of methanol intoxication, and hyperosmolar nonketotic coma.[70]

The residual effects of hypotension or hypoxia upon vital organs, such as heart, brain, liver, and kidney, must be borne in mind when ordering fluid therapy and medications postoperatively.

Several findings suggest prolonged recovery-room care with endotracheal intubation and controlled ventilation and perhaps indicate that the patient should be kept under intensive care for longer than the usual postanesthesia surveillance. These findings include the following:

1. Clinical evidence of inability to cough and raise secretions.
2. Clinical evidence of progressive fatigue.
3. Progressive dyspnea.
4. Respiratory rate of 40 or more per minute.

5. Arterial Po_2 of 60 mm Hg or less on 30 to 40% oxygen.

6. Increase in arterial Pco_2 to 50 mm Hg or greater.

7. Vital capacity less than 2 to 3 times tidal volume.

8. Infiltrates revealed by chest roentgenogram.

The anesthesiologist also can render valuable service in the field of postoperative analgesia. The anesthesiologist should be prepared to administer intravenous narcotics judiciously when the situation demands and to monitor their effects closely. Occasionally, the anesthesiologist may be called upon to perform local nerve blocks, such as intercostal nerve blocks following thoracotomy or laparotomy and continuous epidural blocks for lower extremity pain relief.

References

1. Campbell, D.: Immediate hospital care of the injured. Br. J. Anaesth., *49*:6723, 1977.
2. Jenkins, M. T., and Giesecke, A. H.: Anesthesia considerations. *In* Care of the Trauma Patient. Edited by G. T. Shires. New York, McGraw-Hill, 1966.
3. Crighton, H. C., and Giesecke, A. H.: One year's experience in the anesthetic management of trauma: 1964. Anesth. Analg. (Cleve.), *45*:835, 1966.
4. Baskett, P. J. F.: Uses of anesthesia: the anesthetist in the accident and emergency service. Br. Med. J., *281*:287, 1980.
5. Raj, P. P., Montgomery, S. J., and Bradley, V. H.: Agents and techniques. *In* Clinical Anesthesia. Vol. 11, Anesthesia for the Surgery of Trauma. Edited by A. H. Giesecke, Jr. Philadelphia, F. A. Davis, 1976.
6. Giesecke, A. H., Hodgson, R. M. H., and Raj, P. P.: Anesthesia for severely injured patients. Orthop. Clin. North Am., *1*:21, 1970.
7. Trowbridge, A. M., and Giesecke, A. H.: Multiple injuries. *In* Clinical Anesthesia. Vol. 11, Anesthesia for the Surgery of Trauma. Edited by A. H. Giesecke, Jr. Philadelphia, F. A. Davis, 1976.
8. Rubin, E., and Lieber, C. S.: Alcoholism, alcohol, and drugs. Science, *172*:1097, 1971.
9. Waller, J. A.: Holiday drinking and highway fatalities. J.A.M.A., *206*:2693, 1968.
10. Finkle, B. S., Biasotti, M. C., and Bradford, L. W.: The occurrence of some drugs and toxic agents encountered in drinking driver investigations. J. Forensic Sci., *13*:236, 1968.
11. Brock-Utne, J. G., et al.: The effect of glycopyrrolate (Robinul) on the lower esophageal sphincter. Can. Anaesth. Soc. J., *25*:144, 1978.
12. Wheatley, R. G., Kallus, F. T., Reynolds, R. C., and Giesecke, A. H.: Milk of magnesia is an effective preinduction antacid in obstetric anesthesia. Anesthesiology, *50*:514, 1979.
13. Bynum, L. J., and Pierce, A. K.: Pulmonary aspiration of gastric contents. Am. Rev. Respir. Dis., *114*:1129, 1976.
14. Holmes, C. M.: Intravenous regional analgesia: a useful method of producing analgesia of the limbs. Lancet, *1*:245, 1963.
15. Bedford, R. F., and Wollman, H. W.: Complications of percutaneous radial-artery cannulation: an objective prospective study in man. Anesthesiology, *38*:228, 1973.
16. Bedford, R. F., and Major, M. C.: Percutaneous radial-artery cannulation—increased safety using Teflon catheters. Anesthesiology, *42*:219, 1975.
17. Salem, M. R., Yacoub, M. H., and Holaday, D. A.: Interpretations of central venous pressure measurements. *In* Clinical Anesthesia. Vol. 3, Common and Uncommon Problems in Anesthesiology. Edited by M. T. Jenkins. Philadelphia, F. A. Davis, 1968.
18. Poole-Wilson, P. A.: Interpretation of haemodynamic measurements. Br. J. Hosp. Med., *22*:371, 1978.
19. Blitt, C. D., Wright, W. A., Petty, W. C., and Webster, T. A.: Central venous catheterization via the external jugular vein. J.A.M.A., *229*:817, 1974.
20. Fairley, H. B.: Anesthesia for massive trauma. *In* 25th Annual ASA Refresher Course. Chicago, American Society of Anesthesiologists, 1978.
21. Salem, M. R.: Anesthetic management of patients with "a full stomach": a critical review. Anesth. Analg. (Cleve.), *49*:47, 1970.
22. Satiani, B., Bonner, J. T., and Stone, H. H.: Factors influencing intraoperative gastric regurgitation. Arch. Surg., *113*:721, 1978.
23. Sellick, B. A.: Cricoid pressure to control regurgitation of stomach contents during induction of anaesthesia. Lancet, *2*:404, 1961.
24. Barr, A. M., and Thornley, B. A.: Thiopentone and suxamethonium crash induction. Anaesthesia, *31*:23, 1976.
25. Dundee, J. W.: Clinical studies of induction agents. Br. J. Anaesth, *35*:784, 1963.
26. Virtue, R. W., et al.: An anesthetic agent: 2-orthochlorophenyl, 2-methylamino cyclohexanone HCI (CI-581). Anesthesiology, *28*:823, 1967.
27. Tweed, W. A., Minuck, M., and Mymin, D.: Circulatory responses to ketamine anesthesia. Anesthesiology, *37*:613, 1972.
28. Vaughan, R. S., and Lunn, J N.: Potassium and the anaesthetist. Anaesthesia. *28*:118, 1973.
29. Kelman, G. R., and Kennedy, B. R.: Cardiovascular effects of pancuronium in man. Br. J. Anaesth., *43*:335, 1971.
30. Eisele, J. H., and Smith, N. T.: Cardiovascular effects of 40 percent nitrous oxide in man. Anesth. Analg. (Cleve.), *51*:9056, 1972.
31. Giesecke, A. H.: Perioperative fluid therapy. *In* Anesthesia. Edited by R. D. Miller. New York, Churchill-Livingstone, 1981.
32. Gruber, U. F., and Rittman, W. W.: Hypovolaemic shock—therapy of hypovolaemia and respiratory insufficiency. Triangle, *13*:91, 1974.
33. Giesecke, A. H.: Colloid-crystalloid controversy. *In* 27th Annual ASA Refresher Course. Chicago, American Society of Anesthesiologists, 1980.
34. Baxter, C. R., Zedlitz, W. H., and Shires, G. T.: High output acute renal failure complicating traumatic injury. J. Trauma, *4*:567, 1967.
35. Carey, L. C., Lowery, B. D., and Cloutier, C. T.: Alterations resulting from hemorrhage and trauma. *In* Current

Problems in Surgery. Chicago, Yearbook Publishers, 1971.
36. Horovitz, J. H., Carrico, D. J., and Shires, G. T.: Pulmonary response to major injury. Arch. Surg., *108*:349, 1974.
37. Tinker, J.: Shock: a pharmacological approach to the treatment of shock. Br. J. Hosp. Med., *21*:3, 1979.
38. Litwin, M. S., Smith, L. L., and Moore, F. D.: Metabolic alkalosis following massive transfusion. Surgery, *45*:806, 1959.
39. Ellison, N.: Diagnosis and management of bleeding disorders. Anesthesiology, *47*:171, 1977.
40. Miller, R. D.: Complications of massive blood transfusions. Anesthesiology, *39*:82, 1973.
41. Braunstein, P. W.: Medical aspects of automotive crash injury research. J.A.M.A., *163*:249, 1957.
42. Bricker, D. L., Upton, J., and Telford, J. R.: Blunt trauma to the chest. Tex. Med., *68*:74, 1972.
43. Bond, A. C., and Davies, C. K.: Ketamine and pancuronium for the shocked patient. Anaesthesia, *29*:59, 1974.
44. Chasapakis, G., Kekis, M., Sakkalis, C., and Kolios, D.: Use of ketamine and pancuronium for anesthesia for patients in hemorrhagic shock. Anesth. Analg. (Cleve.), *52*:82, 1973.
45. Shapiro, H. M.: Intracranial hypertension: therapeutic and anesthetic considerations. Anesthesiology, *43*:445, 1975.
46. Bruce, D. A., Gennarelli, T. A., and Longfitt, T. W.: Resuscitation from coma due to head injury. Crit. Care Med., *6*:254, 1978.
47. Gray, R. C., and Coppel, D. L.: Surgery of violence: intensive care of patient with bomb blast and gunshot injuries. Br. Med. J., *1*:502, 1975.
48. Seed, R. F.: Traumatic injury to the larynx and trachea. Anaesthesia, *26*:55, 1971.
49. Walters, F. J. M., and Nott, M. R.: The hazards of anaesthesia in the injured patient. Br. J. Anaesth., *49*:707, 1977.
50. Lopez, G., and James, N. R.: Mechanical problems of the airway. *In* Clinical Anesthesia. Vol. 3, Common and Uncommon Problems in Anesthesiology. Edited by M. T. Jenkins. Philadelphia, F. A. Davis, 1968.
51. Desmond, J.: Paraplegia: problems confronting the anaesthesiologist. Can. Anaesth. Soc. J., *17*:435, 1970.
52. Gronert, G. A., and Theye, R. A.: Pathophysiology of hyperkalemia induced by succinylcholine. Anesthesiology, *43*:1, 1975.
53. Verrill, P. J.: Anaesthesia in upper respiratory obstruction. Br. J. Anaesth., *35*:237, 1963.
54. Jenkins. M. T., and Giesecke, A. H.: Anesthesia considerations. *In* Care of the Trauma Patient. Edited by G. T. Shires. New York, McGraw-Hill, 1966.
55. Sims, J. K., and Giesecke, A. H.: Airway management. *In* Clinical Anesthesia. Vol 11, Anesthesia for the Surgery of Trauma. Edited by A. H. Giesecke, Jr. Philadelphia, F. A. Davis, 1976.
56. Raj, P. P., et al.: Technics for fiberoptic laryngoscopy in anesthesia. Anesth. Analg. (Cleve.), *53*:708, 1974.
57. Jacoby, J. J., et al.: Transtracheal resuscitation. J.A.M.A., *162*:625, 1956.
58. Singer, M. M., and Lee, J.: Management of thoracic injuries. Int. Anesthesiol. Clin., *9*:117, 1971.
59. Stein, L., Shubin, H., and Weil, M. H.: Recognition and management of pericardial tamponade. J.A.M.A., *225*:503, 1973.
60. Paton, B. C., Elliott, D. P., Taubman, J. O., and Owens, J. C.: Acute treatment of traumatic aortic rupture. J. Trauma, *11*:1, 1971.
61. Blair, E., Topuzlu, C., and Davis, J. H.: Delayed or missed diagnosis in blunt chest trauma. J. Trauma, *11*:129, 1971.
62. Watson, R. L., Muldoon, S. M., and Doblar, D. D.: The mechanisms of action and utility of epidurally administered morphine. *In* 27th Annual ASA Refresher Course. Chicago, American Society of Anesthesiologists, 1980.
63. Carrico, C. J., and Horovitz, J. H.: Post injury acute pulmonary failure. *In* Care of the Trauma Patient. 2nd Edition. Edited by G. T. Shires. New York, McGraw-Hill, 1979.
64. Adams, A. K., and Jones, R. M.: Anaesthesia for eye surgery: general considerations. Br. J. Anaesth., *52*:663, 1980.
65. Barr, A. M., and Thornley, B. A.: Thiopentone and pancuronium crash induction. Anaesthesia, *33*:25, 1978.
66. Achauer, B. M., Allyn, P. A., Furnas, D. W., and Bartlett, R. H.: Pulmonary complications of burns: the major threat to the burn patient. Ann. Surg., *177*:311, 1972.
67. Lee, J. F., Giesecke, A. H., and Jenkins, M. T.: Anesthetic management of trauma: influence of alcohol ingestion. South. Med. J., *60*:1240, 1967.
68. Watson, T. D., and Lee, J. F.: Intoxication and trauma. *In* Clinical Anesthesia. Vol. 11, Anesthesia for the Surgery of Trauma. Edited by A. H. Giesecke. Philadelphia, F. A. Davis, 1976.
69. Jenkins, L. C.: Anaesthetic problems due to drug abuse and dependence. Can. Anaesth. Soc. J., *19*:461, 1972.
70. Giesecke, A. H., and Jenkin, M. T.: Anesthesia considerations. *In* Care of the Trauma Patient. 2nd Edition. Edited by G. T. Shires. New York, McGraw-Hill, 1976.

Chapter 11 Open Fractures with Major Skin and Bone Defects

RICHARD E. JONES

A fracture is defined as open if a defect in the skin and soft tissue communicates with the fracture or its hematoma. The cutaneous wound sets the open fracture apart from the closed fracture. The soft-tissue wound makes the fracture management more complex by providing complicating variables to the management of the osseous wound: bacteria are introduced, devitalized soft tissue compromises the ability of the host to respond to bacterial contamination, the soft-tissue injury compromises the ability of the osseous tissue to respond to the fracture insult, and stabilization of the fracture is more difficult because of the loss of soft-tissue support. Consequently, the complex open fracture presents a difficult management problem. The reported outcome of treatment of open fractures shows a significantly higher incidence of infection, delayed union, nonunion, and sundry other wound-healing disturbances.

Our modern society, with its modes of high-velocity transportation, heavy industry, and increasing population, has seen a rise in the volume of patients with severe trauma. Trauma and severe open fractures in such volume previously had been restricted to times of war. However, trauma and accident surgery is falling more and more into the providence of specialists who deal primarily with the severely injured patient.

In the past, each generation of surgeons had to learn how to best manage the complex open fracture, which was an inevitable result of war. At present, the tenor of society has made warlike injuries commonplace in the civilian population.

Historical Background

The history of open fracture management is intertwined with the history of wound surgery during times of war. The use of cautery, which was introduced by Hippocrates (460-377 B.C.), persisted until Pare (1510-1590 A.D.) recognized the deleterious effect of the thermal insult and discontinued the use of boiling oil in open wounds. The modern era of treatment of open fracture wounds was heralded by deSault (1744-1795) when he introduced the concept of debridement. For deSault, debridement was a deep incision made to explore and drain the wound and exposed damaged tissue as well as to excise dead tissue. Dominique Jean Larrey (1766-1842) was a student of deSault and accompanied Napoleon on his battle campaigns. After one battle, Larrey performed or supervised 200 amputations in 24 hours for fractures complicated by severe skin loss. The mortality rate for injuries during this period was 75 to 90%.

Pasteur (1822-1895) determined that disease was caused by bacteria, and Lister (1827-1912) developed antiseptic technique to help to prevent infection. Aseptic technique was made possible by vonBergmann (1836-1907), who introduced steam sterilization in 1886. Winnett Orr, toward the end of World War I, renewed a technique, introduced by Ollier (1825-1900), of resting the injured part. Orr's goal was to provide immobilization and adequate open drainage by a closed plaster treatment for open fracture wounds after initial decompression and open wound drainage. During the Spanish Civil War, Trueta turned to a true debridement: "The removal of the tissue medium favorable to bacterial growth is the fundamental principle on which the whole treatment is based."[1] Trueta's work served as the basis for the theater-wide management of open fracture wounds during World War II.

The practice of early debridement and immobilization followed by delayed primary closure by suture or graft 4 to 6 days post-injury evolved next. Antibiotics were introduced about this time, and the percentage of amputations and the percentage of infections in these war wounds reduced dramatically. In World War I, post-open fracture osteomyelitis occurred at a rate of 80%; in World War II the rate dropped to 25%. During the Viet Nam conflict, rapid helicopter transport and sophisticated forward surgical units enabled further refinement of open fracture wound management with a reduction in morbidity.

Recent advancements in plastic surgery, such as the rediscovery of axial flaps and the microsurgical techniques for one-stage transfer of distant flaps, have brought about innovations in the care of patients with severe open fracture wounds complicated by soft-tissue or osseous-tissue loss.

Classification

Open fractures have been classified on the basis of the kinetic energy required to create the wound, on the basis of the radiographic fracture pattern, which is reflective of the energy absorbed at failure, and on the basis of the appearance of the soft-tissue wound associated with the open fracture. The classification of the open fracture wound presented in Table 11-1 combines all three factors. The more severe the fracture, the less predictable the good outcome. Grade IIIA is a new classification with an even worse prognosis than that for grade III.[2] The grade IIIA classification includes injuries that can cause extensive soft-tissue damage and devitalization.

Special mention should be made of injuries that are characterized by profound bacterial contamination. Open fractures sustained during a tornado are inoculated by unusual, soil-borne, pathogenic bacteria. Open fracture wounds sustained by a rotary power-mower blade are similar to those sustained during a tornado. Open fracture wounds with contiguous bowel injury are likewise severely contaminated. The choice of antibiotic and method of wound care should be made by placing emphasis on open, expectant treatment.

Table 11-1. *Classification of the Open Fracture Wound.*

Grade I	Low energy forces cause spiral or oblique fracture pattern with skin laceration less than 2 cm; relatively clean
Grade II	Moderate energy forces cause comminuted or displaced fracture pattern with skin laceration more than 2 cm; moderate adjacent skin contusion and muscle damage
Grade III	High energy forces cause significantly displaced fracture pattern with severe comminution, segmental fracture, or bone defect with extensive skin loss and muscle damage
Grade IIIA	Vascular injury requiring repair, high-velocity gun shot or shotgun wound, history of crush or degloving injury

Concept

The concept of the open fracture as a wound complex is fundamental to the understanding of wound healing in these injuries. Thus, the open fracture wound involves the skin, the fascia, the muscle, the periosteum, and the bone. Progress toward healing of the fracture depends on progressive healing of the soft-tissue injury. A brief review of the interrelated healing process follows.

Adequate nutrition is necessary for the progression of each phase of wound repair after the initial lag phase. Inflammation, migration, proliferation, secretion, and, finally, maturation are steps usually described. Adequate oxygen potentials are required for collagen cross-linking and remodeling. If the wound tissue becomes hypoxic at this time, e.g., with continued motion at the fracture site, infection or excessive edema and avascular cicatrix result instead of the production of a matrix. Adequate wound nutrition and a good mesenchymal milieu cause the conversion of the matrix into fibrocartilage, hyaline cartilage, or bone by the appropriate stimulus. When the soft-tissue requirements are met, stabilization of the skeletal portion of the open fracture wound results in the production of bone. Rhinelander showed that both the bone and the surrounding soft tissue shared numerous microanastomoses.[3] In displaced fractures with interruption of the endosteal blood supply, early fracture wound healing occurred through proliferation of the muscle supplied periosteal vessels to accommodate callus formation. Holden performed an osteotomy on the rabbit radius and placed circumferential suture around the muscle and periosteum to cause ischemia and to mimic massive trauma.[4] Before fracture wound healing could proceed, muscle and periosteum had to be revascularized. The healing process then was started by neovascular growth from the muscle/periosteum into the cortical bone. The lag time for initiation of fracture callus formation in Holden's experimental model was approximately 3 to 4 weeks.

Therefore, in the complex open fracture with grade II or grade III soft-tissue injury, the restoration of a viable soft-tissue envelope must be accomplished before bone healing can progress. Thinking of the open fracture as a hard- and soft-tissue wound helps to emphasize the need for subscribing to the basic tenets of wound healing for a good end result.

Initial Management

Management of the open fracture wound strives to obtain primary healing of both the soft and hard tissues. Upon arrival of the patient in the emergency room, complete inspection of the limb should be performed. This inspection includes the portion of the limb that lies in a splint or on the examining table, since significant wounds in this area frequently are overlooked. Tissue wound cultures should be obtained for later correlation if infection should ensue. Semi-reduction of the fractured limb to help to align the tissues and to provide decompression in many marginally vascularized areas is maintained by splints.

Tetanus prophylaxis should be augmented by 250 to 500 units of human-immune globulin in high-jeopardy wounds with extensive devitalization and contamination. Parenteral antibiotics used to treat the contaminated wound should be initiated in the emergency suite before the patient is taken to the x-ray department. Cephalosporin-type antibiotics are the usual drug of choice, and we currently recommend 2 g of cefamandole administered through piggyback intravenous methods every 6 hours. Antibiotics are continued for approximately 5 days if no complications ensue. Antibiotics should be discontinued 24 hours after delayed primary closure or when the open fracture wound has remained clean.

The patient then is taken to the operating room, where radical debridement and copious jet-lavage irrigation are performed. The surgeon should not be tentative during debridement since coverage of the wound can be provided by the newer soft-tissue plastic surgical techniques.

A question of viable versus nonviable skin frequently occurs in grade IIIA injuries. Fluorescein (5 to 10 mg/kg administered intravenously, with the higher doses used in dark-skinned patients) can be used to assess the integument.[5] The Wood's light can be used to indicate fluorescence of viable skin 15 minutes after IV injection. Determination of viable muscle cannot be made with the fluorescein techniques because the fluorescein leaks out and covers the surface of muscle, thereby giving a false-positive fluorescence. Skin that does not fluoresce or that is apparently devitalized should be excised.

The patient's history of injury, or the account of any available witness, should be taken, particularly in pedestrian-auto accidents, motorcycle accidents, and close-range, high-energy missile wounds, which cause profound soft-tissue trauma and should be classified as grade IIIA injuries. Such identification of grade III injuries can help to alert the surgeon that aggressive, extensive primary debridement will be necessary and that redebridement at 2-to-3 day intervals will be imperative to ensure removal of all foreign material and devitalized tissue.

Grade I

The osseous tissue of both grade I open fracture wounds and grade I intra-articular open fracture wounds should be stabilized by the surgeon's method of choice. The minimally damaged grade I soft-tissue wound should be converted to a clean surgical wound in which the skin can be closed. If the surgeon doubts that the wound has been converted to a clean surgical wound, primary closure should not be performed. Delayed primary closure by suture or skin graft is a method of choice in such situations. If closure of either an open fracture wound or an intra-articular open fracture wound is undertaken, suction drainage should be provided for the postoperative period.

Most grade I open fractures can be managed by the same means usually employed for closed fractures with the same fracture pattern. Occasionally, external plaster immobilization must be supplemented by internal stabilization if the fracture pattern is inherently unstable.

Grade II

Treatment of grade II open fracture wounds and grade II intra-articular open fracture wounds is somewhat more controversial. After the initial management steps have been taken, the extent of soft-tissue damage determines which form of bony stabilization is best indicated. For patients with a minimal cutaneous interruption, management can approximate that for grade I open fracture wounds. Essentially, the treatment regimen is similar to that for a patient with a closed fracture in the same situation. External skeletal fixation is indicated for more extensive soft-tissue damage that requires access for daily wound care, repeat debridement, and possible secondary closure procedures.

Grade II intra-articular fracture wounds need debridement of the joint and, usually, open reduction and interfragmentary fixation of the articular fragments and primary closure of the joint over drains. If there is severe comminution of the intra-articular fragement that is not amenable to internal fixation, external-fixation frames should be constructed. The fractures should be treated with traction to regain length with semireduction and the joint should be placed in a functional position before mounting the external anchoring frame.

Grade II injuries carry a greater risk when primary closure is attempted. Because of the more extensive soft-tissue wound, complete debridement may not be accomplished. Therefore, delayed primary closure by suture or skin graft is indicated at 3 to 5 days post-injury if the wound remains clean.

Grade III

By definition, grade III open fracture wounds are characterized by profound soft-tissue trauma with large muscle and integumentary wounds and periosteal stripping. Furthermore, the fracture pattern often is accompanied by segmental fractures or frank loss of bone substance. The initial management of the grade III open fracture wound is more difficult because of the more extensive debridement required, and extensive reconstructive procedures often are necessary to restore the limb to a functional status.

The initial evaluation and operative handling of the soft tissues in grade III open fracture wounds are similiar to those of grades I and II wounds. Special emphasis should be placed on assessing the viability of skin by performing the IV fluorescein test. Evaluation of muscle is more difficult because it frequently is damaged at a site distant from the actual wound as a result of transference of kinetic energy. As Gregory observed, residual devitalized muscle left in a wound offers "most salubrious pablum for bacterial growth."[6] Gregory also noted that decisions on the viability of muscle should be based on color, consistency, contractility, and capacity to bleed.

Special circumstances that may alter the state of the muscle include hypovolemic shock, proximal damage to a major artery, or intrinsic small-vessel occlusive disease.

If there is any doubt as to the thoroughness of a debridement, a second look always is indicated. At 2 to 3 days after the time of acute injury, the patient should be returned to the operating room for a repeat debridement and evaluation under anesthesia. This procedure better delineates muscle that is damaged, discovers retained foreign bodies or detritus, and allows further jet-lavage irrigation.

Methods of treatment of complex open fractures are difficult to compare since the data base for each paper on the subject appears to be different. Open fractures of the tibia are reviewed most extensively. Nicoll determined that comminution, wound size, contamination, infection, displacement, and bone loss were the fundamental factors to assess when attempting to predict outcomes of treatment.[7] Edwards showed a clear relationship between soft-tissue injury, especially skin necrosis, and infection in the prognosis of fracture healing.[8] The literature, however, does not offer a clear delineation of the grading of open tibial fractures to determine the severity of the trauma and, therefore, the predictability of the outcome. A high percentage of wound-healing disturbances is described in the studies of Ruedi, Rosenthal,[9] Tonnesen, and Karlstrom and Olerud.[10] Infection, delayed union, nonunion, and fixation failure are commonplace in grade III injuries, particularly when rigid internal stabilization by plates is attempted. The Olerud and Karlstrom group changed from internal plate fixation to external fixation management of grades II and III fractures because of a 34% incidence of severe wound-healing disturbances.[10] Tonnesen correlated the incidence of hard-tissue healing disturbances directly with the incidence of skin necrosis. He suggested that stable external fixation supplemented by myoplasty would be a good alternative treatment for grades II and III open tibial fractures.

Rigid stabilization clearly is necessary to obtain the best chance of healing. Further rigid stabilization enables the limb to handle any superinfection better.[11] Basically, rigid internal fixation requires extensive soft-tissue stripping for plate placement, and further devitalization of bone may occur. Internal plates create dead space in which bacteria may be harbored. Therefore, most grade III open fractures that carry a high risk of wound-healing disturbances, such as infection or the chance of delayed union or nonunion, require rigid external skeletal fixation. This type of treatment enhances observation of the wound, allows access to the wound for dressing changes or repeat debridements, and facilitates secondary soft- and hard-tissue reconstructive procedures.

Interfragmentary compression obtained in comminuted fractures at the time of the initial debridement can help to render overall stability to the limb. The placement of screws for interfragmentary compression does not involve further stripping of soft tissue from the bone. Occasionally, application of rigid-plate internal fixation can be accomplished, again without further stripping. Provision for coverage of the plate should be made according to the following principles.

Associated Neurovascular or Tendinous Injury

The diagnosis of associated vascular injury with grade III open fracture wounds requires a high index of suspicion. Popliteal artery injury with knee dislocation can occur without obvious primary signs of ischemia.[12] If the limb distal to a fracture shows signs of ischemia, such as decreased temperature, absence of the pulse, slow capillary refill, or significant hemorrhage, arteriography is indicated. If prompt arteriography cannot be performed, operative exploration of the vascular tree should be undertaken.

Re-establishment of distal perfusion must be performed within 8 to 10 hours after the original injury to enhance limb salvage. Distal fasciotomy always is indicated after arterial repair to diminish the chance of compartment syndrome of the limb. Compartment syndrome can cause extensive soft-tissue damage, and pain with passive muscular stretch is usually the first indication of its onset.

Grade III open fracture wounds with associated proximal arterial damage are notorious for bone-healing disturbances, probably because the soft-tissue envelope about the bone has marginal vascular supply[2] and cannot contribute to fracture healing in the early phase. Such injuries should be followed closely and selected for union enhancement by bone grafting if there is no progress toward healing.

Assessment for peripheral nerve damage always should be performed. Primary nerve repair rarely is indicated in association with grade III open fracture wounds. The full extent of the nerve damage usually cannot be determined at the first debridement. Additionally, the sophisticated reconstructive procedures involved in peripheral nerve microsurgery and/or nerve grafting should be accomplished only by a well-rested team skilled in such repair surgery. The same guidelines hold true for delayed tendon repair.

Naturally, stabilization of the bone is necessary to protect the vascular and neural anastomoses. External fixation is the preferred method of treatment. Use of an interarterial shunt to re-establish distal perfusion frequently is helpful when debridement and fracture stabilization might prolong re-establishment of vascular flow beyond the 8- to 10-hour deadline.

Indications for Primary Amputation

Usually, the limb with the combination of extensive peripheral nerve damage and extensive, irreparable, vascular injury should be considered for primary amputation. Limb salvage in these extensive injuries requires prolonged treatment and, usually, multiple reconstructive procedures; therefore, patient compliance is essential. Older patients with small-vessel occlusive disease, cardiovascular disease, chronic venous stasis, or history of drug or alcohol abuse[10] are poor candidates for such reconstructive procedures.

Soft-Tissue Reconstruction

The treatment options available for soft-tissue coverage of open fracture wounds include debridement and stimulation of secondary granulation tissue, relaxing incisions, local rotational flaps, split-thickness skin graft, local muscle or myocutaneous flaps, cross-leg flaps, and distant free flaps. The concept of closure is to convert the open fracture to a closed fracture wound when the tissues of the wound are ready to accept closure. Attempts at closure before the wound is clean and thoroughly debrided to viable soft tissue only invite wound breakdown and the establishment of a persistent infection.

Brown and Erbin showed excellent coverage by secondary intention granulation tissue in a series of combat injuries produced by high-velocity projectiles or fragmentation mines.[13] Although these injuries cause destruction of muscles and bone, they usually are associated with minimal skin loss, thus leaving an envelope of skin around the limb to undergo spontaneous secondary closure. If extensive skin damage has occurred as the result of high-kinetic-energy pedestrian-auto accidents, motorcycle accidents, or the like, closure of such defects is less reliable.

Split-thickness skin grafts can be applied to bone that has developed granulation tissue. However, cortical bone that may be denuded of its periosteum does not accept split-thickness skin grafts. When a split-thickness skin graft takes, it usually provides an unstable scar that is adherent to bone and bone multibreakdown when exposed to direct trauma. This situation frequently occurs in tibia fractures where the bone is directly subcutaneous. Hicks followed 54 open tibia fractures with skin breakdown over the anterior medial surface treated by either skin grafting or secondary granulation healing over bone.[14] Of these limbs, 90% showed successful wound healing in the short term, but at 10-year follow-up, only 60% of the limbs had remained healed. The incidence of hard-tissue healing disturbances has been correlated directly with the incidence of skin necrosis.

Rotational flaps can be used on occasion. However, the fluorescein test should be used both before and after the flap is rotated to ensure that the skin is viable. Moreover, the rotational flap can only cover a relatively small defect, and its use usually is not advisable in areas of significant cutaneous loss.

Pedicled Flaps

Pedicled muscle flaps appear to offer the best solution to the problem of soft-tissue coverage of grade III open fracture wounds. Such a flap consists of a strip of skin (cutaneous flap), a strip of muscle (muscle flap), or a strip of muscle and its surface skin (a myocutaneous flap) based on a single or multiple arterial pedicle (foot-like root). Such flaps can be provided for the grade III open fracture wound with a major skin loss when the wound is clean. If debridement is radical and judgment is good, this procedure can be performed at the time of a primary debridement. Because of the extensive injury caused by these wounds, however, a second look should be performed at 48 to 72 hours post-injury to allow any further debridement. Additionally, any organisms cultured at the initial debridement and found resistant to the antibiotic used for treatment can have proper antibiotic coverage provided at this time.

Rosenthal, et al., clearly established the importance of a skin cover and a viable envelope of soft tissue around severe open tibial fractures to prevent nonunion.[9] This finding further emphasizes the open-fracture-wound concept of a unified healing process between the soft and the hard tissues. Transposition of flaps accomplishes coverage of exposed bone, tendons, joint, or neurovascular structures while introducing a richly vascularized, soft-tissue envelope to the area of the fracture. Such an envelope promotes accelerated healing of the bone because it bypasses the usual lag phase required for the initiation of the healing response.[2]

A revolution in flap surgery has taken place over the past 10 years. The application of arterial flaps, the transfer of free flaps by microvascular anastomosis, and the expanding clinical applications of muscle flaps and myocutaneous flaps have vastly improved treatment outcomes and decreased periods of disability.

A major step in the execution of the flap includes an outline of the flap large enough to cover the defect. A local one-stage flap is preferred whenever possible. If flap viability might be in jeopardy, an arterial or myocutaneous flap should be used.

A number of free flaps with microvascular anastomosis have been described for soft-tissue cover.[15,16] However, 85% of the open fracture wounds that involve major skin loss are incurred about the tibia. A description of the most commonly used local flaps for crural coverage follows.

Muscle Flaps for Skin Defects about the Tibia (Table 11-2)

Either the medial (Fig. 11-1) or the lateral (Fig. 11-2) head of the gastrocnemius muscle may be transposed as a muscle flap or a musculocutaneous flap to cover the proximal or middle third of the tibia. Because the technical performance of executing a myocutaneous flap is no more taxing than that needed for executing a

TABLE 11-2. *Crural Myoplasty/Myocutaneous Coverage.*

Site of Soft-Tissue Defect	*Site from which Soft Tissue Transposed*
Tibia-proximal third	Gastrocnemius medial or lateral; soleus
Tibia-proximal/middle junction	Gastrocnemius medial or lateral; soleus
Tibia-middle third	Soleus, flexor digitorum longus
Tibia-middle/distal junction	Soleus, flexor digitorum longus
Tibia-distal third	Flexor digitorum longus; peroneus; distal based soleus

muscle flap, the compound unit usually is preferred. The skin directly overlying the muscle bellies is supplied by segmental blood vessels that penetrate from the underlying muscle fascia. McGraw, et al., established that the gastrocnemius myocutaneous flaps can further carry a random cutaneous flap distal to the muscle belly for about the same length as the width of the muscle (Fig. 11-3).[17]

The individual muscle belly, as well as the antero-posterior and distal borders of the skin flap, should be outlined with a skin marker. The incision is made along these lines without tourniquet control. The distal segment of skin should be elevated to keep intact its deep fascia and skived directly off the Achilles tendon. Medially, the saphenous nerve and vein must be identified while the sural nerve is protected laterally. Dissection should be continued proximally to isolate the gastrocnemius muscle from the soleus muscle. Identification of the gastrocnemius-soleus plane is performed more readily at the proximal level of the wound. Stay sutures should be placed at the muscle-fascia margins and into the subcutaneous tissue to prevent separation of the tissues and compromise of the skin vascularity. At the proximal posterior midline, the sural nerve helps to identify the area of separation of the medial and lateral heads. The vascular pedicle to both heads of the gastrocnemius (Fig. 11-4) usually comes out at or above the level of the tibial tubercle and should be protected as dissection is carried proximally. When the unit has been mobilized, the flap should be rotated into place, taking care not to kink the vascular pedicle. The flap then is sutured into the freshened skin edges of the skin defect. The donor defect is grafted immediately with meshed split-thickness skin.

The medial gastrocnemius myocutaneous flap covers the proximal and middle thirds of the tibia

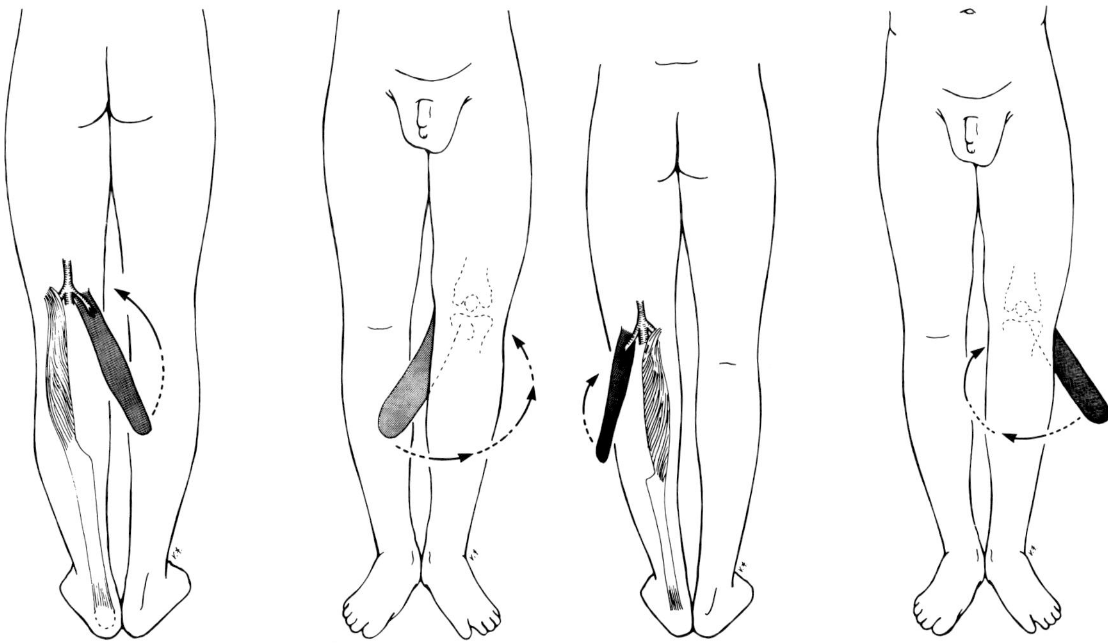

FIG. 11-1. Coverage arc, medial gastrocnemius.

FIG. 11-2. Coverage arc, lateral gastrocnemius.

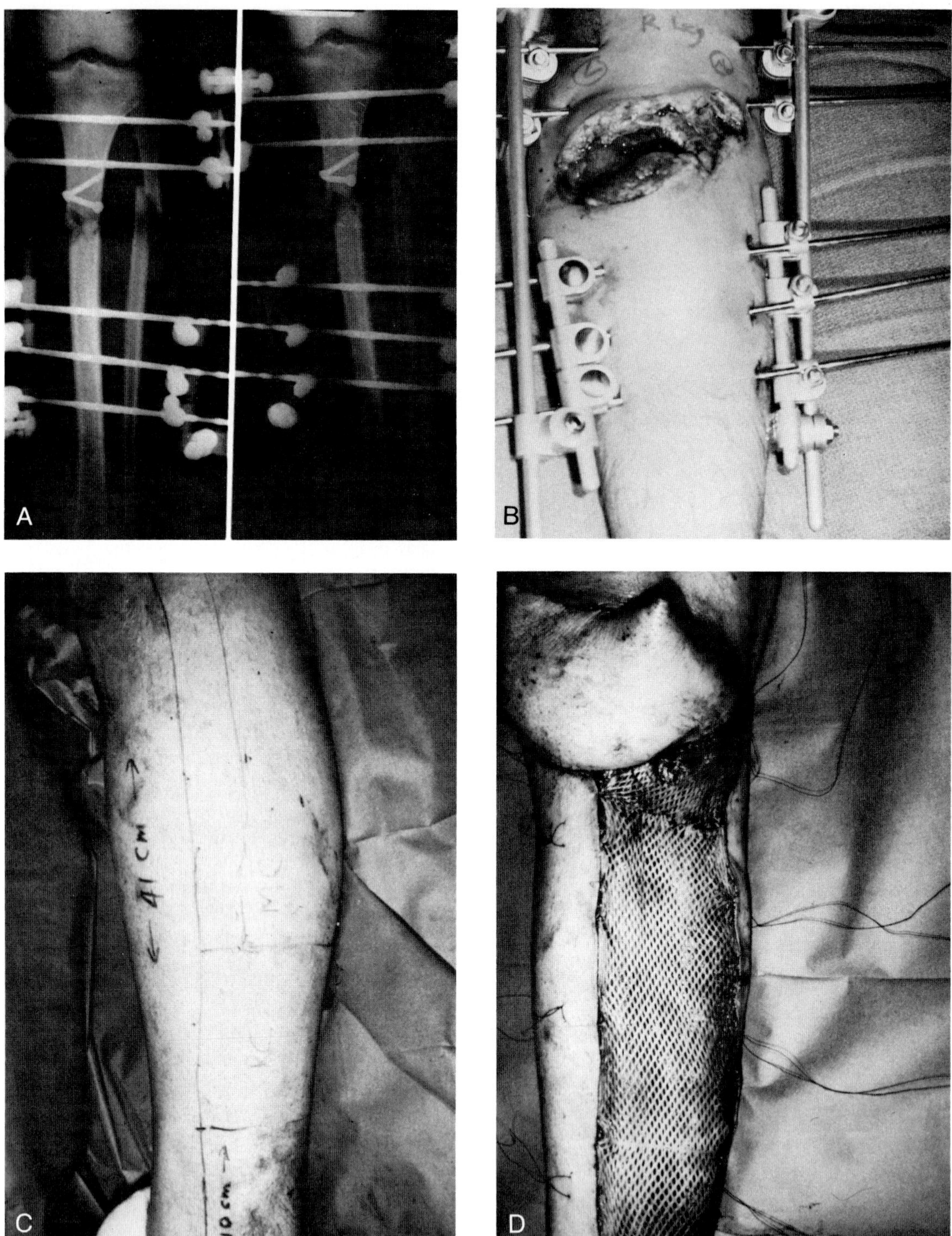

Fig. 11-3. *A*, Grade III open fracture wound managed with interfragmentary lag screws and external fix. *B*, Clinical appearance after second debridement 3 days after injury. *C*, Skin outlined for lateral gastrocnemius myocutaneous flap. *D*, Flap rotated to cover soft-tissue defect. Meshed split-thickness skin graft applied to donor site. *E*, Clinical appearance at 3 weeks after flap. *F*, Clinical appearance at 3 months after flap. (Continued on top of facing page.)

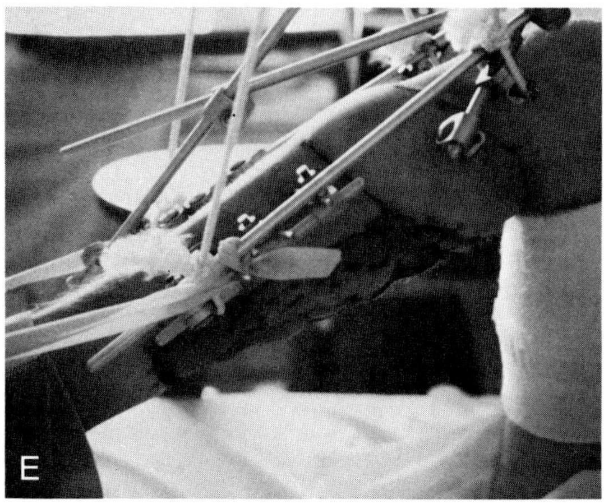

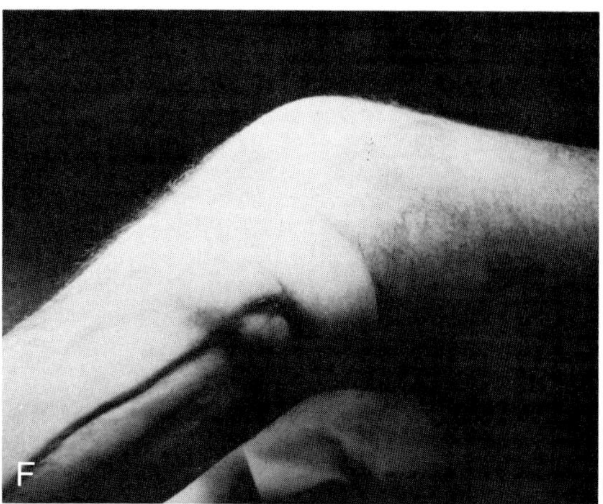

Fig. 11-3. *E, F.*

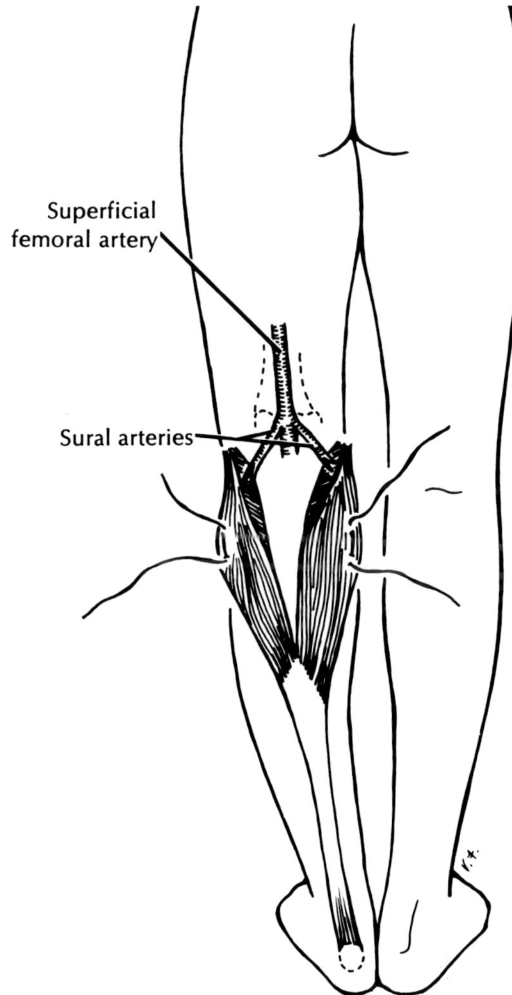

Fig. 11-4. Vascular hilae of gastrocnemius muscle.

on the medial side and resurfaces as much as 15 cm proximal to the knee joint itself. The lateral gastrocnemius myocutaneous flap is not quite as long as the medial gastrocnemius myocutaneous flap and may have some difficulty reaching lateral defects at the middle distal junction of the tibia. Its upward mobility reaches only 10 cm above the knee joint.

The gastrocnemius, as previously stated, also can be taken as a muscle flap. In this situation, exposure of the muscle is performed through a longitudinal posterior medial incision, which passes between the posterior medial border of the tibia and the medial border of the calcaneal tendon and extends from the tibial tubercle down to the distal third of the limb. Proximally, the medial head of the gastrocnemius is superficial to the soleus and just lateral to the plantaris tendon. The muscle belly is transected distally at the musculotendinous junction. Transposition of the muscle is accomplished through a direct cutaneous path by incision or by fashioning a subcutaneous tunnel through which the muscle can be passed anteriorly. Direct connection is preferred because the skin may be marginally vascularized and the underlying fascial segmental blood supply is disrupted when the subcutaneous tunnel is formed.

The soleus muscle is approached for myoplasty in a fashion similar to that for the medial gastrocnemius (Fig. 11-5). The soleus is identified deep to the medial head of the gastrocnemius, and its fibers are dissected sharply from the deep surface of the Achilles tendon. The muscle then is retracted laterally, and the distal arterial pedicles from the posterior tibial artery are li-

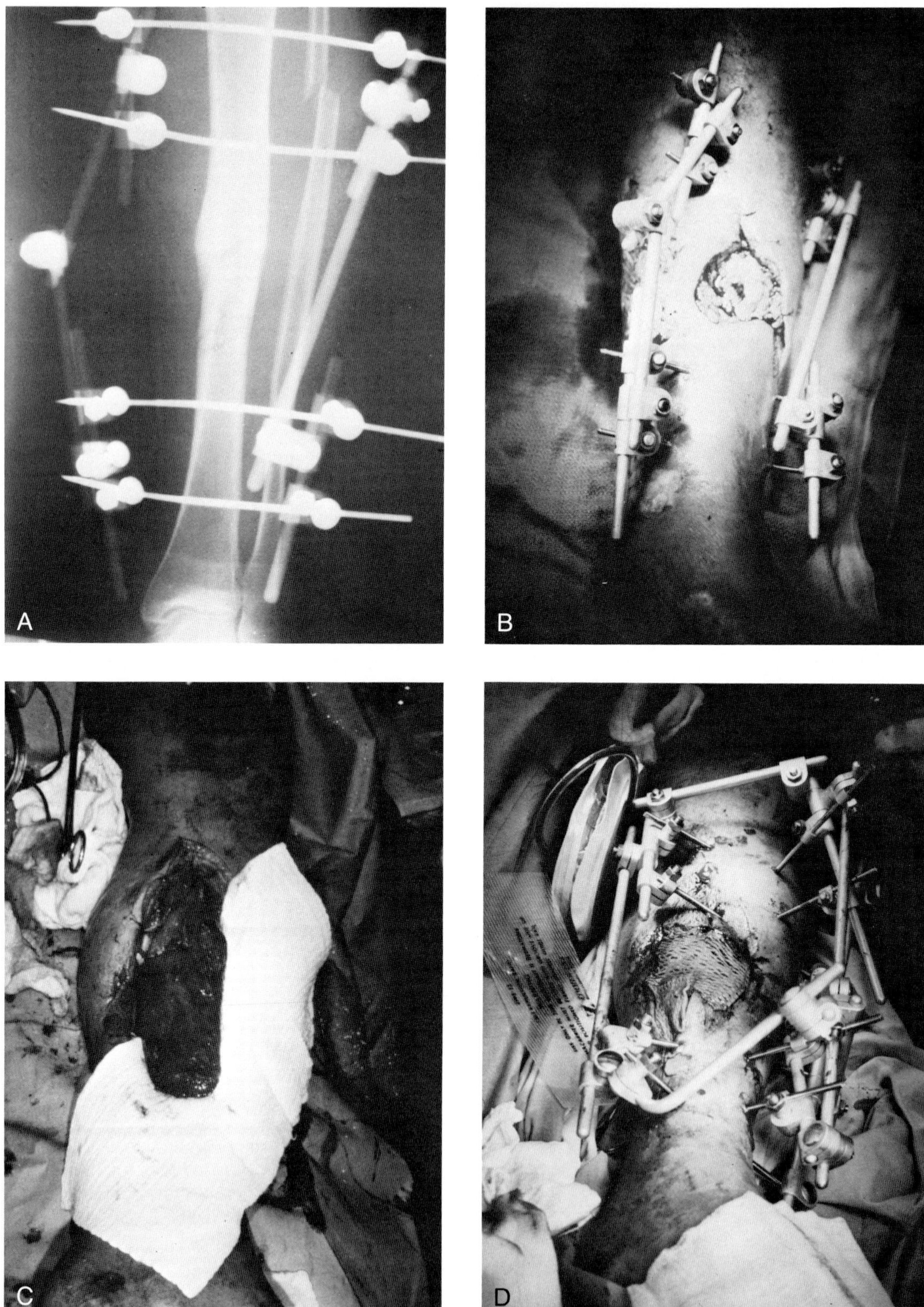

Fig. 11-5. *A* through *D*. (Continued on facing page.)

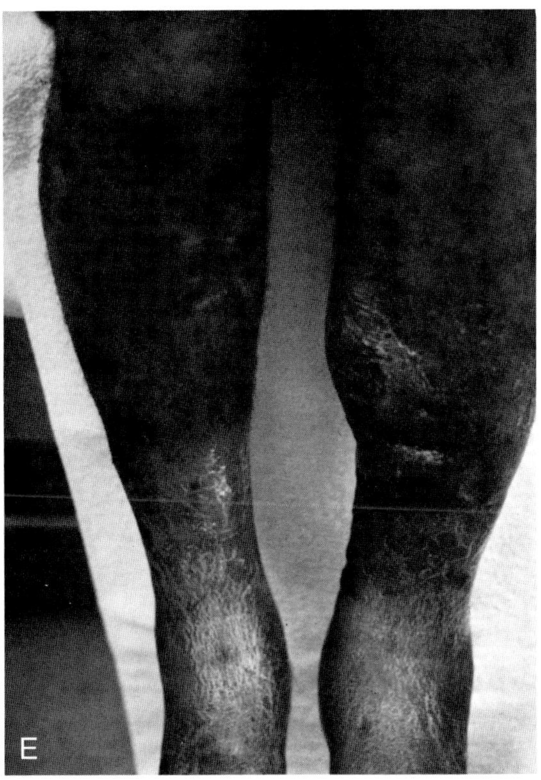

FIG. 11-5. *A*, Grade III open fracture wound in limb compromised by previous but healed grade II open fracture in same segment of tibia. *B*, Clinical appearance at time of soleus myoplasty, 5 days after injury. *C*, Soleus flap dissected out (proximal base). *D*, Soleus flap covered with meshed split-thickness skin graft. *E*, Clinical appearance 3 months after myoplasty.

gated and divided. Stay sutures help to prevent fraying of the lower end of the muscle. The anterior border of the muscle then should be defined as dissection proceeds from distal to proximal. The muscle length is tested continually, and when enough soleus has been mobilized, it is rotated forward into the defect. After hemostasis has been accomplished, suturing is performed into the freshened skin edges of the defect. Usually, the donor area can be closed primarily. Meshed split-thickness skin graft can be applied immediately. Alternatively, skin graft can be harvested and applied 3 to 4 days later after a secondary debridement of the muscle.

The soleus also serves as the best alternative for coverage of the distal third of the tibia. If there is a failure of management in cutaneous cover of the severe open fracture wound or in exposed and dead cortical bone, tendinous or neurovascular structures severely compromise the treatment outcome. A soleus has a unique segmental blood supply that comes from the posterior tibial artery (Fig. 11-6), and a distally based soleus flap has been described.[18] McGraw has described an 18% failure rate overall.[16] The distal-based flap is less predictable than the proximal-based flap and, therefore, is best undertaken after the acute management phase of the injury has passed. Additionally, preoperative arteriography should be performed to demonstrate good feeder vessels to the soleus from the posterior tibial artery. The muscle is exposed with a posteromedial incision. Special care must be taken to preserve the segmental arteries when isolating the undersurface of the soleus. At least three distal segmental vessels should be preserved before the muscle is transected proximally. The flap is rotated through a direct incision or through elevation of a subcutaneous tunnel and can reach the medial malleolus. Skin grafting is performed acutely with meshed skin or at 3 to 5 days postoperatively when a second look is undertaken. Because the distal-based soleus flap is the least pre-

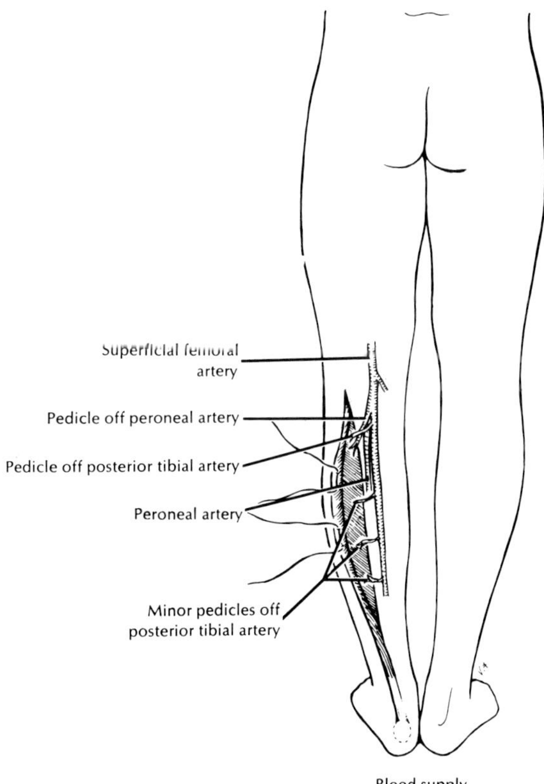

FIG. 11-6. Segmental vascular supply to soleus muscle.

dictable of the flaps described, the graft should be harvested at the initial operation and applied at a second-look procedure 2 to 3 days postoperatively. If any muscle at the tip has necrosed during this time period, it can be debrided back to viable muscle and the skin graft applied thereafter.

Distant Flaps

Cross-leg pedicle flaps can be useful when the ipsilateral open fracture wound is caused by circumferential crush or blast injury or when there is associated proximal arterial injury. In these situations, the local muscle has poor or marginal blood supply and should not be transposed. Cross-leg flaps are best moved as myocutaneous units to establish the best vascular envelope (Fig. 11-7).

The most versatile of the free flaps developed for skin cover is the latissimus dorsi free flap (Fig. 11-8).[19] Microvascular anastomosis is required for such distant free transfers. Bone/soft-tissue composite flaps are discussed in the following section.

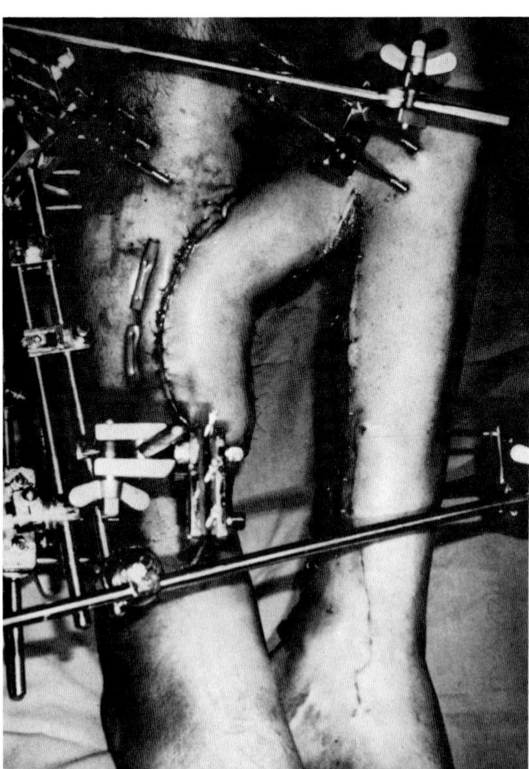

Fig. 11-7. Gastrocnemius cross-leg myocutaneous flap.

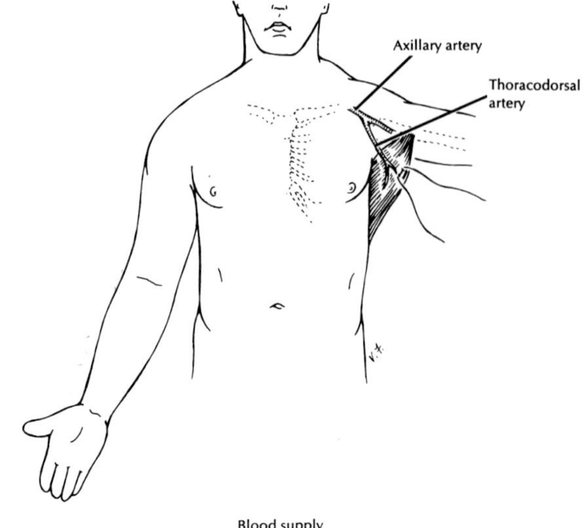

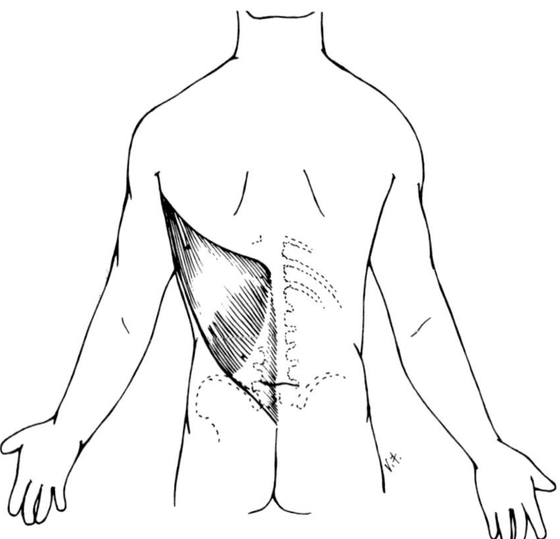

Fig. 11-8. *A*, Vascular supply to latissimus dorsi. *B*, Latissimus dorsi free flap.

Bone Reconstruction

The treatment options available for reconstruction of bone defects associated with open fractures include autogenous, cortical, or cancellous bone, local transfer of whole bone segments,[20] allografted bone transplants,[21] pedicled bone grafts,[22] and free vascularized bone grafts. Each of these techniques presents problems that may compromise the end result. Autogenous, cortical, or cortical-cancellous grafts and allografts become dead segments of bone that require replacement by creeping apposition from the viable bone at each end. By and large, such grafts should be used only as a late reconstructive option. They should not be used in the acute management of open fracture wounds with large bony defects because such grafts have a high propensity to infection or resorption.

Autogenous cancellous bone can serve as a scaffolding for bone repair and seems to be resistant to infection when grafted into open or previously infected fractures.[23] When the bone defect is less than 3 cm in size, or when the limb can be shortened to create a bone defect of 3 cm or less, autogenous cancellous bone can be used to span the defect. If possible, the wound should be clean when the cancellous bone is applied. A circumferential vascular soft-tissue cuff gives the best results, and, consequently, pedicled myoplasty flaps should be turned for coverage instead of leaving the graft exposed.

Frequently, a defect encompasses only part of the total circumference of a bone, e.g., an anterior tibial defect. When there is bone continuity but not full bone volume, the cancellous, autogenous graft can be placed into the cavity. Care should be taken to ensure that the bone surrounding the cavity is viable. Since this procedure should be done as a reconstructive operation in the post-trauma phase, determination of bone viability can be performed. The patient is given 500 mg of tetracycline every 6 hours by mouth for 3 days prior to the contemplated operation. Dead cortical bone can be identified in the operating room by its nonfluorescence to the Wood's light. Autogenous cancellous bone that fills such saucer defects undergoes skin wound healing by secondary intention. Alternatively viable autogenous cancellous bone grafts accept split-thickness skin. However, there remains a problem of adherent, relatively unstable skin coverage, which is subject to repetitive trauma and breakdown. Myoplastic coverage obviates such late breakdown problems.

Freeland and Mutz have reported excellent results with posterior lateral bone grafting for infected nonunions of the tibia.[24] A fibula protibia can be fashioned for acute defects of the tibia by using cancellous bone graft to establish a tibia-fibula synostosis. Such an operation in the acute limb injury is not as predictable as in the chronic, nonunited tibia fracture.

Pedicled bone grafts have been described in the lower limb[25] and in the forearm.[26] In the lower limb, a fibular segment of appropriate length can be taken by osteotomy and isolated on its nutrient blood supply from the feeding peroneal vessels along with a sleeve of muscle. The graft then is positioned next to the tibia, and lag screws are used to fix the proximal and distal ends. Supplemental external skeletal stabilization should be used to protect the tibiofibular synostosis in the early stages. External fixation should be discontinued after early stability is achieved to allow functional stressing of the bone-healing mechanism and to encourage hypertrophy of the fibular graft.

Microsurgical techniques have expanded the application of free vascularized bone grafts, which are particularly useful when a large segmental defect is not close to a bone suitable for pedicle bone grafting. Taylor has described such a free, fibular, vascularized bone graft.[27] Arteriography is required to evaluate the status of the blood supply to both the fibula that will be transferred and the extremity with the defect. This reconstructive procedure is technically demanding. The fibula is isolated along with a circumferential sleeve of muscle and taken with its vascular tree. It is then anastomosed by microvascular techniques to the feeder vessel of the recipient limb. Fixation may be obtained by doweling of the medullary canals with supplemental screw fixation. Again, external skeletal fixation is required in the early phases for supplementation.

When both osseous and cutaneous defects are present, the composite, osteocutaneous free graft is preferred.[28] Because of the inherent curve in the iliac crest, defects larger than 10 cm cannot be spanned by this type of graft. The composite groin flap is based on the superficial circumflex iliac artery, and again, preoperative arteriography is necessary to delineate both the donor and the recipient arterial trees (Fig. 11-9).

The desired result of long-term viability and stability for functional reconstruction of a limb with complex open fracture and bone defect is long in coming. Initially, external skeletal fixation is required to give the entire limb with a bony defect stability for the healing process between the recipient bone and its donor graft. Gradual increases of the functional stressing of the bone cause remodeling and reconstitution, but strength comes late. These limbs should be protected for as long as a year by appropriate casts or functional orthotic devices.

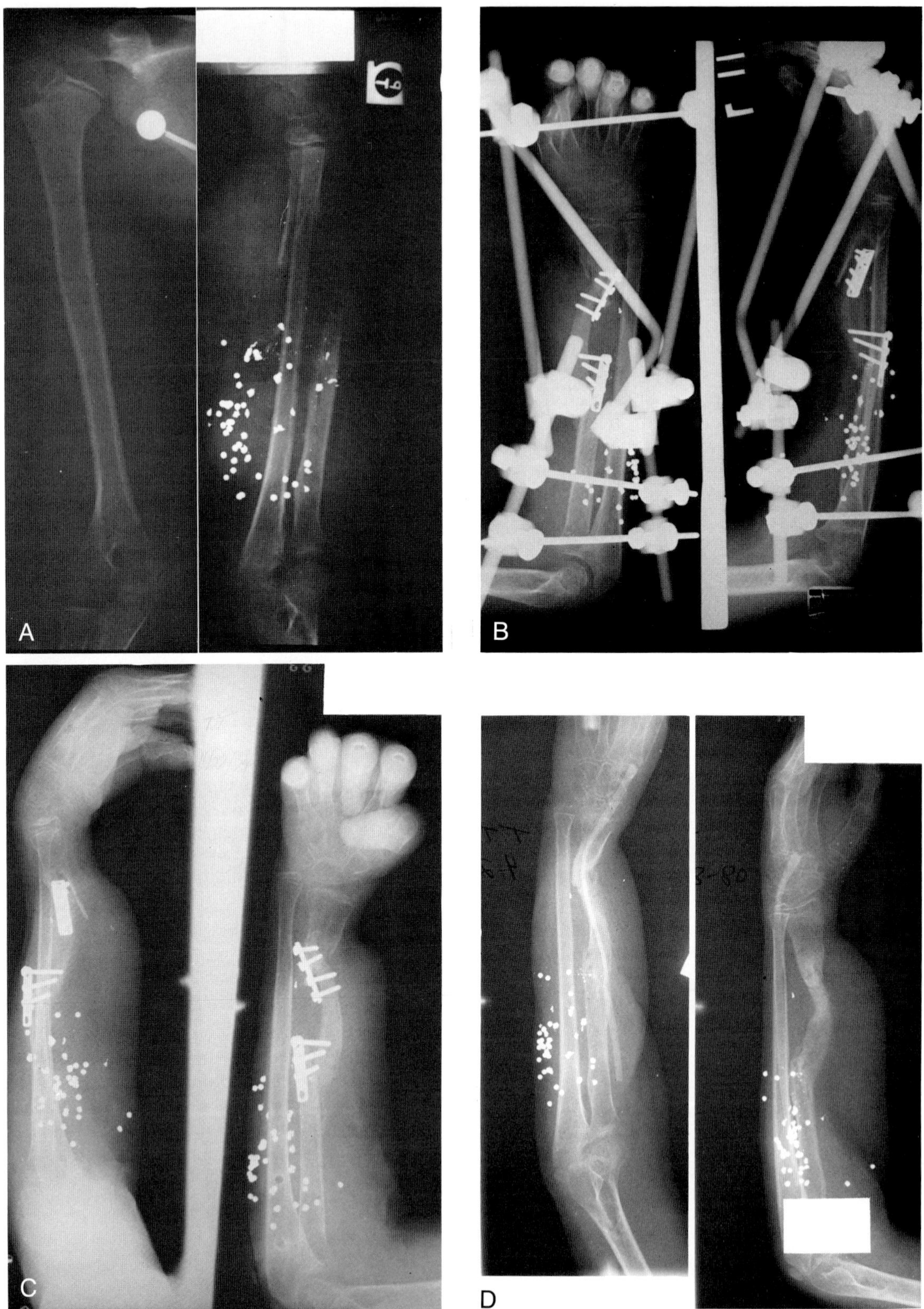

Fig. 11-9. *A* through *D*. (Continued on facing page.)

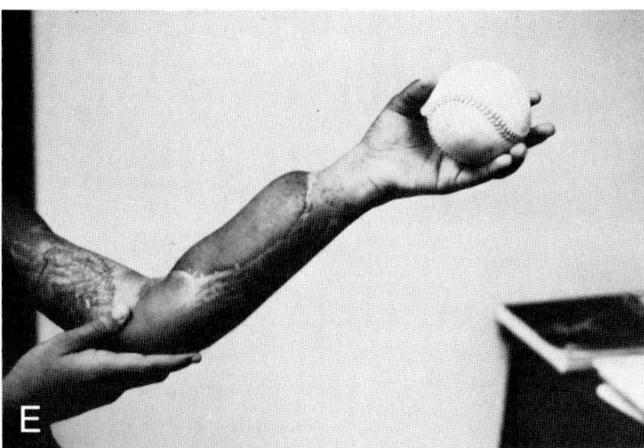

Fig. 11-9. *A*, Close-range grade III shotgun open fracture wound managed by external fixation in 11-year-old male. *B*, Composite iliac crest graft with microvascular anastamosis 2 months after injury. External fixation used to supplement plate internal splintage. *C*, External fixation removed 6 weeks after graft when bony consolidation apparent. Internal fixation removed 3 months after graft. *D*, Radiologic appearance 9 months after injury. *E*, Clinical appearance 9 months after injury.

References

1. Trueta, J.: Treatment of War Wounds and Fractures. London, Hamish-Hamilton, 1939.
2. Jones, R. E., Cierny, G. C., and Byrd, H. S.: External fixation and pedicle muscle flaps for complex open tibia fractures. *In* Current Concepts of External Fixation of Fractures. Edited by H. K. Uhtoff. Berlin, Springer-Verlag, 1982.
3. Rhinelander, F. W.: Tibial blood supply in relation to fracture healing. Clin. Orthop., *105*:34, 1974.
4. Holden, C. E.: The role of blood supply to soft tissues in the healing diaphyseal fractures. J. Bone Joint Surg., *54A*:993, 1972.
5. McGraw, J. B., Meyers, B., and Shanklin, K. D.: The value of fluorescein in predicting the viability of arterialized flaps. Plast. Reconstr. Surg., *60*:710, 1977.
6. Gregory, C. F.: Open fractures. *In* Fractures. Edited by C. A. Rockwood and D. P. Green. Philadelphia, J. B. Lippincott, 1975.
7. Nicoll, E. A.: Fractures of the shaft of the tibia. Acta Orthop. Scand. [Suppl.], *76*:1, 1965.
8. Edwards, P.: Fracture of the shaft of the tibia. Acta Orthop. Scand. [Suppl.] *76*:1, 1965.
9. Rosenthal, R. E., et al.: Non-union and open tibial fractures: analysis of reasons for failure of treatment. J. Bone Joint Surg., *59A*:244, 1977.
10. Karlstrom, G., and Olerud, S.: The management of tibial fractures in alcoholics and mentally disturbed patients. J. Bone Joint Surg., *56B*:730, 1974.
11. Friedrich, B., and Klaue, P.: Mechanical stability and post-traumatic osteitis. Injury, *9*:23, 1977.
12. Jones, R. E., Smith, E. C., and Bone, G.: Vascular and orthopedic complications of the knee dislocation. Surg. Gynecol. Obstet., *149*:554, 1979.
13. Brown, P. W., and Erbin, J. G.: Early weight bearing treatment of open fractures of the tibia. J. Bone Joint Surg., *51A*:59, 1969.
14. Hicks, J. H.: Long-term follow up of a series of infected fractures of the tibia. Injury, *7*:2, 1975.
15. Daniel, R. K., and Taylor, G. I.: Distant transfer of an island flap by microvascular anastomosis. Plast. Reconstr. Surg., *52*:111, 1973.
16. McGraw, J. P., and Dibbell, D. G.: Experimental definition of independent myocutaneous vascular territories. Plast. Reconstr. Surg., *60*:212, 1977.
17. McGraw, J. B., et al.: The versatile gastrocnemius myocutaneous flap. Plast. Reconstr. Surg., *62*:15, 1978.
18. Townsend, P. L. G.: An inferiorly based soleus muscle flap. Br. J. Plast. Surg., *31*:210, 1978.
19. McGraw, J. B., Penix, J. O., and Baker, J. W.: Repair of major defects of the chest wall and spine with latissimus dorsi myocutaneous flap. Plast. Reconstr. Surg., *62*:197, 1978.
20. McMaster, P. E., and Hohl, M.: Tibio-fibular cross leg grafting. J. Bone Joint Surg., *47A*:1146, 1965.
21. Mankin, H. J., et al.: Massive resection and allograft transplantation and the treatment of malignant bone tumors. N. Engl. J. Med., *124*:1247, 1976.
22. Medgyesis, P.: Observations of pedicled bone grafts in goats. Scand. J. Plast. Reconstr. Surg., *7*:110, 1973.
23. Burri, C., Passler, H. H., and Henkeneyer, H.: Treatment of post traumatic osteomyelitis with bone, soft tissue and skin defects. J. Trauma, *13*:799, 1973.
24. Freeland, A. E., and Mutz, S. B.: Posterior bone grafting for infected, ununited fractures of the tibia. J. Bone Joint Surg., *58A*:653, 1976.
25. Weinberg, H., et al.: Early fibular bypass procedures (tibiofibular synostosis) for massive bone loss and war injuries. J. Trauma, *19*:177, 1979.
26. Haddad, R. J., and Drez, D.: Salvage procedures for defects in the forearm bones. Clin. Orthop., *104*:183, 1974.
27. Taylor, G. I.: Microvascular free bone transfer. Orthop. Clin. North Am., *8*:425, 1977.
28. Taylor, G. I., and Watson, N.: One-stage repair of compound leg defects with free revascularized flaps of groin skin and iliac bone. Plast. Reconstr. Surg., *61*:494, 1978.

Chapter 12 Recognition and Treatment of Nutritional Deficits in the Multiply Injured Patient

TAYLOR K. SMITH

With the advent of better methods of providing patients with supplemental nutrition in the form of enteral and parenteral hyperalimentation, there has been renewed interest in the effects of nutrition on wound healing and immunocompetence, particularly among physicians caring for the multiply injured patient. Several studies have indicated that a large number of hospitalized patients show evidence of malnutrition.[1-3] A significant number of these patients are admitted to the hospital in a malnourished state, but even more dramatic is the development of malnutrition in patients undergoing care for surgical conditions, especially trauma. The type of malnutrition exhibited by these hospitalized patients often is subtle and may be missed easily when only the usual parameters, such as height, weight, and physical appearance, are considered.

The metabolic needs of a patient who has been injured can be quite considerable, much greater than those of the unstressed, starving individual. A 70-kg person lying quietly in bed, not moving except to blink his eyes and sustain his bodily functions, utilizes about 600 calories per day. An active individual putting in a full day's work may require 2500 calories per day. A severely injured patient with fractures and burns may need as many as 10,000 calories per day. A patient with several long-bone fractures, lying quietly in bed in traction, requires far more calories and protein per day than does a marathon runner in active training. When these excessive needs for calories and protein are not met, the traumatized patient quickly develops a state of antianabolism or catabolism in which vital functional proteins are broken down to provide for life-sustaining glucose and energy. When the calories and proteins ingested or infused into a patient are inadequate to meet his increased metabolic needs, the patient begins to call upon his body tissues for nourishment, thus jeopardizing his ability to combat infection and heal injuries.

Energy Stores in the Body

Three components of the body can be catabolized for energy. Carbohydrates, mainly in the form of glycogen, provide about 1 or 2 calories per gram. Only about 80 calories of circulating glucose are available within the body. The remainder of these carbohydrates are stored in the liver and muscle glycogen deposits. Liver glycogen can be utilized readily and, in the average patient, provides up to 300 calories of available glucose.[4] Although there is twice as much muscle glycogen as liver glycogen, it cannot be utilized because muscle lacks the enzyme, glucose-6-phosphatase, that is necessary to release muscle glycogen for systemic use. For these reasons, the small stores of carbohydrates within the body are depleted quickly in starvation and stress states. Within 18 to 24 hours, a starved individual has utilized all his available glycogen stores.

Glucose is essential and is the only substrate that can be used for energy by certain organ systems. The central nervous system, the erythrocytes, and the kidney need a continuous source of glucose to maintain their function and viability. The central nervous system can utilize ketones to support some of its function; however, other organ systems, such as red cells of blood, do not have mitochondria and, therefore, cannot oxidize fatty acids for sources of energy.

In anaerobic areas, such as the leading edges of wounds, areas of necrosis and infection, and large areas of tumor, glucose is also the only energy substrate that can be used in the anaerobic metabolic pathway. There is, therefore, a constant demand for glucose in the body. Glucose, when not provided, is derived from other areas, primarily the amino-acid pool.

Fat stores within the body provide about 9 calories of energy per gram of fat. The neutralized fat stores are, however, poor sources of energy during physiologic stress because the body cannot and does not readily use these fat stores under such conditions. The fatty acids cannot be converted into glucose, but instead are oxidized for energy within the mitochondria of certain cells. In a starvation state, the body utilizes fat for 87% of its caloric needs, but 13% of the calories needed must still come from the breakdown of amino acids by gluconeogenesis.

When sufficient exogenous sources of calories and glucose are not provided, the body turns to its amino-acid pool for its source of energy. Amino acids can be converted readily to glucose. Within the body, protein is continuously broken down into its amino-acid components, and new protein is continuously formed from this available pool of amino acid. There is some inefficiency in this constant breakdown and reformation of protein, and in the normal individual, about .4 g of protein per kilogram of body weight is lost per day. This loss is compensated for easily by the ingestion of proteins in a normal diet. When the body's need for glucose is greater than its available stores and the amount of glucose ingested into the system, the amino-acid pool is tapped as a source for glucose. Consequently, the available amino acids needed for reformation of proteins are depleted rapidly from the amino-acid pool. As there is no stored, unutilized protein within the body, the removal of amino acids from this pool has a direct effect on the body's ability to function.

The effects of hypoproteinemia have been noted for years. Impaired wound strength and dehiscence were noted by Mecray, et al.,[5] who believed that such effects were related to the interstitial edema that occurs with lowering of the tissue osmotic pressure. Blood-volume decreases occur with hypoproteinemia, and response to blood loss can be jeopardized. Rhoads noted that poor callus formation in experimental fractures occurred in hypoproteinemic dogs.[6] Antibody production has been noted to be deficient in the hypoproteinemic patient, and the relationship of deficient antibody production to increased sepsis has been studied.[7]

The effects of hypoproteinemia on pulmonary function can be quite profound. Most starvation victims die of pneumonia. It has been postulated that the interstitial edema that occurs with hypoproteinemia, combined with the lassitude of the catabolic patient and the weakness of respiratory skeletal muscles caused by depletion of the skeletal muscle mass, leads to poor pulmonary toilet and the development of pneumonia.

Proteins within the body can be divided into two components. The somatic protein compartment is mainly skeletal muscle; the visceral protein compartment is composed of the blood components, visceral organs, and enzymes that perform vital functions in the body. Utilization of the somatic protein is manifested by wasting and weakness of muscle. When visceral protein is depleted, the various vital organ systems lose their ability to function. The loss of cardiac muscle mass is manifested by atrophy of the myocardium, a decrease in electrical activity as seen on electrocardiograms, and a decrease in the cardiac reserve found in the healthy heart. The transport mechanisms and the various blood components, including white cells and their activities, are affected. The total lymphocyte count decreases. The level of complement, antibodies, and other immune mechanisms are interfered with, and the patient's immunocompetence is jeopardized. The mucosa of the gut becomes atrophic, and the ability to absorb enteral nutrition is decreased. The numerous enzyme systems within the body are composed of proteins that normally turn over rapidly, some with half-lives in the range of minutes. When these enzyme systems begin to fail, the organism's ability to respond in any manner is jeopardized.

An unstressed individual on a starvation diet has several mechanisms that can be used to spare protein and to utilize endogenous carbohydrate and fat. Ketone bodies from fat are utilized readily as sources of calories, and about 70% of the daily energy requirements come from breakdown of fatty tissues. The unstressed, starved individual also decreases his metabolic rate considerably, thus sparing protein by cutting down on metabolic needs. With the onset of lethargy, the activity level of skeletal muscle decreases, the body temperature may fall, amenorrhea may develop, and various other organ systems cut back on their activities and utilization of calories. In a nonstress, starvation state, death results after about 40% of body weight is lost. A starved individual, even with all the protein-sparing mechanisms in force, usually dies of protein deficiency, even when unused reserve fat stores are present at death.

The injured patient, on the other hand, markedly increases his metabolic needs and is not able to bring his protein-sparing mechanisms into play. Proteins vital to the maintenance of function are utilized for fuel, as mentioned previously, and deterioration of organ systems results. Death results in the stressed individual with only a 25 to 30% loss of body weight.

During simple, unstressed starvation, a 70-kg man loses 5 to 7 g of nitrogen per day. During post-traumatic catabolism, 15 to 40 g of nitrogen may be lost each day by a 70-kg man. This nitrogen loss represents 250 g of protein or 1250 g of muscle tissue lost per day. Additional loss of protein from hemorrhage, plasma loss, and direct tissue loss can result in the loss of 3 pounds of muscle, or its equivalent, per day in the injured patient.[8]

Effect of Trauma

A large number of complicating factors increase the metabolic needs of the traumatized patient and decrease the patient's ability to meet these needs. Burns, fractures, and soft-tissue injuries markedly increase metabolic needs since repair of these injuries greatly taxes the pool of available protein and calories. Fever increases the metabolic needs of the patient by about 8% for each rise in temperature of 1°F. When sepsis develops, the polymorphonuclear leukocyte activity greatly taxes the available glucose pool because the anaerobic metabolism relied upon by this white cell needs the glucose to function.

Most traumatized individuals undergo a period of time during which the intake of adequate amounts of protein and calories is interfered with by treatment procedures. Patients held NPO for diagnostic and surgical procedures can lose a great deal of nourishment. In the past, physicians deluded themselves into thinking that they were replacing their patients' caloric needs by administering "maintenance" amounts of 5% dextrose solutions. Three liters of 5% dextrose solution per day provide only 600 calories of energy per day. Consequently, a trauma victim with multiple injuries, fever, and sepsis, who is not taking in adequate amounts of nutrition, rapidly depletes his protein and caloric stores and may develop complications.

Nutritional Assessment

The trauma surgeon must anticipate, recognize, and treat nutritional deficits in patients. A fairly standard nutritional-assessment profile has been formulated over a period of time to give an objective appraisal of the patient's nutritional status. This appraisal consists of anthropometric measurements, laboratory measurements of various parameters, and assessments of the patient's immune response.

The anthropometric studies that we conduct are measurements of height and weight, measurement of the triceps skin fold, and measurement of the arm circumference. By utilizing the following formula, standard charts of height, weight, circumference of triceps skin fold, and circumference of arm muscle have been derived and percent of normal can be calculated.

$$\text{Arm muscle circumference} = \text{Midarm circumference} - (0.314 \times \text{triceps skin fold})$$

Laboratory tests mainly provide insight into the visceral-protein-compartment status. The serum albumin is a gross and somewhat delayed indicator of visceral-protein status as serum albumin has a half-life of about 20 days. A low serum-albumin level indicates a prolonged malnutrition state. (This study may be inaccurate if there has been a recent infusion of blood transfusions or if edema is present.) A more accurate assessment of the serum proteins can be obtained by using the serum-transferrin level. Serum transferrin has a shorter half-life than albumin, measuring only 8.8 days, and is measured by the radial immunodiffusion technique. Proteins with an even shorter half-life are being investigated at this time to give us a more minute-by-minute assessment of the visceral-protein compartment's response to treatment.

The urinary creatinine is measured for 24 hours, and the creatinine height index is calculated by the following formula:

$$\text{Creatinine/height} = \frac{\text{actual urinary creatinine}}{\text{ideal urinary creatinine}} \times 100$$

The nitrogen balance is derived by measuring the protein intake and the urinary urea nitrogen. It is derived by the following formula:

$$\text{Nitrogen balance} = \frac{\text{protein intake in grams}}{6.25} - (\text{urine urea nitrogen in grams} + 4)$$

The function of the immunologic system can be estimated by several measurements. The total lymphocyte count, which is derived by using the following formula, has been a sensitive indicator of the patient's ability to respond to stress.

$$\text{Total lymphocyte count} = \frac{\text{percent lymphocytes} \times \text{WBC}}{100}$$

Skin antigen testing is carried out with .1 mm each of dermatophytin, candida, varidase, mumps, and intermediate purified derivative (PPD). The skin-test response is recorded at 24 and 48 hours; a positive reaction is present if an induration of at least 5 mm in diameter is apparent at 48 hours. The presence of anergy to all the five skin tests carries an increased risk for sepsis and death, and may be indicative of a severe depletion of visceral protein stores.

No test of nutritional status is meaningful by itself; the whole battery of tests must be considered when deciding the nutritional status of a patient. Of even more importance is the change in the nutritional-assessment parameters as the course of the patient's recovery from trauma unfolds. If a patient shows depletion of somatic protein and fat stores by decreases in triceps-skinfold and arm-muscle circumference measurements, shows evidence of visceral protein depletion by a decrease in laboratory parameters of albumin, transferrin, total lymphocyte count, and creatinine height index, is in severe negative balance, and shows a development of anergy to repeated skin testing, he is likely to develop complications during recovery from trauma. This patient more than likely would benefit from the use of hyperalimentation, and elective procedures, such as skin grafting and internal fixation of fractures, perhaps should be postponed until nutritional status is improved. One must be careful not to judge a patient's nutritional status by only one of several of the indices. We have found that a single patient rarely exhibits abnormalities in all areas, even in the presence of severe protein and caloric malnutrition; however, the overall nutritional-assessment profile and the trends it is taking are of great importance.

Hyperalimentation

Hyperalimentation is the provision of nutrition to an individual in amounts greater than he normally consumes. Hyperalimentation in trauma patients is utilized when the nutritional deficits experienced by the patient obviously will jeopardize his ability to recover from injuries. Throughout the ages, mankind has seen the need for adequate nourishment in recovery from disease and injury. Chicken soup, between-meal snacks, and supplementary foods, such as eggs in milk shakes, have been used for many years in an attempt to increase the caloric and protein intake of patients under physical stress.

Intravenous fluid and electrolyte and glucose replacements have been used for decades, but the development of more adequate methods of measuring caloric and protein needs has shown that much greater amounts of nutrients than could be infused through a peripheral vein were needed. As mentioned previously, 3 L per day of 5% glucose only provide 600 calories. Higher concentrations of glucose cause injury to the intima of the peripheral veins, and greater amounts of fluid cause fluid overloading. In 1968, Dudrick and associates demonstrated the clinical and experimental practicality of infusing hypertonic dextrose and amino-acid solution directly into the central venous system.[9] They were able to sustain normal growth and development in puppies, and later in infants, by meeting the need for calories, protein, trace elements, vitamins, and essential fats. This method of intravenous hyperalimentation currently is used to maintain positive nitrogen balance in many types of malnourished patients.

The earliest and simplest method of providing hyperalimentation to patients who could not, or would not, ingest food, but who had normal gastrointestinal tracts, was to infuse nutriments directly into the stomach through a nasogastric tube or a gastrostomy tube, or directly into the jejunum through a jejunostomy tube. These routes still are preferable to that of intravenous hyperalimentation through a central venous line because of the possible complications of sepsis with the central venous line.

If the decision to provide hyperalimentation is made following assessment of the patient's needs, an attempt should be made to use an enteral route, if possible. At the time of laparotomy for other injuries, such as liver lacerations and splenectomy, a gastrostomy or jejunostomy tube may be inserted and brought up through the skin for later use to avoid the anticipated malnutrition. These tubes usually can be removed without a separate operative procedure, and their likelihood of getting infected or being a source of sepsis is quite low.

Enteral routes for hyperalimentation can be utilized in conjunction with parenteral hyperalimentation in cases of severe injury in which the protein and caloric needs of the patient tax the abilities of either route alone. By lessening the load of supplemental nutrition by either route, the complications of administration are decreased.

When intravenous hyperalimentation becomes necessary, great care must be exercised in planning and carrying out the placement of the intravenous catheter as well as in caring for the catheter during intravenous hyperalimentation. The placement of the catheter is carried out under strict aseptic techniques, preferably in the operating room. The patient is placed in a slight Trendelenburg position during the procedure so that positive pressure in the subclavian vein can be maintained. The skin over the clavicle, shoulder, neck, and upper chest is shaved, prepared with a solvent to remove skin oil, and scrubbed and treated with a povidine-iodine solution. The supraclavicular area is widely draped with sterile towels. Local anesthesia is infiltrated into the skin and subcutaneous tissue just beneath the midpoint of the clavicle. A 2-inch, 14-gauge needle attached to a 3-ml syringe is inserted bevel down into the skin and advanced beneath the inferior margin of the clavicle, aiming across the body to the anterior margin of the trachea at the level of the suprasternal notch. During this procedure, the head is turned to the opposite side. A slight negative pressure is maintained on the syringe, and when the needle penetrates the subclavian vein, a flow of venous blood will be encountered. If air is aspirated into the syringe, the needle should be withdrawn and the presence of a pneumothorax ruled out by chest roentgenogram. Bright red blood filling the syringe may indicate that the subclavian artery has been entered; the needle must be backed out and pressure must be applied over the subclavian artery area until bleeding stops.

When the subclavian vein is entered, the needle is advanced slightly into the lumen of the vein, and then is carefully held in place with a hemostat. While the patient performs Valsalva's maneuver to prevent an air embolism, an 8-inch, 16-gauge radiopaque catheter is threaded through the needle and into the vein. The patient should rotate his head back to neutral or to the side of the needle puncture to reduce the possibility of the passage of the catheter into the jugular vein. The catheter should slide easily into the lumen of the vein, and if difficulty is encountered in threading the catheter through the needle, the entire catheter and needle should be removed as a unit. The catheter must not be removed through the lumen of the needle while it is in place because the bevel of the needle may cut the catheter, thereby inciting an embolism in the central venous system. After the catheter is fully threaded into the needle, the catheter is connected to a solution of sterile intravenous fluid and is flushed. The needle then is withdrawn carefully, and the catheter is sutured in place at the skin puncture site. Free flow of the catheter fluid can be checked by lowering the container of solution below the patient's heart level to check for free backflow of blood into the catheter.

An antimicrobial or antiseptic ointment is applied around the puncture site, and an occlusive sterile dressing is fixed to the skin. The intravenous tubing attached to the catheter is looped over the dressing and secured again with tape to prevent traction on the catheter. Chest roentgenograms should be performed immediately to determine the site of the tip of the catheter as well as to rule out the presence of a pneumothorax.

Specific physicians and nurses should be responsible for caring for the catheters used for intravenous hyperalimentation. Meticulous sterile dressing changes should be carried out every 2 days; the intravenous administration tubing should be changed at that time also. The exit site is cleansed with a solvent, and additional antimicrobial or antiseptic ointment is applied around the catheter site. The sterile occlusive dressing is replaced. This catheter should not be used for drawing blood for laboratory studies nor should it be used for the infusion of blood products, bolus medication or other drugs. Finally, this catheter should not be used for central venous pressure monitoring.

If sepsis develops, the central venous catheter

must be removed, appropriate cultures of the catheter tip and puncture site taken, and appropriate antibiotics begun. If parenteral hyperalimentation is to be continued, another puncture site can be used after removal of the infected catheter. If the patient is systemically septic from other causes, such as burns or pulmonary infections, the catheter site should be changed every 2 or 3 days, as colonization of bacteria on the catheter quickly leads to catheter sepsis. If the patient does not develop sepsis and is tolerating the intravenous hyperalimentation without difficulty, the catheter should be changed every month until treatment is completed.

This chapter will not describe in detail the formulation of hyperalimentation solutions. The composition of the hyperalimentation solutions should be individualized to each patient and should be tailored according to the response of the patient to nutritional supplementation (indicated by the nutritional-assessment parameters). Most intravenous hypertonic nutrient solutions consist of 20 to 25% dextrose, 4 to 5% crystalline amino acids or protein hydrolysates, and 1 to 3% of trace minerals and multiple vitamins. Each unit of solution provides about 5.25 to 6 g of nitrogen and 900 to 1000 calories per 1100 ml of solution. The electrolyte concentrations are altered according to the patient's needs. Sodium administration is decreased in patients with congestive heart failure or liver failure, and amounts of potassium, phosphorus, and magnesium often are omitted in patients with decreased renal function. Acidosis can be compounded by the use of amino acids that are prepared as salts of chloride and hydrochloride ions, but acetate salts can be substituted to avoid hyperchloremic metabolic acidosis.

The level of glucose in the solution should be monitored carefully because excessive blood glucose levels result in osmotic diuresis. The addition of insulin to the intravenous infusion may facilitate the utilization of glucose, especially in patients with diabetes mellitus. The development of hyperglycemia may herald the onset of sepsis or may indicate hypercatabolism, as seen with abscess formation.

Summary

The physician who treats patients with multiple injuries should be aware that the metabolic needs of polytrauma patients are far in excess of basal metabolic needs and that various factors can increase the patient's likelihood of developing malnutrition. By utilizing the nutritional-assessment profile, the presence of malnutrition and the response of the patient to nutritional supplementation therapy can be evaluated. Of far greater importance, of course, is the recognition that these patients need supplementation to counteract the severe protein and caloric deficiencies they develop and that these treatment modalities should be instituted early in the course of the patient's care. Various routes and compositions of hyperalimentation are available, and the physician should attempt to choose those most appropriate for the patient.

References

1. Bistrian, B. R., Blackburn, G. L., Hallowell, E., and Heddle, R.: Protein status of general surgical patients. J.A.M.A., *230*:858, 1974.
2. Bistrian, B. R., et al.: Prevalence of malnutrition in general medical patients. J.A.M.A., *235*:1567, 1976.
3. Hill, G. L., et al.: Malnutrition in surgical patients—an unrecognized problem. Lancet, *1*:689, 1977.
4. Cahill, G. F.: Starvation in man. N. Engl. J. Med., *282*:668, 1970.
5. Mecray, P. M., Barden, R. P., and Ravdin, I. S.: Nutritional edema: its effects on gastric emptying time before and after gastric operations. Surgery, *1*:53, 1937.
6. Rhoads, J. E., and Kasinskas, W.: Influence of hypoproteinemia on the formation of callus in experimental fracture. Surgery, *11*:38, 1942.
7. Wohl, M. D., Reinholt, J. G., and Rose, S. B.: Antibody response in patients with hypoproteinemia. Arch. Intern. Med., *83*:402, 1949.
8. Dudrick, S. J., and Rhoads, J. E.: Metabolism in surgical patients. *In* Textbook of Surgery. Edited by D. C. Sabiston. Philadelphia, W. B. Saunders, 1977.
9. Dudrick, S. J., Wilmore, D. W., Vars, H. M., and Rhoads, J. E.: Long-term total parenteral nutrition with growth, development and positive nitrogen balance. Surgery, *64*:134, 1968.

Chapter 13 Extremity Fractures in Head Injured Adults

DOUGLAS E. GARLAND
ROBERT L. WATERS

Although the total number of adults with acute brain injuries is decreasing, the number of survivors is increasing as the result of advances in emergency care and the establishment of trauma centers and specialized intensive-care facilities.[1] These survivors are generally males who are less than 25 years of age.[2] The injury is frequently the result of a high-velocity accident—a moving vehicle or a fall from a height (Table 13-1).[1] Multiple injuries are common.

These patients pose considerable diagnostic and therapeutic challenges to the orthopaedic surgeon. Life-saving resuscitation often detracts from complete physical and radiographic evaluation of associated musculoskeletal injuries. Clinically significant injuries usually are painful, and the patient with an intact sensorium directs the physician's attention to them. The comatose or disoriented patient with brain injury, however, cannot assist in the history or physical examination. Even when a musculoskeletal injury is recognized, an uncertainty regarding the proper course of treatment often prevails because of the lack of understanding of the patient's prognosis for neurologic recovery from the head injury.

TABLE 13-1. *Type of Trauma and Age Group in 121 Consecutive Patients at Adult Head Trauma Unit—Rancho Los Amigos Hospital.*[8]

Injury	*Age Groups*				
Major Trauma	*18–29*	*30–39*	*40–49*	*>50*	*Total*
Automobile	38	5	7	5	55
Motorcycle	20	1	1	—	22
Auto-pedestrian	5	1	2	1	9
Train-auto	1	—	—	—	1
Fall from height	4	—	—	—	4
Localized Head Trauma					
Blunt object	4	4	3	3	14
Fall	—	—	2	8	10
Unknown	—	1	3	2	6
Total	72	12	18	19	121

Neurologic and medical instability, poor patient compliance, spasticity, and heterotopic ossification complicate fracture management in patients with head injuries. Certain general principles for overall fracture care are applicable, and specific guidelines aid in the treatment of individual fractures.

General Treatment

Five basic principles were formulated from a 2-year review of 99 skeletal injuries to aid in the prevention of complications in fracture treatment.[3,4] The value of these rules has since been verified in the treatment of a large number of acute fractures in the patient with head injuries. These rules are: (1) establish the diagnosis; (2) base treatment on the assumption that the patient who survives will make a good neurologic recovery; (3) do not cast joints in a flexed position; (4) avoid traction methods, either skin or skeletal, for prolonged fracture management; and (5) anticipate uncontrolled limb motion and poor patient compliance.

Delayed Recognition of Trauma

One of the most common reasons for unsatisfactory healing of a fracture is the delayed recognition of the injury. Two separate reviews of patients with head injuries treated at Rancho Los Amigos Hospital, undertaken approximately 5 years apart, demonstrated a 10% incidence of missed orthopaedic injuries (Table 13-2).[3,5] The first study revealed that mainly spine or hip injuries were overlooked, whereas the second study identified a large number of missed peripheral nerve palsies. After the first review we recommended that a patient who is comatose following a high-velocity accident should undergo anteroposterior and lateral radiographic examination of the cervical and thoracolumbar spine. Pedestrian victims of auto accidents should be screened for injuries to the pelvis, hips, and knees by an anteroposterior roentgenogram of the pelvis, including the hips, and an anteroposterior radiograph of the knees.

In the second review, 29 of 254 patients demonstrated 39 unrecognized injuries.[5] These 29 patients sustained 72 fractures or dislocations. Twenty-nine neuropathies were discovered and generally were associated with fractures. Some neuropathies were primary, whereas others were secondary to nerve compression. The most commonly missed neuropathies involved the peroneal, ulnar, and median nerves. Neuropathies always should be suspected in the vicinity of a fracture, and the limb should be evaluated periodically for their occurrence.

Prognosis

Early prediction of survival and neurologic recovery after injury is difficult. When possible, prognostication of survival greatly enhances acute care of extremity injuries. Many methods of prediction are available based on clinical and laboratory data. We are at present utilizing the Glasgow Coma Scale, as defined by Teasdale and Jennett, and have found this method useful in aiding fracture care and in predicting successful rehabilitation candidates (Table 13-3).[6] The scale examines three aspects of the behavior of a pa-

TABLE 13-3. *Glasgow Coma Scale.*[(6)]

Eye opening	Spontaneous	4
	Speech	3
	Pain	2
	None	1
Motor response	Obeys	6
	Localize	5
	Withdrawal	4
	Abnormal flexion	3
	Extension	2
	None	1
Verbal response	Oriented	5
	Confused conversation	4
	Inappropriate	3
	Incomprehensible	2
	None	1
Responsiveness or coma sum = 1–15 points		

TABLE 13-2. *Missed Injuries.*

1970 Review		*1976 Review*			
Fracture	*Total*	*Fracture*	*Total*	*Neuropathy*	*Total*
Cervical spine	4	Tibial spine	1	Ulnar	9
Lumbar spine	1	Tibial plateau	1	Peroneal	9
Hip fracture or dislocation	3	Acetabulum	1	Median	6
Tibial plateau	1	Ulna	1	Brachial plexus	3
Olecranon	1	Greater multangular	1	Radial	1
Carpal navicular	1	Acromioclavicular dislocation	2	Anterior interosseous	1
Knee-ligament injury	1	Radius, distal	3		

tient—eye opening, motor response, and verbal response. These behaviors are given numeric values according to a hierarchy of responses. The range of responses is 3 to 15 points. By making a profile of repeated observations at 24 hours, 2 to 3 days, and 4 to 7 days, the physician can predict with accuracy the assessments of survival and neurologic recovery.[7]

Two reliable and useful indicators of survival and neurologic outcome are readily applicable—age and duration of coma.[7,8] Age is related directly to survival and neurologic recovery. Generally, the younger the patient when injured, the better the chance for survival and neurologic recovery. Patients under 20 years of age have a 25% mortality and at least a 60% chance of becoming independent in activities of daily living. Patients over 60 years of age have only a slight chance for survival, and physical and severe cognitive disabilities are common.[7] The duration of coma is related inversely to the neurologic outcome; consequently, the longer the patient is in coma, the poorer the chance for functional recovery. The patient in coma for more than 1 month has minimal opportunity for a good neurologic recovery.

If survival is anticipated, patients should be treated as if they will gain a substantial neurologic return, especially when they are young. Fewer than 5% of survivors remain in a persistent vegetative state.[7] A 2-year review of our patients demonstrated that two thirds became ambulatory and independent in self-care activities.[8] Even if neurologic recovery is incomplete, all fractures should be treated adequately since skeletal disability perceived as insignificant for a neurologically intact individual may be incapacitating to the person with neurologic impairment.

Anesthesia

Neurosurgeons often are reluctant to authorize anesthesia for comatose patients since neurologic status cannot be monitored. Most anesthetic agents are cerebral vasodilators, which are contraindicated during the acute phase of cerebral swelling. Carbon dioxide is also a potent cerebral vasodilator. During intubation, an increase in intracranial pressure may occur from hypercarbia. Hypercarbia or anesthetic agents can increase intracranial pressure, thereby causing uncal herniation or decreased cerebral perfusion producing cortical damage on an ischemic basis.

If general anesthesia is required, certain guidelines should be followed:

(1) Any patient with evidence of post-traumatic encephalopathy or altered states of consciousness should undergo computerized axial tomography. Approximately 25% of adults with head injuries have increased intracranial pressure without mass effect and are still "at-risk." The intracranial pressures of such patients now may be obtained directly through ventricular monitoring and can be monitored during surgery if necessary.

(2) The patient should be neurologically stable. Most neurosurgeons recommend that general anesthesia be delayed until the neurologic status is stable or has not worsened over a 24-hour period.

(3) The anesthesiologist must be familiar with basic principles of neuroanesthesia. Controlled hyperventilation should be employed to prevent hypercarbia, and the anesthetic agent with the least effect on cerebral blood flow should be selected. Blood should be replaced with blood and dextrose, and water must be avoided.

Most deaths following head injury occur during the first month (Table 13-4). Death during the first week generally occurs as a direct consequence of the brain injury or multiple injuries. Death in the second and third week is related to secondary medical complications, such as metabolic abnormalities, stress ulcers, or pneumonia. These patients frequently are unsuitable for orthopaedic procedures. Cerebral edema appears within 24 hours of injury. Maximal edema is reached 3 to 5 days after injury and generally subsides in 7 to 10 days. Generally, risks of cerebral damage from anesthesia are small after this time.

Since anesthetic risk is minimized, most elective orthopaedic procedures may be undertaken safely at 10 to 14 days if no major medical complication is present. A review of 90 consecutive

TABLE 13-4. *Number of Deaths and Number Expiration Days from Injury in 123 Consecutive Patients with Severe Head Injuries.*[(23)]

Days from Injury	*Total Deaths*
1	1
2–3	10
4–7	9
8–14	12
15–28	19
>30	9
	60

patients with head injuries at Rancho Los Amigos Hospital who underwent general anesthesia for fracture repair later than 2 weeks after injury failed to demonstrate any neurologic deterioration postoperatively.[9]

Plaster

The use of circular plaster casts in patients with acquired spasticity has been condemned or employed with guarded caution.[10-12] Our experience has demonstrated that circular plaster casts may be used advantageously in the subacute period after the initial swelling has started to subside. Disoriented brain-injured patients tend to remove splints. When hypertonicity is severe, sufficient limb motion may occur within the splint, thereby causing pressure sores, as well as allowing loss of reduction. Circular plaster casts aid not only in controlling the fracture but also in preventing joint contractures resulting from hypertonic muscles. Circular plaster casts also decrease hypertonic muscle activity (Fig. 13-1, *A* and *B*). The joints above and below the fracture should be incorporated into the plaster cast to aid in the control of muscles and joints, as well as of the fracture (Fig. 13-1, *C*).

Patients with head trauma generally are not capable of expressing pain caused by a snug cast. Neurovascular compression may ensue and must be anticipated. Therefore, circumferential plaster casts should be used with caution to treat acute injuries. Our preference for fractures with significant soft-tissue injury is the use of a circular plaster cast that is immediately split or bivalved. When swelling subsides, a new circular cast is applied.

MAXIMUM ANKLE DORSIFLEXION
(PRE PLASTER)

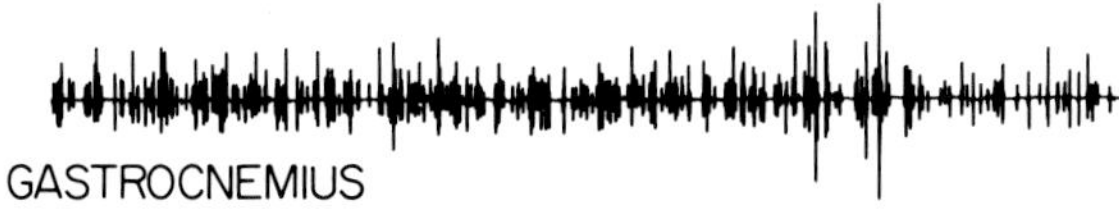

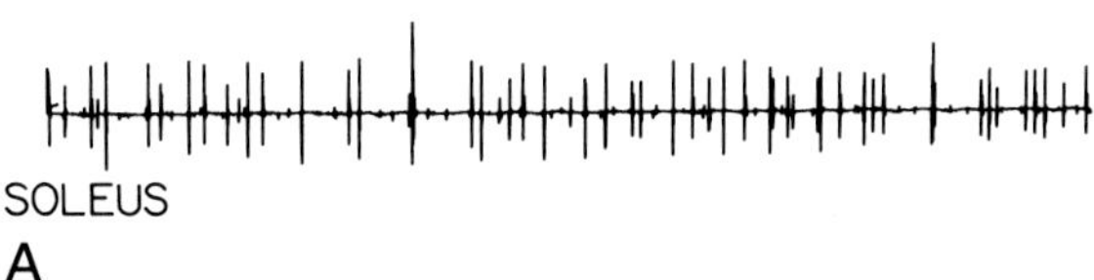

MAXIMUM ANKLE DORSIFLEXION
IN PLASTER

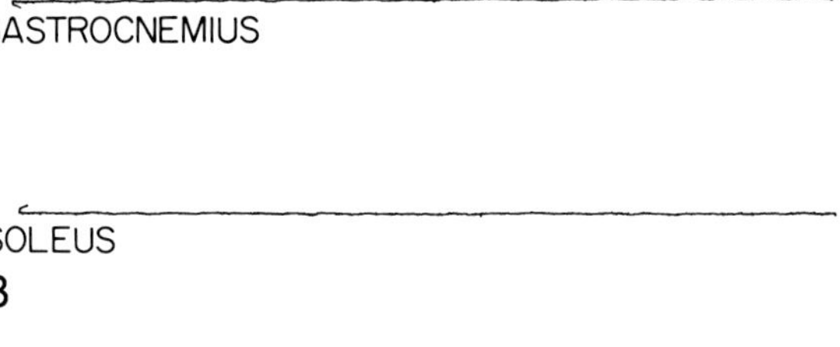

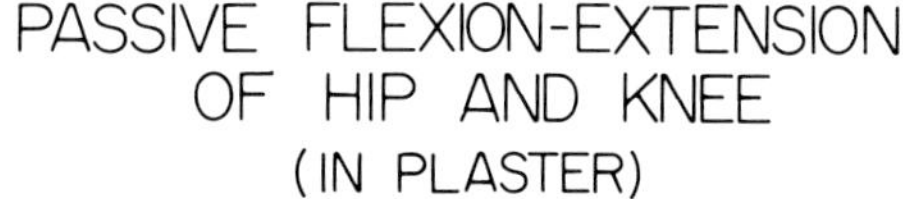

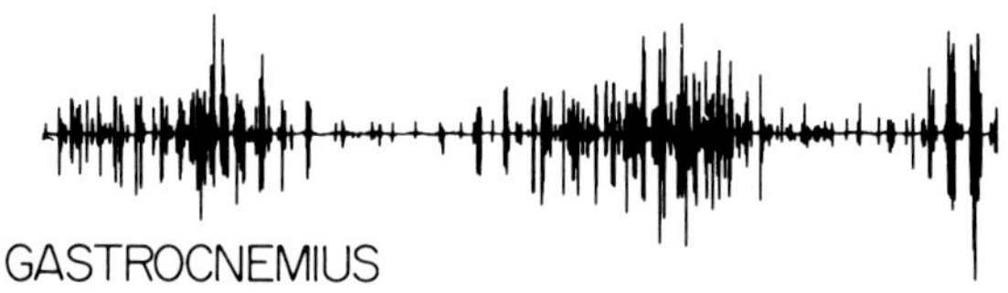

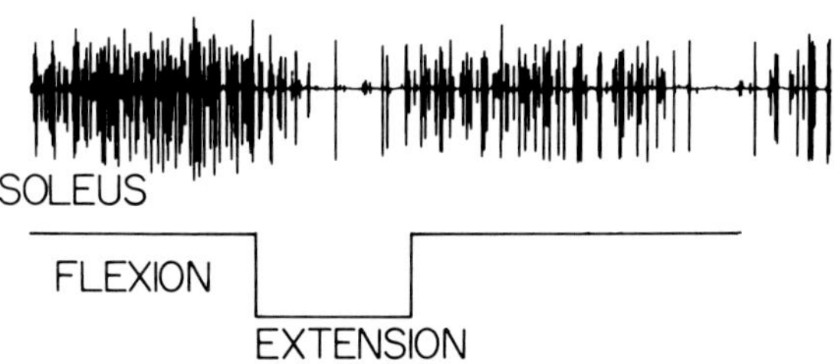

Fig. 13-1. *A*, A dynamic electromyogram of a head injured patient with spastic hemiplegia. Electrodes have been inserted into the gastrocnemius and soleus muscles, and the ankle is positioned passively in maximum dorsiflexion. *B*, A short-leg circular plaster cast has been applied with the ankle maintained in the same position. Muscle activity has ceased. *C*, The short-leg cast is still in place. The hip and knee are ranged passively. Muscle activity (synergy) now is elicited in the gastrocnemius and soleus muscles. Extension of the cast above the knee further decreases this activity.

Closed reduction is not always easy to achieve in the brain-injured patient. Joints often are placed in flexion to aid in reduction. After the fracture develops some internal stability, the cast should be changed to place the joints in more functional positions. Otherwise, the fracture may heal in normal alignment, but a joint contracture may persist. In the upper extremity, the elbow is immobilized at 45°, the wrist at 0°, the metacarpal phalangeal joints at 45 to 60°, the interphalangeal joints at 0°, and the thumb is extended and abducted. In the lower extremity, the hip, knee, and ankle should be immobilized in a neutral position.

Traction

Traction methods, either skin or skeletal, frequently prove unsatisfactory for prolonged fracture management. Traction in the medically unstable or agitated-restless patient greatly complicates nursing care. Transportation for diagnostic testing is facilitated when the patient is not in traction. Finally, mental and physical rehabilitation may be initiated earlier if the patient can be mobilized.

Traction is indicated mainly for certain pelvic and acetabular fractures that cannot be treated by other methods and for the early treatment of femur fractures. Skeletal traction is preferable to skin traction. Traction that employs minimal ropes and pulleys is preferable since the patients often are located in intensive-care units or general or neurosurgical floors. We prefer cast traction or modified Neufeld roller traction[13] for early treatment of femur fractures because of its ease of application, simplicity of traction and suspension system, ease of control of the femur when out of bed, and ease of nursing care. Lastly, this plaster method aids in the control of spasticity and maintains the knee and ankle in a neutral position.

Cast traction is applied in the following manner. A threaded 5/32-inch Steinmann's pin is inserted into the distal femur or preferably the proximal tibia. A short-leg cast is applied incorporating the pin. When the cast has hardened, reduction of the fracture is attempted by distal traction. A thigh plaster cast is added while maintaining fracture reduction. Wooden dowels are incorporated anteriorly over the thigh and posteriorly at the Achilles tendon. Rubber tubing is attached to the distal dowel and a post on the end of the bed (Fig. 13-2). Traction is increased by wrapping the tubing around the dowel. The amount of traction required for suspension of the leg usually is sufficient for maintenance of fracture reduction. Rubber tubing is applied to the proximal dowel only as necessary. Its application

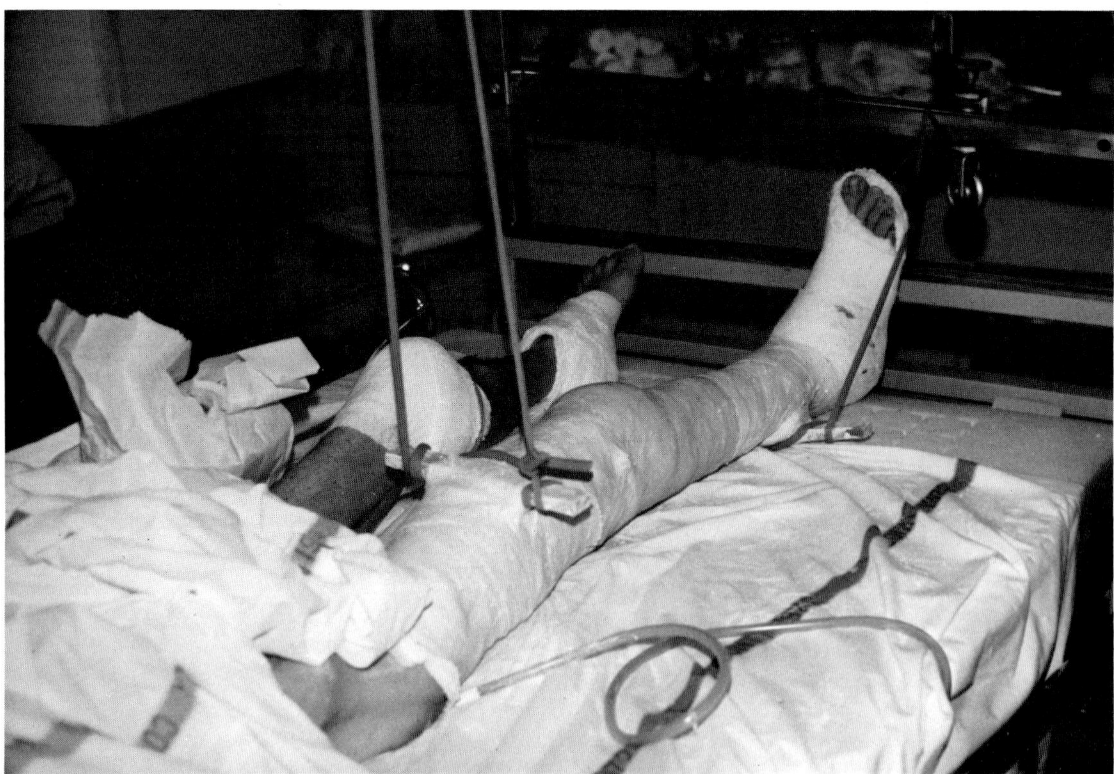

FIG. 13-2. Cast traction. A femoral skeletal pin has been incorporated in a long-leg plaster cast. Traction is applied through the distal rubber tubing. The proximal tubing aids in suspension.

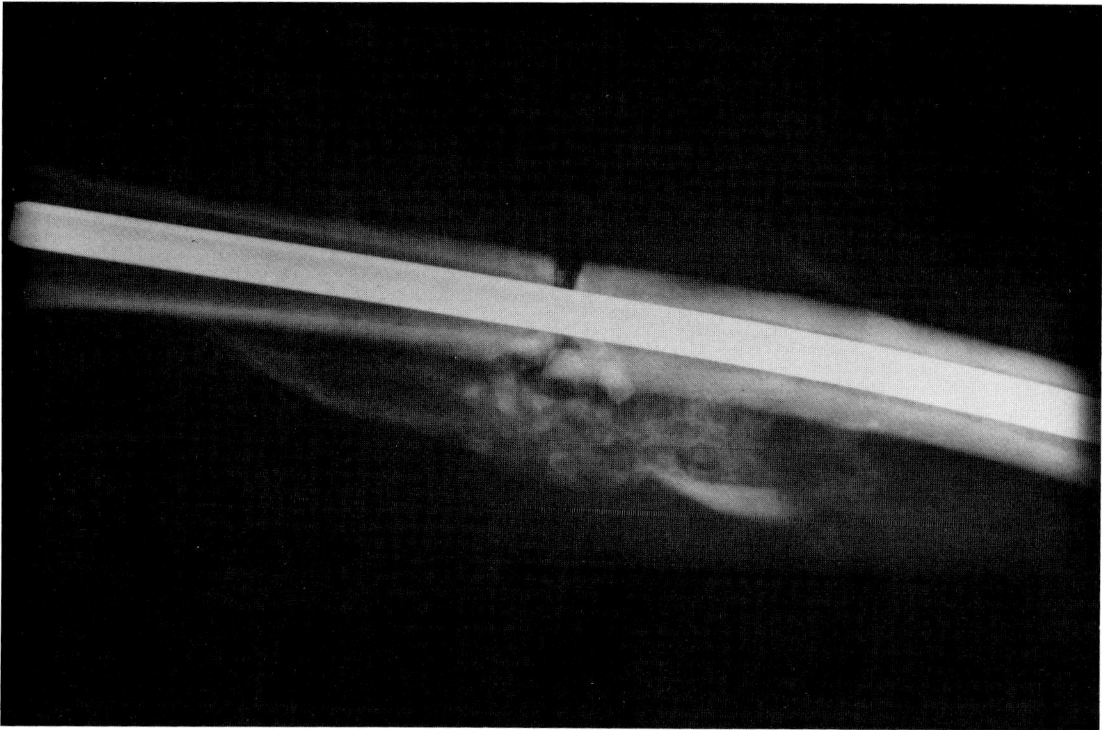

Fig. 13-3. Lateral radiographs of a femur fracture that was treated by an open intramedullary nailing. Excessive callus, which we believe represents myositis ossificans, is present in all planes of the femur.

aids in suspension of the leg, which assists bed, bowel, and bladder care, and in the control of occasional posterior angulation at the fracture site.

Fracture Healing

A general belief exists that fractures unite more rapidly and with increased frequency in the patient with head injuries. Our review of 47 tibia fractures in patients with head injuries demonstrated an average time to union of 5.6 months and a 4% incidence of nonunion;[14] a survey of 68 fractured femurs in patients with head injuries demonstrated that all united at 4 months.[15] We concluded that the healing rate of fractures in patients with head injuries is essentially the same as that in the normal population.

Exuberant callus occurs in fractures in the neurologically involved patient.[10-12] We did not identify exuberant callus in our review of tibia fractures. Our survey of femur fractures did demonstrate some femurs with excessive callus. Many patients who underwent open reduction and internal fixation of femur fractures developed exuberant callus (Fig. 13-3), which, we believe, results from surgical trauma to muscles and represents a form of myositis ossificans. Few of the femurs not operated on developed excessive callus. Amounts of callus greater than those normally expected occasionally occurred in the agitated patient who thrashed about, in the functionally braced femur, or in the infected, often debrided fracture. We did not identify a relationship between exuberant callus and early clinical union and, consequently, believe that exuberant callus, when it does occur, is of minimal clinical significance.

The effect of spasticity on fracture healing may be examined more closely in hemiplegic patients. In our review of tibia fractures, the time to union was the same for the fracture occurring on the hemiplegic limb as for the fracture on the normal extremity.[14] In our study of femurs, clinical union was prolonged 1 month for the fracture occurring on the hemiplegic extremity versus the fracture on the normal extremity.[15] Exuberant callus was uncommon on both the normal and hemiplegic limb. We concluded from our observation of hemiplegic patients that brain injury and spasticity do not influence directly the formation of excessive callus nor do they accelerate fracture healing.

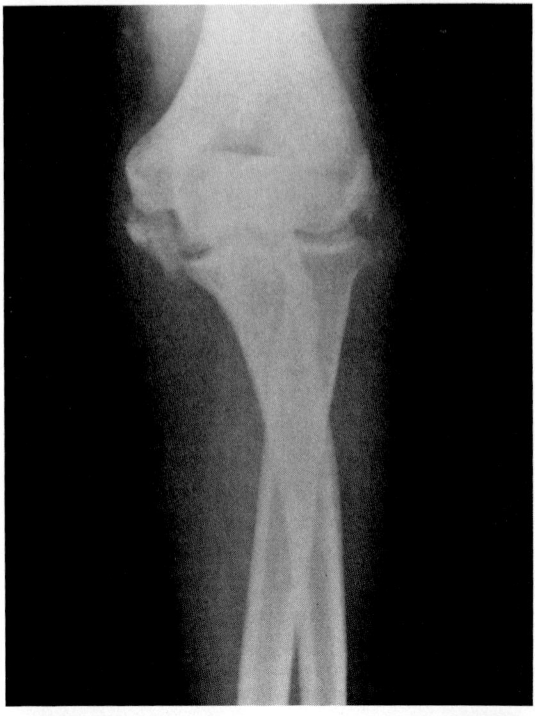

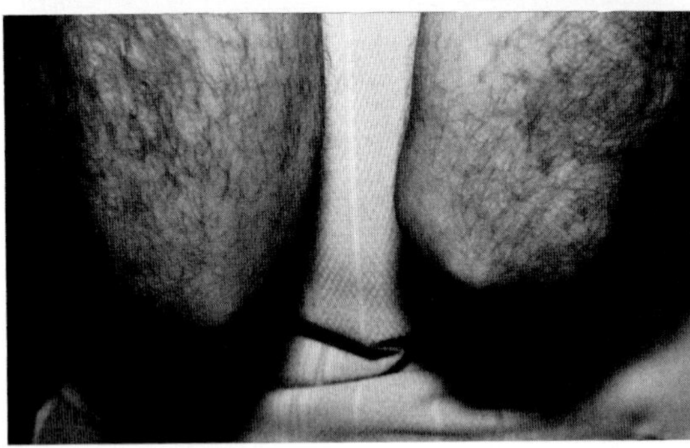

Fig. 13-4. *A*, Anterior radiograph of a previously dislocated elbow. Heterotopic ossification is present medially and laterally. This ossification in the medial location may compromise the ulnar groove. *B*, Left elbow, when compared to the right elbow, demonstrates an increased mass medially and laterally caused by heterotopic ossification. The medial heterotopic ossification plus external compression led to tardy ulnar palsy.

Specific Treatment

Upper Extremity Fractures

In the patient with head injuries, upper extremity injuries are not as common as lower extremity injuries;[3] multiple fractures in the upper limb are not as common as multiple fractures in the lower extremity. Significant injuries in the upper extremity usually are detected by physical examination. The most commonly missed skeletal fractures are injuries about the shoulder girdle and the minimally displaced distal radius fractures. Frequently these injuries are the only musculoskeletal insult, and when unrecognized, the orthopaedist is not called to evaluate the patient. The injuries most commonly delayed in recognition are peripheral nerve injuries, especially to the median and ulnar nerves (see Table 13-2).

Shoulder Girdle (Clavicle, Scapula, Acromioclavicular Joint)

In the patient with head injuries, the shoulder girdle is the most common site of injury in the upper extremity. Many injuries may be detected on the routine chest roentgenogram. Specific radiographs of the shoulder should be obtained when signs of trauma are present. These fractures generally do not pose significant treatment obstacles, and standard orthopaedic care is applicable. Brachial plexus injuries commonly result from a motorcycle accident in which the rider has landed simultaneously on the head and shoulder, thereby distracting the plexus.[16] An underlying brachial plexus palsy should be suspected until proved otherwise in the adult with head injuries and a flail upper extremity.

Humerus

Although fractures of the humeral shaft are not common in the neurologically impaired patient, they may pose treatment dilemmas. Radial nerve function may be difficult, if not impossible, to evaluate. Treatment of these fractures with traction is not desirable since patient mobility is decreased and nursing care is increased. Furthermore, traction to the arm during the agitation phase of neurologic recovery may allow initial or further injury to the radial nerve. Other standard methods of treatment of this fracture may not apply. The principles of the hanging-arm cast cannot be applied to the bedridden population. These patients often are able to remove coaptation splints or an orthotic device, thus, these devices should be employed with caution. Consequently, we believe that open reduction and internal fixation of the fracture with radial nerve exploration are more frequently indicated in patients with head injuries than in the general population. Internal fixation also allows passive range of motion postoperatively by the therapist, aids in prevention of contractures, and prevents damage to the radial nerve by the fracture.

Elbow

The elbow poses significant treatment difficulties resulting from spasticity about the joint, potential heterotopic bone formation, and ulnar neuropathy. If the decision is made to treat the elbow by closed methods, the elbow should be casted in 45° of flexion. If flexor spasticity is present, or develops later, this position aids in preventing a flexion contracture, which becomes apparent when the fracture has healed. Open reduction, if technically possible, is the preferred treatment. Operative techniques that afford the best fixation should be employed to allow early motion postoperatively. Passive range of motion, even in severely impaired patients, is important in preventing flexion contracture of the elbow. Traumatic dislocations of the elbow, which have a high incidence of heterotopic bone formation after reduction, require early mobilization to prevent ankylosis.

The incidence of heterotopic bone in fractures and dislocations about the elbow is more frequent in neurologically impaired patients than in the general population and approaches 90% of all injuries (Fig. 13-4, *A*). When heterotopic bone develops, the elbow becomes painful, sometimes swollen and warm, and often results in loss of motion. Whereas idiopathic periarticular heterotopic ossification usually forms anterior or posterior to the elbow, traumatic heterotopic bone may form in all or any areas—medial, lateral, anterior, or posterior.[16a] Furthermore, although idiopathic heterotopic bone usually is associated with spasticity about the joint, traumatic ossification occurs with equal frequency in extremities with no neurologic involvement. Manipulation of the elbow under general anesthesia, when possible without disturbing the fracture site, may be beneficial in preventing ankylosis.[17]

Ulnar neuropathy may result in the initial injury or later from impingement of the nerve by heterotopic bone in its canal (Fig. 13-4, *B*). The neuropathy frequently is not diagnosed for several weeks until sufficient recovery of the central nervous system has occurred so that physical signs are present. The nerve is transposed anteriorly.

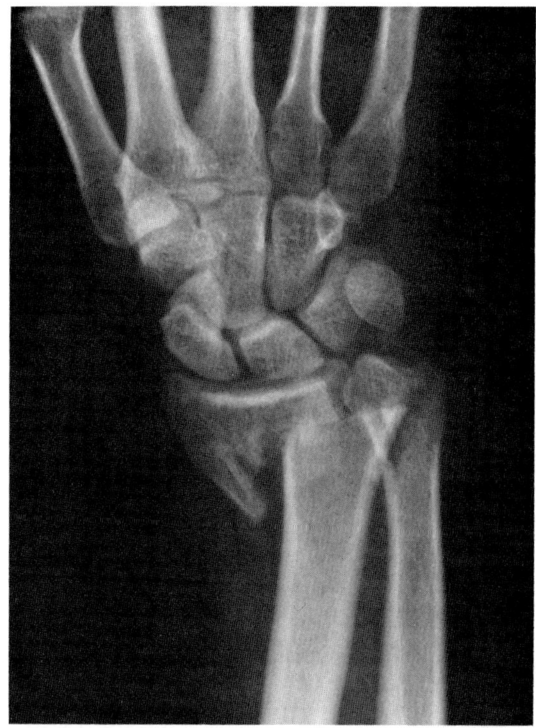

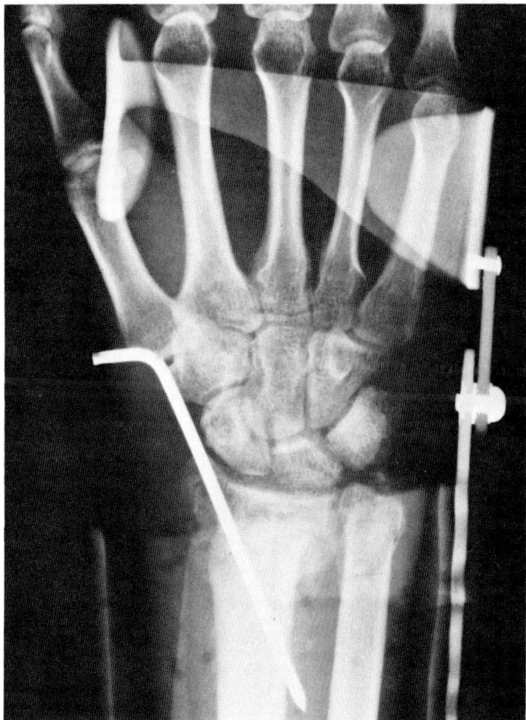

Fig. 13-5. *A*, Appearance of an unreduced distal radius fracture 1 month after injury upon the patient's transfer to Rancho Los Amigos Hospital. *B*, Anterior roentgenogram taken after open reduction and internal fixation were performed.

Forearm

Forearm fractures pose significant treatment dilemmas in the brain-injured patient. Fractures can be reduced with closed methods, but normal alignment is difficult to maintain. Severe restriction of pronation and supination is common following closed treatment methods. Single-bone fractures with minimal displacement sometimes may be treated by nonoperative methods. Open reduction and internal fixation are often necessary for single-bone fractures to allow anatomic reduction, initiation of range of motion, and prevention of contracture by the patient or the therapist. The rate of union and complications from open reduction and internal fixation of single-bone fractures in the patient with head injuries are similar to those for the general population. Both bone fractures often are accompanied by injury to the interosseous membrane. This injury, plus the surgical insult of open reduction and internal fixation, leads to a 50% incidence of calcification of the interosseous membrane with a 33% complete ankylosis rate in patients with head injuries. These percentages of incidence of calcification of the interosseous membrane and ankylosis are greatly increased over the ankylosis rate of 5% in the general population.[10,18,19]

To minimize the likelihood of interosseous calcification and ankylosis, we prefer to fix these fractures by closed intramedullary techniques if deemed technically possible for reduction and secure fixation. If reduction and fixation cannot be performed by closed techniques, we prefer to make a small incision over the fracture site to aid in reduction. Surgical exposure and dissection are minimized with this procedure when compared to the exposure and dissection resulting from plating. If intramedullary fixation is not deemed possible, open reduction and plate fixation are necessary. A careful and meticulous dissection that avoids the interosseous membrane is important. The fixation must be secure so that pronation and supination exercises can be initiated soon after surgery to prevent ankylosis. Bone grafting, even for late repairs, rarely is indicated since it seems to hasten ossification of the interosseous membrane.

Surgical resection of the ankylosis site generally is not indicated if hemiplegia is present on the same side as the forearm that is ankylosed in pronation. When the forearm is in an unacceptable position, the fixation device is removed after union and the ankylosis site is resected. The forearm is placed in the desired position and is maintained with plaster casts. A large gain in motion is uncommon unless some voluntary control is present. Maintenance of motion depends on physiotherapy following resection. The recurrence rate of ankylosis is high, and splinting in the most functional position is recommended.

When ankylosis occurs and a normal neurologic return ensues, the fixation device is removed after union and the ankylosis site is resected. Although considerable bone may be present along the interosseous membrane, only the site of ankylosis is removed. We have not been inserting a silastic membrane in the resected area nor employing disphosphonates postoperatively. Satisfactory motion generally is achieved.

Distal Radius

Adequate fracture care is not always rendered to the distal radius fracture because of the uncertainty of the patient's neurologic outcome and the assumption that this disability would be of little consequence (Fig. 13-5, *A* and *B*). At times, a good neurologic return occurs, and the patient is left with a significant deformity (Fig. 13-6, *A*, *B*, and *C*).

Median neuropathy should be anticipated when circular casts are employed, especially in the unreduced fracture. We prefer reduction of the fracture followed by application of sugar-tong splints or a circular plaster cast, which is later bivalved. Poor reduction, swelling, and circular plaster casts increase the risk of compression of the median nerve and, occasionally, of the ulnar nerve at the wrist. Since the patient cannot complain of dysesthesia, the neuropathy frequently is not diagnosed until after the plaster cast is removed and physical signs are evident. When the diagnosis is established, carpal tunnel release is performed. If the radial deformity is severe and pronation and supination motion is limited, a Darrach procedure is performed at the same time. Since most patients with this injury are young, significant remodeling of the fracture site may occur and near-normal flexion-extension may be achieved (Fig. 13-6, *D*, *E*, *F*, and *G*). A Darrich procedure, if indicated, allows near-normal pronation and supination.

Lower Extremity Fractures

In patients with head injuries, fractures occur more often in the lower extremity than in the upper extremity. Concomitant fractures in the same extremity are common. Complications of fracture care occur more frequently in the lower extremity than in the upper extremity.

Fig. 13-6. *A*, Early wrist deformity from distal radius fracture. Median and ulnar neuropathies were present. *B* and *C*, Anterior and lateral radiographs of wrist.

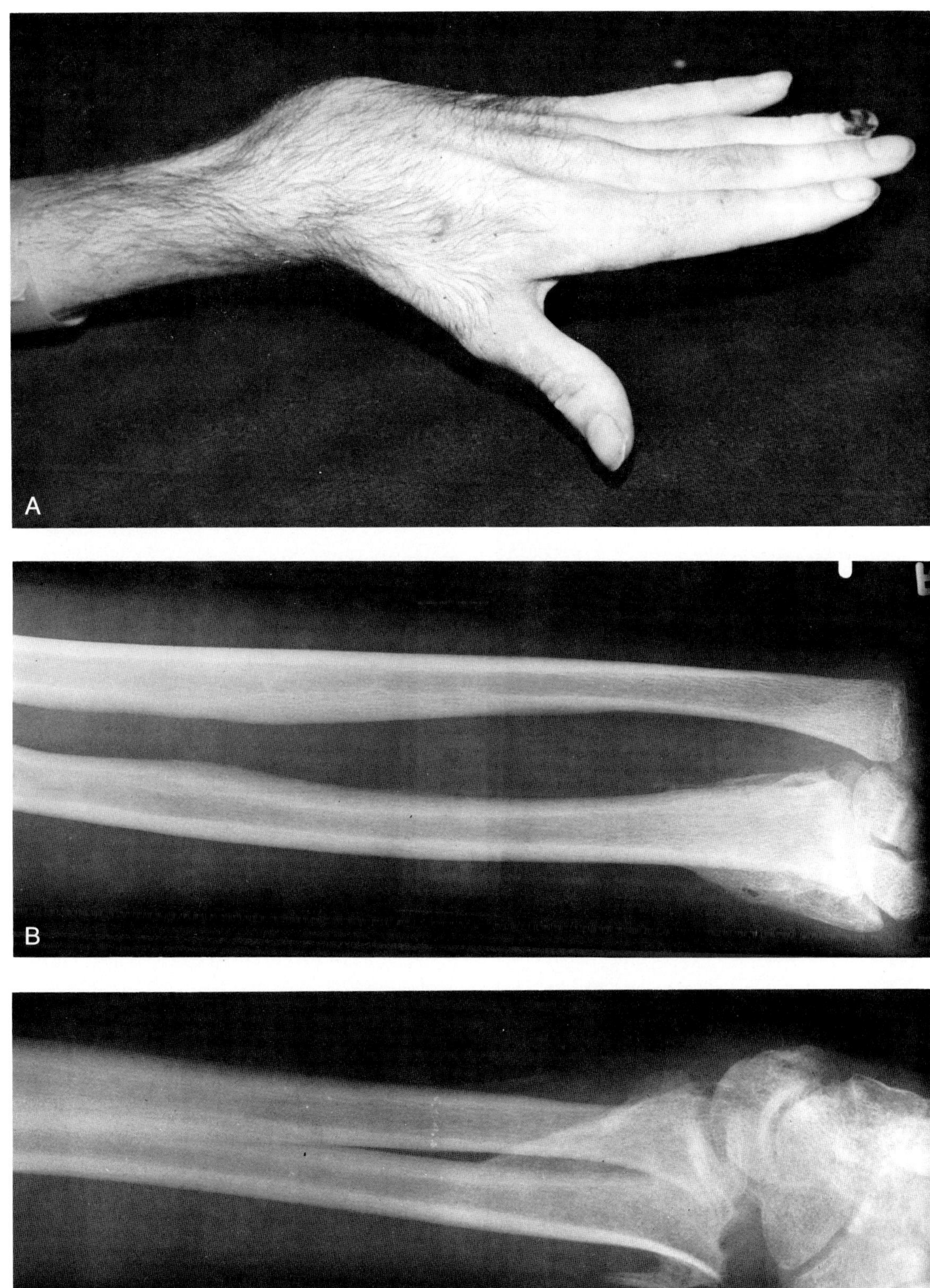
A
B
C

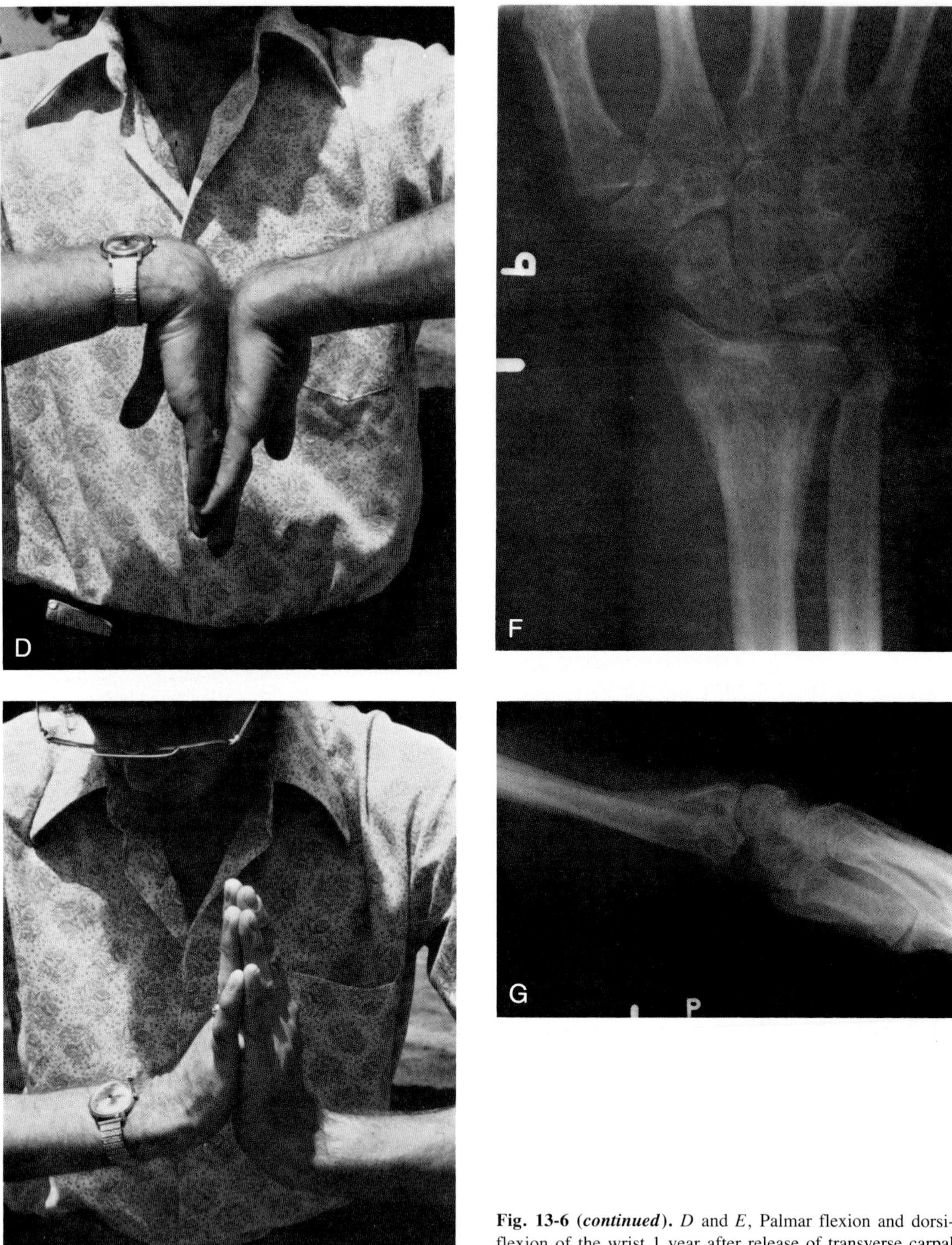

Fig. 13-6 (*continued*). *D* and *E*, Palmar flexion and dorsiflexion of the wrist 1 year after release of transverse carpal ligament and Guyon's canal and Darrich procedure. The patient also sustained an injury to his right wrist. *F* and *G*, Anteroposterior and lateral radiographs taken 1 year after injury. Considerable remodeling of the fracture site has occurred.

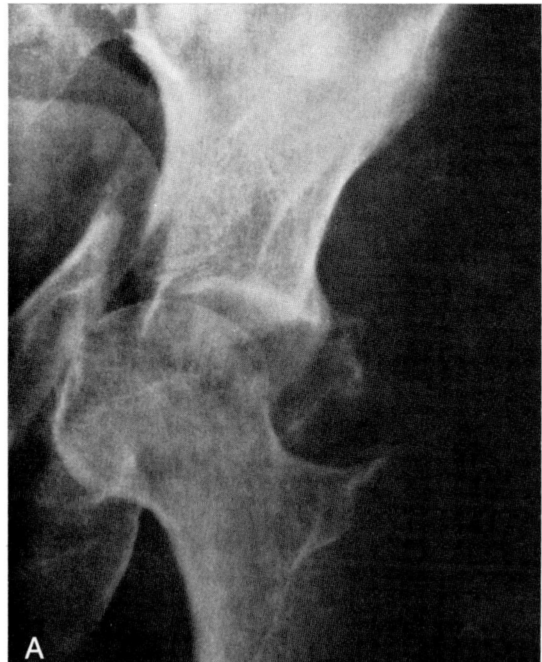

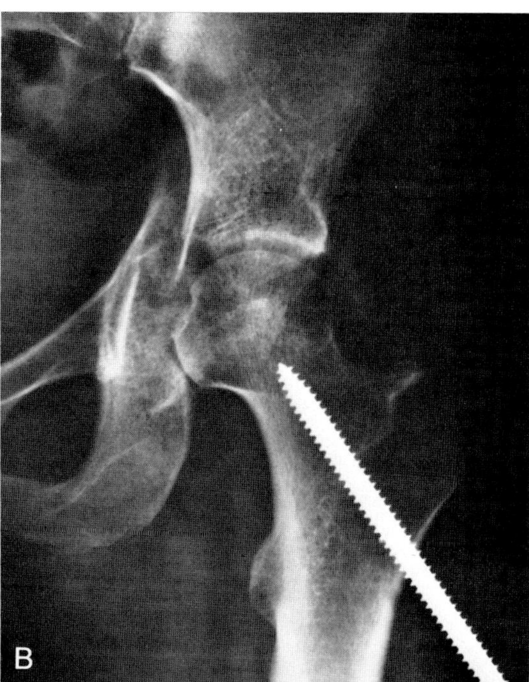

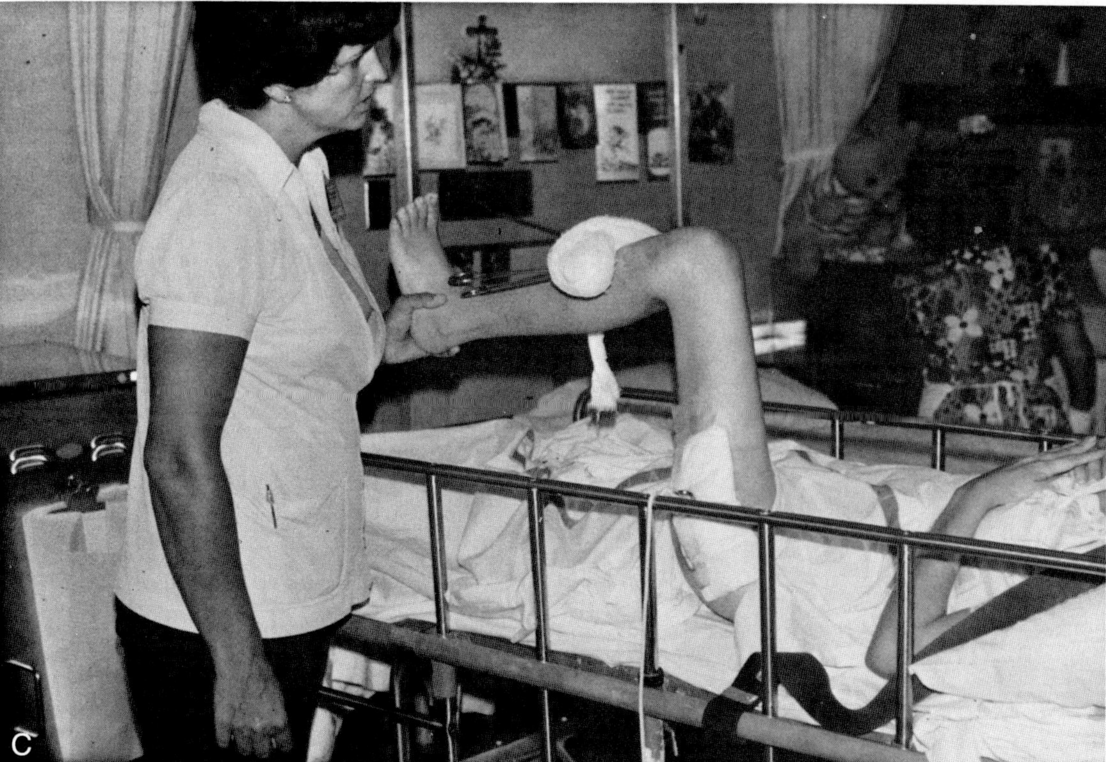

Fig. 13-7. *A*, Central fracture-dislocation of the acetabulum 9 weeks after injury. Heterotopic ossification is already present. *B*, The fracture-dislocation has been reduced with lateral femoral and proximal tibia skeletal traction. *C*, Ranging of the hip is performed while lateral skeletal traction is maintained. Distal traction is reapplied when the ranging exercises have been completed.

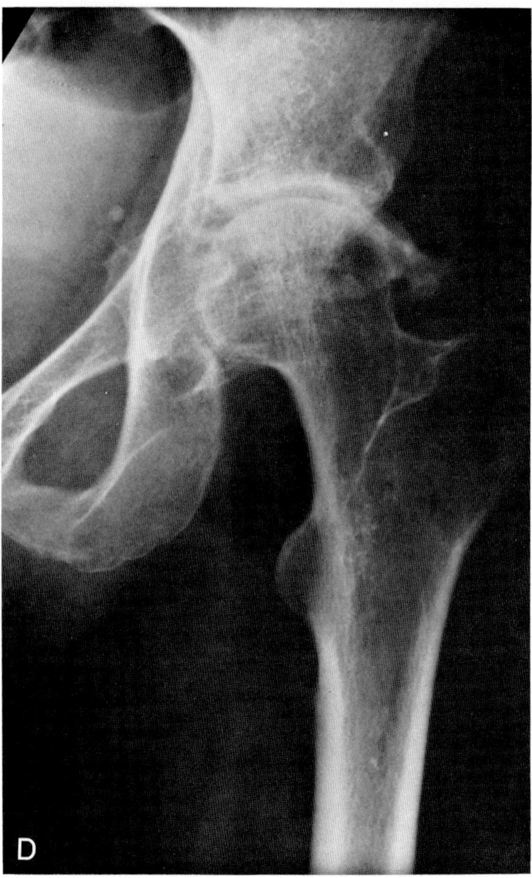

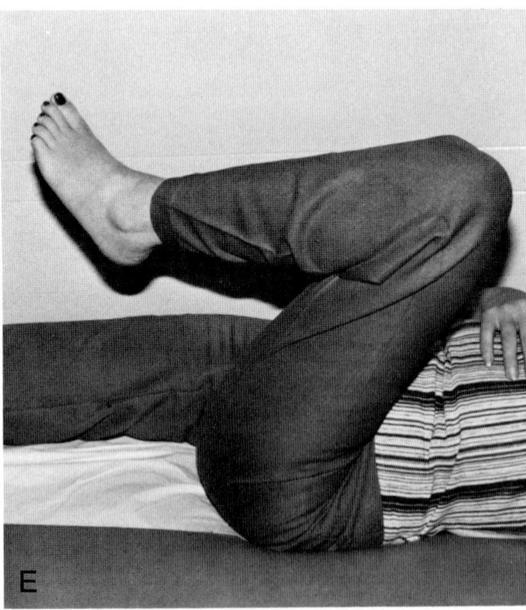

Fig. 13-7 (*continued*). *D*, Radiograph taken 1 year after injury. Traction time was 6 weeks. *E*, Final hip flexion at 1 year. Hip extension was neutral.

Pelvis

Diagnosis of the pelvic fracture in the brain-injured patient is important as a source of undetected blood loss and shock as well as for its treatment. This fracture always should be suspected in patients involved in auto-pedestrian accidents. Routine radiographs of the pelvis that include the hips usually establish the diagnosis. Our review of surviving victims who were struck by automobiles, which correlates closely with autopsy material, demonstrated that three fourths of these patients had pelvic and lower extremity fractures.[20] The victims had a 50% incidence of lower extremity fracture and a 50% incidence of pelvic fracture. Combined injuries of the lower extremity and pelvis occurred in one fourth of the patients.

Pelvic fractures generally heal rapidly. Fractures that disturb the pelvic ring often require traction. The sacroiliac joint and symphysis pubis often ossify rapidly after injury, and this type of injury usually does not require prolonged traction.

Acetabulum

The acetabular fracture poses significant treatment dilemmas in the neurologically impaired patient. Many fractures require traction for reduction or maintenance of reduction. Open reduction and internal fixation lead to myositis ossificans and eventual decreased joint motion, especially when extensive soft-tissue dissection is involved. These fractures may develop heterotopic bone about the joint when treated by closed methods, but generally not to the degree developed with the operated acetabulum.

We prefer nonoperative treatment, even if traction is necessary, unless extensive exposure is not required, such as with fixation of the posterior lip of the acetabulum in a posterior fracture-dislocation of the hip (Fig. 13-7, *A* and *B*). Prolonged traction usually is not required since many of the fractures develop heterotopic bone and early stability.[19,21] We institute an early, vigorous ranging program while the patient is in traction (Fig. 13-7, *C*, *D*, and *E*). At times, motion is difficult to gain and maintain since these patients often experience significant pain and voluntary muscle guarding, especially if heterotopic bone is developing. If the fracture is healed and motion is decreasing as a result of heterotopic ossification, manipulation under anesthesia is performed. Considerable increase in motion, especially flexion, can be achieved.[17]

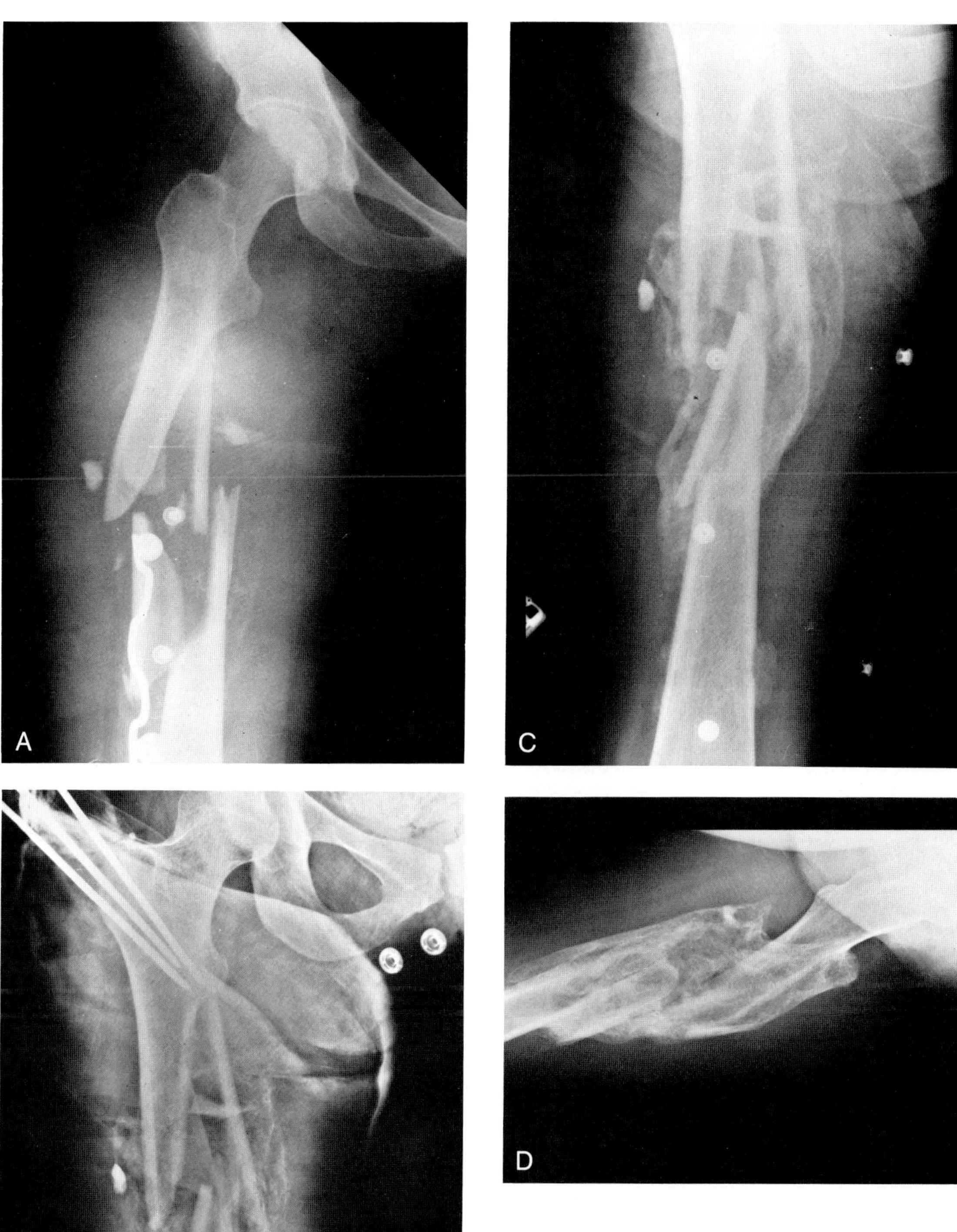

FIG. 13-8. *A*, Subtrochanteric fracture with comminution. *B*, One month after injury, percutaneous pins were inserted proximally and a through-and-through pin was inserted distally. The pins were incorporated into a thigh plaster cast. The fracture is now out to length. *C* and *D*, Final result after 2 months of treatment. The patient was out of bed, and gait training was initiated at the time of removal of pins and plaster.

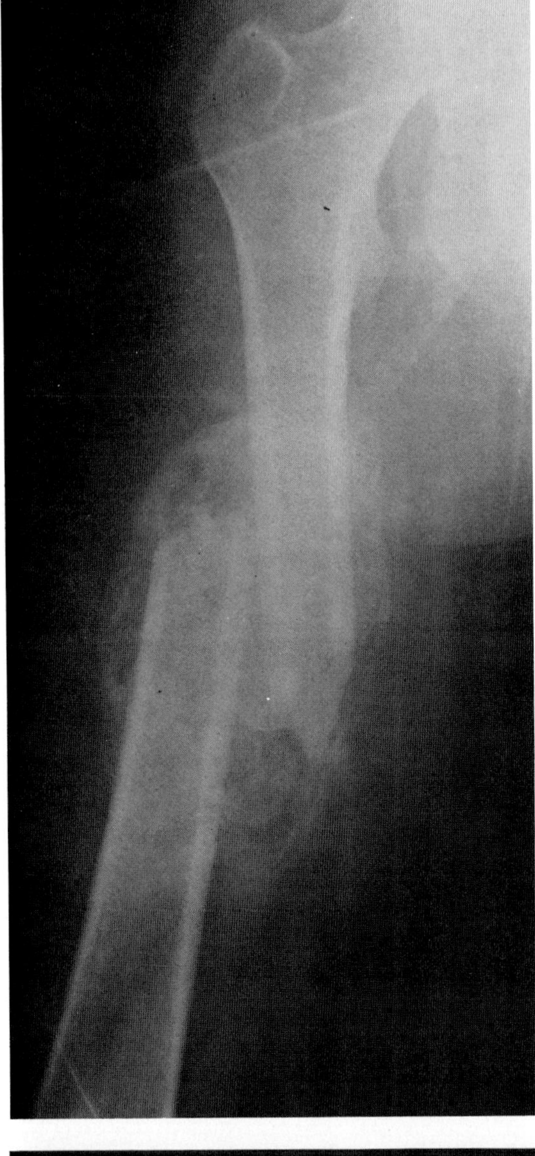

Hip

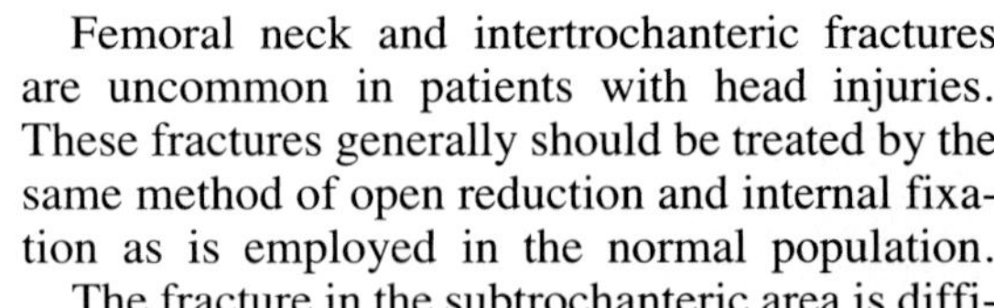

Femoral neck and intertrochanteric fractures are uncommon in patients with head injuries. These fractures generally should be treated by the same method of open reduction and internal fixation as is employed in the normal population.

The fracture in the subtrochanteric area is difficult to treat in the normal population as well as in the population with head injuries. Open reduction and internal fixation of this fracture may require prolonged operative time, involve significant blood-volume changes, and may require protected movement postoperatively. Our preference for treating the comminuted fracture in the young, potentially functional patient is with the use of pins incorporated in a thigh plaster cast (Fig. 13-8, *A, B, C,* and *D*). We have demonstrated that these fractures can be controlled satisfactorily by this method, and prolonged traction is not required prior to the pins-in-plaster application.[22] No blood loss occurs, and the patient may bear weight to tolerance after application.

The patient is taken to the operating room for application of pins in a plaster cast when medically and neurologically stable or after 7 to 10 days of skeletal traction. After anesthetic induction, the patient is placed on a fracture table. Traction is applied through a distal tibial pin. Under radiographic control, two or three 5/32-inch threaded Steinmann's pins are inserted from

Fig. 13-9. *A*, Midshaft femur fracture after treatment with skeletal traction and a hip spica cast. Shortening is greater than 1 inch. Valgus angulation, which was secondary to adductor hypertonicity, is present. *B*, Lateral radiograph of femur. Anterior angulation, which was secondary to hamstring spasticity, is present. Note the position of the proximal tibia.

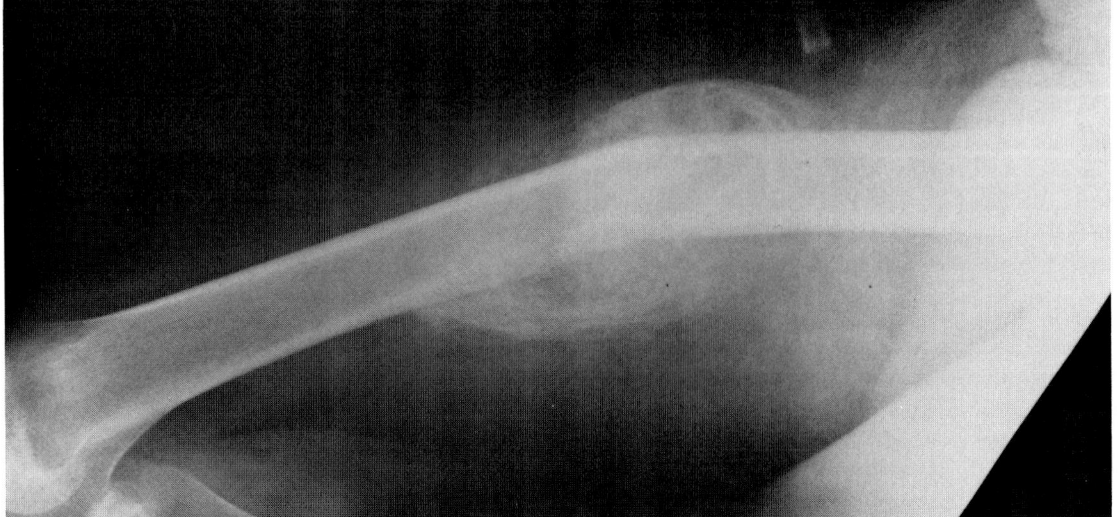

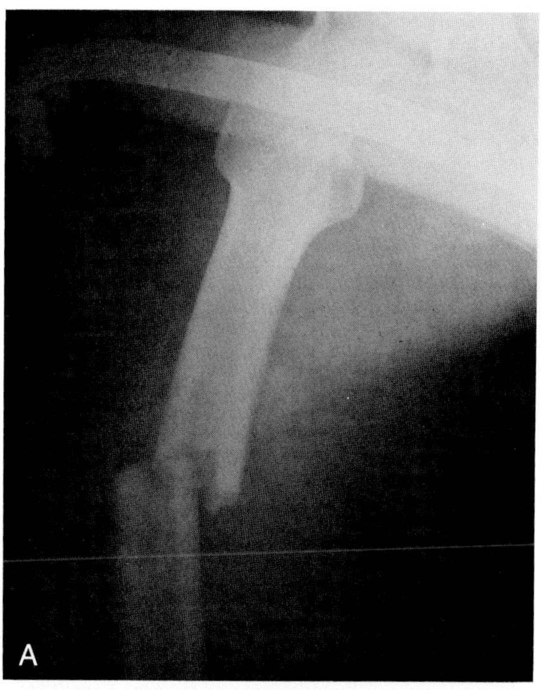

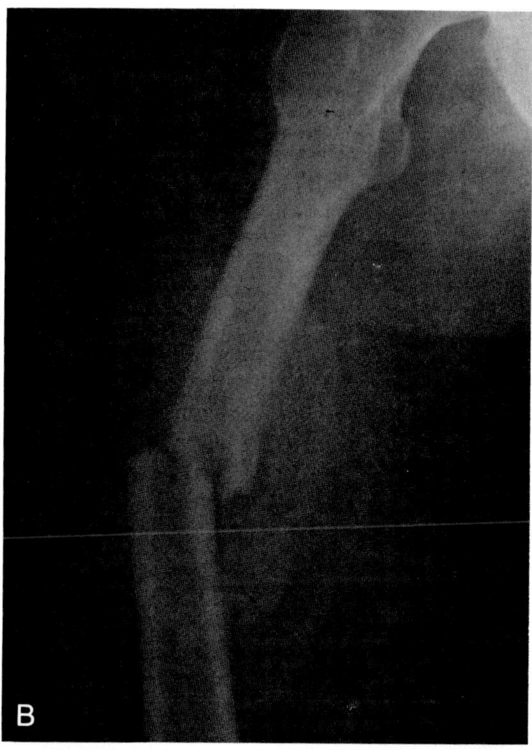

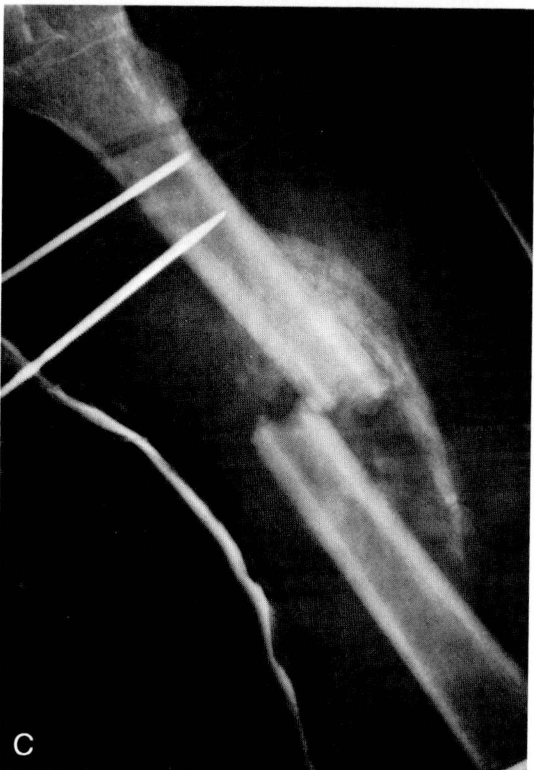

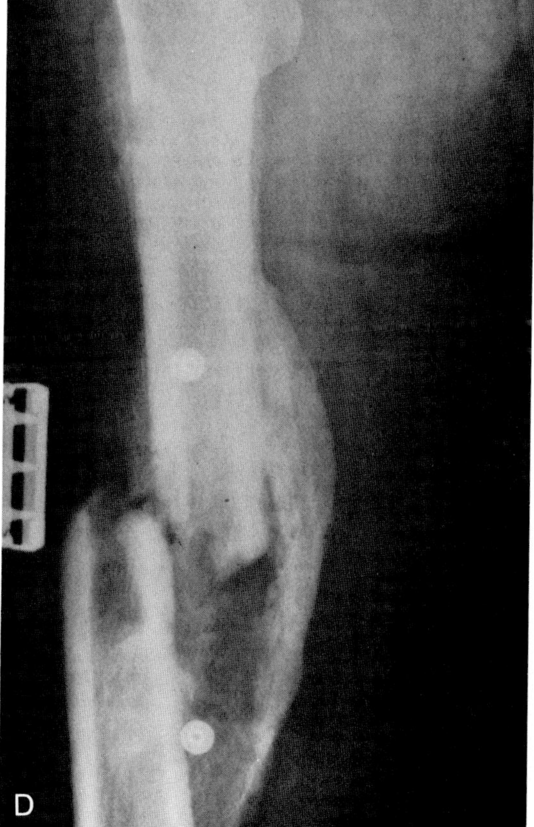

Fig. 13-10. *A*, This patient had sustained an open femur fracture. A mild amount of drainage was present at transfer. Callus already is visible, and maintenance of normal alignment is difficult with the standard cast-brace. *B*, A routine cast-brace had been applied. Varus angulation increased. *C*, Percutaneous pins have been incorporated into a thigh plaster cast. Lateral molding is necessary to aid in prevention of the recurring varus angulation. *D*, Final alignment of femur after 2 months of treatment with pins and a thigh plaster cast.

the greater trochanter toward the lesser trochanter, stopping after piercing the medial cortex. One distal through-and-through 5/32-inch threaded pin is inserted in the distal femur. A circular thigh plaster cast, applied over cast padding, incorporates the pins. A neutral or slight valgus position is achieved by lateral molding of the plaster cast at the fracture site. The patient is allowed to bear weight to tolerance.

Femur

Femur fractures are the most common lower extremity injury. Prolonged traction followed by application of a hip spica cast has limited use in the patient with head injuries. Nursing care and rehabilitation are difficult with this method of treatment. Fractures treated in this manner often display a shortening of greater than 1 inch. Valgus angulation of 10° or more is common and results from uncontrolled adductor spasticity. Anterior angulation also is common and results from hamstring hypertonicity (Fig. 13-9). Neutralization of these muscle forces and consequent angular deformities are difficult to control with traction and spica-cast treatment.

Our preferred method of treatment is cast or roller traction followed by closed intramedullary nailing. The intramedullary nail should firmly engage both proximal and distal fracture sites. Hypertonic muscle groups have the potential to rotate the fragments on the nail unless fixation is firm. Open intramedullary nailing often leads to myositis ossificans (See Fig. 13-3). Approximately 50% of open nailings and platings develop this process.[15] If open techniques are employed, knee motion may be compromised if the myositic process involves a significant amount of the quadriceps muscles. Postoperative ranging of the knee must be instituted soon after the operation. The incidence of wound infections in our patients with head injuries was increased over that for the normal population. Increased wound infection most likely occurs from local reasons since patients with head injuries are usually bowel and bladder incontinent and often manipulate the incision site.

Recently we have been treating nonoperative candidates with the cast-brace. The results are satisfactory to date, and the cast-brace appears to be a viable treatment alternative when an operation is contraindicated. The cast-brace consists of a thigh plaster cast, polypropylene hinges, and a short-leg cast. The ankle may be left free if normal motor function is present and if a skeletal pin is in place. Although early ambulation may not be possible, satisfactory healing occurs. Shortening has not been difficult to control, and only 1 patient with shortening of 1 inch has been encountered. Varus angulation in patients with head injuries does not occur with the same frequency as in normal patients because of adductor spasticity, which promotes valgus angulation. Knee flexion, which sometimes is difficult to obtain in the normal population, may be enhanced by hamstring spasticity. Flexing the knee decreases the deforming forces of the spastic hamstring muscles, and anterior angulation of the fracture is less common in patients treated with the cast-brace than in the population treated with the spica cast.

One small group of femur fractures poses considerable treatment difficulties. This troublesome fracture is open or comminuted, or occurs in a patient who remains medically unstable and is treated with prolonged traction. The fracture is not always adequately reduced in traction and may begin to unite in malposition (Fig. 13-10). Although reduction may be achieved with closed means, the fracture so treated displays a tendency to drift toward the original healing position. If a cast-brace is employed, percutaneous pins inserted into the femur must be incorporated into the thigh plaster cast to aid in preventing a return to the previous position. Even then, the proper alignment of these fractures is often difficult to maintain. If possible, this fracture is best treated by open reduction and internal fixation.

Knee

Surgical indications for repair of intra-articular fractures about the distal femur and the proximal tibia are similar for the patient with head injuries and the normal population (Fig. 13-11). If a long-leg plaster cast is employed, the knee should be neutral. A cast-brace applied postoperatively is a good adjuvant for obtaining stability and protection and for gaining knee motion. Heterotopic bone about the knee is uncommon.

Knee Ligament. Although primary repair is recommended for normal patients with ligamentous injury about the knee, primary repair is not always indicated in patients with head injuries. Despite plaster immobilization, the repair may not be maintained in patients with head injuries because of hamstring spasticity. After primary repair, the knee is placed in a position of flexion,

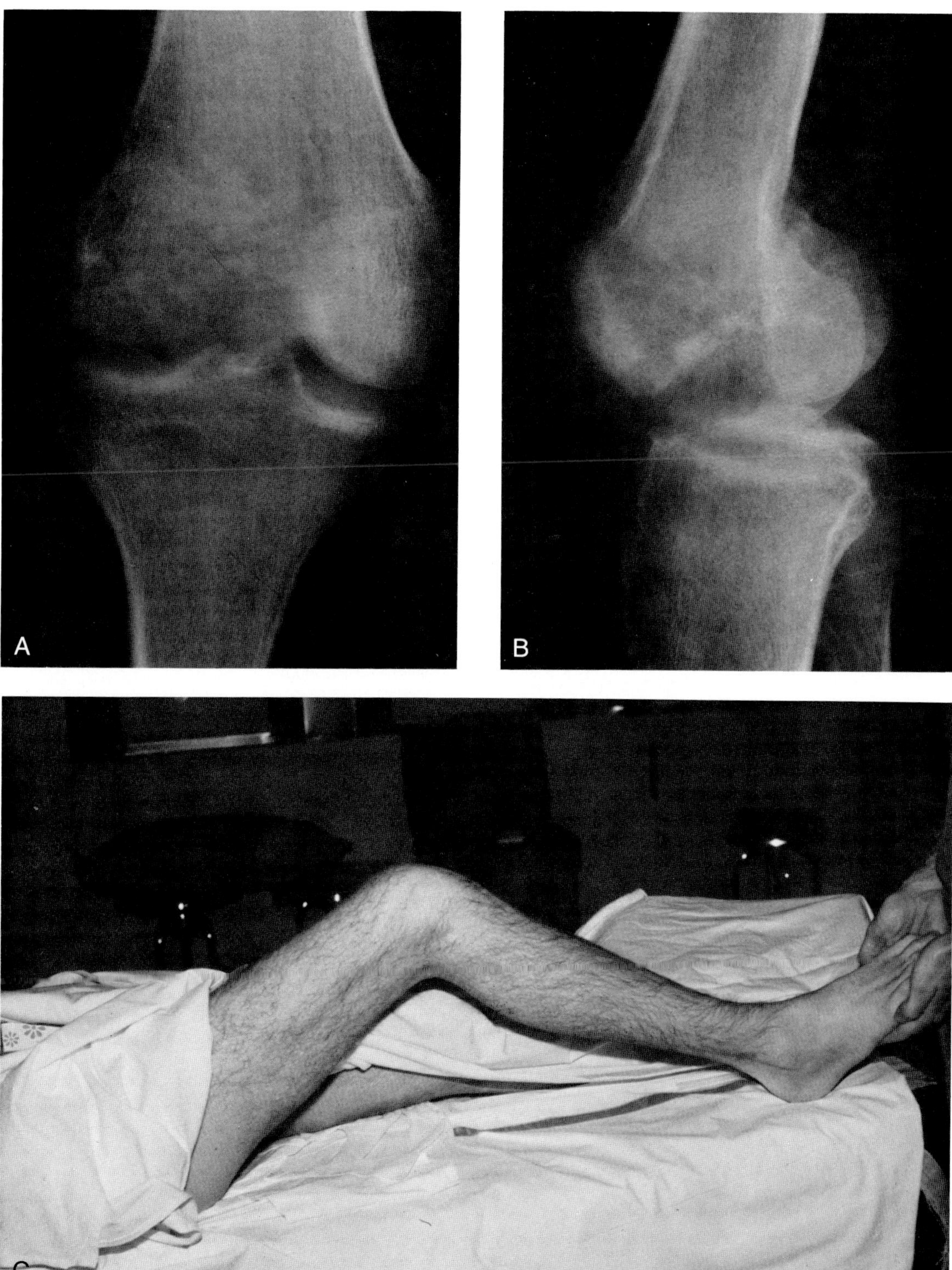

Fig. 13-11. *A* and *B*, Anterior and lateral radiographs of displaced lateral femoral condyle. The patient was treated with a posterior plaster splint. *C*, Preoperative knee flexion 6 weeks after injury.

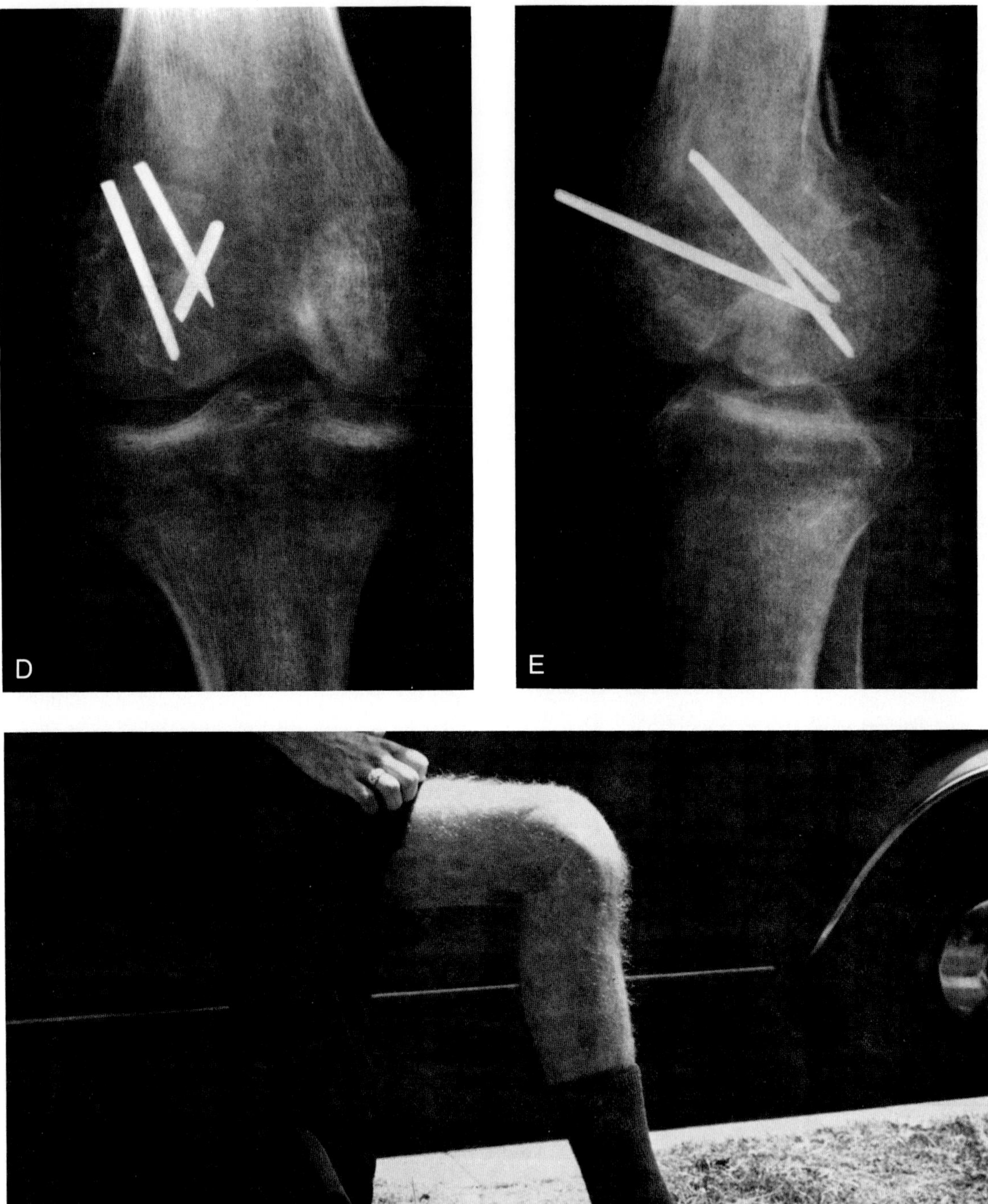

Fig. 13-11 (*continued*). *D* and *E*, Anterior and lateral radiographs taken after open reduction and internal fixation had been performed. Union had occurred. *F*, Knee flexion 1 year after open reduction and internal fixation were performed.

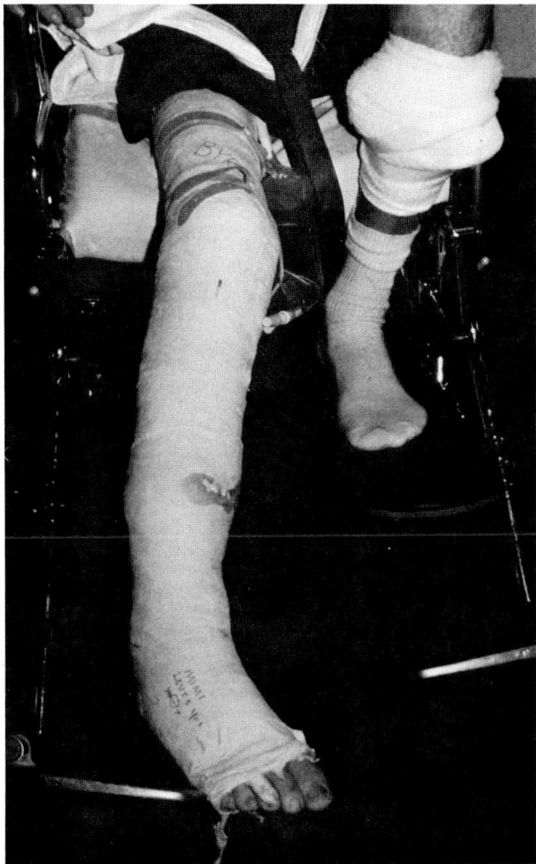

Fig. 13-12. An open tibia fracture was placed in this long-leg plaster cast. The knee is flexed, and the ankle is in an equinovarus position. This type of cast encourages flexion contractures of the knee and ankle. The cast was changed to a long-leg plaster cast with the ankle and knee in neutral position.

which is not desirable for such persons since it encourages the formation of a flexion contracture. With ligamentous repair of the knee, these patients can be rendered nonambulatory with a contralateral hemiplegia. After repair and casting, regaining strength in the quadriceps muscles is difficult to achieve in the patient with central-nervous-system damage. Since these patients do not return to competitive athletics, the stability achieved by cast immobilization usually is sufficient for their needs. Reconstructive surgery can be performed later in patients who become symptomatic and has achieved satisfactory results thus far.

Tibia

Although tibia fractures are the second most common fracture of the lower extremity, they generally pose no significant treatment problems for the patient with head injuries. Our review of 47 tibial shaft fractures demonstrated a union rate of 93.5%. Time to union was 5.6 months.[14] The fractures responded to conventional plaster-cast methods. Initially, the knee and ankle should be positioned in a neutral position in a long-leg cast (Fig. 13-12). The cast may be changed to a patellar tendon weight-bearing plaster cast or a short-leg cast when the patient becomes mobile and the fracture can be controlled adequately. Functional bracing usually is not employed since many patients tend to remove the brace. Furthermore, a circular plaster cast affords better control of the ankle and foot, thereby helping to prevent equinus, which occurs when the gastrocnemius and soleus are hyperactive. A complication of plaster-cast treatment is pressure paralysis of the peroneal nerve.[5,14] Extra padding over the fibular head and neck should be employed when applying the cast. Evaluation of nerve function should be performed periodically.

Open tibia fractures are common and accounted for 50% of our tibial fractures. A temptation exists to treat many of these open fractures with the external fixation device. We prefer the use of percutaneous pins in a plaster cast when treating the open fracture or the comminuted fracture, which is difficult to control. The ankle and knee can be best positioned and maintained at a neutral position with this method. The patient with head injuries may endanger himself with the protruding pins of the external fixation device during the agitation phase of recovery. Patients with head trauma are sensitive to pain; the more pins that penetrate skin and muscles, the greater the amount of pain. The patient or the therapist may have difficulty ranging the joint nearest the fixation device because of this pain, and flexion contractures may result (Fig. 13-13).

Ankle and Foot

Fractures about the ankle in patients with head injuries generally follow the same surgical indications as do those that occur in the general population. The ankle always should be placed in a neutral position when treated with a plaster cast.

References

1. Caveness, W. F.: Incidence of Craniocerebral Trauma in the United States in 1976 with Trend from 1970 to 1975. *In* Advances in Neurology. Vol. 22. Edited by Thompson and Green. New York, Raven Press, 1979.

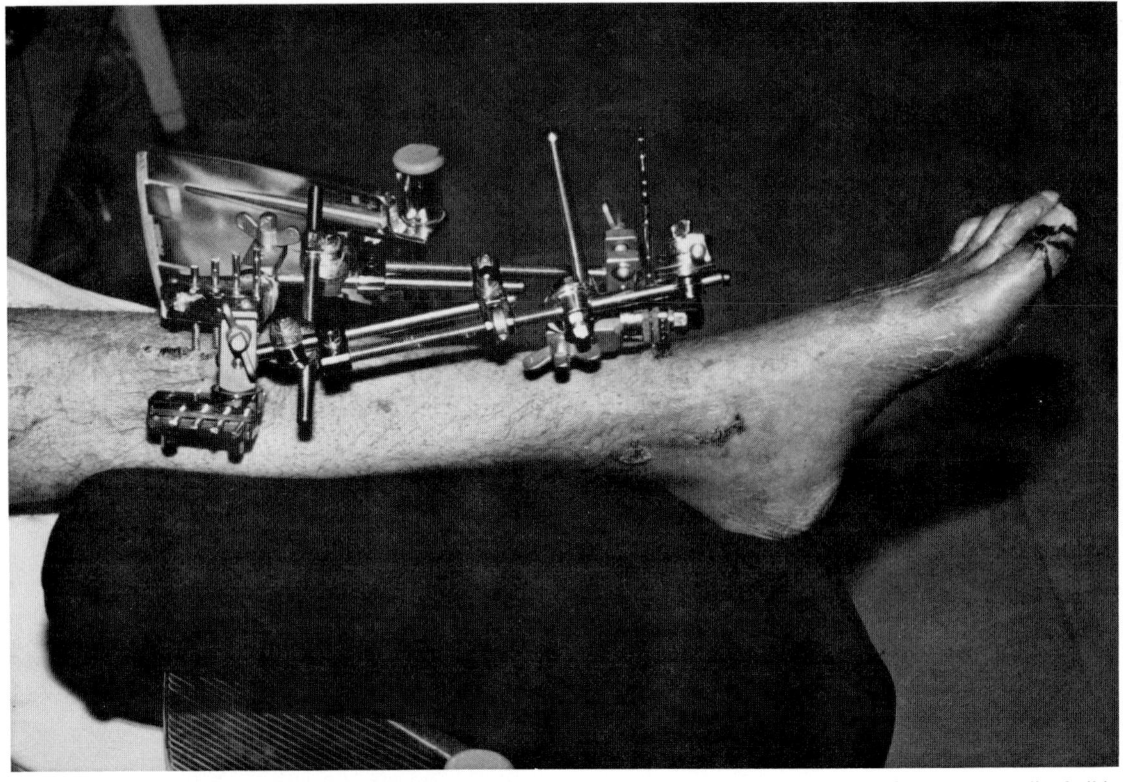

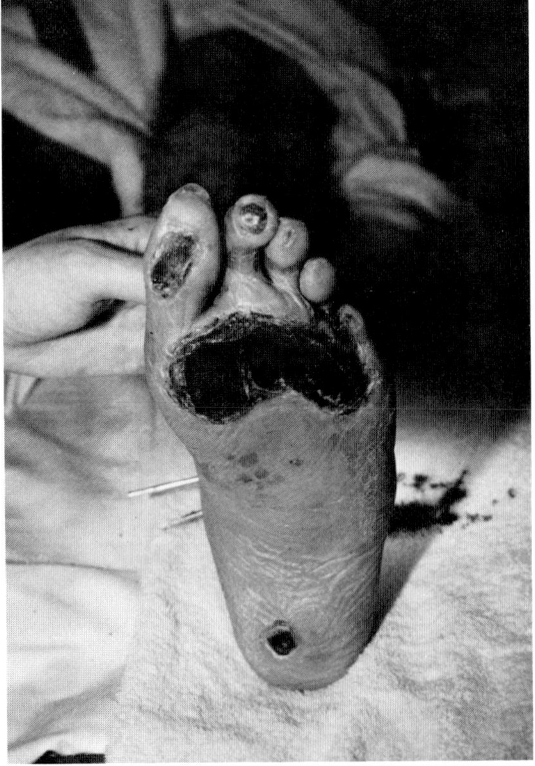

Fig. 13-13. *A*, This patient sustained an open distal tibia fracture. An external fixation device was applied. The patient could not dorsiflex his foot actively because of inadequate muscle control and pain caused by the pin. An equinus contracture developed. *B*, The patient developed this pressure sore from his inability to dorsiflex and from the placement of a strap to prevent equinus.

2. Kraus, J. F.: Epidemiologic features of head and spinal cord injury. *In* Advances in Neurology. Vol. 19. Edited by Schoenberg. New York, Raven Press, 1978.
3. Garland, D. E., and Rhoades, M. E.: Orthopedic management of brain injured adults. Clin. Orthop., *131*:111, 1978.
4. Garland, D. E.: Head injuries in adults. *In* Orthopedic Rehabilitation. Edited by Nickel. New York, Churchill Livingstone. N.Y. 1982.
5. Garland, D. E., and Bailey, S.: Undetected injuries in head injured adults. Clin. Orthop., *155*:162, 1981.
6. Teasdale, G., and Jennett, B.: Assessment of coma and impaired consciousness. A practical scale. Lancet, *2*:81, 1974.
7. Heiden, J. S., et al.: Severe head injury and outcome: a prospective study. *In* Neural Trauma. Edited by Popp. New York, Raven Press, 1979.
8. Rhoades, M. E., and Garland, D. E.: Orthopedic prognosis of brain injured adults. Clin. Orthop., *131*:104, 1978.
9. Garland, D. E., Capen, D., and Waters, R. L.: Surgical morbidity in patients with neurologic dysfunction. Clin. Orthop., *145*:189, 1979.

10. Comarr, A. E., Hutchinson, R. H., and Bors, E.: Extremity fractures of patients with spinal cord injuries. Am. J. Surg., *103*:732, 1962.
11. Eichenholtz, S. N.: Management of long-bone fractures in paraplegic patients. J. Bone Joint Surg., *45A*:299, 1963.
12. Freehafer, A. A., and Mast, W. A.: Lower extremity fractures in patients with spinal cord injury. J. Bone Joint Surg., *47A*:683, 1965.
13. Neufeld, A. J., Mays, J. J., and Naden, C. J.: A dynamic method of treating femoral shaft fractures. Orthop. Rev., *1*:19, 1972.
14. Garland, D. E., and Toder, L.: Fractures of the tibial diaphysis in head injured adults. Clin. Orthop., *150*:198, 1980.
15. Garland, D. E., Rothi, B., and Waters, R. L.: Treatment of femur fractures in head injured adults. Clin. Orthop., *166*:219, 1982.
16. Fletcher, K.: Traction lesions of the brachial plexus. Hand, *1*:129, 1969.
16a. Garland, D. E., Blum, C. E., and Waters, R. L.: Periarticular heterotopic ossification in head-injured adults. Incidence and location. J. Bone Joint Surg., *62-A*:1143, 1980.
17. Garland, D. E., Razza, B., and Waters, R. L.: Manipulation of joints with heterotopic ossification in head injured adults. Clin. Orthop., *169*:133, 1982.
18. Anderson, L. D., Sisk, D. T., Tooms, R. E., and Park, W. I.: Compression plate fixation in acute diaphyseal fractures of the radius and ulna. J. Bone Joint Surg., *57A*:287, 1975.
19. Carnesale, P. G., Stewart, M. J., and Barnes, S. N.: Acetabular disruption and central fracture-dislocation of the hip. J. Bone Joint Surg., *57A*:1054, 1975.
20. Garland, D. E., Glogovac, S. V., and Waters, R. L.: Orthopedic aspects of pedestrian victims of automobile accidents. Orthopedics, *2*:242, 1979.
21. Tipton, W. W., D'ambrosia, R. D., and Ryle, G. P.: Non-operative management of central fracture-dislocation of the hip. J. Bone Joint Surg., *57A*:888, 1975.
22. Garland, D. E., Chick, R., Taylor, J. and Salisbury, R. B.: Treatment of proximal-third femur fractures with pins and thigh plaster. Clin. Orthop., *160*:86, 1981.
23. Heiden, J. S.: Personal communication, unpublished data.

Chapter 14 Fractures and Major Nerve Injuries in the Fractured Extremity

GEORGE E. OMER, JR.

The incidence of major nerve injuries associated with fractures is unknown. A humeral fracture, however, is the most likely fracture to have an associated nerve injury.[1] Approximately 12% of fractures of the shaft of the humerus are complicated by immediate radial nerve paralysis.[2–5] An estimated 237,000 humeral fractures occur each year in the United States in persons between the ages of 17 and 64 years.[6] In our personal practice, approximately 75% of adult humeral fractures involve the shaft, which means by deductive reasoning that there are more than 21,000 radial palsies each year associated with fractures of the shaft of the humerus. Approximately 5% of supracondylar fractures of the humerus are complicated by immediate nerve injuries,[7–9] of which about 40% are radial neuropathies. An estimated 134,000 humeral fractures occur each year in the United States in children below the age of 16 years.[6] In our personal practice, approximately 50% of humeral fractures in children involve the supracondylar area, which means by deductive reasoning that there are more than 3000 nerve injuries of the elbow each year involving the ulnar, radial, and median nerves. Collected series of nerve injuries associated with fractures and fracture-dislocations indicate the following percentages of total nerve injuries;[10–12] radial nerve, 60%; ulnar nerve, 18%; common peroneal nerve, 15%; and median nerve, 6%. These figures suggest an annual incidence of more than 35,000 nerve injuries associated with fractures and fracture-dislocations. This extraordinary number emphasizes that spontaneous recovery of these injuries is the rule. Seddon recorded 91% spontaneous recovery in 211 upper-limb nerve injuries caused by skeletal damage.[13]

Classification for Prognosis

A clinical classification can be related to the cause of the nerve injury:

1. Primary injury by the displaced bony fragments
   a. physiologic interruption—the most common injury
   b. anatomic interruption
      1. laceration
      2. stretch or traction related to dislocations and anatomic fixation of the nerve. For example, the peroneal nerve is angulated and relatively fixed at the neck of the fibula so that dislocation of the knee joint provides a deforming force that is not dissipated over a long length of the nerve.

2. Secondary injury
   a. manipulation or traction
   b. pressure
      1. internal caused by expanding hematoma or displaced bone from a dislocation
      2. external, such as a constricting circular plaster cast
3. Delayed injury
   a. ischemia from injury to vessels
   b. infection
   c. involvement in scar tissue or callus collar with slow compression, stretch, or friction. The tardy ulnar palsy that follows a fracture-dislocation of the elbow joint is a good example.

During World War II,[14] Seddon introduced a simple classification of traumatic nerve injuries. In this classification, minimal injury is termed neurapraxia and may be secondary to localized ischemic demyelination. Moderate injury is termed axonotmesis. It is characterized by interruption of the axons and their myelin sheath; the endoneurial tubes remain intact and guide the regenerating axons to their appropriate peripheral connections. Severe injury, termed neurotmesis, involves a nerve that either has been completely severed or is so seriously disorganized that spontaneous regneration is impossible. Most traumatic injuries, including fractures, dislocations, and traction injuries, can result in any of the three types of injury.

Sunderland has provided the following classification in relation to the internal structure of the nerve trunk:[15] (1) first degree—loss of axon conduction; (2) second degree—transection of the axon with an intact endoneurial sheath; (3) third degree—transection of axon and endoneurial sheath inside an intact perineurium; (4) fourth degree—transection of many axons with their endoneurial sheath and the perineurium; nerve trunk continuity is maintained by epineurial tissue; and (5) fifth degree—transection of the entire nerve trunk. Injuries may not be of uniform severity, either across or along the length of the nerve trunk. Partial and mixed lesions are produced by varying combinations of the first four degrees of injury.

The prognosis is different for open and closed injuries, and is related to the severity of damage to the extremity. Seddon reported 83.5% spontaneous recovery in 109 cases of closed fracture of the upper extremity with nerve injury, but spontaneous recovery was seen in only 65% of 37 open fractures.[16] Omer reported a prospective study of 46 fractures and 7 stretch injuries; 83% of these fractures demonstrated spontaneous return of function.[17] The time scale for spontaneous recovery of nerve function following fractures was 1 to 4 months. Stretch injuries that have spontaneous recovery may be either a neurapraxia or an axonotmesis injury; the time scale for spontaneous recovery was 3 to 6 months. The more severe the extremity injury, the more likely that the nerve lesion is an axonotmesis or a neurotmesis lesion, and the less likely that spontaneous recovery will occur.

The more extensive and severe the injury to the involved extremity, the longer the time required for homeostasis of all tissues. Severe vascular insufficiency, chronic osteomyelitis, and articular incongruity contribute to fibrotic infiltration and decreased function. Nerves are only as functional as are the pertinent sensory receptors and muscle-tendon motors. Multiple nerve involvement is a more serious complication to functional recovery of the entire extremity than is an isolated nerve injury.

Major Nerve Injuries and Fracture Combinations

Shoulder

Brachial plexus injuries from torsional strains on the shoulder or neck are serious problems. A fractured clavicle allows increased distraction and related traction between the head and shoulder, and usually results in a supraclavicular (nerve roots and divisions) injury rather than a more favorable infraclavicular (nerve cords and terminal branches) injury. The patient with a supraclavicular injury often has Horner's syndrome, avulsion fractures of the transverse processes of the cervical vertebrae, and a fractured clavicle.[18] Diagnosis is made with the use of early radiographs and voluntary muscle tests. Approximately 1 month after injury, an evaluation should be made using electromyography, sensory nerve conduction, and Tinel's sign. Electrodiagnostic studies should be repeated at monthly intervals. If no recovery has been demonstrated at 3 months, myelography and tests of axon responses are performed. Most patients with plexus injuries caused by stretch or contusion recover spontaneously within 3 to 6 months.[19] Microsurgical repair of lesions distal to the nerve roots is appropriate when the clavicle has lacerated the plexus.[20] Excessive callus from a healing fractured clavicle may exert compression on the brachial plexus, thus requiring external neurolysis.[21]

The axillary nerve is injured most frequently in glenohumeral dislocations. Any combination of fractures and dislocation may result in infraclavicular brachial plexus palsy. Except for isolated circumflex nerve injuries, the prognosis generally is good for infraclavicular injuries.[22] Although prognosis for nerve recovery is generally good, functional recovery may be impaired seriously by stiff joints or muscle atrophy. The period required for recovery of the intrinsic muscles of the hand may be more than 2 years. Joints must remain mobile.

Arm

The radial nerve is injured more frequently than any other major nerve and is particularly vulnerable to fractures of the mid-third of the shaft of the humerus.[23] Approximately 12% of fractures of the shaft of the humerus are complicated by immediate radial nerve paralysis,[2–5] the incidence of which is related to the close relationship between the bone and the nerve. Spontaneous recovery is recorded in 70% or more of these nerve injuries.[24] The time for recovery of function in complete lesions is 8 to 16 weeks.[3] Garcia and Maeck reported a series of 23 immediate explorations of radial palsy during which the nerve was found to be divided in only 1 case.[2] Gurdjian and Smathers reported elective exploration of the radial nerve in 32 patients; 5 nerves were divided, and 3 were sutured.[11] All sutured nerves demonstrated recovery.

Holstein and Lewis emphasize the danger of a spiral fracture involving the distal third of the shaft of the humerus with radial angulation at the fracture site.[25] The radial nerve in such fractures was found caught between the bone ends. This particular spiral fracture was found in 7 of 341 humeral fractures. If suspected, open reduction should be performed.

Shaw and Sakellarides note the prognostic difference between primary (immediate) and secondary (manipulative) radial palsy associated with fracture of the humerus.[26] Spontaneous recovery occurred in only 40% of 31 primary paralyses. Spontaneous recovery occurred in all 14 patients in whom there was a secondary paralysis resulting from manipulation or open reduction of the fracture.

If there is gross instability of the humeral fracture and evidence of interposition of the radial nerve between the fracture fragments, surgical correction is indicated to remove the nerve from the fracture site and stabilize the fracture. Epps and Cotler report 3 patients seen 6 months to 3 years after injury with no return of function.[27] At exploration, the radial nerve was totally entrapped in callus and, thus, had never achieved return of function. An intact functioning nerve seems to have some resistance to compression from callus.

Elbow

The median, radial, and ulnar nerves are in close relationship to the bones of the elbow joint. Approximately 5% of supracondylar fractures of the humerus have primary (immediate) nerve palsy.[7–9,28] Spitzer and Paterson recorded 200 supracondylar fractures; 25% were complicated by nerve injuries, and in 64% of these, the median nerve was affected. In 4%, there was absence of a radial pulse, which always was combined with a median nerve lesion. All the palsies recovered spontaneously in an average of 5 months. Fowles and Kassab reported 127 supracondylar fractures divided into 110 extension and 17 flexion cases.[5] Eighteen percent of the extension fractures had complications involving the brachial artery, the radial nerve, or the median nerve. Of the 17 flexion fractures, 3 had ulnar neuropathy. In addition, six postreduction palsies occurred as a result of the additional trauma of the manipulative procedures. All the nerve lesions had spontaneous recovery. If the rare diagnosis of an entrapped median nerve is made, early surgical release is required for an optimum result.[30]

The ulnar nerve has the highest incidence of injury related to dislocations of the elbow.[11] Cubitus valgus resulting from trauma is the major cause of delayed ulnar palsy at the elbow. Surgical intervention has been the accepted treatment of an established ulnar palsy at the elbow. In all cases, the ulnar nerve must be released from tight fibrous bands, such as the medial intermuscular septum. The aponeurotic roof of the cubital tunnel should be incised and the area inspected. We prefer to leave the ulnar nerve attached to the soft tissue in the depth of the groove, providing this vinculum-like tissue is elastic and not fibrotic. If the ulnar nerve does not dislocate from the condylar groove, but does compress against the medial epicondyle on flexion, a medial epicondylectomy is indicated.[31] Anterior transposition of the ulnar nerve is indicated when severe hypertrophic osteoarthritis is present or when the nerve displaces completely across and anterior to the medial epicondyle when the elbow is flexed completely.[32] The potential for full motor recovery after operation is reduced greatly in patients in whom neuropathy symptoms have been present for more than a year.

Most radial nerve injuries at the elbow are associated with Monteggia's fracture-dislocations, and the majority have spontaneous recovery of function. Boyd and Boals reported neurologic deficits in 5 of 159 Monteggia's lesions with total spontaneous recovery.[33]

Hip

The sciatic nerve is injured in approximately 13% of patients with posterior fracture-dislocations of the hip. Epstein noted this 13% incidence in 282 cases; two thirds involved only the peroneal division and one third involved both components of the sciatic nerve.[34] He also recorded a 6% incidence of neuropathy following posterior dislocations. Hunter reported 83% spontaneous recovery of sciatic nerve lesions,[35] but Seddon recorded that only 73% had normal or slightly impaired function.[36] Prompt reduction of the dislocation is the primary treatment of a sciatic paralysis. Postreduction radiographs of fracture-dislocations are essential to ascertain the position of all the acetabular fragments. If neuropathy persists and a fragment remains posteriorly or medially displaced, early operative intervention is indicated to reduce the dislocation, stabilize the fragments, and decompress the nerve. Secondary sciatic neuropathy may result when traction is applied to a dislocation without reduction. Neuropathy may develop within 24 to 72 hours and requires immediate intervention.[37] Delayed paresis can result from heterotopic bone formation. Improvement can be expected following thorough and meticulous removal of the bone and surrounding scar. Exploration of the clinically complete neuropathy resulting from fracture-dislocation is appropriate at 3 to 4 months.

Obturator nerve injury is rare in anterior dislocations of the hip, and no specific treatment beyond reduction is indicated.

Fractures through the shaft of the femur are not commonly associated with nerve injury because the nerves are well protected by muscle mass. Peroneal nerve injury sometimes is associated with femoral traction.[38] If the leg is maintained in external rotation to align fractures, the peroneal nerve may be compressed at the head of the fibula.

Knee

The incidence of nerve injury is higher in dislocations and stretch injuries than in fractures. Nerve problems occur in approximately 18% of knee dislocations (usually traction injuries that vary from neurapraxia to neurotmesis).[39] Peroneal nerve palsy has an even greater incidence in an injury to the knee with disruption damage to the lateral ligamentous structures. Towne and co-authors recorded a 56% rate of injury to the peroneal nerve in 18 knees with lateral compartment syndromes.[40] Highet and Holmes reported eight cases of traction peroneal palsy; four had complete rupture and four had macroscopic changes.[41] Only one of six neurorrhaphies regained any function. However, White described 6 cases in which 2 nerves were sutured with functional recovery; the other 4 nerves had spontaneous recovery with onset between 2 and 6 months and complete function between 4 and 12 months. When neurotmesis has occurred, the prognosis is poor. Meyers and co-authors recorded 14 peroneal palsies in 53 cases; 12 nerves did not regain function.[43] Ottolenghi and Traversa described 22 cases in which the common peroneal nerve was injured; 12 did not regain function.[44] Ligamentous injuries should undergo early operative repair. When the ligamentous injury is sutured, the damaged nerve should be explored and freed.

Coincidental Fractures

A fracture often is caused by the same wounding agent that causes the nerve injury. The fracture does not produce the nerve injury in this instance.

The distinguishing feature of high-velocity gunshot wounds is the pressure disturbance in the tissues, which often results in fractures and loss of neural function, but does not disrupt the peripheral nerves. During the Viet Nam conflict, Omer developed a prospective study of 595 gunshot wounds to determine the percentage of spontaneous recovery.[17] Spontaneous recovery occurred in 227 of 331 (69%) low-velocity gunshot wounds and 183 of 264 (69%) high-velocity gunshot wounds.

Shotgun wounds are more dangerous, have a higher percentage of peripheral nerve injuries, and require thorough debridement with early exploration of neurovascular structures. The rate of spontaneous recovery of shotgun wounds has been reported as only 45%;[45] consequently, low-velocity shotgun wounds result in a higher percentage of peripheral nerve disruption (neurotmesis) than do high-velocity missile wounds.

Management Program

Closed nerve injuries associated with fractures of long bones should be observed for 4 or 5 months because approximately 85% of these lesions have spontaneous recovery. The older the patient and the more severe the trauma, the less likely is spontaneous recovery (e.g., an adult involved in a high-speed vehicle accident resulting in a closed comminuted fracture of the mid-third of the humerus with primary (immediate) onset of radial palsy). When manipulating fractures, one should remember the potential additional injury to nerves, e.g., the spiral fracture with radial angulation involving the distal third of the humerus.

Nerve injuries associated with a dislocated joint or a fracture adjacent to a joint are suspect because fascial envelopes hold the nerves close to the bone near joints. These fracture-dislocation accidents often stretch the nerve, resulting in an axonotmesis lesion with spontaneous recovery that may require 4 to 9 months. The nerve lesion associated with a dislocation is less likely to have spontaneous recovery than is a nerve lesion associated with a fracture.

Open wounds with nerve palsy require debridement. Incisions should be placed to observe the involved neurovascular structures. High-velocity missile wounds with fractures and nerve palsies may be observed for 6 to 9 months because approximately 70% of these nerve lesions have spontaneous recovery within 9 months. Shotgun wounds have a poor prognosis, and the neurovascular structures should be visualized.

The loss of peripheral nerve function also robs the patient of the pain sensation related to compartment ischemia caused by swelling and hematoma. Measurement of the pressure in tissue compartments at risk is indicated in these patients, especially in dislocation injuries, which often have associated vascular problems. The arrangement of skeletal traction should be meticulous for the insensitive extremity or for the patient who has cerebral loss of sensibility to pain.

If expectant treatment is utilized, complete and precise physical examination of peripheral nerve function at the time of injury is the best baseline for management. Electromyographic examination should be delayed until 1 month after injury to allow Wallerian degeneration to occur. The course of clinical recovery then should be recorded monthly with electrodiagnostic studies. Voluntary muscle tests, Tinel's sign tests, and sensory nerve conduction studies should be included.

The proximal (high) injury presents a difficult problem because the site of the nerve lesion may be a considerable distance from the first motor or sensory point to be reinnervated. From the time of injury, there is progressive distortion and degeneration of the distal motor and sensory endorgans, with associated slowing of the regenerative process for axon regrowth. Expectant treatment could be prolonged until suture of a previously unrecognized severed nerve would be without hope of functional recovery.

At 3 to 4 months, exploration of the clinically complete nerve lesion in stretch injuries caused by dislocated joints, severely comminuted fractures, fractures adjacent to joints, and missile wounds above the elbow or knee is appropriate. However, approximately 60% of these nerves have a neuroma-in-continuity,[46] and a decision concerning resection of the neuroma can be difficult to make. Kline has developed an intraoperative technique for stimulating the involved nerve proximal to the neuroma-in-continuity and recording the nerve action potential distally.[47] The nerve action potential is related to axon population and myelin. Significant spontaneous recovery is gained in approximately 90% of such nerves when a nerve action potential is recorded across a neuroma-in-continuity at 3 months after injury.

References

1. Barton, N. J.: Radial nerve lesions. Hand, *3*:200, 1973.
2. Garcia, A., Jr., and Maeck, B. H.: Radial nerve injuries in fractures of the shaft of the humerus. Am. J. Surg., *99*:625, 1960.
3. Kettelkamp, D. B., and Alexander, H.: Clinical review of radial nerve injury. J. Trauma, *7*:424, 1967.
4. Klenerman, L.: Fractures of the shaft of the humerus. J. Bone Joint Surg., *48B*:105, 1966.
5. Mast, J. W., Spiegel, P. G., Harvey, J. P., and Harrison, C.: Fractures of the humeral shaft. A retrospective study of 240 adult fractures. Clin. Orthop., *112*:254, 1975.
6. Kelsey, J. L., et al.: Upper Extremity Disorders. A Sur-

vey of Their Frequency and Cost in the United States. St. Louis, C. V. Mosby, 1980.
7. D'Ambrosia, R. D.: Supracondylar fractures of the humerus—prevention of cubitus varus. J. Bone Joint Surg., *54A*:60, 1972.
8. Fowles, J. V., and Kassab, M. T.: Displaced supracondylar fractures of the elbow in children. J. Bone Joint Surg., *56B*:490, 1974.
9. Keon–Cohen, B. T.: Fractures at the elbow. J. Bone Joint Surg., *48A*:1623, 1966.
10. Goodall, R. J.: Nerve injuries in fresh fractures. Tex. Med., *52*:93, 1956.
11. Gurdjian, E. S., and Smathers, H. M.: Peripheral nerve injury in fractures and dislocations of long bones. J. Neurosurg., *2*:202, 1945.
12. Lewis, D., and Miller, E. M.: Peripheral nerve injuries associated with fractures. Ann. Surg., *76*:528, 1922.
13. Seddon, H. J.: Surgical Disorders of the Peripheral Nerves. 2nd Edition. Edinburgh, Churchill Livingstone, 1975.
14. Seddon, H. J.: Three types of nerve injury. Brain, *66*:237, 1943.
15. Sunderland, S.: A classification of peripheral nerve injuries producing loss of function. Brain, *74*:491, 1951.
16. Seddon, H. J.: Nerve lesions complicating certain closed bone injuries. J.A.M.A., *135*:691, 1947.
17. Omer, G. E., Jr.: Injuries to nerves of the upper extremity. J. Bone Joint Surg., *56A*:1615, 1974.
18. Leffert, R. D.: Brachial-plexus injuries. N. Engl. J. Med., *291*:1059, 1974.
19. Simeone, F. A.: Neurological complications of closed shoulder injuries. Orthop. Clin. North Am., *6*:499, 1975.
20. Leffert, R. D.: Lesions of the brachial plexus, including thoracic outlet syndrome. Instructional course lectures, Am. Acad. Orthop. Surg., *26*:77, 1977.
21. Miller, D. S., and Boswick, J. A., Jr.: Lesions of the brachial plexus associated with fractures of the clavicle. Clin. Orthop., *64*:144, 1969.
22. Leffert, R. D., and Seddon, H.: Infraclavicular brachial plexus injuries. J. Bone Joint Surg., *47B*:9, 1965.
23. Mast, J. W., Spiegel, P. G., Harvey, J. P., Jr., and Harrison, C.: Fractures of the humeral shaft. A retrospective study of 240 adult fractures. Clin. Orthop., *112*:254, 1975.
24. Omer, G. E.: The results of untreated traumatic injuries. *In* Management of Peripheral Nerve Problems. Edited by G. E. Omer, and M. Spinner. Philadelphia, W. B. Saunders, 1980.
25. Holstein, A., and Lewis, G. B.: Fractures of the humerus with radial nerve paralysis. J. Bone Joint Surg., *45A*:1382, 1963.
26. Shaw, J. L., and Sakellarides, H.: Radial-nerve paralysis associated with fractures of the humerus. A review of forty-five cases. J. Bone Joint Surg., *49A*:899, 1967.
27. Epps, C. H., and Cotler, J. M.: Complications of treatment of fractures of the humeral shaft. *In* Complications in Orthopaedic Surgery. Edited by C. H. Epps. Philadelphia, J. B. Lippincott, 1978.
28. Vahvanen, V., and Aalto, K.: Supracondylar fracture of the humerus in children. A long-term follow-up study of 107 cases. Acta Orthop. Scand., *49*:225, 1978.
29. Spitzer, A. G., and Paterson, D. C.: Acute nerve involvement in supracondylar fractures of the humerus in children. Proceedings of Australian Orthopaedic Association. J. Bone Joint Surg., *55B*:227, 1973.
30. Post, M., and Haskell, S. S.: Reconstruction of the median nerve following entrapment in supracondylar fracture of the humerus: a case report. J. Trauma, *14*:252, 1974.
31. Froimson, A. I., and Zahrawi, F.: Treatment of compression neuropathy of the ulnar nerve at the elbow by epicondylectomy and neurolysis. J. Hand Surg., *5*:391, 1980.
32. Omer, G. E., Jr.: The ulnar nerve at the elbow. *In* Difficult Problems in Hand Surgery. Edited by J. W. Strickland, and J. B. Steichen. St. Louis, C. V. Mosby, 1982.
33. Boyd, H. B., and Boals, J. C.: The Monteggia lesion. A review of 159 cases. Clin. Orthop., *66*:94, 1969.
34. Epstein, H. C.: Posterior fracture–dislocations of the hip. J. Bone Joint Surg., *56A*:1103, 1974.
35. Hunter, G. A.: Posterior dislocation and fracture–dislocation of the hip, a review of fifty-seven patients. J. Bone Joint Surg., *51B*:38, 1969.
36. Seddon, H. J.: Surgical Disorders of the Peripheral Nerves. 2nd Edition. Edinburgh, Churchill Livingstone, 1972.
37. Derian, P. S., and Bibighaus, A. J.: Sciatic nerve entrapment by ectopic bone after posterior fracture–dislocation of the hip. South. Med. J., *67*:209, 1974.
38. Simeone, F. A.: Nerve injuries complicating fractures and dislocations. *In* Fracture Treatment and Healing. Edited by R. B. Heppenstall. Philadelphia, W. B. Saunders, 1980.
39. Kennedy, J. C.: Complete dislocation of the knee joint. J. Bone Joint Surg., *45A*:889, 1963.
40. Towne, L. C., Blazina, M. E., Marmor, L., and Lawrence, J. F.: Lateral compartment syndrome of the knee. Clin. Orthop., *76*:160, 1971.
41. Highet, W. B., and Holmes, W.: Traction injuries to the lateral popliteal nerve and traction injuries to peripheral nerves after suture. Br. J. Surg., *30*:212, 1943.
42. White, J.: The results of traction injuries of the common peroneal nerve. J. Bone Joint Surg., *50B*:346, 1968.
43. Meyers, M. H., Moore, T. M., and Harvey, J. P.: Follow-up notes on articles previously published in the Journal: traumatic dislocation of the knee joint. J. Bone Joint Surg., *57A*:430, 1975.
44. Ottolenghi, C. E., and Traversa, C. H.: Vascular and nerve complications in injuries of the knee. Reconstr. Surg. Traumatol., *14*:114, 1974.
45. Luce, E. A., and Griffin, W. O.: Shotgun injuries of the upper extremity. J. Trauma, *18*:487, 1978.
46. Kline, D. G., and Hackett, E. R.: Reappraisal of timing for exploration of civilian peripheral nerve injuries. Surgery, *78*:54, 1975.
47. Kline, D. G.: Evaluation of neuroma-in-continuity. *In* Management of Peripheral Nerve Problems. Edited by G. E. Omer, Jr., and M. Spinner. Philadelphia, W. B. Saunders, 1980.

Chapter 15 Fracture-Dislocations of the Lumbar Spine

E. SHANNON STAUFFER

Victims of severe trauma who suffer injuries to multiple systems may have fractures of the thoracolumbar spine. Such fractures may escape early detection because of the severity of the more obvious and life-threatening injuries. Injudicious handling of the patient by medical personnel who are not aware of a spinal fracture may produce or increase an existing neurologic injury, possibly resulting in permanent paralysis. The presence of a fractured spine modifies the priorities of treatment of the patient's other injuries, and the existence of injuries in other systems may compromise the optimal treatment of the spinal fracture. The spinal fracture, even with paraplegia, does not have the immediate life-threatening potential of other system injuries; however, it may produce the most serious impairment—that of long-term disability after the patient recovers from other system injuries. Therefore, the differential diagnosis of all patients with multiple-system trauma must include a suspicion of fractures of the spine until ruled out by physical examination and appropriate roentgenograms (Fig. 15-1).

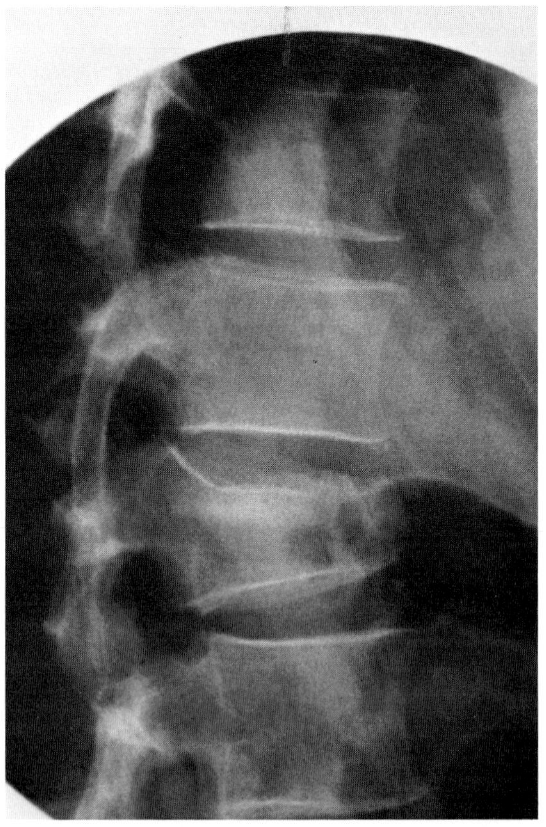

Fig. 15-1. Lateral roentgenogram of a 38-year-old man with back pain following a snowmobile accident demonstrates a fracture of L1.

Diagnosis, Priorities, and Pitfalls

The basis of the diagnosis of a spinal fracture in the multiply injured patient is the history, the physical examination, and the high index of suspicion. An accurate history frequently is difficult to obtain from the patient who is in severe pain, unconscious from a head injury, or in shock. On occasion, the evaluation may be superseded by the necessity for rapid life-saving diagnostic and resuscitative measures. If the history cannot be obtained from the patient, it should be obtained from observers or family members of the patient. Any evidence of a fall from a height, a vehicular accident, or a gunshot wound in the vicinity of the spine should alert the examiner to the possibility of a spinal fracture. The patient's activity immediately following the injury should be documented carefully. Was the patient conscious? Did the patient move his upper and lower extremities? Was the patient able to move himself from the scene of the accident? Specifically, did the patient walk, crawl, or sit up? If conscious, did the patient complain of back pain?

The physical examination of the conscious patient consists of a voluntary muscle survey of the upper and lower extremities. The patient's ability to move his fingers, hands, wrists, elbows, toes, ankles, and knees without movement of the hips or spine, which may cause motion of a potentially unstable spinal fracture site, should be documented. A sensory testing with a pin is then performed to document the presence or absence of sensibility over the patient's extremities and trunk. Signs of other injuries that may be associated with lumbar-spine fractures, such as abdominal contusions from an automobile lap type of seat belt or tenderness and crepitus of the heels signifying os calcis fracture, should be noted. Following splinting of any long-bone fractures that may be present and appropriate dressing of open wounds or bleeding areas, the patient's legs are abducted gently and a rectal examination is performed to ascertain the presence or absence of voluntary sphincter control, a bulbocavernosus reflex, and perception of sharp/dull discriminatory sensation in the perianal area. The physical examination is completed by gently rolling the patient slightly to one side in a "logrolling" fashion and palpating the posterior midline spinous processes. If there is any area of a prominent gibbus or of tenderness or pain, this area should be noted and carefully evaluated on the subsequent roentgenograms.

Reflexes in the lower extremities should be tested at the knees and the ankles with a percussion hammer and compared with upper extremity reflexes. The presence of reflexes is a good sign of neurointegrity; however, decreased or absent reflexes may be due to a peripheral nerve injury, muscle damage, or fractures of the long bones of the lower extremities, as well as to spinal cord or cauda equina injury.

The postinjury history of the patient who is unconscious when first seen by the medical staff is important. Did the patient have a period of consciousness, and if so, what were his observed movements of the extremities? How long was the patient conscious before lapsing into unconsciousness? When testing sensation, one must document whether there is any difference between upper and lower extremities in regard to appreciation of painful stimuli, response to painful stimuli, and reactive withdrawal movements. If the patient has no appreciation of or response to painful stimuli, no perceptible voluntary motion in the upper or lower extremities, no reflex activity, and is completely flaccid, neurologic injury may be due to brain damage or upper cervical spinal cord injury. However, if there is a perceptible difference between reactions in the upper and lower extremities and if the patient has some perception of sensation, withdrawal response, and deep tendon reflexes in the arms but not in the lower extremities, one must tentatively diagnose a thoracic or lumbar spinal cord or cauda equina injury.

Neurologic Evaluation of the Paraplegic Patient

The clinical evaluation of the patient with a neurologic loss associated with a fracture or dislocation of the thoracic or lumbar spine includes establishing the anatomic level of the lesion, differentiating a spinal cord lesion from a nerve root and/or cauda equina lesion, and documenting whether the lesion is complete or incomplete (Fig. 15-2). To establish the functional level of the paraplegia, the examiner documents the lowest normally functioning spinal cord segment as determined by accurate reproducible sharp/dull sensory discrimination and voluntary muscle power at the fair (+3) grade or better. The marginal region of vague sensory perception and trace to poor muscle power adjacent to the normal sensory and motor level is usually the result of edema around the cord lesion or partial nerve root injury. This area of present but poor neurologic function may show progressive improvement of sensation and muscle power adjacent to the level of the neurologic loss when edema recedes or the function of the partially injured nerve root improves.

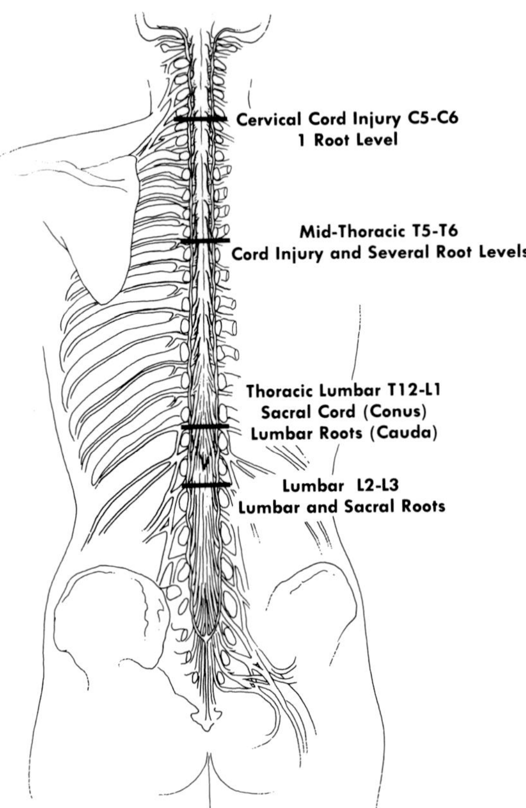

Fig. 15-2. Neurologic injury pattern of various levels of the spine; of particular importance is the T12-L1 area where the sacral segments of the cord and the lumbar roots may be injured.

The diagnosis of a complete spinal cord lesion is best documented by careful examination to determine that there is no sensory or voluntary muscle control from the spinal cord segments caudal to the lowest functioning level. The areas innervated by the sacral cord segments of the conus medullaris, in particular, must be examined carefully in injuries of the thoracic vertebral area. If the patient has some evidence of scattered sensation or muscle control over the lower extremities, feet, perineum, or, specifically, any sensation or muscle power around the anal sphincter, the patient's disorder is diagnosed as an incomplete spinal cord lesion. If, however, there is no perianal sensation or voluntary sphincter control, and no other muscle or sensory innervation is found below the level of the injury, then the patient's disorder is diagnosed as a complete spinal cord lesion. The patient must be evaluated periodically over the first 24 to 48 hours following injury, and if no sign of sensation or voluntary muscle control returns during that time, the lesion is diagnosed as complete. The complete lesion is confirmed with the return of the bulbocavernosus reflex, which indicates the end of spinal shock and the absence of any return of voluntary sensation or muscle control. The bulbocavernosus reflex usually is present within 24 hours following injury.

Incomplete spinal cord injuries have a good prognosis for progressive recovery. Complete spinal cord lesions have virtually no chance of recovery of spinal cord function. Injuries to the intradural nerve roots in the cauda equina, on the other hand, have a variable prognosis for recovery of root function that is difficult to predict.

Clinical Patterns of Paralysis (Table 15-1)

Thoracic Injuries: T1 to T10

A complete lesion is characterized by complete anesthesia and paralysis below the injured level.

The following injuries are the result of partial lesions:

1. Brown-Séquard syndrome. This injury is characterized by partial paralysis with weakness greater in one leg and ipsilateral side of the trunk and sensory loss greater in the contralateral leg and side of the trunk. Prognosis is good for progressive recovery of ambulation and bladder and bowel control.

2. Central cord syndrome. The patient with this injury has profound loss of lower extremity sensation and muscle control, but accurate perception of sensation around the perianal area. The patient may have some voluntary control of the toe flexors or sphincter muscles. This syndrome has a good prognosis for progressive recovery of improved sensation and control of the lower extremities.

3. Anterior cord syndrome. The patient with this injury has complete motor paralysis and loss of sharp/dull discrimination below the level of injury, but maintains preservation of deep pressure sensory modalities in the lower extremities. The patient can tell which leg is being squeezed and may have accurate proprioception sensation. This syndrome has a poor prognosis for recovery of sharp/dull discriminatory sensation and muscle control of the lower extremities.

Thoracolumbar Junction Injuries: T11, T12, and L1

These injuries may involve the sacral segments of the spinal cord (conus medullaris) and any or all of the intradural lumbar innervated spinal

TABLE 15-1. *Neurologic Pattern of Complete Transverse Lesions.*

Fracture-Dislocations	*Initial Functional Level*	*Roots Involved (Recovery?)*	*Injured Cord Segment (Flaccid)*	*Reflex Functioning Cord Below Injury (Spastic)*	*Abdominals*	*Legs*	*Bowel and Bladder*
T1–T9	Vertebral level of injury	One level lower	One or two levels lower	Thoracic, lumbar, and sacral cord segments below lesion	Spastic	Spastic	Spastic
T10	T9	T10 and T11	T12	Lumbar and sacral cord	Flaccid/ voluntary	Spastic	Spastic
T11	T10	T11, T12, and L1	L1 to L2	Lumbar and sacral cord segments	Voluntary	Spastic	Spastic
T12	T11	T12, L1, L2, and L3	L3 and L4	L5 and sacral cord segments	Voluntary	Flaccid/ voluntary	Spastic
L1	T12	L1, L2, L3, L4, and L5	S1, S2, and S3	S4 to S5 segments	—	Flaccid/ voluntary	Flaccid
L2	L1	L2 to L5 and S1 to S5	—	—	—	Flaccid/ voluntary	Flaccid/ voluntary
L3	L2	L3 to L5 and S1 to S5	—	—	—	Flaccid/ voluntary	Flaccid/ voluntary
L4	L3	L4 to L5 and S1 to S5	—	—	—	Voluntary/ flaccid	Flaccid/ voluntary
L5	L4	L5 and S1 to S5	—	—	—	Voluntary	Flaccid/ voluntary

roots (cauda equina). Therefore, the sacrally innervated segments of the skin and muscle should be examined to document any cord lesion, and the lower extremity lumbar innervated skin and muscles must be examined to document any cauda equina injuries.

One must differentiate the neurologic loss from the spinal cord injury (conus medullaris) from the loss that may occur from nerve root (cauda equina) injury. Recovery from paralysis due to spinal cord injury can be predicted fairly accurately, based on the extent and severity of the injury. However, nerve root injury and cauda equina injuries show progressive recovery over a period of 3 to 6 months, the degree of which is difficult to predict. Injuries below the L1 vertebral level do not involve the spinal cord and injure the cauda equina only.

Lumbar Injuries: L2 to L5

Injuries below the L1 level do not involve the spinal cord, and any neurologic loss is due to a cauda equina injury. Even well-documented complete lesions of the cauda equina may show progressive recovery of sensation and motor power as the nerve roots recover from neurapraxia or axonotmesis injuries. The sensory nerve roots have a greater resistance to injury, and there may be widespread sensory sparing with complete motor paralysis, indicating that the ventral motor roots have been injured and the dorsal sensory roots have been spared. This syndrome has a good prognosis for recovery of the motor roots to match the sensory sparing. However, when sensation is completely absent, the sensory (dorsal) nerve roots have the poorest prognosis for recovery because the nerve cell is situated in the dorsal ganglion at the neural foramen distal to the level of injury. The motor roots (ventral) have the best prognosis for recovery since the motor cell body is in the spinal cord proximal to the injury. Progressive motor recovery is rare in the neurologic distribution where permanent sensory loss persists. Therefore, if the patient has a cauda equina lesion with some sensory sparing, motor power can be expected to return to match the sensory sparing. If, however, no sensory sparing is evident after the first 48 hours, motor recovery or sensory recovery in these areas is possible but less likely.

Unilateral Motor Weakness and Sensory Loss

This syndrome indicates that the motor and sensory roots on one side of the cauda equina have been injured to a greater extent than those on the opposite side. In this syndrome, if the sensory loss persists for more than 24 hours (axonotmesis or neurotmesis), sensory recovery is possible but unlikely. However, if sensation does return during the first 24 to 48 hours, the prognosis is good for the return of motor recovery to match the sensory sparing, even though it may take several weeks or months for the motor recovery to occur.

Roentgenographic Evaluation

All initial roentgenograms should be taken in the trauma unit of the emergency department where the patient can be monitored continually. The patient should not be transferred to the radiology department. The initial anteroposterior roentgenograms for evaluation of the chest, abdomen, and pelvis in the multiply injured patient should be observed for any malalignment, associated fractures of the ribs or lumbar transverse processes, or other bony abnormalities. Good-quality lateral roentgenograms of the skull and cervical, thoracic, and lumbar spine should be taken on all patients who suffer multisystem trauma, who have a history or physical indication suspicious of a spinal injury, or who are unconscious with multiple injuries. The lateral roentgenograms taken in the emergency room usually help to diagnose the presence of a fracture, but are not sufficient to determine accurately the amount of bony comminution, displacement, or stability of the fractured area.

In general, the more comminuted displaced fractures are associated with greater neurologic injury; however, the neurologic injury itself cannot be diagnosed by roentgenograms. The neurologic diagnosis depends on the clinical evaluation. If there are no signs of spinal fracture, the patient's other injuries may be managed in the most optimal way. However, if there is a fracture of the thoracolumbar spine area, management of other injuries, such as intrathoracic or intra-abdominal organ injuries or extremity long-bone fractures, must be undertaken with great care to prevent any motion of the spinal fracture site.

When the diagnosis of spinal fracture, with or without neurologic injury, is made, certain aspects of the management fall into different priorities. The acute life-threatening conditions assume first priority, e.g., maintaining an airway for adequate respiration, mechanical ventilation if necessary, control of hemorrhage either externally with pressure dressings or internally by surgical laparotomy, and insertion of chest tubes for intrathoracic injury. Application of traction pins for lower extremity injuries and irrigation and debridement of open fractures also take priority over management of the spinal fracture. These procedures must be done carefully to minimize motion of the spinal fracture site.

Other Diagnostic Tests

Spot films in the anteroposterior and lateral projections of the recognized fracture area and oblique views may improve the understanding of the displacement and comminution of the fracture. Lateral tomograms are useful in determining the amount of dislocation and fracture of the posterior elements (Fig. 15-3). The disadvantage of this examination is that the patient usually must be turned to his side to obtain high-quality lateral tomograms. It is difficult to safely turn the multiply injured patient on his side, particularly if he has a spinal or lower extremity fracture.

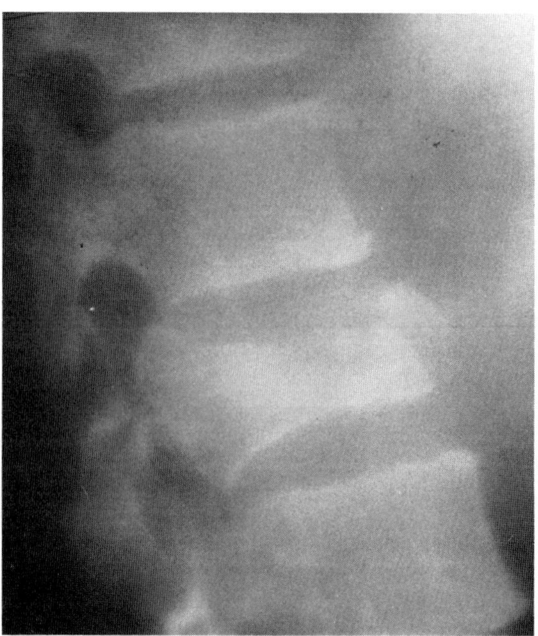

Fig. 15-3. Lateral tomogram of a 45-year-old man injured during a race-car accident. Retropulsion of vertebral body fragments into the spinal canal is demonstrated.

Computerized axial tomography (CAT scan) has allowed major improvements in detecting the amount of comminution of the vertebral body fractures, occult dorsal element fractures, and fractures of bone intruding into the spinal canal. (Fig. 15-4). Persons who have written about spinal cord injury have long believed that the presence of bony fractures merely indicates the amount of trauma expended into the spinal canal at the time of fracture and that the residual fragments in the canal do not add to the neurologic injury. Removal of these fragments has not proved in the past to be neurologically beneficial to the injured spinal cord. At present, great controversy exists regarding the value of removing these bone fragments to facilitate recovery of the nerve roots of the cauda equina. Since the spinal cord ends at the level of L1, most of the contents of the neurocanal in the lumbar area consist entirely of cauda equina nerve-root tissue. The cauda equina has a much greater propensity for progressive recovery from injuries than does the spinal cord, and only future studies will document the value of removing impending bone fragments from the cauda equina to enhance neurologic recovery. Future studies that document the pre- and postoperative CAT scans and the documentation of neurologic recovery will help to clarify this situation.

The myelogram is of negligible value during the initial management period. Because of the hemorrhage in the spinal canal, edema in the subarachnoid space, and disc and bone fragments, virtually all myelograms show a high degree of block. The neurologic injury occurs at the moment of impact, and this residual myelographic picture does no more than confirm the level of subarachnoid injury at the level of the fracture. Patients who have milder injuries with incomplete neurologic deficits have a higher percentage of free-flow myelograms. Patients with severe injuries and profound paraplegia have a higher percentage of block. However, there is no evidence that surgical attempts to unblock the canal improve neurologic recovery of the injured spinal cord.

Stability Versus Instability

In general, stability of the lumbar spine consists of integrity of the anterior and posterior columns adjacent to the spinal canal. If the posterior column is removed, but the anterior vertebral body, disc, annulus, and longitudinal ligaments are intact, spinal stability is not compromised greatly. If the anterior portion of the vertebral body is compressed or removed, but the posterior elements are intact along with the interspinous ligaments, the posterior longitudinal ligaments, and the posterior aspect of the vertebral body, even though the anterior aspect of the vertebral body is comminuted and shattered, spinal stability is not compromised greatly (Fig. 15-5). However, if there is disruption of both the anterior and the posterior columns, in addition to disruptions of facets, the posterior aspect of the vertebral

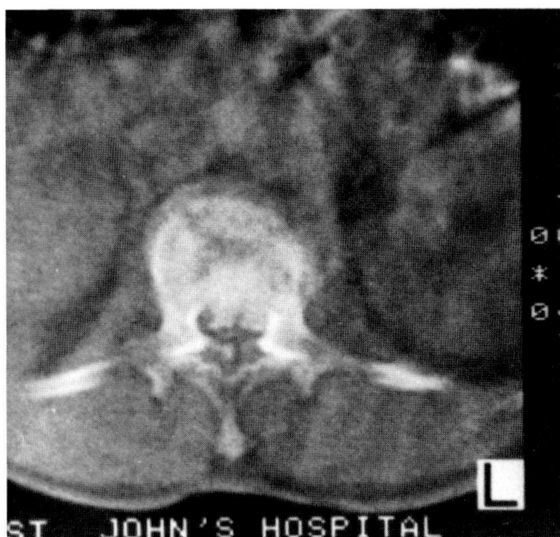

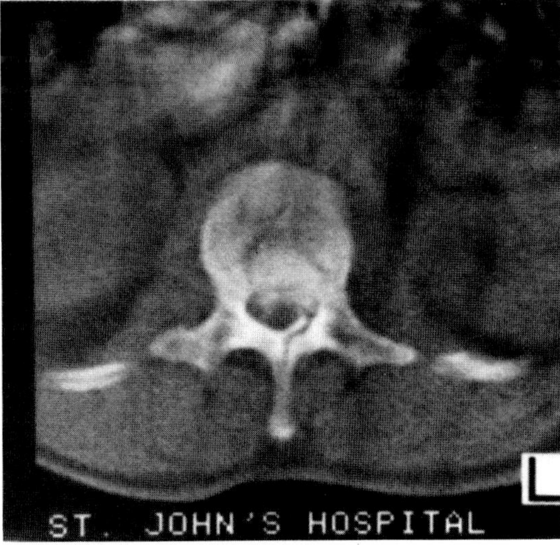

Fig. 15-4. CAT scan of patient in Figure 15-3 shows occlusion of canal and dorsal element fracture.

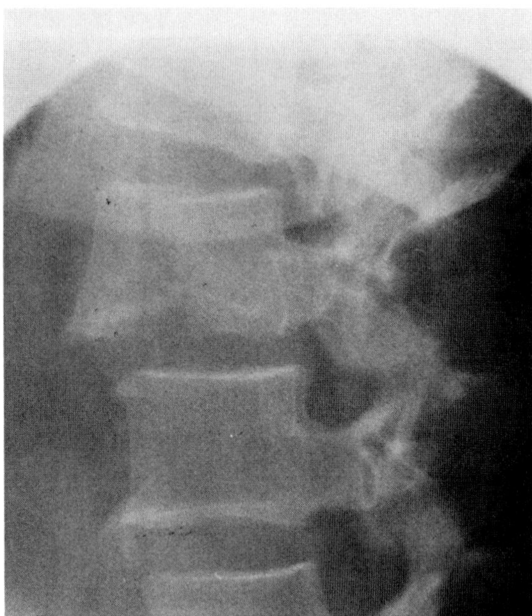

Fig. 15-5. Lateral roentgenogram of a 50-year-old physician/farmer with a 6-week history of back pain following a fall. Posterior elements and intact posterior vertebral body maintain stability.

body, or the posterior longitudinal ligament, the spinal fracture is judged unstable, and the propensity for neurologic damage is much greater (Fig. 15-6).

Pitfalls in Diagnosis

The greatest pitfall in diagnosis is not suspecting a spinal fracture after obtaining the patient's history and not making an adequate physical evaluation of the spine and neurologic examination of the lower extremities. The second pitfall is accepting inadequately exposed roentgenograms as demonstrating no fracture. When the history is reviewed, the physical examination performed, and good-quality roentgenograms demanded, few diagnoses are missed.

The Seat Belt Triad

One of the most commonly missed lumbar fractures occurs in the patient who has been involved in a high-speed vehicular accident while sitting on the passenger side of the front seat and wearing a lap type of seat belt. When the vehicle comes to a sudden stop, the pelvis is restrained by the seat belt and the momentum of the patient's upper torso carries the head, neck, and trunk forward. The lumbar spine is flexed acutely with a distraction force until the head and face strike the windshield or dashboard. The patient then suffers facial or head injuries, may be unconscious, and may also have a ruptured intra-abdominal viscus. These injuries command the immediate attention of the examining physician, and consequently, the lumbar spine is not considered. Additionally, even though the lumbar distraction ("Chance") fracture may be unstable, the patient frequently has no neurologic injury; therefore, the examining physician is misled by the normal neurologic evaluation of the lower extremities, and unless the back is palpated carefully and lateral lumbar-spine roentgenograms obtained, the unstable fracture may be missed for several days (Fig. 15-7). During this time, trips to the operating room for such procedures as laparotomy and facial restruction can jeopardize the neuroelements in the spinal canal as a result of

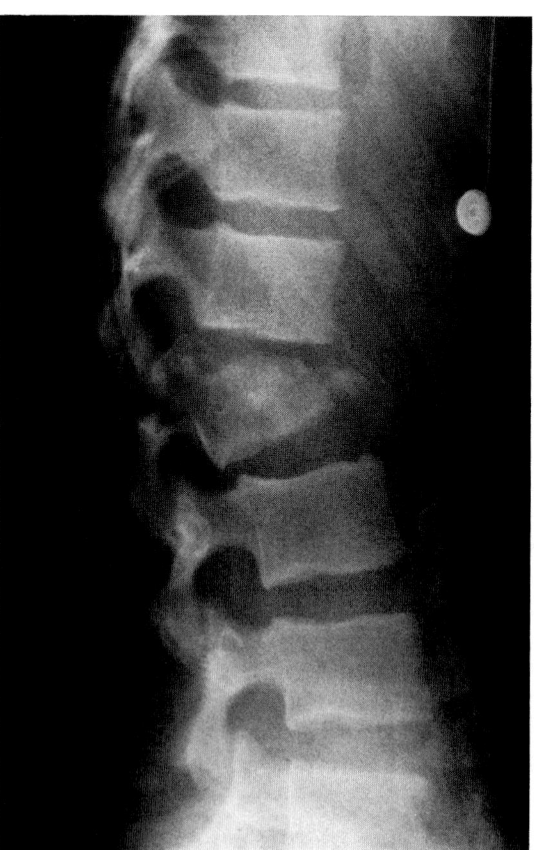

Fig. 15-6. Lateral roentgenogram of a 17-year-old girl injured in a motor-vehicle accident. Anterior and posterior disruption creates gross instability.

injudicious movement while the patient is completely relaxed under anesthesia. Therefore, patient evaluation following an automobile accident in which a lap type of seat belt was used for restraint must include a careful palpation of the lumbar-spine area, neurologic evaluation of the lower extremities, and careful evaluation for a ruptured intra-abdominal viscus.

Initial Management

When the patient has no neurologic deficit, early spinal operation is not indicated. If the patient has a profound paraplegia in the absence of a progressive neurologic deficit, an immediate spinal operation is not indicated. No statistics indicate that acute "decompression" of an acutely traumatized spine reverses the paralysis of a spinal cord injury. Many patients who have severe neurologic deficits show progressive recovery of function when managed nonoperatively. Immediate surgical intervention on the acutely traumatized spine and spinal cord has the potential for disrupting more blood supply to the spinal cord, producing more edema, and increasing the neurologic deficit. Therefore, observation for the first 24 to 48 hours to monitor the patient's overall condition, as well as to observe for neurologic recovery, is my preferred method of management. If the patient develops a progressive loss of neurologic function in the lower extremities, a posterior exploration and appropriate decompression of the neural canal, searching for epidural or subdural hematoma or progressively displacing bone or disc fragments, are indicated. Stabilization of the spine with internal fixation should be accomplished at the same time. Progressive loss of neurologic function may be the result of progressive compression by hematoma and/or bone or disc fragments and may be reversible with surgical decompression. Application of halofemoral traction for displaced fractures that cannot be reduced satisfactorily by postural positioning in the supine position in bed should be considered. Some surgeons believe that the improved reduction with early halofemoral traction may improve neurologic recovery and may facilitate an operative reduction and internal fixation planned for a later date. If the supine positioning has not satisfactorily improved a displaced fracture with a paraplegia, halofemoral traction can be instituted with local anesthesia during the first 24 to 48 hours after injury.

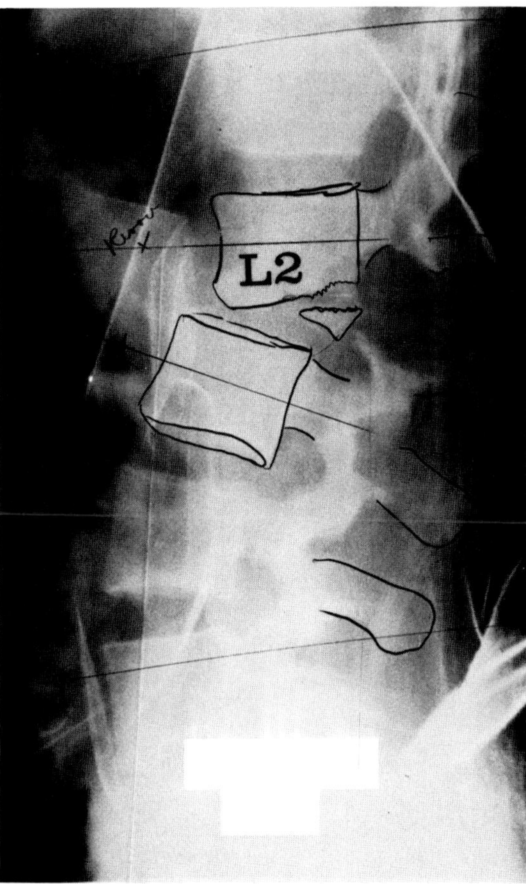

Fig. 15-7. Lateral roentgenogram of a flexion distraction (seat-belt) injury with disruption of posterior elements and fracture through the inferior portion of vertebral body.

During the initial resuscitation period, it is important to instill a urinary bladder catheter to monitor urinary output and a nasogastric tube to prevent distention from an adynamic ileus. The patient should take nothing by mouth until adequate bowel sounds reappear and should have adequate intravenous replacement of fluid losses.

Surgical Indications

When considering surgical treatment of the patient with a fracture-dislocation of the lumbar spine, several assumptions must be accepted based on previous experience, principles of pathophysiology of bone and nerve injury repair, and results of nonoperative treatment as reported in the literature. These assumptions may and should be challenged in hopes of improving neurologic recovery and the care of the paraplegic patient in the future.

The following four assumptions guide principles of treatment:

1. Fractures of the lumbar spine heal with physiologic processes of bone and soft-tissue repair to regain stability when treated in recumbency for 12 weeks, followed by external support (brace) for an additional 12 weeks.[1]
2. The amount of permanent neurologic deficit caused by spinal cord injury, versus progressive recovery, depends on the amount of injury to the neural tissue at the time of impact. Nothing can be done surgically or medically to improve the neurologic recovery rates over those documented with nonsurgical treatment.[1-3]
3. Malunited fractures healed in mild-to-moderate displacement or angulation do not cause any greater future pain or disability than do those healed in the surgically anatomically reduced position.[4]
4. The medical complications experienced by a paraplegic patient at bed rest for 6 to 12 weeks, i.e., pressure sores, urinary-tract infections, muscle atrophy, and joint contracture, can be prevented in the modern, well-equipped, spinal injury unit by expert nursing care and physical therapy performed in the recumbent position in bed, as well as in the upright position sitting in the wheelchair.

Highly respected, world-renowned advocates of the nonoperative approach to lumbar-spine fractures strongly endorse the preceding four assumptions and have documented their recovery rates and patient followups in the literature. They openly challenge the advocates of surgical treatment to impugn these principles and to produce statistically significant results to document improved care by operative methods. Many reports in recent years have attempted to document improved patient care by operative reduction and internal stabilization of thoracic and lumbar fractures. It has been documented statistically that patients who have undergone internal stabilization of their spinal fractures do have shorter periods of recumbency, have shorter periods of hospitalization, enter rehabilitation programs sooner, achieve higher levels of rehabilitation skills sooner, and have straighter spines as seen on roentgenograms.[4-7] However, no well-documented series show that these patients have better neurologic recovery, less pain, or less disability at 1 and 2 years postinjury followup than do those treated nonoperatively.

Surgical Stabilization

The following are indications for surgical stabilization.

1. Stabilization of the unstable displaced fracture for early mobilization is particularly important in the paraplegic patient because it greatly decreases the acute pain in the back, which occurs with turning in bed or on a special frame. Surgical stabilization reduces and stabilizes the spine for early mobility to the upright sitting position so that the patient can begin to learn the necessary techniques of paraplegic rehabilitation, transfer activities, wheelchair propulsion, intermittent self-catheterization, and other self-care techniques that cannot be learned during the 2 to 3 months of enforced bed rest. Muscle atrophy of normal upper extremities is prevented by this procedure, and the patient can be discharged in a wheelchair and followed as an outpatient in much less time than if treated with strict recumbency and restrictive bracing until stability of the spine is assured.[4,7]
2. Fracture-dislocations that cannot be reduced adequately with supine positioning in bed or with halofemoral traction require surgical stabilization. If the posterior facets are dislocated and locked, or if the body is so comminuted that there is displacement of more than 50% or angulation of more than 40° in the lateral or anteroposterior plane, progressive increased displacement and angulation will occur until bony union finally is established. Significant malunion with pelvic obliquity may result, making walking with crutches and braces difficult and producing an asymmetric pelvis, which increases the potential for producing severe ischial pressure sores while sitting unbalanced in the wheelchair.
3. The patient with an incomplete lesion who has progressive improvement for several weeks and then plateaus with a persistent deficit localized to one or more nerve root areas is a candidate for surgical stabilization. This is also an indication for a myelogram. If a significant degree of impingement of the dura correlates with the nerve root deficit, open reduction with decompression of the cauda equina by either an anterior or posterior lateral approach may be indicated in addition to concomitant internal stabilization.

Instrumentation

No universally acceptable instrumentation has been developed for accurate reduction and stabilization of fracture-dislocations of the lumbar spine. Harrington instruments developed for the treatment of scoliosis are the most popular instruments at this time. Because of the kyphosis of the thoracolumbar junction and the lordosis of the lumbar spine, the rods have to be contoured and curved carefully to obtain adequate reduction and to maintain stability in the anatomically correct position.

Distraction Rods. Distraction rods are the most universally satisfactory instruments (Fig. 15-8). The distraction three-point pressure techniques advocated by Dickson and associates are particularly advantageous when there is gross comminution of the dorsal elements or a comminuted burst fracture of the vertebral body.[5] One disadvantage of the distraction rods is that they require a long segment of stabilization at least two motion segments above the fracture-dislocation area and two motion segments below. Some surgeons advocate "long rodding," extending the rods three interspaces above and three interspaces below the fractured area, and claim better reduction and more stable fixation. Another disadvantage of the distraction-rod technique is that the fractured area is completely unloaded of all stresses and, therefore, heals more slowly with a bone union of poorer quality. During this healing period, the gravitational forces of the body weight of the upper trunk, upper extremities, head, and neck are supported by the upper hooks under the facet joints in the thoracic spine. The weight then is supported by the rods and transferred through the lower hooks to the laminae of the lower lumbar vertebrae. The vertebral column itself is unweighted, and the stability of the system depends on the integrity of the hook-bone interface.

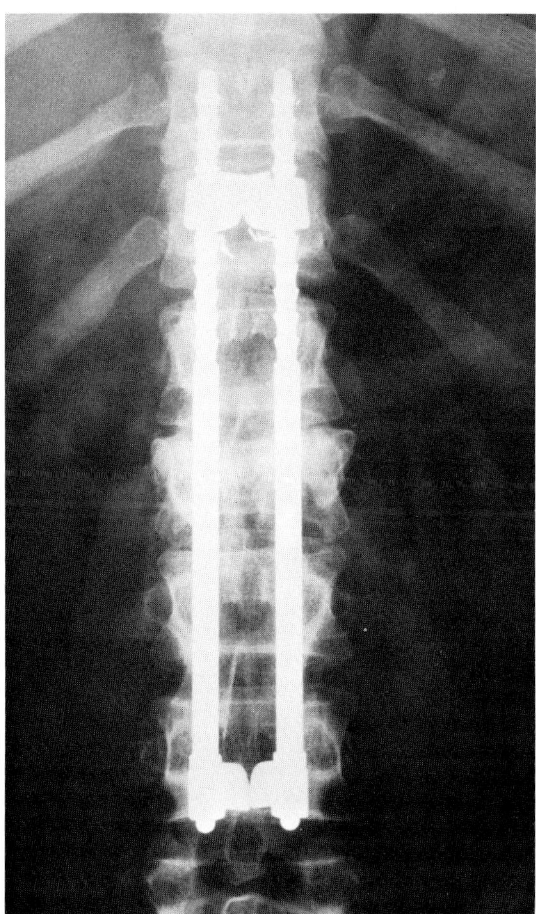

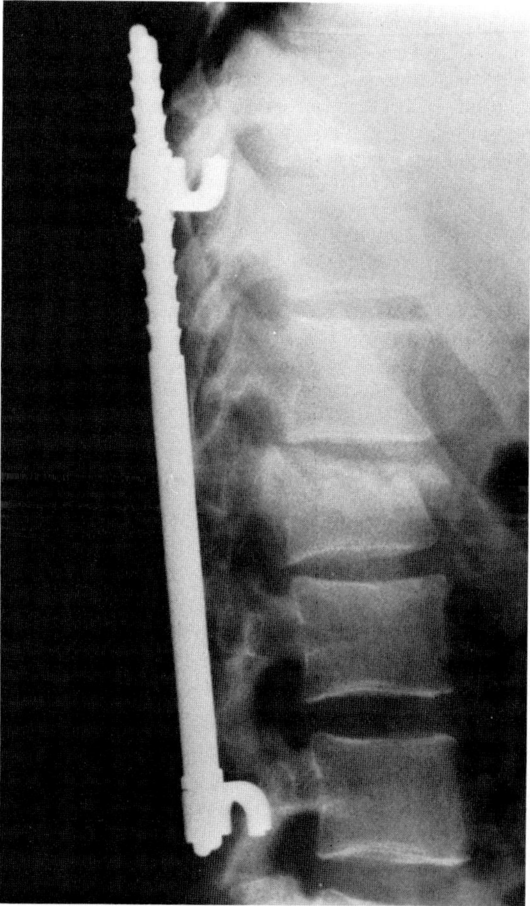

Fig. 15-8. *A* and *B*, Anteroposterior and lateral roentgenograms of double Harrington distraction rod fixation, which stabilizes from two levels above fracture-dislocation to two levels below.

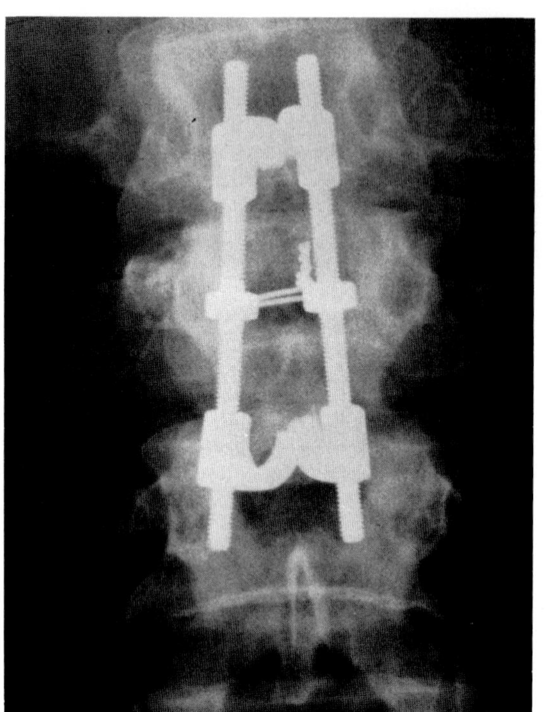

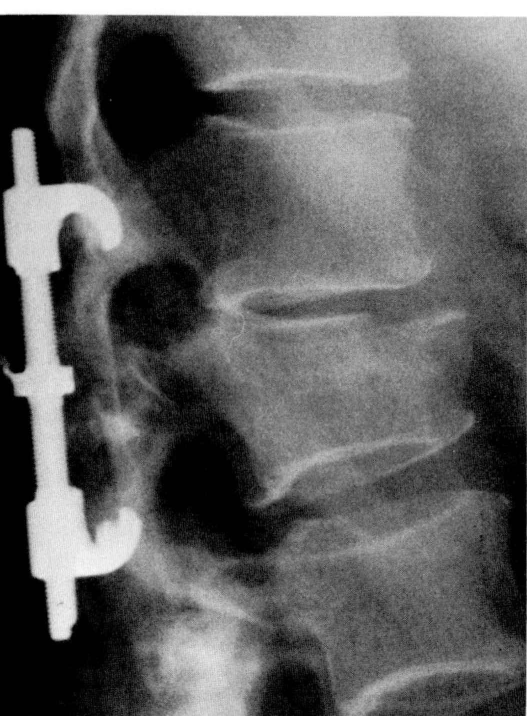

Fig. 15-9. *A* and *B*, Anteroposterior and lateral roentgenograms of double compression rod (Knodt rods) fixation limited to one motion segment.

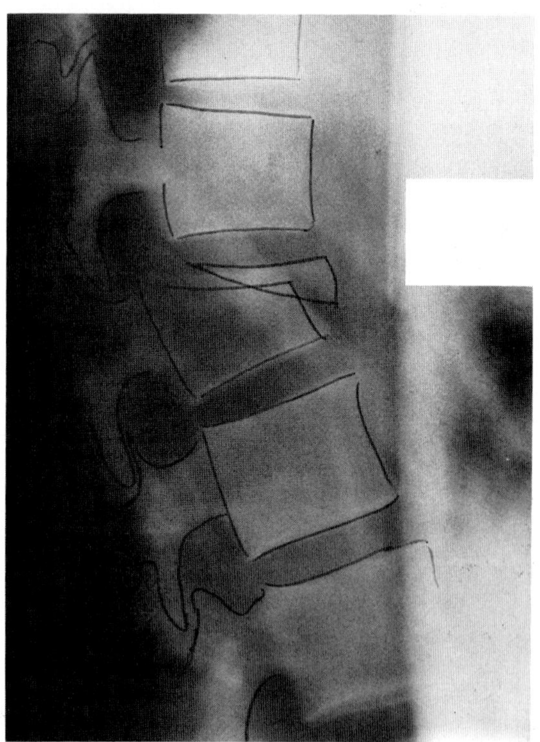

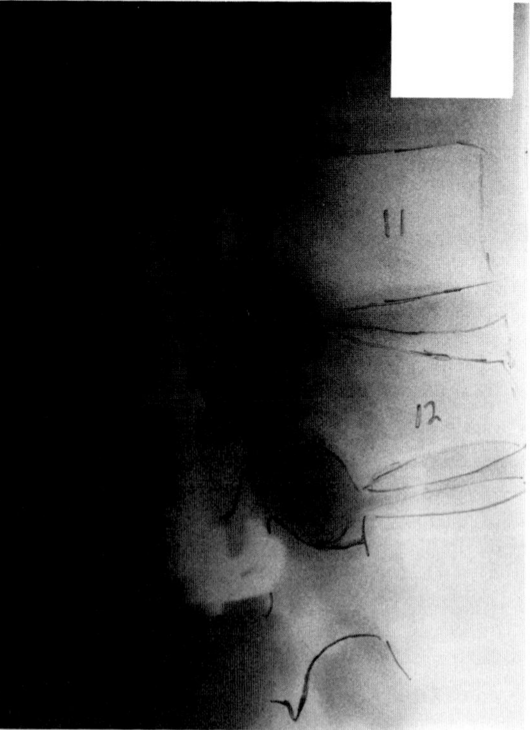

Fig. 15-10. *A*, Lateral roentgenogram of T11-T12 fracture-dislocation with facets "jumped" but intact. *B*, Lateral roentgenogram taken after open reduction and internal fixation were performed by double compression system.

Compression Apparatus. Short compression rods placed posteriorly over one motion segment provide rigid stability if the posterior elements are not comminuted (Fig. 15-9). At the T11-T12 interspace, the facets are in the coronal plane and frequently are "jumped" and locked, but not fractured. At this level, the facets can be reduced and the motion segment stabilized by two short compression rods (Fig. 15-10). The advantage of this system is that, because of the weight of the upper trunk and extremities, the gravitational forces continue to be supported by the reduced fractured vertebrae and the healing bone is more stable.

The seat belt (Chance) fracture, which is a pure bone lesion without ligamentous disruption or comminution, frequently can be stabilized and reduced with the short compression-rod technique, which provides immediate stability and allows early mobilization and ambulation (Fig. 15-11).[8] Chance fractures frequently show progressive displacement by rotation of the vertebrae in the lateral plane caused by the complete disruption of posterior stability. As the patient begins to contract the abdominal muscles, e.g., while moving in bed and attempting to sit up, further displacement of the vertebral fracture occurs. Such displacement is prevented by short posterior-rod stabilization.

Contraindications

Contraindications to surgical stabilization include:

1. Other injuries requiring bed rest. If the patient has fractures of the extremities that will be treated in traction and require bed rest for a specific period of time, spinal stabilization offers little advantage. The spinal fracture heals during the period of bed rest while the other injuries heal.

2. Neurologically normal patients with a fracture of the spine. One should not risk causing increased neurologic insult by open manipulation of the fractured spine if the patient has had a normal neurologic examination. The patient is served best by bed rest until the reaction of trauma subsides. Then, the advantages of open stabilization for early mobilization and accurate reduction versus nonoperative treatment in the supine position with resultant healing in a mild to moderate malunited position can be discussed with the patient. After the best possible reduction can be obtained by positioning or halofemoral traction, surgical stabilization can be performed 10 to 20 days postinjury without manipulation of the spine to assure stability in the reduced position, prevent future angulation, and provide early mobilization.

Prior to operating on a patient who is thought to be neurologically normal, one must document the patient's voluntary control of the sphincters, parasympathetic innervation of the bladder, and sexual function. During the first day following a severe injury to the spine, the patient may have had a Foley catheter inserted into the bladder. He may have had slight atony of the bladder and no penile erections because of the pain of the injury or an occult neurologic injury to the conus medullaris or cauda equina that is not appreciated on gross neurologic examination. This diagnosis must be made and bladder or sexual problems must be documented prior to surgery. If these

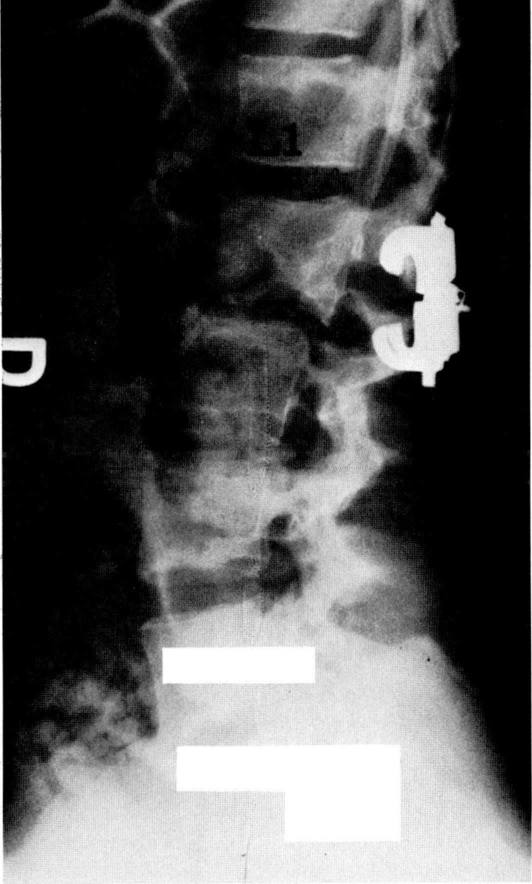

Fig. 15-11. Lateral roentgenogram of internal fixation of fractured dorsal element of L2 in patient in Figure 15-7.

steps are not taken, the patient will have some concern after surgery when the pain is gone, he is walking, and then realizes that he does not have full control of his bladder, cannot have erections, and cannot discontinue use of the Foley catheter or must continue on intermittent catherization. If neurologic injury was not diagnosed prior to the surgical procedure and the physician had reported a normal neurologic examination, there may be some concern.

3. Other life-threatening injuries requiring treatment that supersedes spinal surgery. One should not take the risk of trying to stabilize the spine surgically when concomitant chest or abdominal trauma that needs close monitoring or emergency surgical procedures are present.

Treatment Options

The selection of the appropriate treatment for individual patients is based on a knowledge of the functional changes that occur when bone, ligament, and nerve tissue heal without surgical intervention and of the areas in the healing process that can be improved by surgical intervention. Treatment options depend on the degree of instability of the spine.

The treatment options for stable injuries include:

1. Observation and allowing the patient with a stable injury to resume normal activities when the pain subsides sufficiently.
2. External immobilization with a thoracolumbosacral orthosis.
3. External immobilization with a plaster circular body cast.

The treatment options for unstable displaced injuries include:

1. Bed rest in the supine position with frequent logrolling from side to side.
2. Bed rest in a plaster cast.
3. Closed reduction with manual traction and counterpressure over the gibbous area followed by immobilization.
4. Closed reduction with postural positioning in bed.
5. Closed reduction with halofemoral traction.
6. Open reduction with posterior stabilization with distraction rods.
7. Open reduction with posterior stabilization with compression rods.
8. Open reduction combined with posterolateral decompression of the neurocanal.
9. Anterolateral removal of comminuted vertebral body and cortical strut grafting.
10. Posterior open reduction with internal fixation followed by a second-stage anterior vertebral body and disc removal for decompression of the neurocanal.

My Preferred Methods of Treatment

Stable Fractures. Stable fractures with no neurologic loss (vertebral body compression fractures, transverse process fractures, and isolated dorsal element fractures) are treated with bed rest until symptoms subside. Then, mobilization with the use of a corset or brace, if necessary for symptomatic relief, is undertaken. Spine extensor and abdominal flexion exercises are initiated as soon as possible.

T11-T12 Slice Fracture of Vertebral Body with Dislocation of Posterior Facets Without Dorsal Element Fracture. When such fractures are not accompanied by neurologic loss, observation of the patient at bed rest for 4 to 5 days with attempted postural reduction is my preferred method of treatment. If reduction is not accomplished and the facets still are locked, patients in the older age group, i.e., over 40, can be treated with cast immobilization or brace immobilization until the fracture heals (if the gibbous angular deformity is acceptable). Younger patients, i.e., under 40, should undergo an open posterior reduction and internal fixation with short one-segment compression rods. There is some risk of neurologic injury with this procedure, and intraoperative spinal cord monitoring or the "wake-up test" should be employed.

Patients with neurologic injury should be observed for 24 to 48 hours with attempted postural reduction to determine whether spontaneous neurologic recovery may occur. If neurologic recovery is evident, surgery should be delayed for 5 or 6 days to monitor the recovery. If no recovery is evident within 24 to 48 hours and the lesion is complete, open reduction for stabilization, early mobilization, and rehabilitation should be performed.

Slice Fracture-Dislocation of T12, L1, and L2. Combined fractures of the body of the posterior facet are treated with bed rest, logrolling, and observation. If improvement occurs, operative procedures may be delayed for 10 to 14 days to monitor the recovery period. As long as progressive recovery occurs, there is no urgent indication for surgical intervention. If recovery plateaus within several days, an operation may be performed with less risk to the neurologic tissue after the initial period of edema and surgical trauma is over. If the neurologic injury is complete and remains complete for 24 to 48 hours, the physician must decide to treat with bed rest and logrolling or open reduction and internal stabilization. Surgical stabilization in these injuries is best achieved by distraction rods because of the posterior element fracture as well as the anterior body fracture and instability.

Burst Fractures of L2 and L3. Such fractures are treated in a manner similar to that for the previously described injury, but require contoured, square-ended distraction rods to achieve adequate reduction and stability and to preserve the normal lumbar lordosis.

Fractures of L4 and L5. Such fractures are rare, frequently displaced but usually quite stable, and difficult to reduce by currently available techniques. These fractures are best treated by bed rest until healing occurs. If late instability ensues, bilateral lateral intertransverse process fusion to the sacrum provides the needed stability.

Operating Techniques

Posterior Internal Fixation and Stabilization

The posterior approach is accomplished through a straight midline incision extending from one vertebra above the proposed instrumentation to one vertebra below the level to be instrumented. In the typical T12-L1 fracture-dislocation, the rods should extend from two levels above the disrupted level (under the inferior facets of T10) to two levels below the disrupted level (under the superior laminae of L3). If the spine will be fused the length of the rods, the muscles are elevated carefully by subperiosteal dissection out to the edges of the facet joints and extending lateral to the tips of the transverse processes. The interspinous ligaments and facet capsules are removed carefully. The superior hook site on the left is prepared by resecting the inferior 50% of the inferior facet joint of T10 and by sliding a sharp hook into the facet joint and cutting a notch into the inferior aspect of the pedicle of T10. A dull hook then is impacted firmly against the inferior facet joint into the pedicle. The inferior hook site under the superior laminae of L3 is prepared by removing the ligamentum flavum from the interlaminar space, removing part of the inferior surface of the L2 laminae to facilitate insertion of the hook under the intact superior rim of the L3 laminae. As little as possible of the superior aspect of the L3 laminae should be removed to establish a firm, flat hook site while maintaining the cortical integrity of the lamina. The outrigger then is placed into the hooks to provide some stabilization without overdistraction. The right side of the posterior elements of T10 through L3 then is approached and carefully decorticated with a rongeur and air drill. A sharp spinal gouge may be used to decorticate the spinous processes; however, one must be careful when using a gouge and mallet on the unstable laminae over the injured area of the spinal cord and cauda equina. The cartilaginous facet-joint surfaces are removed with a sharp osteotome. When the laminae are decorticated and the transverse processes are exposed, the hook sites are prepared on the right side in a manner similar to that for the left side. A Harrington distraction rod is placed into the hooks on the right side to provide three-point fixation, effect reduction, and provide stability. The outrigger then is removed from the left side. The left posterior elements are decorticated in a similar fashion, and a straight distraction rod is placed on the left side of the posterior elements into the superior and inferior hooks. Strips of autogenous iliac-crest bone graft then are applied over the decorticated laminae medial and lateral to the Harrington rod out over the transverse processes. The wound is closed over suction drainage.[5]

The long rod/short fusion technique is employed for patients who are not paraplegic and in whom maximum spinal flexibility is desired following healing of the fracture. In this technique, long rods are connected to hooks placed three levels above the fracture-dislocation level to three levels below. The approach is a straight midline incision. The muscles are reflected laterally; however, the interspinous ligament is not removed, and the laminae and facet joints are not decorticated, except for the two contiguous vertebrae at the fracture site, i.e., T12 and L1 in most instances. After subperiosteal exposure of the muscles on the left side, the hooks and outrigger are placed into the inferior facet and pedicle of the third vetebra above the disrupted level (T9) and the third vertebra below the disrupted level (L4). The spinous processes of T12 and L1 then are removed and cut to be used as bone graft. The lateral laminae, rib, and transverse processes on the right of T12 and L1 are decorticated with a very sharp gouge or rongeur and air drill. The upper laminae of T9, T10, and T11 above the fracture and the lower laminae of L2, L3, and L4 below the fracture, as well as the transverse processes, are not exposed or decorticated. A long rod then is inserted on the right side from T9 to L4. The outrigger is removed from the left side, and the dorsal elements are treated in a similar manner with decortication of T12-L1 spinous processes and laminae and transverse processes. This step is followed by insertion of a long rod on the left side. The fragments of the removed spinous processes are then used as local bone grafts. No additional autogenous or homologous grafts are used. The patients develop a one-level fusion at the fracture site, and arrangements should be made to remove the rods at approximately 1 year after injury, or sooner if they become loose or fracture.

Surgical Technique for Use of the Short Compression Rods

If the dislocation of the posterior elements can be reduced and there is no significant posterior fracture or if there is a transverse split fracture of the spinous processes, as frequently occurs with seat belt injuries in which the fracture traverses the pedicles and vertebral body without posterior or anterior comminution or displacement, a short compression rod is placed in the following manner to stabilize the unstable segment. The ligamentum flavum is removed with a sharp, small, curved curette above the upper laminae and below the lower laminae of the vertebra to be stabilized. A previously assembled, short, small compression rod with compression hooks and nuts on both ends is placed beneath the laminae on each side of the spinous process and gradually is tightened until the fractured spinous process, or the dislocated facets are reduced to the desired position. Knodt rods can be used by reversing the distraction hooks to the compression position. Compression then is facilitated by turning the one nut in the center of the Knodt rod.

Postoperative Management

Following the posterior stabilization, the closure of the wound, and the application of sterile dressings, the patient is transferred to a regular hospital bed. He is logrolled from side to side every 2 hours. At 24 to 48 hours, the suction drain is removed. At 10 days, the dressings and sutures are removed and the patient is placed in a plaster body cast. If the patient has no neurologic loss, walking can resume. As soon as the patient is walking safely, he can be discharged and followed as an outpatient. If the patient has a neurologic deficit and cannot walk, the plaster jacket is bivalved to be used only when the patient is in the upright position. The jacket must be removed when the patient is in bed to prevent the formation of pressure ulcers over the bony prominences under the plaster cast. The patient is allowed to be upright in a wheelchair in the plaster cast and can begin transfer activities and wheelchair propulsion. Torso-twisting activities and floor-to-chair and chair-to-bed transfers are not practiced until 6 weeks after surgery. The plaster cast is worn for 8 weeks, at which time the patient begins to increase the exercises, and the cast is discontinued gradually. At 10 weeks, the cast is no longer used; at 12 weeks, the patient usually is independent in function in the wheelchair and arrangements can be made to follow the patient as an outpatient for continued rehabilitation.

In patients who have undergone a short rod/full length fusion procedure, no arrangements are made to remove the rods unless they become loose or fracture. In patients who have undergone a long rod/short fusion procedure, arrangements are made to remove the rods at approximately 1 year after surgery to regain maximum spinal mobility after the fracture has healed.

Anterior Approach to the Thoracolumbar Spine

The anterior approach to the thoracic spine, down to and including L1, is achieved by a standard thoracotomy, preferably through the left side of the chest through the bed of the tenth rib. This incision provides adequate visualization of the lower half of the thoracic vertebra and first lumbar vertebra. The posterior parietal pleura is split carefully, and the segmental vessels traversing the spine of each vertebral level are identified and divided between ligatures or hemostatic clips. The periosteum of the vertebral body and the annulus of the disc then can be elevated subperiosteally to expose the vertebral bodies and disc space. The fractured area is identified, and the comminuted vertebral-body fractured elements, as well as the injured discs above or below the fractured vertebra, are removed with ronguers and gouges. The debridement is carried down to the dura that is exposed, and any bone or disc fragments compressing the dural tube anteriorly then can be removed under direct vision. Replacement bone graft is then fashioned from the fibula or iliac crest to replace the vertebral body (Fig. 15-12). This graft is reinforced with sections of the ribs removed for the thoracotomy. The parietal pleura then is closed over the bone graft site, and the chest is closed with chest-tube drainage for 48 hours.

The lumbar spine from L1 through L4 is exposed through a lateral flank approach similar to the approach for a sympathectomy or nephrectomy. The segmental vessels are identified again and divided between ligatures or hemostatic clips. The fracture vertebral body fragments and disc fragments can be removed under direct vision and the vertebral body replaced with a bone graft fashioned from the fibula or iliac crest. These wounds are closed over suction drainage for 24 to 48 hours.

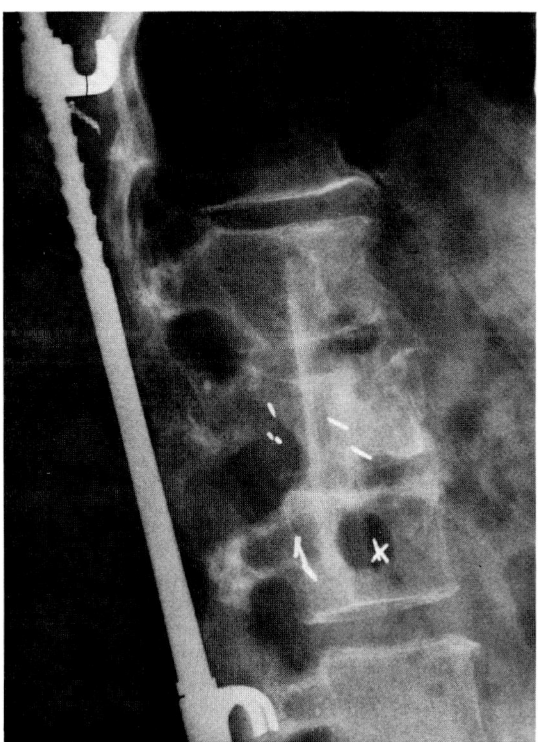

Fig. 15-12. Lateral roentgenogram of second-stage posterior distraction rodding followed by anterior debridement and fibular strut graft.

Anterior Approach to Fractures of L1

Fractures of the L1 vertebra at the thoracolumbar junction often require a combined thoracoabdominal approach to provide adequate visualization of the L1 vertebra and exposure for adequate bone grafting from T12 to L2. This approach is similar to the Dwyer approach to the anterior vertebral bodies and consists of thoracotomy combined with a division of the diaphragm and retroperitoneal abdominal approach. Through this approach, the lower thoracic and upper abdominal vertebrae can be exposed. Upon closure of this incision, suction drainage tubes are left in the retroperitoneal space and chest tubes are left in the chest for 24 to 48 hours. The patient is treated with bed rest for 10 days, after which the sutures are removed and an appropriate body jacket is applied for mobilization to the upright position, either walking or using a wheelchair, depending on the neurologic status of the patient.

Operative Complications

The following complications may ensue during the surgical procedure.

1. Cardiac arrest. Patients with paraplegia may suffer sudden cardiac arrest associated with the use of succinylcholine as an anesthetic muscle relaxant. Therefore, succinylcholine should not be used in the patient with a spinal cord injury. The patient also may suffer sudden cardiac arrest with sudden change of position from bed to the operating table while anesthetized. Therefore, patients with spinal cord injuries must be moved gently and slowly.
2. Facet fracture. Improper laminae, facet, and pedicle preparation may cause fracture of the facet and laminae during reduction and distraction. This complication requires extension of the hook site one level higher.
3. Improper placement of a hook under a rib instead of the facet and inter-rib penetration with a currette or gouge. Such situations may cause a pneumothorax at the time of surgery.
4. Inadequate reduction. A lateral roentgenogram should be taken prior to closure of the wound to verify adequate reduction and rod length. A rodding that is too short or instrumenta-

tion at wrong levels leads to loss of reduction during the postoperative period.

5. Increased neurologic deficit. The placement of the reduction and internal fixation device must be done without adding further trauma to the spine. Increased neurologic deficit and loss of nerve-root-level function have been reported to occur during the procedure. If the patient has voluntary control of his lower extremities, a "wake-up test" should be performed after rods are placed and the reduction is accomplished. Spinal cord monitoring with somatosensory-evoked potentials, if available, is valuable to detect any changes of cauda equina or spinal cord function during the surgical procedure.

Postoperative Complications

The following complications may occur during the postoperative period.

1. Wound infections. Wound infection is rare with posterior spinal surgery, and the spine tolerates infection better than do most bones. When infection does occur, the wound should be opened, irrigated, packed loosely with moist gauze, and allowed to granulate with the rods in place. Secondary closure can be accomplished in 5 to 7 days if the wound is sufficiently clean and there is no sign of sepsis.

2. Postoperative loss of correction. If the levels selected are not accurate, early mobilization may lead to loss of reduction. Early torso-bending activities also may lead to displacement of the upper hook sites.

3. Thrombophlebitis. One must be aware that thrombophlebitis is common in paraplegic patients. Early range of motion of lower extremities is recommended, and the patient must be observed for signs of thrombophlebitis during the early mobilization period.

4. Pressure sores. Pressure sores may occur under plaster jackets or braces if the skin under the cast is not observed carefully every day with a flashlight.

The intraoperative or postoperative complications most frequently seen are due to lack of adequate surgical planning, lack of understanding of the principles of internal fixation, or technical errors made during the surgical procedure.

Results

There has been a great wave of enthusiasm for operative management of fractures and fracture-dislocations of the thoracolumbar spine in recent years. For surgical treatment to be a valid option, the results must be demonstrated to provide better overall patient care than the documented results of the traditional nonoperative techniques. Most authors agree that properly selected patients treated with open reduction and internal fixation can benefit by early mobilization, rapid progression to sitting upright and standing, and ambulatory function. The general physiologic complications that often accompany forced bed rest in the paraplegic patient (i.e., pressure sores, muscle atrophy, psychologic deterioration, urinary tract deterioration, and osteoporosis) are decreased by establishing spinal stability and early mobilization. Although some authors indicate that their early experience suggests better neurologic recovery, their findings have not been statistically documented as yet. The physician must weigh the advantages of the documented results of the nonoperative and operative care versus the potential complications of the nonoperative and operative methods of care before the most beneficial recommendations regarding treatment plans can be made to the patient.

References

1. Guttmann, L.: Spinal deformities in traumatic paraplegics and tetraplegics following surgical procedures. Paraplegia, *7*:38, 1969.
2. Frankel, H. L., et al.: The value of postural reduction in the initial management of closed injuries of the spine with paraplegia and tetraplegia. Paraplegia, *7*:179, 1969.
3. Bedbrook, G. M.: Treatment of thoracolumbar dislocation and fractures with paraplegia. Clin. Orthop., *112*:27, 1975.
4. Osebold, W. R., et al.: Thoracolumbar spine fractures: results of treatment. Spine, *6*:13, 1981.
5. Dickson, H., Harrington, P. R., and Erwin, W. D.: Results of reduction and stabilization of the severely fractured thoracic and lumbar spine. J. Bone Joint Surg., *60A*:799, 1978.
6. Bradford, D. S., Akbarnia, B. A., Winter, B., and Seljeskog, E. L.: Surgical stabilization of fracture and fracture-dislocations of the thoracic spine. Spine, *2*:185, 1977.
7. Jacobs, R. R., et al.: Thoracolumbar spinal injuries, a comparative study of recumbent and operative treatment in 100 patients. Spine, *5*:463, 1980.
8. Chance, G. Q.: Note on a type of flexion fracture of the spine. Br. J. Radiol., *21*:452, 1948.

Chapter 16 Fracture-Dislocations of the Cervical Spine

ROBERT W. BUCHOLZ

The human cervical spine permits a wide range of motion in all planes. As a supporting structure, it is situated between the relatively fixed thoracic spine and the large, free weight of the head. These two factors, hypermobility and precarious location, account for the vulnerability of the cervical spine to indirect injury from high-energy accidents.

While the exact incidence of cervical spine injuries in multiply injured patients has not been well documented, their frequency of occurrence in multiple-trauma fatalities has been studied. Nearly one fourth of all persons who die from polytrauma have cervical fractures or dislocations.[1] The pattern of injury differs from clinical cases. Approximately 80% of fatal injuries occur between the occiput and the axis, and many are associated with brainstem or high cervical-cord lesions incompatible with survival. Atlanto-occipital dislocation is the most common fatal injury and is rarely seen in the surviving polytrauma patient. Other injury patterns, such as bilateral pedicle fractures of the axis and odontoid fractures, are frequently found in both fatal and nonfatal cases. The majority of clinically treated cervical spine fractures, however, are located below the axis.

These statistics attest to the need for thorough evaluation of every polytrauma patient for possible osseous and ligamentous injury to the spine. A cervical spine injury should be presumed in all multiply injured patients until proved otherwise.

Emergency Management

The cervical spine and spinal cord must be protected before and during all initial diagnostic and therapeutic measures. A 10% incidence of worsening of the neurologic status of patients with a cervical fracture subsequent to the time of injury was detected by Rogers.[2] Proper training of emergency medical technicians and emergency room personnel is crucial to avoid this dire complication. Strict immobilization of the head and neck in a neutral position during all maneuvering of the patient usually is sufficient. Cervical traction without knowledge of the injury pattern can be harmful.

Following resuscitation of the polytrauma patient, a detailed effort to elicit any symptoms or signs of cervical spine injury is imperative. If the patient is alert, a history of neck pain, transient neurologic symptoms, or pre-existing spinal problems should be sought. The head and neck are inspected for evidence of external injury, and the neck is palpated gently anteriorly and posteriorly for point tenderness. The preliminary neurologic examination to detect spinal cord and nerve root injury should include sensory and motor testing. Pinprick testing of all dermatomes from C2 to T1 provides a presumptive diagnosis of the level of a spinal cord injury. Light touch, deep pressure, vibratory sense, and proprioception of the lower extremities then should be checked. Systematic motor testing confirms the probable level of injury. Checking rectal tone, voluntary sphincter control, and the bulbocavernosus reflex is especially important when spinal cord injury is suspected. Until spinal shock has resolved, diagnosis of a complete neurologic lesion is impossible. In the patient with an apparently complete spinal cord injury, special attention to long-toe flexor function and perianal sensation is necessary. Presence of either of these two findings implies an incomplete cord lesion and significantly better prognosis than that of a complete cord injury.

A cross-table lateral radiograph of the cervical spine should be taken in all polytraumatized patients. If the head and neck are not in neutral position, radiographic interpretation can be difficult. Adequate visualization of the spine from the occiput to the inferior vertebral end-plate of C7 is essential. Manual traction on both arms at the time of radiography, or requisition of a "swimmer's" view, may be required to expose adequately the entire cervical spine in patients with short necks (Fig. 16-1). Segmental spinal injuries are common, and radiographic evaluation should not be terminated after documentation of what is assumed to be an isolated upper cervical spine injury until the remainder of the spine is visualized.

In most multiple-trauma patients with no history of neck complaints, no significant physical findings, and a normal state of consciousness, a normal lateral radiograph is adequate evaluation. Further radiographic examination is indicated if there is any complaint of neck pain, point tenderness over the spine, or any questionable neurologic deficit. A full cervical-spine series includes lateral, anteroposterior, right and left oblique, and open-mouth odontoid views. Even if these are interpreted as normal, a high index of clinical suspicion demands that flexion-extension lateral views be obtained to rule out an occult ligamentous injury. The prerequisites for flexion-extension views are absolute. They include (1) the absence of any demonstrable neurologic deficit, (2) the absence of an altered state of consciousness, including intoxication, and (3) the ability of the patient to flex and extend his neck actively without assistance. Passive flexion and extension of the neck by the technician or physician are contraindicated. The physician should be present at the time of radiography to ensure that the views are taken properly and that the patient is monitored adequately during the procedure.

In patients with clearly unstable lesions on lateral radiograph, the cervical spine should be sta-

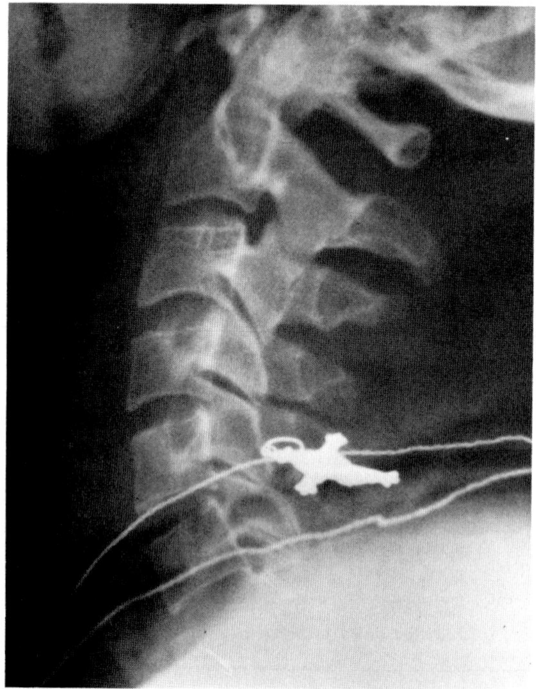

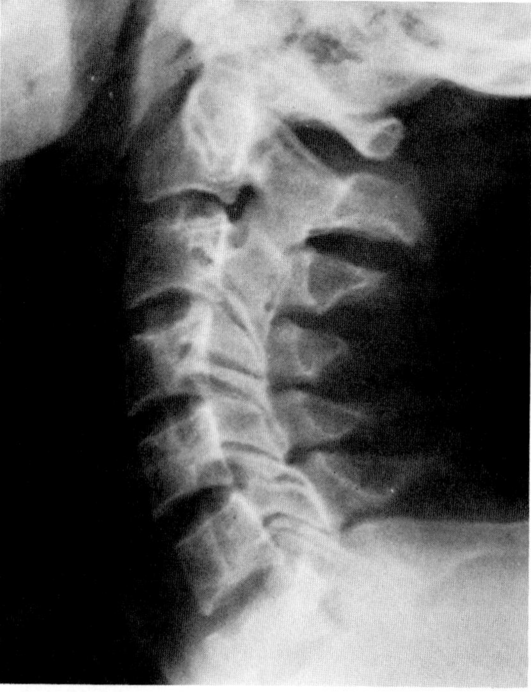

Fig. 16-1. *A*, Standard lateral radiograph of the cervical spine permitted visualization of the spine only to C6. *B*, Compression fracture of the C7 body was detected after traction on the shoulders.

bilized with skull traction, cervical orthosis, or both prior to further radiographic examination. Application of a soft collar alone, especially in the uncooperative patient, is not sufficient. The unconscious patient must be treated with special care. Loss of the normal protective reflex in such patients increases the possibility of displacement of the unstable spinal injury.

Once these initial radiographs are obtained in the emergency department, a decision must be made as to the best way to proceed with the evaluation of the cervical spine.

Diagnostic Evaluation

Plain Radiographs

Familiarity with normal variants can avert overtreatment of incorrectly suspected injuries. The resultant savings to the patient in terms of cost and discomfort can be significant. On the other hand, familiarity with the subtle radiographic signs of occult injury can minimize the chance of missing a potentially serious spinal injury.

There are several common pitfalls in the interpretation of the lateral radiograph. The importance of the loss of the normal cervical lordosis has been overemphasized. A straightening or reversal of the cervical curve can be secondary to the position of the head in a military, chin-down posture or to spasm of the cervical musculature.

The width of the prevertebral soft-tissue shadow is a good indirect indicator of cervical spine injury. A localized increase in the width of the shadow may signify the presence of a fracture or ligamentous injury involving the anterior elements of the spine (Fig. 16-2). The shadow normally is 5 mm or less in anteroposterior breadth from the occiput to C4.[3] Its width increases below C4 and may be quite variable. In children, the soft-tissue shadow may be wider, especially if the child was crying at the time of radiography.

Minor degrees of horizontal translation of one vertebral body on an adjacent vertebra frequently can be seen in the normal cervical spine. This anteroposterior displacement commonly involves multiple segments of the cervical spine, but is usually greatest at the C2-C3 interspace. It corrects on flexion-extension views. Similarly, there may be minor variations in the height of the vertebral bodies from one level to the next. These variants should not be misinterpreted as compression fractures of the vertebra. Differences in the relative heights of the intervertebral discs are also common, especially in the elderly patient.

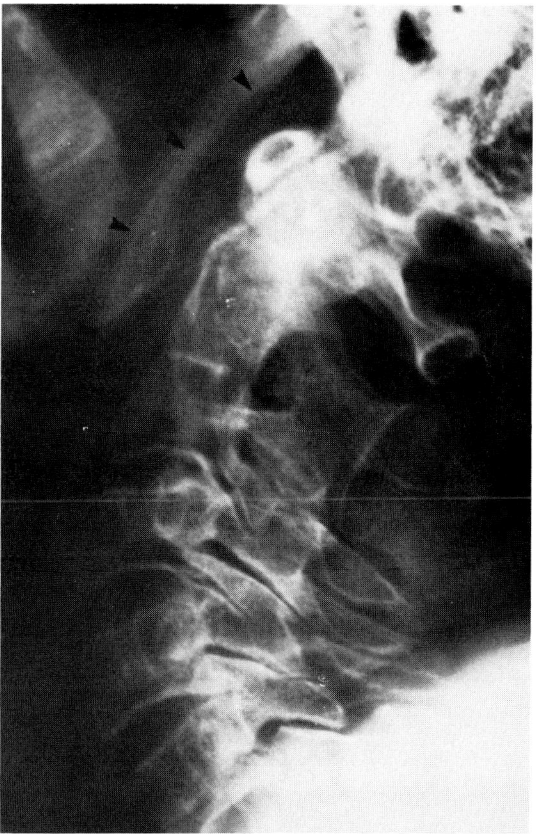

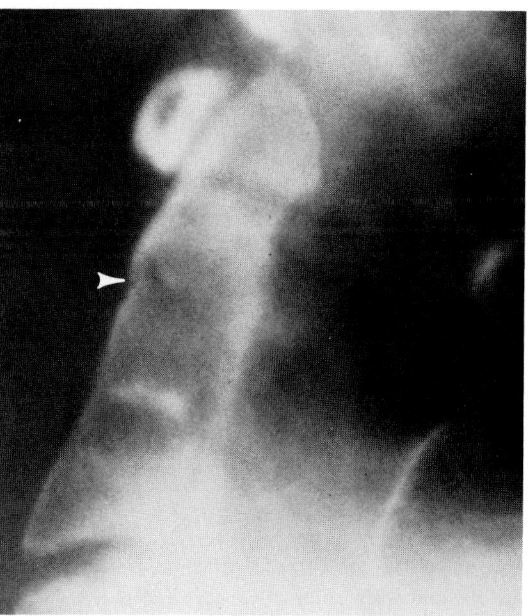

Fig. 16-2. *A*, Localized increase in the width of the prevertebral shadow anterior to a congenitally fused axis and C3 (arrows). No obvious fracture is evident. *B*, Tomography revealed a minimally displaced odontoid fracture (arrow).

Evaluation of the pediatric cervical spine is fraught with many potential radiographic traps. Pseudosubluxation of the upper cervical spine involving mainly the C2-C3 and C3-C4 levels is a frequent normal variant. Under the age of 8 years, half of all children demonstrate some degree of pseudosubluxation on flexion lateral radiographs of the cervical spine.[4] The anterior ring of the atlas similarly may appear to be riding extremely high on the odontoid. This finding is most apparent on an extension view. The distance from the anterior ring of the atlas to the odontoid is greater in children than in adults because of the thicker cartilaginous surface of these structures in children. This distance, which is important in the diagnosis of transverse and alar ligament disruptions, can be increased markedly if the head is rotated at the time of lateral radiography. The normal C1-odontoid distance in children is 4 mm or less.

The multiple synchondroses and secondary centers of ossification also make interpretation of pediatric radiographs perplexing. There also may be absence of uniform angulation between adjacent vertebrae when the neck is in a flexed posture. Knowledge of the spectrum of normal pediatric variants minimizes any overreading of the cervical spine radiographs in children.

Frequent errors also occur in the reading of other radiographic views. The mouth must be opened sufficiently wide on the open-mouth odontoid view to avoid overlapping of the teeth and facial bones. Misinterpretation of the shadows of the facial bones as fracture lines is common. The head must be in a neutral position. Slight rotation to either side results in asymmetry of the lateral masses of the atlas of a normal spine. On oblique radiographs, deviation of the beam from the standard 45° can result in misleading radiographic changes. Individual foramina may appear abnormally narrow, and the apophyseal joints are not clearly visualized. The anteroposterior radiograph generally is the least valuable view, though it allows identification of vertical fractures of the bodies and the lateral masses.

Tomography

Plain radiographs are often technically suboptimal in the multiply injured patient. The need for tomography hinges on the adequacy of the routine views. Although tomographic evaluation of the cervical spine is excellent for delineating the pathologic anatomy of the osseous injury, it aids little in determining any compromise to spinal stability. Specific indications for cervical tomography include (1) suspicious radiographs but no definite evidence of fracture, (2) neurologic deficit without any apparent fracture, and (3) inability to visualize adequately the lower cervical spine by standard techniques.

Tomography is generally more helpful in evaluating lower cervical spine injuries and is more likely to influence therapeutic decisions for injuries in this area. Maravilla and associates reviewed 79 patients with spinal injury studied by plain radiographs followed by tomography.[5] Of these patients, 18% had significant alterations in their treatment plans based on their tomographic findings. Only 41% of all fractures were seen on the plain radiographs. Tomography is particularly useful in patients with unilateral locked facets. Articular fractures of the facets can be evaluated and their size used to anticipate the ease or difficulty in securing a reduction of the joint. Upper cervical spine injuries infrequently necessitate tomography.

Tomography as an adjunctive study is indicated most commonly in the polytrauma patient, the patient with an altered mental status, and in patients in whom flexion-extension views are not feasible. If any doubt exists as to the full extent of a cervical spine injury, tomography can be a safe and useful procedure (Fig. 16-3).

Flexion-Extension Radiographs

In the neurologically intact patient with a cervical spine fracture, treatment decisions are based largely on an assessment of the effect of the injury on spinal stability. A cervical spine is rendered unstable following an injury if there has been sufficient osseous or ligamentous disruption to cause damage to the spinal cord or cervical nerve roots when under physiologic loads. This is a qualitative definition. Attempts to quantitate spinal stability have necessarily had to center on various experimental models. The study of the cadaver spine performed by White and associates concluded with the following criteria of instability.[6]

1. When either all the anterior elements or all the posterior elements are destroyed or unable to function.

2. When more than 3.5 mm of horizontal displacement of one vertebra is present in relation to an adjacent vertebra, anteriorly or posteriorly, measured on resting lateral or flexion-extension roentgenograms of the spine (Fig. 16-4).

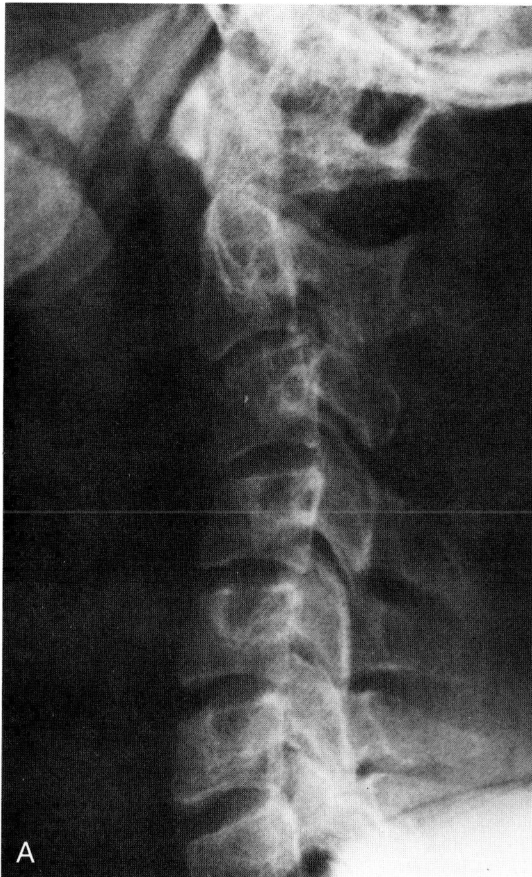

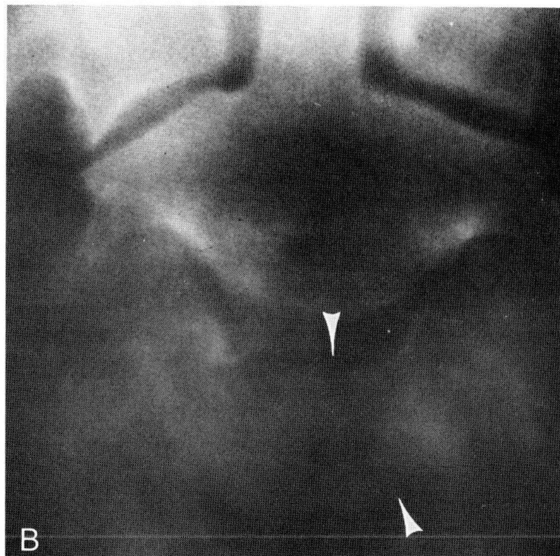

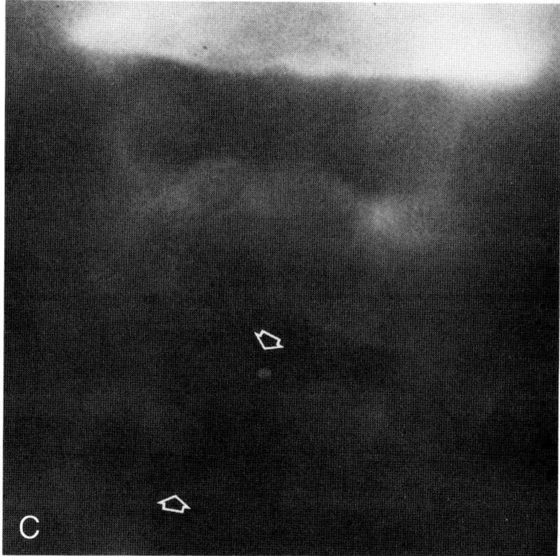

Fig. 16-3. *A*, Lateral cervical radiograph showing sharp reversal of normal cervical curvature at the C3-C4 segment, but no clearly delineated fracture lines. *B*, Anterior tomographic cut demonstrates a vertical fracture of the C3 body (arrows). *C*, Posterior tomographic cut reveals a comminuted C3 laminar fracture extending into the right facet (arrows).

3. When more than 11° of angulatory difference exists when compared with that of either adjacent vertebra, measured on a resting lateral or flexion-extension roentgenogram (Fig. 16-5).

These criteria apply only to the cervical spine segments below C3. Their application to any specific clinical case should be done with caution, but in general terms, they provide reasonable objective measures for spinal stability.

Evaluation of spinal stability demands a dynamic study of spinal motion. Neither plain radiographs nor tomography provide such information. Unless there is gross displacement of a spinal segment on the resting lateral radiograph, which is diagnostic of instability, flexion-extension radiographs are indispensable. As mentioned previously, there are multiple prerequisites for procuring such views. Technically superior radiographs are obtained when the patient is standing or sitting erect during the flexion and extension of the neck. The presence of a supervising physician during the radiography is desirable. Flexion-extension lateral radiographs are particularly useful in detecting occult posterior ligamentous disruptions. On the flexion view, accurate assessment of the status of the interspinous and capsular ligaments is ordinarily possible (Fig. 16-6). The anterior cervical spine in children is largely cartilagenous, and thus, flexion-extension views similarly may be essential for eliciting otherwise subtle lesions.

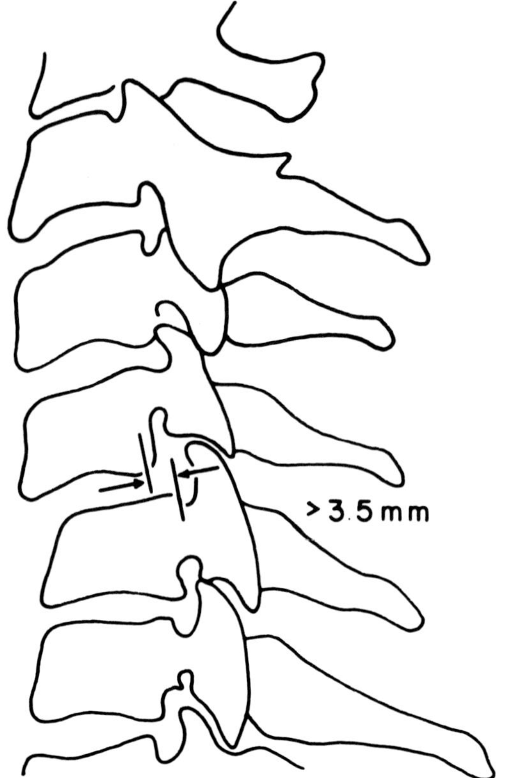

Fig. 16-4. Spine instability is suggested when horizontal translation is greater than 3.5 mm. (From White, A., Johnson, R., Panjabi, M., and Southwick, W.: Biomechanical analysis of clinical stability in the cervical spine. Clin. Orthop., *109*:85, 1975.)

The major limitation of such radiographs is the inability to obtain an adequate study. Muscular spasm may restrict active cervical motion sufficiently to cause a false-negative result. If any doubt exists as to the adequacy of the views, rigid immobilization of the neck for several weeks is the best method of treatment. As soon as the spasm has subsided, the radiographs should be repeated.

Myelography

The primary indication for cervical myelography following spinal injury is in patients in whom the neurologic deficit is more profound than would be expected by the apparent osseous and ligamentous disruption. Localized discal compression of the cord occasionally can be diagnosed. Myelography has much more limited use in cervical subluxations or dislocations with either partial or complete neurologic loss. Differentiation of cord hemorrhage and edema from possible cord compression by osseous or discal tissue is difficult. The principal disadvantages of myelography include the risks of positioning a patient for the study and the misleading results causing unwarranted surgical "decompression" of an acute injury.

Computer Assisted Tomography

The ultimate role of computer assisted tomography in the evaluation of acute spinal injuries has not yet been defined. This study provides an excellent three-dimensional view of the vertebral canal, but its potential superiority over plain radiographs and regular tomography in analyzing spinal fractures has not been proved. In the upper cervical spine, computer assisted tomography is useful in diagnosing atlantal ring fractures and atlantoaxial rotatory subluxation (Fig. 16-7). Neural arch and facet fractures in the lower cervical spine can be outlined exactly. Computer assisted tomography also is helpful in studying the size and shape of the vertebral canal, any osseous fragments and foreign bodies within the canal, the paravertebral soft-tissue structures, and the cervicothoracic junction.

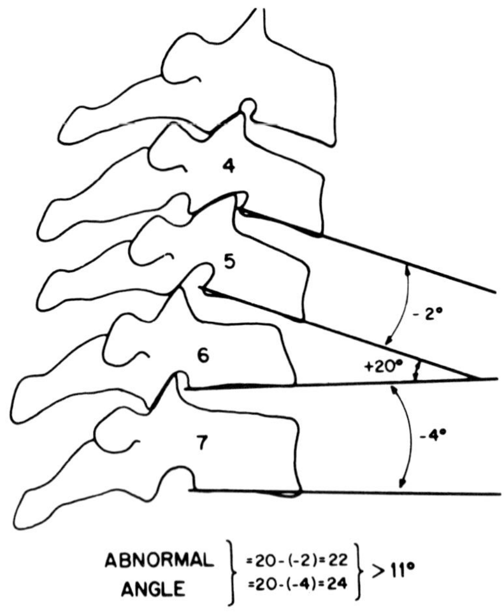

Fig. 16-5. Angulatory displacement of a spinal segment of greater than 11° when compared to adjacent segments also implies spinal instability. (From White, A., Johnson, R., Panjabi, M., and Southwick, W.: Biomechanical analysis of clinical stability in the cervical spine. Clin. Orthop., *109*:85, 1975.)

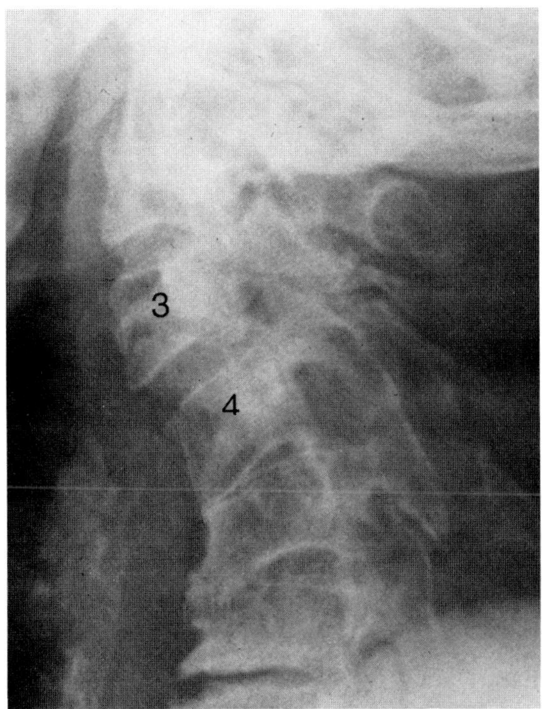

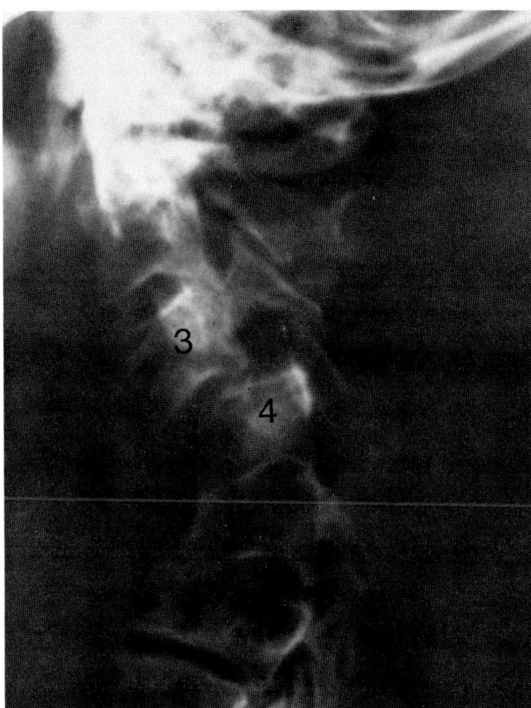

FIG. 16-6. *A*, A C3-C4 fracture in an elderly patient with pre-existing cervical spondylosis. Initial displacement of C3 on C4 is minimal. *B*, Flexion lateral radiograph documents marked horizontal translation of the C3 body on C4, thus implying severe posterior ligamentous and osseous injury.

Patterns of Cervical Spine Injuries

Fractures of the Atlas

Fractures of the ring of the atlas are relatively uncommon in the polytrauma patient. Isolated fractures of the posterior ring are the most frequent pattern. These hyperextension injuries may be associated with bilateral pedicle fractures of the axis. Posterior ring injuries are stable lesions, and their treatment merely involves cervical immobilization for patient comfort.

Burst fractures of the atlas were first described in detail by Jefferson.[7] Simultaneous fractures both anterior and posterior to the lateral masses are caused by an axial load to the vertex of the skull. Because of the oblique inclination of the

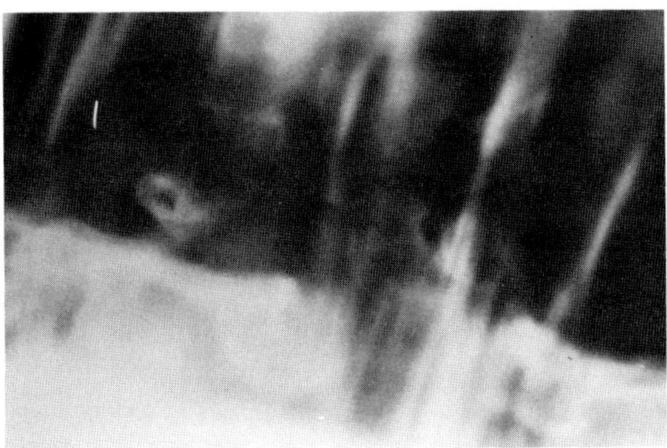

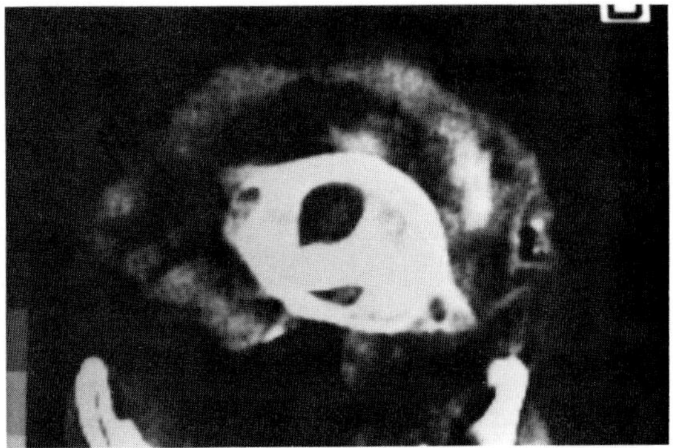

FIG. 16-7. *A*, Anteroposterior tomogram of a child with a post-traumatic fixed torticollis. *B*, Computer assisted tomography of the same child clearly demonstrates a fixed C1-C2 rotatory subluxation (Courtesy of Drs. Ono and Okada, Osaka University).

atlanto-occipital joint, the transmitted forces result in multiple fractures. The lateral masses of the atlas are displaced laterally in relation to the occiput and the axis. Jefferson fractures rarely are associated with any neurologic deficit because the vertebral canal is widened by the injury.

The diagnosis of a burst fracture of the atlas is impossible to make based on the lateral radiograph alone. Posterior ring fractures may be evident, but an open-mouth odontoid view is necessary to identify the entire injury. The lateral masses of the atlas are displaced bilaterally on the superior articulations of the axis (Fig. 16-8). Such bilateral displacement can occur only with both anterior and posterior fractures. Tomography and flexion-extension views are usually of no diagnostic value. The degree of displacement of the lateral masses must be measured to detect possible disruption of the transverse ligament. Experimental work suggests that a total spread of the masses of greater than 7 mm is indicative of a torn transverse ligament.[8]

The majority of atlantal burst fractures can be treated solely with external immobilization. A halo device or intermediate-class orthosis is sufficient, and the choice of immobilization depends largely on the patient and his associated injuries. In patients with wide spreading of the lateral masses, halo immobilization is required until the fracture is healed. At approximately 3 to 4 months, the patient must be evaluated for atlanto-axial instability. If atlanto-axial subluxation is present as a result of a torn or attenuated transverse ligament, posterior atlanto-axial arthrodesis is indicated. The fusion is simpler and less extensive if performed following healing of the atlantal fractures than if performed immediately after the injury.

Odontoid Fractures

The odontoid process or dens is the keystone to the stability of the mobile atlanto-axial articulation. Either a fracture of the odontoid or a rupture of the transverse ligament can result in potential

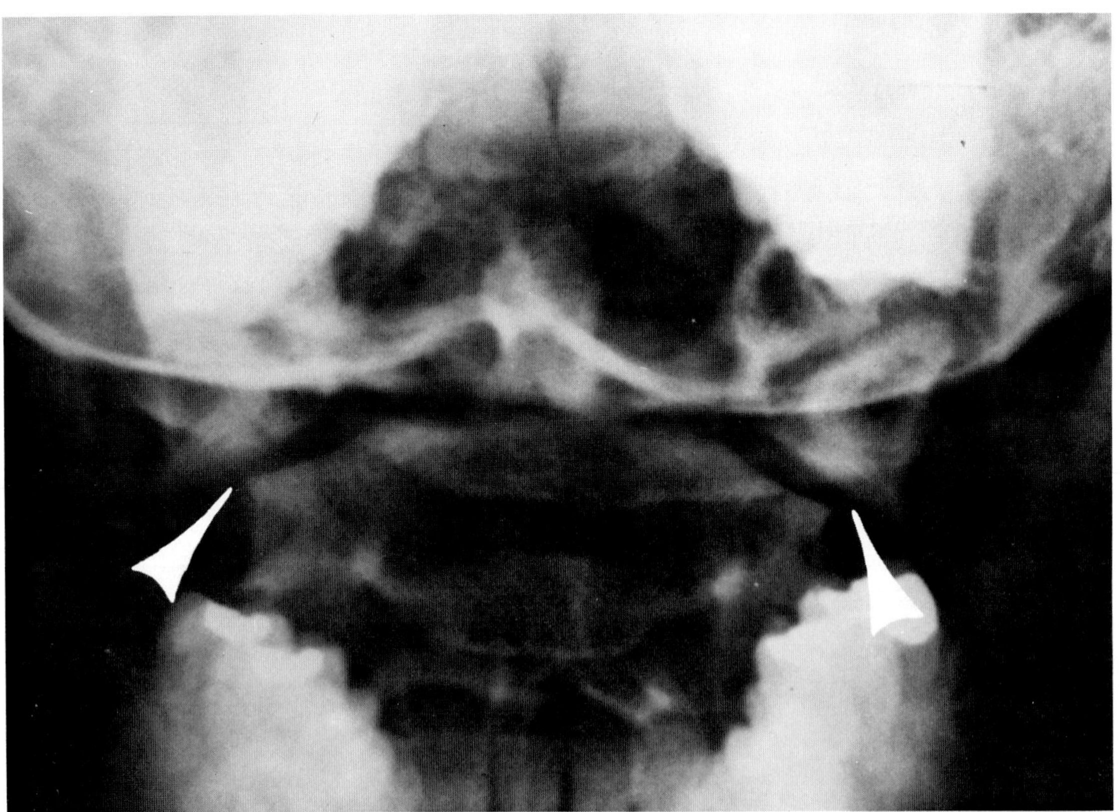

Fig. 16-8. Jefferson fracture shown on open-mouth odontoid radiograph. Arrows point to bilateral displacement of the lateral masses of the atlas.

instability. Most odontoid fractures are probably hyperflexion injuries, though shear forces occasionally may be involved. The vertebral canal is fortunately quite spacious at this level, and neurologic compromise rarely is encountered in clinical cases. Odontoid fractures, however, are also a common fatal pattern of injury.

Fractures of the odontoid are seen frequently in multiply injured patients. In a series of 49 odontoid fractures, Anderson and D'Alonzo reported 4 associated cervical spine fractures and 10 patients with extremity fractures.[9] Schatzker and associates noted a lower incidence of multiple trauma.[10]

Of the many classification schemes of odontoid fractures, that of Anderson and D'Alonzo seems to have the greatest prognostic significance. The rare type I fracture represents an avulsion fracture by the alar ligament off the tip of the odontoid process. It occurs above the level of the transverse ligament and, thus, does not compromise the stability of the articulation. The type II injury through the body or base of the odontoid is the most common pattern. The fracture is usually at the level of the superior articular surfaces of the axis. The fracture line of the type III injury passes into the cancellous bone of the body of the axis. The fracture is usually at the level of the superior articular surfaces of the axis. Displacement is normally less in the type III fractures than in the type II fractures.

The fracture site may be obscured on the lateral radiograph because of the overlapping shadows of the lateral masses of the atlas. An open-mouth odontoid view is, therefore, necessary for both the diagnosis and classification of the fracture. Flexion-extension views are not indicated, and tomography is useful only when there is a questionable fracture that cannot be defined on plain radiographs. The diagnostic radiographs should be of adequate quality to determine both the level of the fracture and its degree of displacement.

The type I fractures require a cervical orthosis for comfort only. Of the type III fractures, 90% unite with proper external immobilization. A halo jacket or vest provides the best rigid fixation. Controversy surrounds the treatment of the type II injuries.[11] A 20 to 60% nonunion rate can be expected with any form of external immobilization. For this reason, many authors recommend early atlanto-axial fusion (Fig. 16-9). The trade-offs of the treatments involve prolonged halo immobilization with a significant chance of nonunion versus the risks of surgery and loss of atlanto-axial motion with fusion. If early fusion is chosen, a posterior atlanto-axial arthrodesis is preferred.[12] Extension of the fusion to the occiput or C3 is not necessary unless there are other upper cervical spine fractures. Nonunion of the odontoid is an unacceptable clinical result because of the risk of reinjury and the possibility of developing a late myelopathy.

The occurrence of isolated transverse ligament ruptures is rare compared to that of odontoid fractures.[13] On the lateral radiograph, the diagnosis is made by measuring the distance between the anterior ring of the atlas and the anterior border of the odontoid (Fig. 16-10). A distance of greater than 3 mm in adults and 4 mm in children is suggestive of a ligamentous injury. Flexion-extension views help to confirm the presence of the lesion. In all well-documented cases, posterior atlanto-axial fusion is indicated because of the expectant poor healing of the ligament and the potential for chronic atlanto-axial instability.

Bilateral Pedicle Fractures of the Axis

Bilateral pedicle fractures of C2 also are referred to as traumatic spondylolisthesis of the axis and hangman's fracture. Most such injuries are secondary to hyperextension of the upper cervical spine with or without axial compression. With the superior articular processes of the axis located anteriorly and the inferior facets situated posteriorly, hyperextension forces are concentrated at the level of the pedicles. Bilateral pedicle fractures are a common clinical and fatal pattern.[1] A whole spectrum of injuries can occur, ranging from the isolated nondisplaced pedicle fractures to the fatal fracture-dislocation. The severity of the injury depends on the degree of associated soft-tissue disruption, specifically of the anterior longitudinal ligament, the C2-C3 disc, the posterior longitudinal ligament, and the posterior atlanto-axial membrane.

In their series of 29 bilateral pedicle fractures of the axis, Brashear and associates reported 4 segmental cervical spine injuries and 6 patients with major polytrauma.[14] Neurologic loss is encountered in less than 10% of clinical cases.

The simplest classification differentiates stable from unstable lesions. Stability implies minimal associated ligamentous and discal injury. With unstable injuries, there is sufficient soft-tissue disruption to cause displacement of the cervicocranium on the rest of the cervical spine under physiologic loads, resulting in neurologic damage

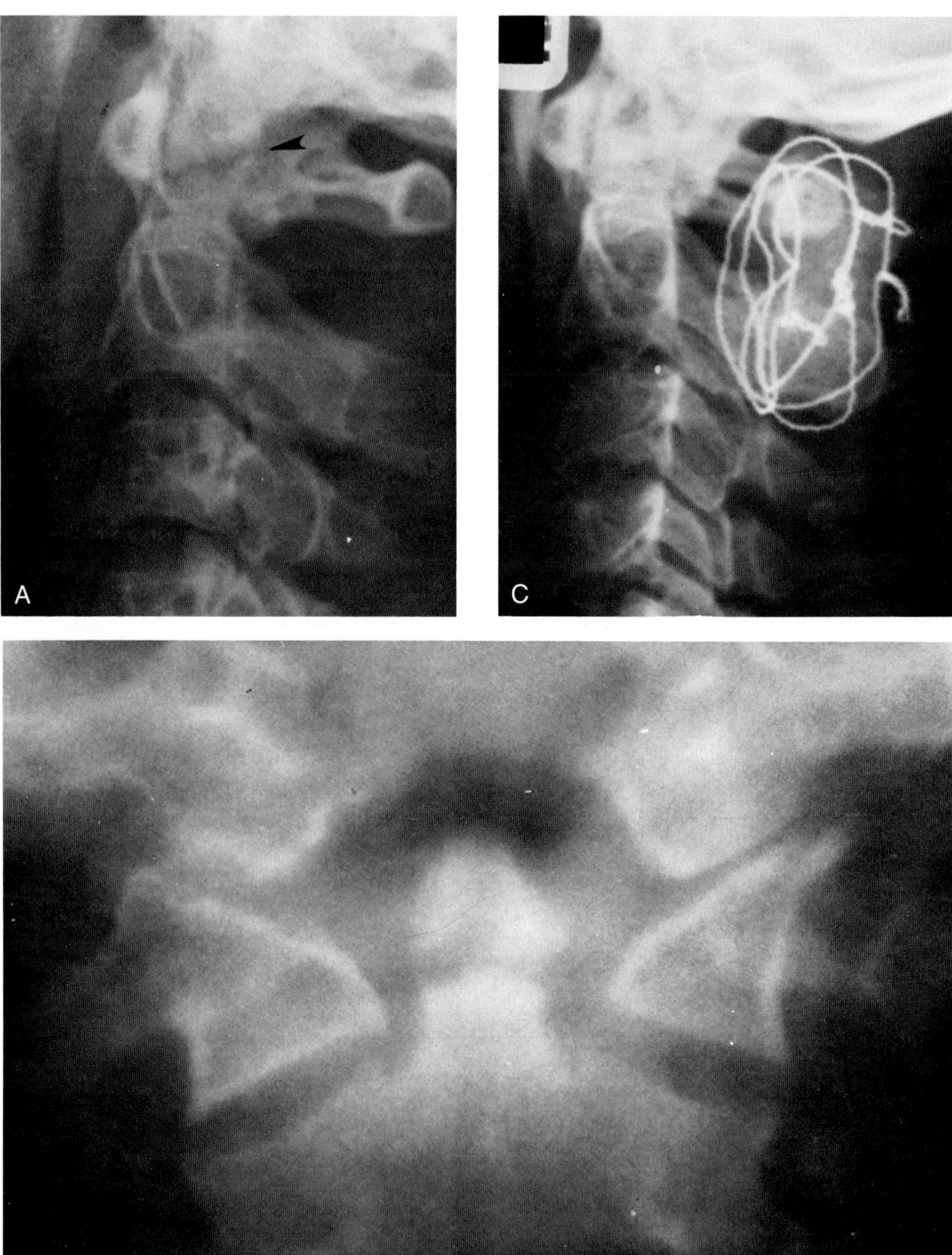

Fig. 16-9. *A*, Lateral radiograph of a polytrauma patient showing a minimally displaced odontoid fracture (arrow). *B*, Anteroposterior tomogram reveals that the fracture is a high type II variant. *C*, Because of a high probability of a nonunion of the fracture, a primary posterior atlantoaxial fusion was performed.

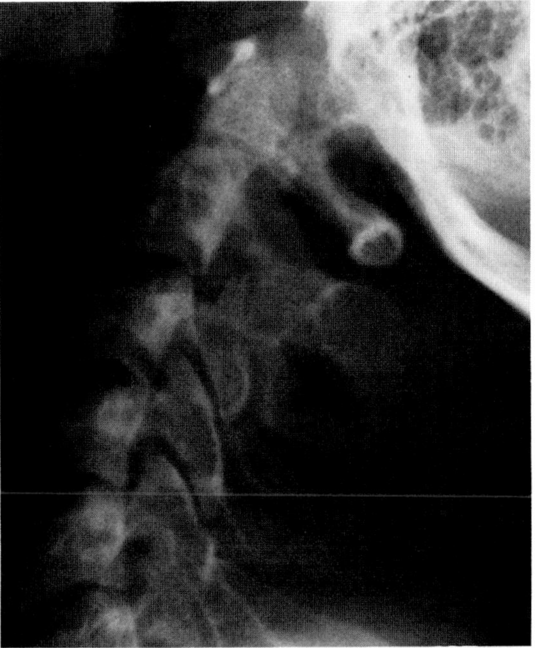

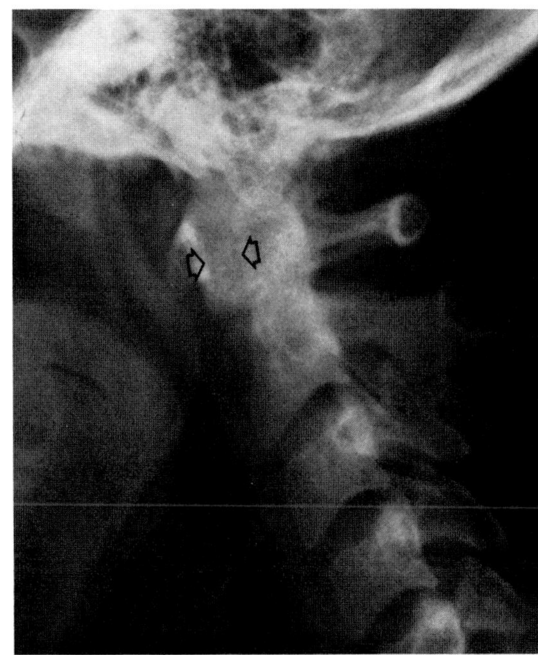

Fig. 16-10. *A*, Extension lateral radiograph of a patient who sustained a blow to the occiput. *B*, Flexion lateral radiograph of the same patient showing a 6-mm displacement of the C1 anterior ring on the odontoid (arrows). This degree of subluxation suggests a complete transverse ligament rupture.

(Fig. 16-11). No quantitative measure of stability of bilateral pedicle fractures of the axis exists.

The diagnosis is usually obvious on the lateral radiograph. If the neck is extended slightly at the time of radiography, however, the pedicle fracture lines may be subtle. Fractures with gross diastasis or angulation of the axis on C3 are assumed to be unstable and should be treated appropriately. Minimally displaced fractures may be stable or unstable. If the prerequisites for flexion-extension views are satisfied, these radiographs can be helpful in confirming the structural integrity of the supporting soft-tissue structures.

All bilateral pedicle fractures of the axis should be treated as unstable upper cervical spine injuries until proved otherwise. If a minimally displaced fracture is shown to be stable on adequate flexion-extension radiographs, treatment with an intermediate-class cervical orthosis, such as a Yale, SOMI, or four-poster brace, suffices. If a bilateral pedicle fracture demonstrates sufficient angulatory or translatory displacement to suggest complete soft-tissue disruption, traction or halo immobilization is imperative. If traction is elected, overdistraction of the fracture fragments must be avoided. Other variants of ring fractures of the axis, including fractures that extend into the C2-C3 facet, are occasionally sustained and are usually stable. The prognosis for union and full recovery of function following most bilateral pedicle fractures is excellent. In the series of Brashear and associates, all patients regained stability of the spine by healing of the fractures or spontaneous fusion between C3 and the axis. Surgical intervention is not warranted except in cases of established nonunion.

Flexion Injuries to the Lower Cervical Spine

Most fractures of the lower cervical spine are caused by a combination of forces in different planes of motion. Pure flexion injuries are of two types—wedge compression fracture of the vertebral body and posterior ligamentous disruption with or without a slice fracture off the vertebral body. The injury pattern depends on the location of the center of motion of the flexion force. Wedge compression fractures of a vertebral body are managed easily. Following confirmation of posterior ligamentous integrity by flexion-extension radiographs, treatment consists of short-term immobilization of the neck for comfort.

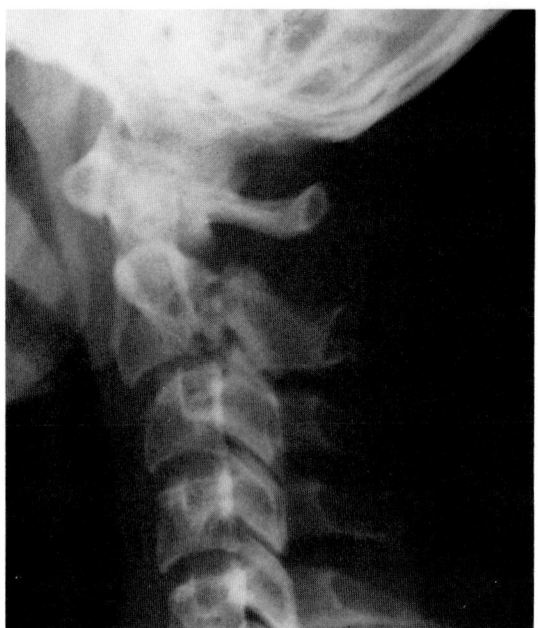

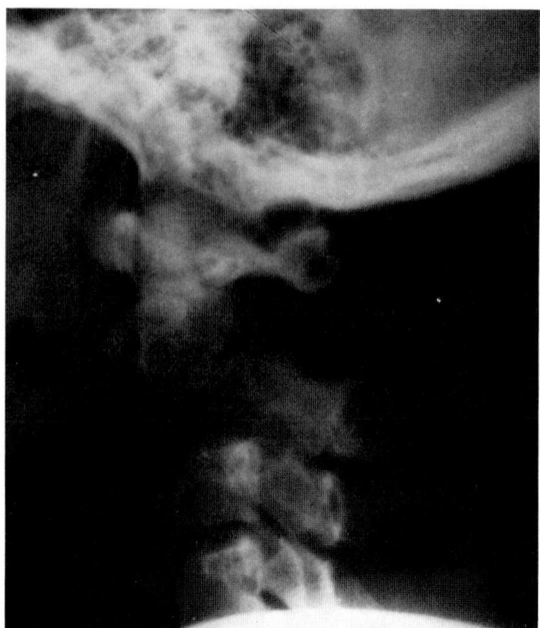

FIG. 16-11. Stable (*A*) and unstable (*B*) bilateral pedicle fractures of the axis.

Posterior ligamentous injuries represent more of a diagnostic and therapeutic challenge. Plain radiographs often are deceiving since the vertebral subluxation may be reduced with the neck in a neutral or extended position. If flexion-extension views are not performed, the patient is assumed to have no injury or a trivial avulsion fracture of the vertebral body. A satisfactory flexion radiograph demonstrates abnormal angulation at the vertebral segment, widening of the interspinous distance, and subluxation of the facets if the facet capsules and ligaments are torn. A comparison with adjacent spinal levels usually discloses the extent of the soft-tissue injury. The stability criteria of White and associates aid in the recognition of an unstable lesion.[6]

Cervical spine ligaments frequently do not regain their normal tensile strength following complete rupture. Late segmental instability may result. In the patient with documented complete posterior ligamentous disruption, posterior stabilization and fusion are therefore recommended. An interspinous wiring with autogenous bone graft of the type described by Rogers is preferred.[2] If surgery is contraindicated by other injuries or for unrelated reasons, maintenance of the cervical spine in a reduced position is mandatory to maximize the chance for adequate ligamentous healing.

Unilateral Locked Facet

Unilateral locked facet or unilateral rotatory subluxation is a frequently overlooked fracture pattern of the lower cervical spine. The C5-C6 and C6-C7 levels are the most common sites of injury. The mechanism of injury is simultaneous flexion and rotation resulting in primarily unilateral posterior ligamentous disorder. The facet capsule on the side opposite to the direction of rotation and the interspinous ligament are torn uniformly with variable disruption of the posterior longitudinal ligament, anterior longitudinal ligament, and disc. In the majority of cases, these latter ligaments are only attenuated, and spinal stability is not severely compromised.[15] There may be an associated compression fracture of the lower adjacent vertebral body.

The clinical presentation may vary from minimal neck discomfort to a complete quadriplegia. Of the 37 unilateral locked facets reported by Braakman and Vinken, 15 had a delay in diagnosis of more than 2 weeks.[16] Minimal cervical complaints, which delayed the patient's consultation with a physician, were the cause of this disorder in many of his patients. Of the 37 patients, 3 had a total transverse lesion of the spinal cord. Radicular symptoms secondary to cervical nerve root compression at the intervertebral foramen are common.

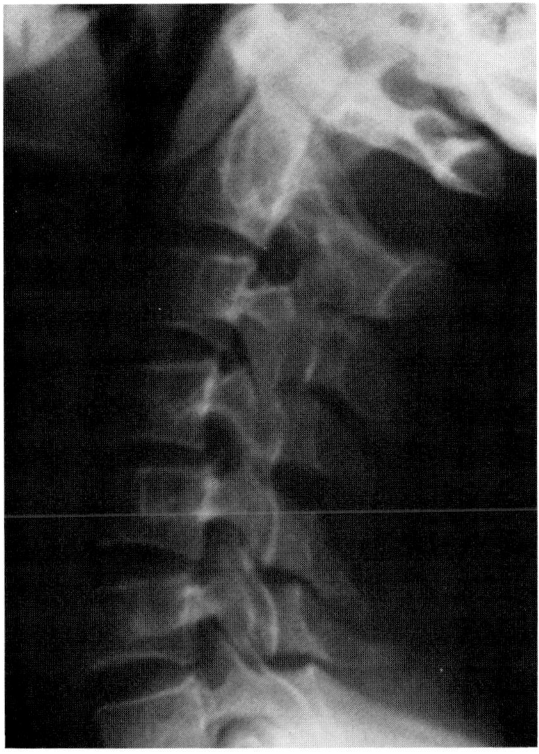

Fig. 16-12. *A*, Translatory displacement of C4 on C5 suggests a unilateral locked facet. Note widening of interspinous distance. *B*, Tomography demonstrates a unilateral subluxated facet associated with fracture of the superior articular process of C5 (arrow).

The diagnosis is usually apparent from the lateral radiograph. Radiographic changes include displacement of one facet joint, approximately 25% horizontal translation anteriorly of the superior vertebral body, and visible rotation of the upper cervical segments above the level of injury. On the anteroposterior radiograph, there is malalignment of the spinous processes with the processes superior to the level of injury being displaced toward the side of the locked facet. The locking of the facet is evident on the oblique view. The specific pathologic anatomy, including fractures of the superior or inferior articular processes, may be verified by lateral tomography (Fig. 16-12).

All acutely locked facets should be reduced and stabilized. Although reduction may not be absolutely necessary, some authors believe that it decreases the likelihood of persistent radicular symptoms.[16] Reduction can be achieved by traction or manipulation. Skeletal traction by halo or tongs of up to 30 to 40 pounds is a standard requirement. Under good radiographic control, the traction weight should be increased by 5-pound increments every 30 to 60 minutes. When the dislocated facet is disengaged, the neck is extended and rotated gently to the involved side to secure the reduction. Manipulative reductions, which are popular in Europe, should be attempted only by the experienced surgeon. Surgical reductions are indicated only when nonoperative techniques fail.

Stabilization may be accomplished by a halo apparatus or Minerva cast. Prolonged traction and surgical fusion are less desirable alternatives. The use of less rigid cervical orthoses is not recommended because of the difficulty in maintaining the reduction, especially in patients with associated fractures of the articular processes. Minor recurrent subluxation in locked facets with fractures of the articular processes is frequent but not significant because of the tendency for spontaneous late fusion in such cases. Reduction of a unilateral locked facet of greater than 6 to 8 weeks of age should not be attempted.

Bilateral Locked Facets

Vertebral dislocation with bilateral locked facets results from a combination of flexion, rotation, and distraction forces. In contrast to the unilateral locked facet injury, bilateral locked facets involve a much more extensive disruption of the supporting structures of a spinal segment. With the usual pattern of injury, all posterior ligaments, the posterior longitudinal ligament, and the disc are disrupted, and the anterior longitudinal ligament is attenuated or stripped off the inferior vertebral body. There may also be a slice fracture of the lower vertebral body.

Neurologic deficits are invariably more profound with bilateral locked facets than with unilateral locked facets. Over one half of these injuries have complete spinal cord lesions.[17] Fracture of the vertebral arch of the superior vertebra occasionally decompresses the canal and, thus, lessens the severity of the neurologic loss.

The lateral radiograph is diagnostic. Radiographic findings include an increase in the interspinous distance, obvious displacement of the facets, and a greater than 50% anterior horizontal translation of the superior vertebral body. Tomography is useful in detecting associated articular facet fractures that may influence the optimal treatment of a dislocation.

Reduction techniques for bilateral locked facets are similar to those utilized for unilateral locked facets. Reduction should be accomplished on an emergency basis since the most effective decompression of the vertebral canal can be attained by rapid restoration of spinal alignment. Because of the complete disruption of most supporting ligaments, reduction can be achieved easily by traction. Manipulative reduction is controversial.

If the posterior injury is purely ligamentous, fusion is preferable to prolonged immobilization in traction or a halo device. The probability of late segmental instability after nonoperative management is high. The fusion can be performed electively as long as an adequate reduction is maintained preoperatively. Posterior fusion using the Rogers wiring technique provides the best immediate stabilization when the articular facets are intact. When the facets are fractured, some form of interfacet wiring may be required.

Routine laminectomy has no place in the enlightened care of spinal cord injuries. The rare indications for cervical laminectomy include cord compression from a laminar fracture, certain open injuries to the spinal cord, and the cervical dislocation with a progressive neurologic deficit despite a satisfactory reduction.[18] Laminectomy is not justified solely on the basis of satisfying the patient and family that "everything possible has been done." The risk of further compromise to spinal stability is greater than the dubious value of a decompressive laminectomy.[19]

Extension Injuries

Hyperextension forces applied to the lower cervical spine may result in osseous, ligamentous, and discal injuries. Some fracture patterns, such as an isolated unilateral fracture of the lateral column, are relatively insignificant. Other extension injuries may cause profound neurologic loss despite minimal displacement of the spine. Acute central cord syndrome is the most common neurologic pattern. The cord damage is thought to be due to compression between the lamina and ligamentum flavum posteriorly and the bulging disc anteriorly. In a series of 51 extension injuries, Burke classified 36 as extension disruption without dislocation.[20] The average age of these patients was 56 years, and the majority had moderately severe changes of cervical spondylosis. All series of hyperextension injuries similarly cite a relative vulnerability of the spondylotic spine to this form of injury.

The nature of the injury may be concealed by spontaneous reduction of the fracture-subluxation. A variable degree of retrolisthesis of the superior vertebral body on the lower adjacent body is frequently evident on the lateral radiograph. A small chip of bone often is avulsed off the anterosuperior or anteroinferior edge of a vertebral body at the site of rupture of the anterior longitudinal ligament. Alternatively there may be a fracture of a spondylolytic osteophyte. Careful examination of good-quality plain radiographs is all that normally is needed to localize the level of injury. Tomography is useful in any questionable case. In the younger patient with a demonstrable neurologic loss and normal radiographs, a hyperextension injury with central herniation of a disc should be suspected. Myelography is essential to confirm the diagnosis and localize the level of herniation.

Following reduction, spinal stability is ordinarily not a problem. The intact posterior longitudinal ligament and posterior structures preclude significant redisplacement of the spine. External immobilization with the head in neutral or slight flexion is sufficient to maintain alignment during healing.[21] Spontaneous anterior fusion at the injured vertebral interspace often occurs. Immobilization should be maintained for 2 to 3 months. Spinal cord recovery is variable, but at least partial return of function generally can be expected. The prognosis of the spinal cord injury is worse in patients with cervical spondylosis and ankylosing spondylitis than it is for patients with normal spines sustaining hyperextension injuries.

Burst Fractures

Compression injuries to the lower cervical spine are caused by an axial load applied to the vertex of the head. A history of diving into a shallow pool often is given. The most common pattern of injury is a burst fracture of the body of the fifth or sixth vertebra. When combined with major flexion forces, wedge compression fractures with or without posterior ligamentous injury may also be present.

With severe fragmentation of the body and retropulsion of the fracture fragments, quadriparesis or quadriplegia is the rule. Patients with wide anteroposterior diameters of their vertebral canals occasionally escape neurologic injury despite significant retrolisthesis of the vertebral body.

Radiographically, the body appears crushed with the posterior cortex retropulsed into the canal (Fig. 16-13). A teardrop fracture is seen anteriorly. The anteroposterior radiograph commonly demonstrates a vertical fracture through the center of the body. Tomography is helpful in disclosing the degree of compromise of the canal, especially when the C7 vertebra is involved.

There is no unanimity of opinion regarding the optimal treatment of burst fractures. The two main alternatives are (1) alignment and external immobilization and (2) early decompression with vertebrectomy and anterior fusion.[22] The former is adequate for all neurologically intact cases. For patients with nerve root or spinal cord symptoms and signs, the choice of treatment is controversial. Unfortunately, the importance of displaced bone fragments and discal tissue posteriorly into the canal on the prognosis for cord and nerve root return has never been documented clearly. When a definite, complete, spinal cord injury is sustained, vertebrectomy does not alter the dismal prognosis. The most convincing argument for early anterior debridement and fusion is its potential benefit in decompressing the nerve root at the level of injury. This theoretic advantage must be weighed against the increased morbidity and mortality of a major surgical procedure in a frequently polytraumatized patient. Late instability following either the use of external immobilization or vertebrectomy with anterior fusion is uncommon.

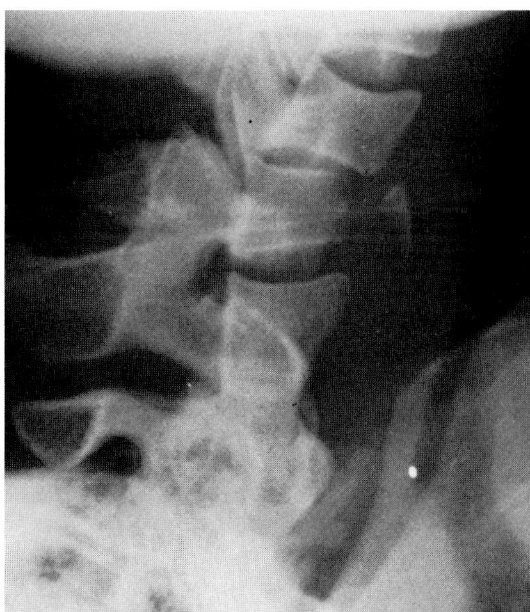

FIG. 16-13. Burst fracture of C3 with only slight retrolisthesis of the vertebral body and moderate posterior ligamentous disruption. The patient was intact neurologically.

Penetrating Wounds to the Cervical Spine

Direct rather than indirect forces occasionally inflict substantial damage to the cervical spine. Of the various types of penetrating trauma to the spine, the most frequent are low-velocity gunshot, shrapnel, and knife wounds. The vast majority of such wounds result in minimal structural damage to the spinal elements. The soft-tissue injury, especially vascular and neural, is of paramount importance. The spine generally can be managed with only an orthosis for patient comfort. If there is any suggestion of a compromise to spinal stability, flexion-extension radiographs are indicated.

One variant of penetrating trauma with a higher incidence of spinal complications is the transpharyngeal gunshot wound to the cervical spine. Cervical osteomyelitis is a common sequela of such injuries when they are inadequately treated.[23] Aggressive treatment is necessary to avoid chronic infection with pharyngeal flora. Once cervical spine involvement and a transpharyngeal course of the missile are substantiated, exploration of the spine is indicated. Thorough soft-tissue and bony debridement, closure of pharyngoesophageal wounds, and adequate drainage are recommended. Appropriate antibiotics and cervical spine immobilization should be continued postoperatively.

Special Problems in the Polytrauma Patient

Cervical spine injuries often complicate and limit the standard diagnostic and therapeutic measures to be taken in the management of the polytrauma patient. Spinal cord injuries may mask the customary signs and symptoms of various intra-abdominal and pelvic injuries. The presence of spinal shock can confuse the routine evaluation of the polytrauma patient's blood loss. A temporary sympathectomy of the trunk and legs occurs following traumatic quadriplegia. It can be distinguished from hypovolemic shock by the presence of hypotension without an elevation in the pulse rate. An unstable cervical fracture or subluxation also may diminish the ease and safety with which various diagnostic tests can be performed.

Restraints on the use of many therapeutic modalities are even greater. Anesthesia for emergency surgical procedures poses a special problem. In the patient with a potentially unstable cervical spine injury, standard hyperextension and manipulation of the neck during intubation are contraindicated. The spine should be immobilized in a neutral position using skull traction or a halo device.[24] Awake nasotracheal or orotracheal intubation is preferable with quick postintubation testing of neurologic function prior to the administration of the general anesthetic. If a change in neurologic status is noted, anesthetic induction is stopped, and the spine is re-evaluated radiographically. When an operation is performed electively on a patient in a halo cast or vest, certain precautions are warranted. Nasotracheal intubation is usually necessary. When cardiac arrest occurs intraoperatively, all essential equipment for quick removal of the halo cast or vest to permit closed- or open-chest massage must be available. Postoperative extubation should be delayed routinely until the patient is fully alert.

Early stabilization of all fractures and rapid mobilization out of bed are desirable goals in most polytrauma patients. Cervical spine injuries frequently alter the ideal early management of these patients. Although skull traction allows safe turning of the patient on an appropriate bed or frame, it may preclude the successful use of traction for lower or upper extremity fractures.

Because of the risk of skin breakdown in the patient with neurologic loss, traction and circumferential casts for extremity fractures should be applied with more than the usual care and should be checked frequently. Early open reduction and internal fixation of extremity fractures expedite mobilization and rehabilitation and greatly facilitate pulmonary care.

All multiply injured patients with cervical spine fractures amenable to external bracing using a halo apparatus, Minerva cast, or intermediate-class cervical brace should be mobilized in the appropriate orthosis as soon as possible. Serial radiographs are necessary to check for loss of the spinal reduction. Even in the halo apparatus, spinal motion and loss of reduction can occur.[25,26] Good nursing care is important to prevent skin breakdown beneath the orthosis.

References

1. Bucholz, R.: Unstable hangman's fractures. Clin. Orthop., *154*:119, 1981.
2. Rogers, W.: Fractures and dislocation of the cervical spine—An end result study. J. Bone Joint Surg., *39A*:341, 1957.
3. Weir, D.: Roentgenographic signs of cervical injury. Clin. Orthop., *109*:9, 1975.
4. Cattell, H., and Filtzer, D.: Pseudosubluxation and other normal variations in the cervical spine in children—A study of 160 children. J. Bone Joint Surg., *47A*:1295, 1965.
5. Maravilla, K., Cooper, P., and Sklar, F.: The influence of thin section tomography on the treatment of cervical spine injuries. Radiology, *127*:131, 1978.
6. White, A., Johnson, R., Panjabi, M., and Southwick, W.: Biomechanical analysis of clinical stability in the cervical spine. Clin. Orthop., *109*:85, 1975.
7. Jefferson, G.: Fractures of the atlas vertebrae: report of 4 cases and a review of those previously recorded. Br. J. Surg., *7*:407, 1920.
8. Spence, K. F., Decker, S., and Sell, K.: Bursting atlantal fracture associated with rupture of the transverse ligament. J. Bone Joint Surg., *52A*:543, 1970.
9. Anderson, L., D'Alonzo, R.: Fractures of the odontoid process of the axis. J. Bone Joint Surg., *56A*:1663, 1974.
10. Schatzker, J., Rorabeck, C., and Waddell, J.: Fractures of the dens—An analysis of 37 cases. J. Bone Joint Surg., *53B*:392, 1971.
11. Southwick, W.: Management of fractures of the dens (odontoid process). J. Bone Joint Surg., *62A*:482, 1980.
12. Fielding, J. W., Hawkins, R., and Ratzan, S.: Spine fusion of atlanto-axial instability. J. Bone Joint Surg., *58A*:400, 1976.
13. Fielding, J. W., Van Cochran, G., Lawsing, J. F., and Hohl, M.: Tears of the transverse ligament of the atlas. J. Bone Joint Surg., *56A*:1683, 1974.
14. Brashear, H. R., Venters, G., and Preston, E.: Fractures of the neural arch of the axis—A report of 29 cases. J. Bone Joint Surg., *57A*:879, 1975.
15. Beatson, T.: Fractures and dislocation of the cervical spine. J. Bone Joint Surg., *45B*:21, 1963.
16. Braakman, R., and Vinken, P.: Unilateral facet interlocking in the lower cervical spine. J. Bone Joint Surg., *49B*:249, 1967.

17. Braakman, R., and Penning, L.: Injuries of the Cervical Spine. Amsterdam, Excerpta Medica, 1971.
18. Jacobs, B.: Cervical fractures and dislocations. Clin. Orthop., *109*:18, 1975.
19. Bohlman, H.: The pathology and current treatment concepts of cervical spine injuries: A critical review of 300 cases. J. Bone Joint Surg., *54A*:1353, 1972.
20. Burke, D.: Hyperextension injuries of the spine. J. Bone Joint Surg., *53B*:3, 1971.
21. Forsyth, H. F.: Extension injuries of the cervical spine. J. Bone Joint Surg., *46A*:1792, 1964.
22. Bailey, R., and Badgley, C.: Stabilization of the cervical spine by anterior fusion. J. Bone Joint Surg., *42A*:565, 1960.
23. Jones, R., et al.: Cervical osteomyelitis complicating transpharyngeal gunshot wounds to the neck. J. Trauma, *19*:630, 1979.
24. Nickel, V., Perry, J., Garrett, A., and Heppenstall, M.: The halo: A spinal skeletal traction fixation device. J. Bone Joint Surg., *50A*:1400, 1968.
25. Johnson, R., et al.: Cervical orthoses. J. Bone Joint Surg., *59A*:332, 1977.
26. Koch, R., and Nickel, V.: The halo vest—An evaluation of motion and forces across the neck. Spine, *3*:103, 1978.

Chapter 17 Complex Fractures of the Pelvis

ROBERT W. BUCHOLZ
BERND CLAUDI

Pelvic injuries constitute a major source of morbidity and mortality in modern automotive societies. The steadily decreasing mortality rates of patients with treated pelvic fracture-dislocations over the last 100 years is more a reflection of early recognition and improved management than of diminished severity of the injuries. A high incidence of occult fatal injuries has been reported,[1,2] and a recent study of 150 multiple-trauma fatality victims yielded a frequency of pelvic injuries of nearly 1 in 3.[3] The mortality rate from complications of recognized pelvic fractures still remains between 10 to 20%.[4–7] The potential for late disability from such injuries also persists despite improvements in the understanding of their pathogenesis.[8–10] Pelvic fractures and dislocations clearly do not deserve to be placed at the bottom of the treatment priority list of injuries in the multiply traumatized patient. Past experience attests to the need for early recognition of both acute and late complications of such injuries.

Classification of Pelvic Fracture-Dislocations

Many different detailed classification schemes have been devised in an attempt to distinguish between minor and major fracture patterns.[5,7,11–13] Minor fractures include:

1. Fractures of individual bones without a break in the continuity of the pelvic ring.
   A. Avulsion fractures.
   B. Fracture of the pubis or ischium.
   C. Fracture of the wing of the ilium.
   D. Fracture of the sacrum.
   E. Fracture of the coccyx.
2. Single break in the pelvic ring.
   A. Fracture of two ipsilateral rami.
   B. Fracture near, or subluxation of, the symphysis pubis.
   C. Fracture near, or subluxation of, the sacroiliac joint.[12]

These stable fracture patterns are relatively uncommon in the multiply traumatized patient. Most result from a low-energy and/or well-localized injury force applied to the pelvis. Significant hemorrhage and long-term sequelae from such injuries are experienced infrequently. Except for the rare associated visceral or neurologic injury, these stable fractures do not alter the general treatment plan for the patient. These minor fractures of the pelvis will not be further considered.

Three major pelvic injury patterns commonly are encountered in the polytrauma patient:

1. Double break in the pelvic ring.
   A. Malgaigne's hemipelvis fracture-dislocations.
   B. Straddle fractures.
   C. Combined hemipelvis fractures.

All large series of pelvic injuries implicate these three groups as responsible for the vast majority of early and late complications.[4–7,14] Complex acetabular fractures, including rim, column, and central fractures, present unique diagnostic and therapeutic challenges and will be covered under a separate heading.

Malgaigne's hemipelvis fracture-dislocations involve double vertical breaks in the pelvic ring. The anterior break may include fractures of the pubic or ischial rami and/or a disruption of the pubic symphysis. The posterior break occurs posterior to the hip joint and may involve a vertical or oblique fracture of the ilium or sacrum, or, frequently, a disruption of the sacroiliac joint. The resulting free hemipelvis fragment may be displaced in three different planes. With sacroiliac disruptions, the hemipelvis rotates externally in the axial plane, resulting in a variable diastasis of the pubic symphysis or displacement of rami fractures (Fig. 17-1). This opening up of the pelvis like an oyster shell is often a result of the isolated tearing of the anterior sacroiliac ligaments with preservation of the stronger posterior and superior ligament complex.[3,15] With more extensive ligament or osseous injury posteriorly, the hemipelvis also can displace cephalad and posteriorly (Fig. 17-2). The amount of cephalad migration is easy to detect radiographically, but the posterior displacement often is unrecognized.

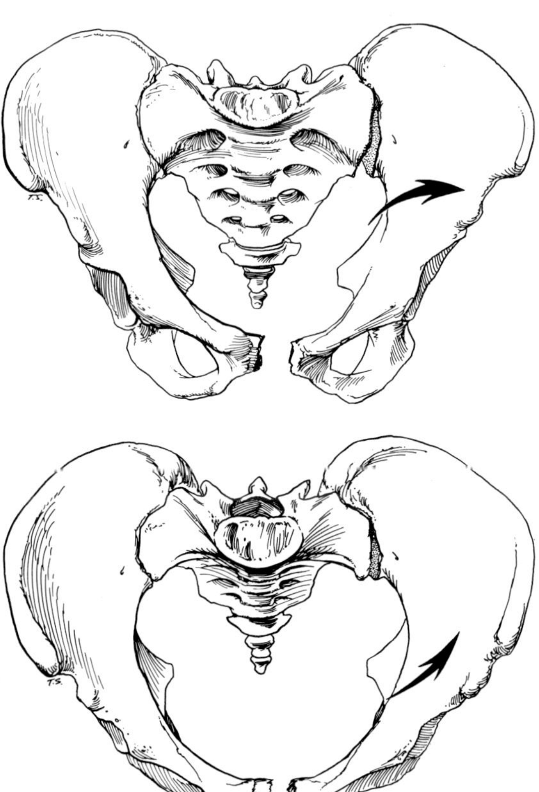

FIG. 17-1. *A*, Stable hemipelvis disruption with tearing of the anterior sacroiliac ligaments and pubic ligaments but preservation of the posterosuperior sacroiliac ligament complex. *B*, Axial view of stable pattern demonstrating external rotation of hemipelvis.

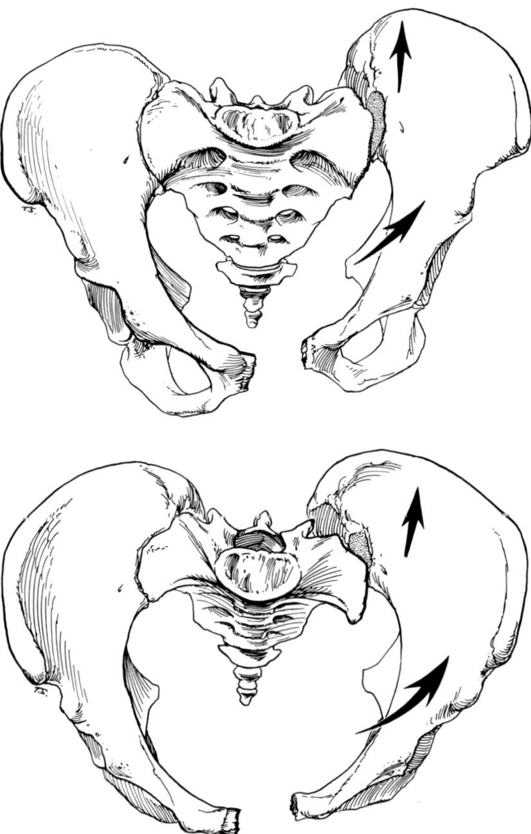

FIG. 17-2. *A*, Unstable hemipelvis disruption with complete sacroiliac dislocation and cephalad displacement of the hemipelvis. *B*, Axial view of unstable pattern showing posterior displacement of the hemipelvis.

Bilateral superior and inferior rami fractures are also called straddle fractures. Unlike Malgaigne's fracture-dislocations and central fracture-dislocations of the acetabulum, straddle fractures do not include an interruption of the normal line of weight transmission through the pelvis. The straddle injury, however, deserves the classification of a major fracture pattern because of its high rate of associated complications, especially lower urinary tract injuries.[4,7] A significant proportion of such straddle injuries may also have subtle, radiographically inconspicuous injury to the sacroiliac joint.[3] Mixed pelvic injuries consisting of combinations of these three major patterns and the minor fracture patterns are sustained occasionally (Fig. 17-3).

Emergency Management and Diagnostic Procedures

A systematic approach to the evaluation of a multiply injured patient with a suspected pelvic fracture aids in the detection of all potential injuries and complications. Conolly and Hedberg have outlined an excellent plan for the early evaluation and management of fractures of the pelvis (Table 17-1).[4]

Routine radiographs, including the anteroposterior, inlet, and tilt views, often are suboptimal in quality. The extent of posterior ring injury and displacement is especially difficult to judge.[16] The recent introduction of computer assisted tomography has aided in the delineation of specific injury patterns.

The emergency care of the polytrauma patient does not end with resuscitation and diagnosis of all injuries. The multiply injured patient is in the best medical condition for reparative surgery immediately after emergency stabilization. After several days of bed rest, pulmonary insufficiency often develops on the basis of pulmonary contusion, sedation from analgesics, fat embolism, sepsis, or a combination of several of these factors. A major surgical procedure performed at

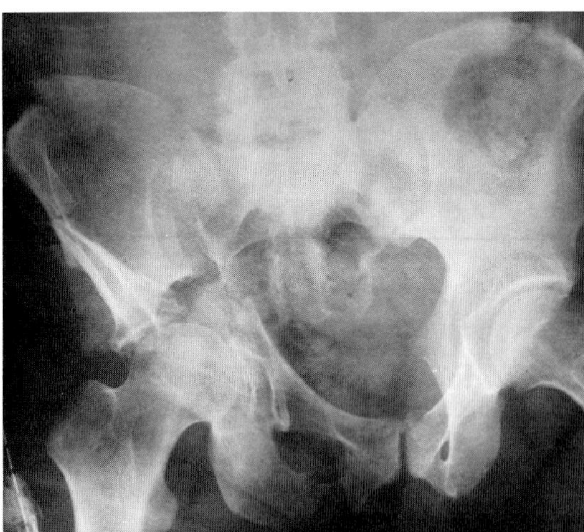

Fig. 17-3. Mixed pelvic injury with fractures of the pubic symphysis, pubic rami, right iliac wing, and dome and central portions of the acetabulum. The right hip and sacroiliac joints are dislocated.

Table 17-1. *Emergency Management of Pelvic Fracture-Dislocations. (Modified from Conolly and Hedberg[4].)*

Procedure for Immediate Management of Fracture of the Pelvis

I. History—Note:
   A. The time, direction, and nature of the trauma.
   B. The time the patient passed urine. If he has not voided, urge him not to void.
   C. The time and amount of food and drink taken prior to the injury.
   D. The symptoms of associated injury, e.g., other sites of pain, loss of consciousness.

II. Examination
   A. General
      1. Record the pulse, blood pressure, respiration, and adequacy of airway.
      2. Rapidly survey all potential sites of injury. Remove all clothing and examine front and back, head, spine, thorax, abdomen, and limbs.
   B. Local
      1. Inspect the perineum for ecchymosis, swelling, extravasation of urine.
      2. Determine the instability of the pelvic rim by palpating the symphysis pubis and rami and compressing and distracting the wings of the ilium. Palpate posteriorly over the sacroiliac joint to detect radiographically occult sacroiliac disruptions.
      3. Perform a rectal examination to feel a displaced prostate (in case of ruptured urethra) or tenderness over a fractured sacrum.
      4. Test carefully for any neurologic loss in either lower extremity.

III. Investigations
   A. Plain roentgenograms are taken of the pelvis, chest, and other regions of suspected injury. The pelvic roentgenogram, supplemented by physical findings, determines whether the fracture is major or minor. Internal and external oblique radiographs are required in all cases of central fracture-dislocation of the acetabulum. Inlet and tilt views of the pelvis are useful in delineating the planes of displacement of Malgaigne's injuries.
   B. Catheterization. If the patient had a full bladder at the time of injury, or if he suffered a bilateral fracture of the pubic rami, lower urinary tract damage should be suspected. A urethrogram is necessary prior to attempts at catheterization in men with blood in the urethral meatus, a high-riding prostate, hematuria, or an inability to void. In all other cases, make one attempt at clean catheterization. If the attempt is successful, complete urethral rupture is virtually excluded. If catheterization is not successful, cystostomy is indicated, but an intravenous pyelogram and urethrocystogram provide valuable information.
   C. A midline abdominal tap above the level of the umbilicus is indicated in all cases of suspected ruptured viscus and in all unconscious or severely shocked patients.

TABLE 17-1 *(continued)*

D. Indications for diagnostic angiography are infrequent, but should be recognized early if present. Indications include absent distal pulses, a pulsatile hematoma, and a bruit over the fracture.

---

that time may carry a prohibitive anesthetic risk. Colonization of open lacerations and abrasions of the peripelvic region may postpone further a necessary operation. Soft-tissue contractures occur rapidly in the pelvic area, and reduction of displaced fractures or dislocations becomes more difficult with each passing day. Delayed and inadequate reduction of a pelvic disruption can increase the potential for developing any of several residual abnormalities, including leg-length discrepancy, degenerative arthritis, gait disturbance, and narrowing of the pelvic outlet in females.[10,17,18]

The optimal time for the reduction of the pelvic fracture and a decision on the method of definitive orthopaedic management of the injury is immediately following the resuscitation of the patient and the completion of initial diagnostic procedures.

Orthopaedic Management of Major Pelvic Fracture-Dislocations

The wide spectrum of different treatment modalities reflects the inadequacies of any one technique in the management of all pelvic disruptions. Each type of treatment has its relative advantages and disadvantages in minimizing possible acute and long-term complications.

Bed Rest

Bed rest, followed by gradual mobilization when the patient is comfortable, remains the standard of treatment for all stable minor pelvic fractures. It is also the preferred treatment for straddle injuries in which the normal line of weightbearing through the pelvis is not broken. Results are uniformly good because of the potential for early mobilization within several days of injury and the low incidence of late disability even with significant displacement of these fracture patterns. Clinically significant deep venous thrombosis and pulmonary embolism are infrequent complications of these pelvic fractures except in patients with protracted pain necessitating prolonged bed rest.

Postural Reductions and Casting

Described by Watson-Jones in 1938,[13] this technique is now seldom indicated for major pelvic fracture-dislocations in the polytrauma patient. In Malgaigne's disruptions in which the hemipelvis is rotated externally (see Fig. 17-1), the extended hips of the patient lying supine act as a deforming force. Lateral recumbency does facilitate the reduction, and a well-molded hip spica cast can prevent recurrent displacement of the hemipelvis. The attainment and maintenance of an anatomic reduction in the other possible planes of displacement (usually cephalad and posterior) are accomplished much less readily. Hip spica casts are cumbersome and often hinder treatment of associated soft-tissue and lower extremity injuries.

Traction and Pelvic Slings

Devised by Ashley Cooper and popularized by Holdsworth,[6] the use of pelvic slings supplemented with longitudinal lower extremity traction remains a useful treatment method. Skeletal traction via a distal femoral or proximal tibia Steinmann's pin is applied to the leg on the side of the injury. Bilateral skeletal traction through distal femoral pins may be required in significantly displaced bilateral Malgaigne's injuries. The pelvic sling can be positioned to exert compressive forces on both iliac crests, thereby closing any diastasis of the symphysis or rami fractures. Traction and pelvic slings are the preferred treatment for minimally displaced Malgaigne's fractures and for patients with isolated pelvic injuries who are not at high risk for secondary organ failure during bed rest. It is a useful technique for temporary partial immobilization of the pelvis during early diagnostic evaluation of the patient. It is also helpful in the rare Malgaigne's fracture-dislocation in the pediatric patient.[19,20]

Several problems are commonly encountered in the use of this technique. Maintenance of the pelvic sling in its correct position is not easy. It often tends to slip cephalad, restricting respiratory function, and thus requires frequent adjustments. The reduction of a Malgaigne's dislocation displaced in any plane other than pure external rotation can be difficult with the use of traction and slings alone. Nursing care of a patient in slings and traction is taxing, and access to soft-tissue wounds of the perineum and buttocks is hindered. The management of associated lower extremity injuries may be complicated. Finally, this method of treatment has all the disadvantages of prolonged bed rest and immobilization.

Other Nonoperative Techniques

These treatment modalities are largely of historical interest only. They include the use of a turnbuckle cast, a modification of well-leg traction,[21] and traction applied through hooks in the iliac crests.[22]

Reduction and External Fixation

With the resurgence of interest over the last decade in the external fixation of fractures, its application to the treatment of Malgaigne's type of pelvic injuries has gained wide popularity. A variety of different external fixation devices have been utilized. The most extensive experience has been with the Hoffmann external fixation apparatus.[23–26] Preliminary results have been encouraging, and the complication rate has been consistently low. Success at obtaining an ''anatomic reduction'' is, however, variable. Other external fixation devices currently being tested are the Anderson splint, the epoxy tube system, the Wagner apparatus,[27] and a more complex system using a hemiloop with full crest transfixion pins.[28]

Most devices involve the use of three half pins inserted into each iliac crest (Fig. 17-4, *A*). A small incision made adjacent to the pin sites during insertion is often helpful in ensuring accurate placement of the pins into the thin crests (Fig. 17-4, *B*). Satisfactory reduction usually can be obtained by a combination of longitudinal traction on a fracture table, internal rotation of the hips, lateral compression on the iliac crests, and direct manipulation of the displaced hemipelvis (Fig. 17-4, *C* and *D*). Fluoroscopy of the pelvis in the operating room is helpful in determining which manipulative maneuvers optimize the reduction. All cephalad and posterior displacement of the hemipelvis must be corrected prior to the use of any lateral compression. The external fixation usually is applied in a trapezoidal or quadrilateral configuration. The Hoffmann device allows for further compression of the pelvis as needed.

Reduction and external fixation is an attractive treatment alternative for unstable Malgaigne's fracture-dislocations. Application is easy, and complications are few. Hemorrhage at the pelvic fracture site is decreased, and pain relief is impressive. Although fracture reduction is often far from anatomic,[29] it is usually better than that which can be obtained by other nonsurgical techniques. Reduction is most easily accomplished when attempted within several days of the injury. Rigid stabilization allows early mobilization of the patient to a sitting position and enhances pulmonary care.[30] Pin tract infections are common, but rarely result in osteomyelitis of the ilium. Haraharju and Slatis recommend removing the frame and pins at 6 weeks.[24]

The current state of the art of external fixation accepts less than anatomic reduction of many pelvic injuries in return for the benefits that the technique provides, namely rapid immobilization of the fracture and early mobilization of the patient. As more experience with reduction and external fixation of pelvic fracture-dislocations accrues, many of the potential long-term sequelae of malunion may be avoided. In the interim, there may be a movement toward more aggressive surgical management of such injuries.

Open Reduction and Internal Fixation

The risks of uncontrollable hemorrhage, pelvic infections, and inexperience with operative approaches have limited attempts to surgically reduce and stabilize Malgaigne's fracture-dislocations. Taylor reviewed the disappointing results of various authors attempting direct surgical management using internal fixation with Lane's plates, wires, bone graft, Parham bands, silk, or tendons.[31] No series yielded predictable success using any particular technique. Jenkins and Young recently emphasized the potential benefits of rigid stabilization of these injuries, including a shortened hospital stay, freedom from pain, and restoration of the pelvic anatomy.[32] Their use of a single compression plate at the symphysis, however, may not provide the assurance of anatomic reduction and rigid fixation in Malgaigne's dislocations with triplane displacement. A separate posterior approach with reduction and plate fixation may be required in such cases. The advisability of open reduction and internal fixation of unstable pelvic dislocations awaits the long-term results of both nonoperatively treated and externally fixed injuries. This approach should be used only by surgeons experienced in pelvic surgery and current techniques of internal fixation.

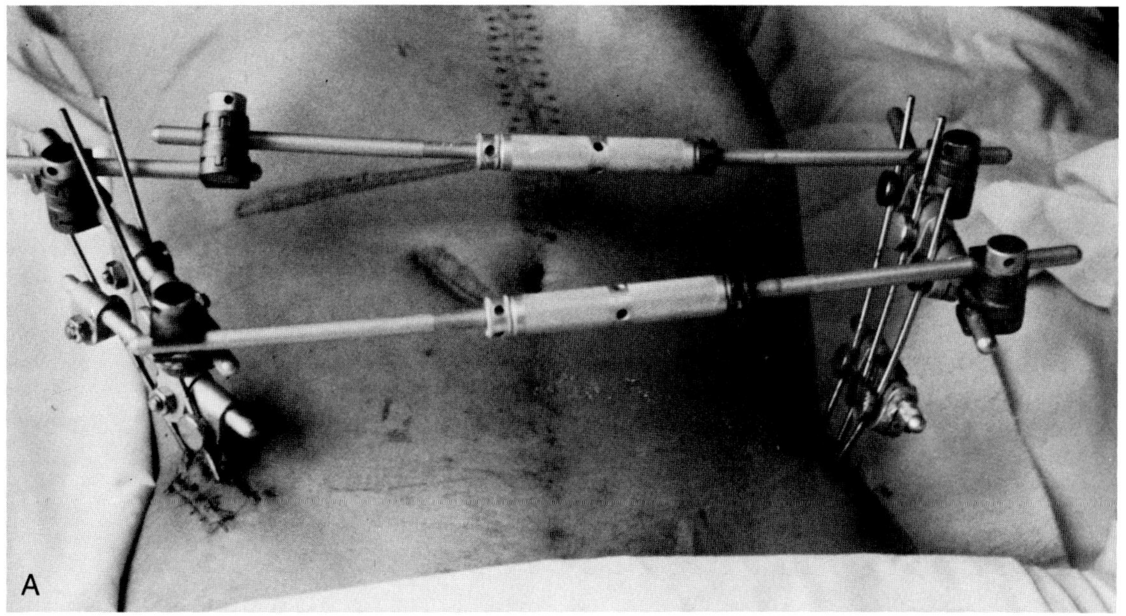

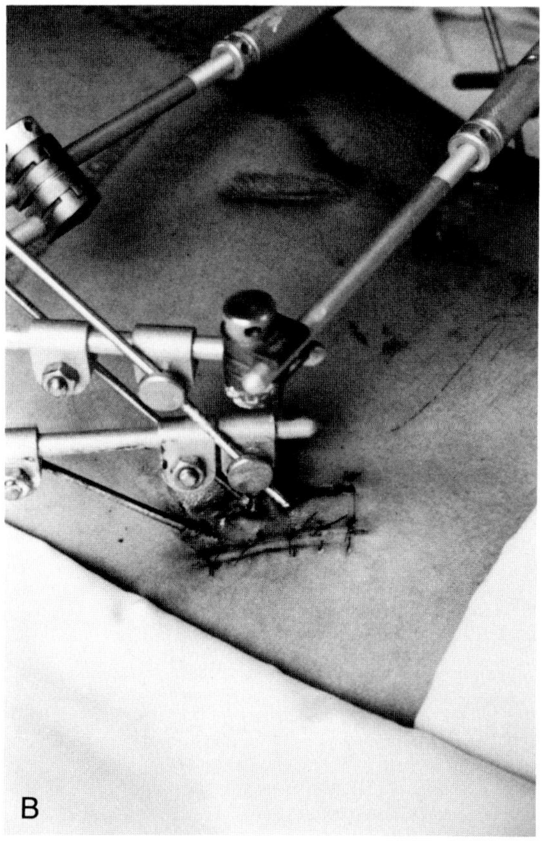

Treatment of Central Fracture-Dislocations of the Acetabulum

Central fracture-dislocations of the acetabulum are most frequently secondary to a major impact force on the greater trochanter or to a force transmitted through the femur from the knee while the hip is flexed and abducted. Central protrusion of the femoral head into the pelvis usually implies fractures of both the anterior and posterior columns of the acetabulum.[11] Comminution of the fracture, as well as femoral head and acetabular cartilage damage, is often present. Avascular necrosis of the femoral head is an infrequent sequela of this injury in comparison with posterior fracture-dislocation of the hip.

Accurate preoperative radiographic evaluation of the acetabulum is important. The status of the anterior and posterior columns, as well as of the dome of the acetabulum, is determined by multiple radiographic views, including anteroposterior and internal and external obliques.[33] Specific osseous landmarks should be scrutinized in each view to detect all bony injuries. Computerized tomography is an especially useful adjunctive study for localizing all acetabular fractures.

Fig. 17-4. *A*, Roger-Andersen external fixation using three half pins in each iliac crest. *B*, A 5-cm incision adjacent to pin sites allows for identification of outer table of iliac crest and accurate placement of the half pins.

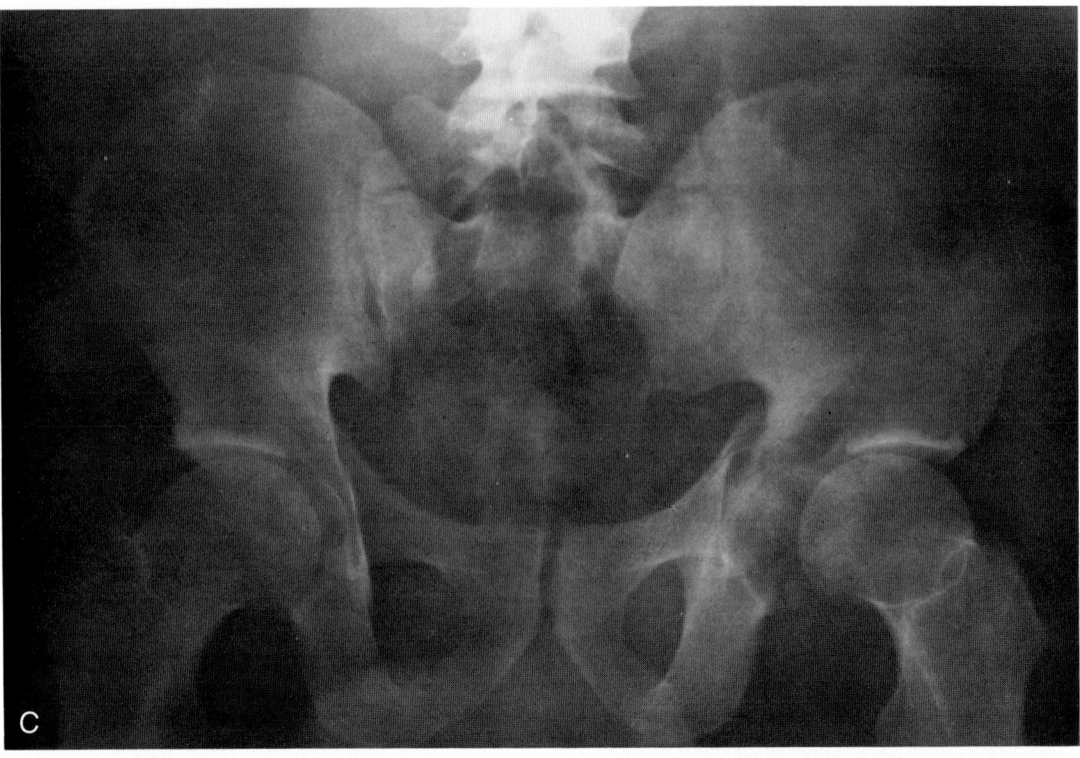

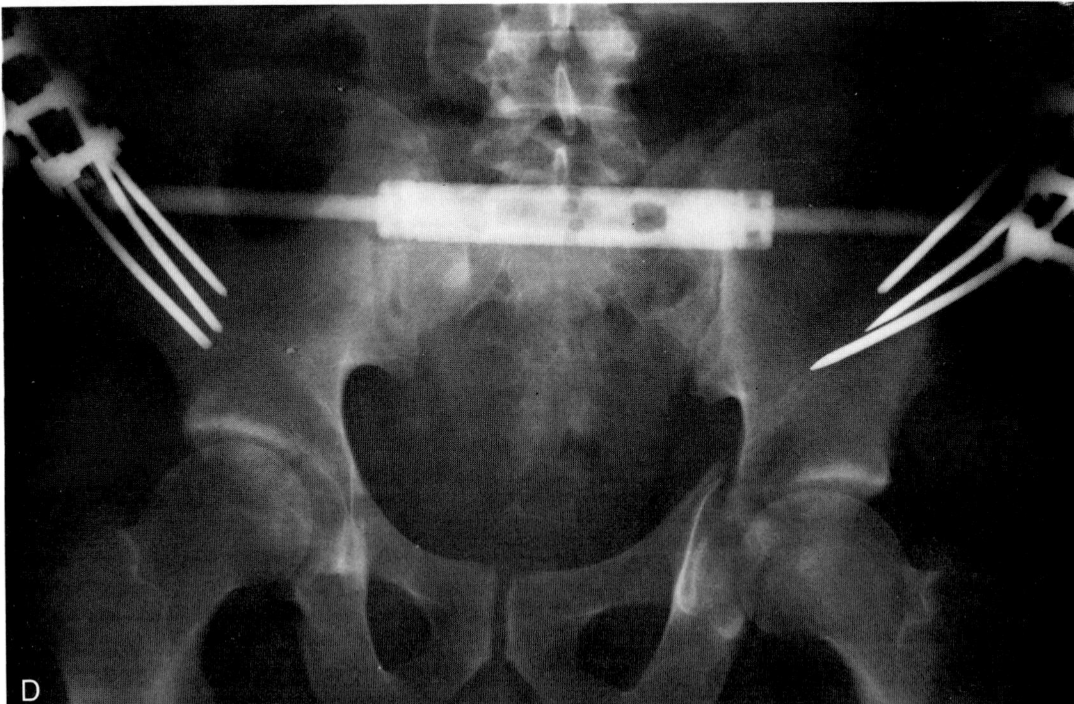

Fig. 17-4 (*continued*). *C*, Prereduction radiograph showing left sacroiliac disruption, central acetabular fracture, and external rotation of left hemipelvis. *D*, External fixation device significantly improves the external rotatory displacement of the hemipelvis. Further reduction and supplemental plate fixation of the central acetabular fracture are normally indicated in such an injury.

Central fracture-dislocation of the acetabulum is an intra-articular fracture of a weightbearing joint. Orthopaedic principles of anatomic reduction, fixation, and early motion are, therefore, applicable to this injury. Because of the difficulty of surgical approaches, the frequently discouraging degree of comminution, and the recent development of a predictably good salvage procedure in total hip replacement, surgeons traditionally have compromised their orthopaedic principles in the handling of these intra-articular fractures. A consistently poor prognosis has been reported by many authors.[34,35]

Longitudinal skeletal traction supplemented as necessary by lateral traction through trochanteric pins is the standard method of treatment in most medical centers. Despite a poor radiographic appearance, the long-term functional results were found to be good or satisfactory in 50 to 60% of cases reported by Tipton and associates[36] and Carnesale and associates.[37] Sparing of the superior weightbearing dome of the acetabulum increases the probability of a satisfactory result as long as the femoral head is well centered beneath the dome. Fracture comminution of the superior dome leads to a predictably poor clinical result. Traction for a minimum of 12 weeks is recommended.

In the polytrauma patient with severe associated injuries, alternative treatments permitting rapid mobilization have been proposed. External fixation, alone or in combination with open reduction and internal fixation, has been attempted.[23,28] Extensive experience with external fixation devices is a prerequisite for anyone undertaking such a treatment. Direct operative reduction and stabilization similarly require specialized skills and understanding of pelvic anatomy.

The surgical approach to a central fracture-dislocation depends on an accurate preoperative radiographic interpretation of the fracture anatomy. Any surgeon undertaking an operative stabilization of a central acetabular fracture must have a thorough knowledge of the radiographic and surgical principles outlined by Judet and Letournel.[11,33] Either an anterior or posterior approach or both may be necessary depending on which columns of the acetabulum are involved in the injury. The posterior column is exposed easily by a straight posterior approach to the hip. Following division of the short external rotators and identification and protection of the sciatic nerve, the posterior column can be manipulated both intrapelvicly and extrapelvicly. The accuracy of reduction can be judged by direct inspection of the acetabular surface through a small capsulotomy. Reduction and stabilization of the anterior column often do not require further exposure but merely may be secured by lag-screw fixation from the posterior exposure. If reduction of the anterior column is incomplete, further exposure can be obtained by a separate Smith-Petersen incision or by osteotomy of the greater trochanter.[38] Anatomic reduction may be formidable, especially if surgery is postponed for more than several days. Comminution is the rule, and debridement of all fracture fragments that cannot be stabilized is necessary.

When open reduction and rigid internal fixation are feasible, many benefits can be realized (Fig. 17-5). The patient can be mobilized rapidly so long as other lower extremity injuries are amenable to stabilization. By restoring the congruity of the acetabulum and debriding all free osteochondral fracture fragments from the joint, the probability of developing post-traumatic arthritis is decreased. If a late reconstructive or salvage procedure is required, the restored osseous structure of the acetabulum makes such a procedure technically easier and perhaps more predictably successful.

Treatment of Posterior Fracture-Dislocations of the Hip

Posterior dislocation of the hip, with or without an acetabular rim fracture, usually is sustained from a dashboard injury. The force of impact is transmitted through the knee and femur to the flexed hip. The degree of adduction or abduction of the hip dictates the size of the acetabular fragment.

Traumatic dislocation of the hip is an orthopaedic emergency. Following resuscitation of the patient, examination of neurovascular loss, and radiographic documentation of the dislocation, closed reduction should be attempted. The majority of pure dislocations and dislocations with a small acetabular lip fracture are stable after concentric reduction. Early mobilization of the patient and protected weightbearing are possible in such cases.

The indications for open reduction and internal fixation of these fracture-dislocations include irreducibility of the hip by closed manipulation, nonconcentric reduction secondary to interposed osseous or soft tissue, and instability of the hip

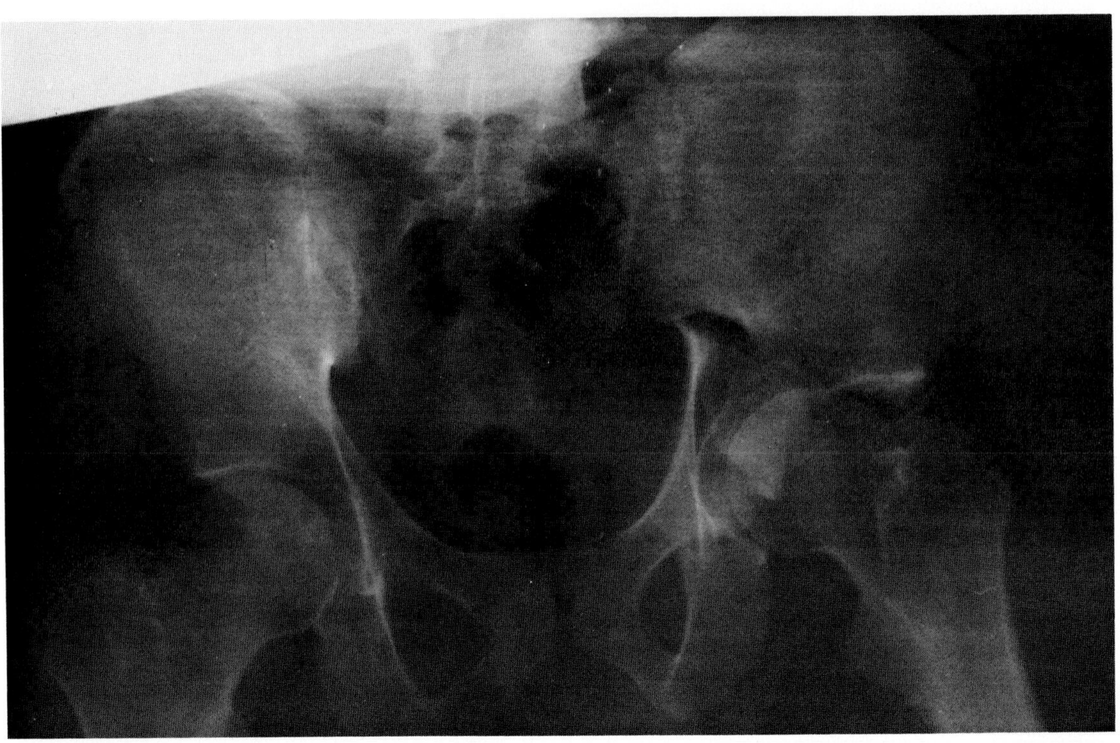

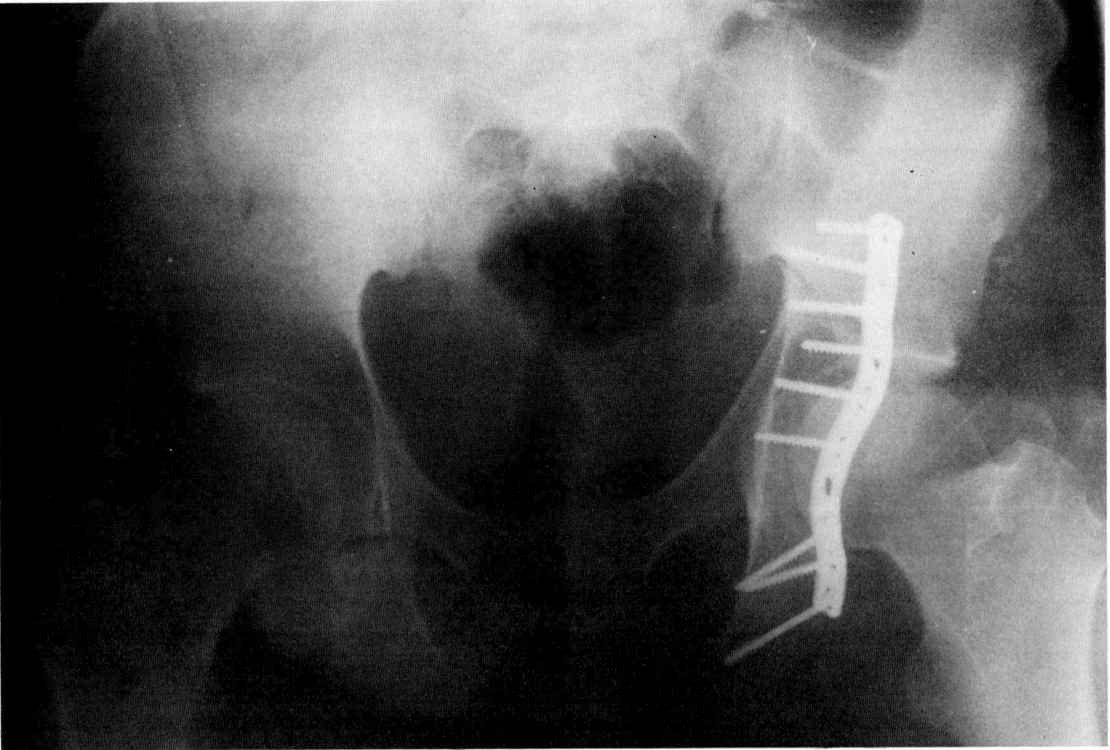

Fig. 17-5. *A*, Central fracture-dislocation of the left hip. *B*, Reduction and posterior plate stabilization restored the congruity of the hip joint.

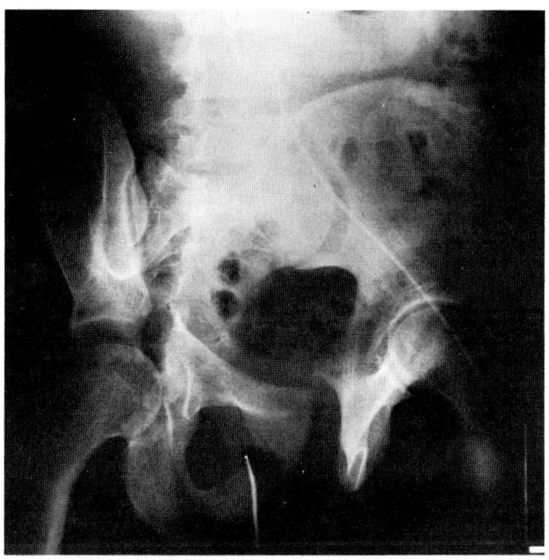

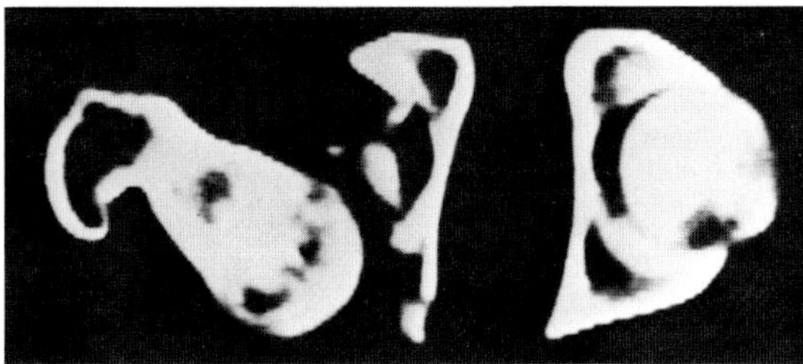

Fig. 17-6. *A*, Right hip dislocation associated with posterior rim and central acetabular fractures. *B*, Computerized tomography reveals multiple interposed osteochondral fragments within the joint.

after successful reduction. When reduction is attempted with the patient adequately relaxed with a general anesthetic, irreducibility of the hip is rare. Ipsilateral femoral shaft fracture may make closed manipulations impractical. Nonconcentric reductions from interposed tissues in the acetabulum are diagnosed by careful evaluation of the postreduction radiograph for widening of the joint space. Routine tomography or computerized tomography of the hip may be useful in the borderline case to detect small osteochondral fragments (Fig. 17-6). Following a successful reduction, the hip always should be ranged gently through 90° of flexion. If the joint subluxes or redislocates through this arc of motion, the hip is unstable, and operative fixation of the acetabular fracture is necessary.

The hip should be approached posteriorly. All capsular and osseous tissues are preserved carefully to allow for optimal reconstruction. Acetabular rim fractures should not be devitalized by total release of their soft-tissue attachments. The hip is redislocated gently and all free debris within the joint removed. Posterosuperior acetabular rim fragments frequently are locked in the joint, and extraction may be difficult. The fragments are attached to a thick capsular and iliofemoral ligamentous pedicle, which is twisted superiorly and anteriorly over the femoral neck. Extraction of the fragments is accomplished by spinning the fragments and pedicle superiorly over the neck. Care must be taken not to devitalize the fragments. Fixation is secured by multiple cortical or cancellous screws inserted to give interfragmental compression (Fig. 17-7). Plate fixation is needed occasionally in patients with associated posterior-column fractures or extensive rim comminution. All operative procedures to stabilize posterior rim or column fractures should be done with the ipsilateral knee kept in a flexed position to avoid additional damage to the sciatic nerve.

Late sequelae of posterior dislocations of the hip include avascular necrosis of the femoral head and post-traumatic arthritis. These complications are avoided best by early, concentric reduction of the dislocation.

Special Problems in the Multiply Injured Patient

Hemorrhage

The estimated blood loss from pelvic fractures as reflected in the blood-volume replacement required to maintain a normal blood count varies in different large series.[5,39] The amount of hemorrhage, however, is clearly a function of the severity of the fracture pattern. The average number of transfusions for displaced Malgaigne's fracture-dislocations was calculated by Hauser and Perry as 7.4 units per patient.[5] Whole-blood replacement and early stabilization of the pelvis are the keystones to the treatment of hemorrhage from pelvic injuries. The appearance of shock usually is slow to develop in most patients and, therefore, allows sufficient time for safe, effective blood replacement. Manipulation of the patient during diagnostic procedures should be kept to a minimum. Early stabilization of the pelvic fracture by the use of a pelvic sling, G-suit, or external fixation device prevents further aggravation of the hemorrhage. In a small percentage of patients these maneuvers are not adequate in con-

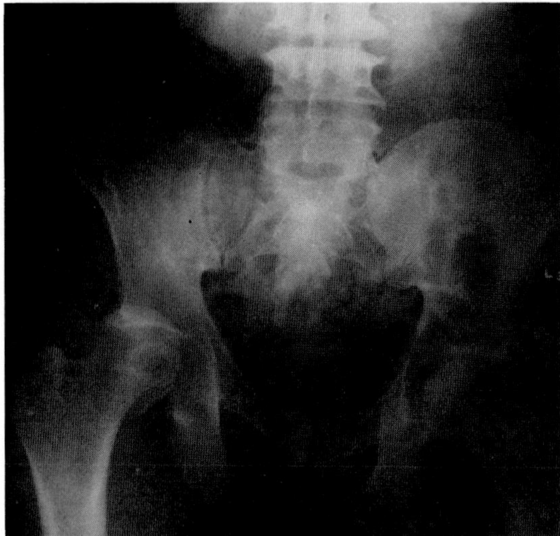
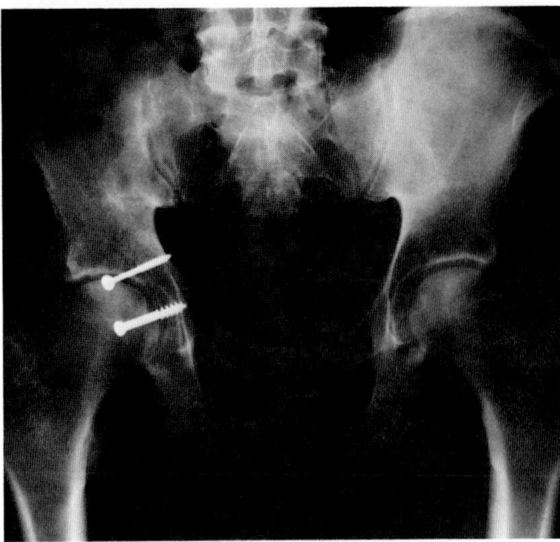

Fig. 17-7. *A*, Posterior fracture-dislocation of the right hip with a large interposed posterosuperior acetabular rim fracture. *B*, Careful preservation of soft-tissue attachments of the fragment and anatomic reduction with screw fixation restored the stability of the joint.

trolling hemorrhage, and one of the following techniques may have to be employed.

Various modifications of external counterpressure suits are now commonly used as adjunctive treatment in emergency patients with pelvic and lower extremity trauma.[40,41] Flint and associates stressed not only the tamponade effect of the suit but also its added advantage of immobilization of the pelvic fracture.[41] It is contraindicated in patients with pulmonary edema, impaired pulmonary function, cerebral edema, and lower extremity injuries with a high likelihood of developing a compartment syndrome. Extreme caution is indicated during the deflation of the suit to avoid sudden changes in blood pressure.

During the last 10 years, angiography and embolization of bleeding, traumatized vessels have been popularized. Selective transcatheter arterial embolization is valuable when greater than 10 to 12 units of blood loss from a pelvic fracture occurs over a 24-hour period.[42,43] A variety of materials, including autologous clot, muscle homogenate, Gelfoam particles, silicone spheres, and steel coils, have been used as emboli. Gelfoam is the preferred agent for long-term occlusion.[42]

The results of laparotomy and ligation of the internal iliac artery are unpredictable. Although some authors report satisfactory control of the hemorrhage by internal iliac ligation,[5,44] others implicate the tremendous arterial collateral circulation of the pelvis in the usual failure of the technique.[14,45,46] Attempts at direct control of bleeding by ligation, cautery, packing, and hemostatic agents can similarly be unrewarding. Kane noted only a 1% incidence of major arterial bleeding.[47] Such a major arterial injury usually can be suspected preoperatively by the presence of decreased pulses, a bruit, or a pulsatile hematoma and can be documented by an angiogram. Multiple small bleeding sites are encountered more frequently when the retroperitoneal hematoma is evacuated. Adequate exposure is difficult. Both Riskin and associates[48] and Hawkins and co-workers[49] described direct operative control of retroperitoneal hemorrhage as successful and life saving in a significant number of their cases. The mortality rate is high, however, and an average of 30 units of blood are transfused intraoperatively and postoperatively.[48] Most general surgeons consider such heroic surgery as a last-resort technique.

Need for Early Mobilization of the Patient

All large series of major pelvic fracture-dislocations reveal a much higher mortality rate in the subclass of cases with multiple associated injuries. Of the 72 deaths from pelvic fractures studied by Rothenberger and associates,[14] 71 had a high concomitant injury rate. Pulmonary injuries and complications resulting in respiratory insufficiency are largely responsible for the increased mortality in the multiply injured patient. Of the

186 patients with pelvic fractures reported by Peltier,[7] 25% had also sustained chest injuries. The incidence was highest in patients with Malgaigne's injuries, straddle fractures, and central fracture-dislocations of the acetabulum. In Hauser and Perry's series of 196 pelvic fractures,[5] associated chest trauma was present in 33 patients, 15 of whom died from their injuries. In addition to the obvious harmful effects of rib fractures, pulmonary contusion, hemothorax, and pneumothorax on respiratory function, pulmonary insufficiency may be induced by a variety of other factors. Fat embolism arising from long-bone fractures or other crush injuries, oversedation from heavy use of analgesia, sepsis, and diaphragmatic splinting following laparotomy may contribute to the pulmonary insufficiency in the polytrauma patient.

The goal in the multiply injured patient with a major pelvic fracture-dislocation should be early mobilization to minimize the adverse mechanical factors and to improve the pulmonary toilet. More aggressive management of the pelvic injury, including the use of external fixation or open reduction and internal fixation, is indicated in patients in the higher-risk categories.

Early mobilization also may diminish the hazards of thrombophlebitis and pulmonary embolism. Anticoagulation of the polytrauma patient with a major pelvic injury usually must be delayed for 7 to 10 days to avoid the risks of further hemorrhage.

Concomitant Spinal and Extremity Injuries

Spinal trauma occurs in approximately 2 to 4% of patients who sustain major pelvic injuries.[5,7] Fractures of the lumbar spine and the thoracolumbar junction occur most frequently. Neurologic loss may or may not be present, and its origin may be confused with possible traction injuries to the lumbosacral-plexus that occasionally accompany pelvic dislocations.[10,50] Management decisions about the spinal injury in the neurologically intact patient center on a judgment of the effects of the injury on spinal stability. If spinal stability has not been compromised, as judged by plain radiographs, spinal tomography, and carefully controlled flexion and extension views, an appropriate orthosis usually is sufficient. The patient with neurologic injury and/or an apparent unstable spinal lesion revealed by radiographs requires more aggressive treatment.

As with spinal injuries, the presence of concomitant lower extremity fractures often alters the ideal treatment of a given pelvic fracture. Ipsilateral femur fracture and hemipelvis dislocation make traction treatment of one or both injuries impractical. Stabilization of the extremity with rigid external or internal fixation of all fractures simplifies management and allows for early patient mobilization. Tibial and ankle fractures are less likely to influence the optimal treatment of the pelvic injury.

Associated Abdominal and Urologic Injuries

Abdominal visceral injuries are sustained in approximately 5 to 10% of patients with pelvic fractures.[4,5,7,20] Standard diagnostic procedures for intra-abdominal disorders, including serial examinations, radiography, and abdominal paracentesis, dictate the need for laparotomy. Abdominal taps below the level of the umbilicus may be false-positive as a result of anterior extension of the retroperitoneal hematoma. Hawkins, Pomerantz, and Eiseman listed several findings they consider as absolute or relative indications for laparotomy.[49] They include (1) classic evidence of free intraperitoneal bleeding or visceral perforation, (2) bladder perforation into the peritoneal cavity, (3) a large, palpable, expanding suprapubic hematoma, (4) radiographic evidence of bony fragments driven into the pelvis, and (5) blood loss exceeding 2.5 L that cannot be ascribed to associated injuries. Exploratory laparotomy in the patient with a suspicious abdominal injury may be life saving and should not be delayed. When only an isolated retroperitoneal hematoma is identified, it should not be disturbed.

Injuries to the lower urinary tract occur in 10 to 15% of patients with pelvic fractures. Physical signs suggestive of urologic injury include blood at the urethral meatus, hematuria, inability to void, a high-riding prostate, and marked suprapubic tenderness. Proper emergency evaluation of the lower urinary tract assists in the detection of all injuries and minimizes the potential for late complications from occult lesions. Retrograde urethrography should precede any attempt at catheterization in men with possible urethral damage. When urethral injury is ruled out, a cystogram is performed using a minimum of 300 to 400 ml of water-soluble contrast material. Following static and delayed drainage films, an intravenous pyelogram must be performed to detect upper urinary tract injury. Contingent on the findings of these preliminary radiographs, further diagnostic tests may be warranted. The treatment of special urologic injuries has been well outlined by many authors.[12,51] The presence of a urologic injury rarely alters the preferred orthopaedic management of a given pelvic fracture.

Open Pelvic Fractures

Direct communication between a pelvic fracture and a skin, vaginal, or rectal laceration defines an open pelvic fracture. This subclass of pelvic fractures is associated with higher-velocity injuries, massive hemorrhage, increased risk of pelvic infection, and a mortality rate that may approach 50%. Rothenberger and associates found the pelvic fracture to be the primary cause of death in 8 of 11 patients with an open fracture.[52] Of these 8 patients, 4 had a deep pelvic infection at the time of death.

Standard surgical and orthopaedic principles should be used in managing these fractures. Resuscitation may include the need for massive transfusions of greater than 20 units of blood. Exploratory laparotomy for large-vessel and visceral-injury repair is performed as needed. Diverting colostomy is mandatory in all cases of rectal, vaginal, or perineal laceration. The open fracture should be debrided and all potential dead space drained. The wound may be packed open and closed secondarily or may be closed with soft-tube drainage. Intravenous antibiotics are started at the time of resuscitation.

Rectal or vaginal lacerations communicating with pelvic fractures are rare, and few surgeons have extensive experience with their management. Awareness of the higher incidence of such lacerations in crushing injuries to the pelvis,[53] detection of vaginal bleeding in a patient who is not menstruating,[54] and performance of adequate rectal and vaginal examinations ensure the early recognition of such injuries. Treatment includes thorough debridement, diverting colostomy for all anal or vaginal tears, repair of the lacerations, and intravenous antibiotics.

Open fractures secondary to gunshot wounds similarly carry a high risk of chronic sepsis. Exploratory laparotomy is indicated almost universally, and diversion of fecal or urinary streams is often necessary. Lucas, in his study of 20 pelvic fractures from gunshot wounds, strongly recommended leaving all wounds open to ensure adequate drainage.[55] Deep-seated chronic sepsis was still an unfortunate frequent complication.

References

1. Braunstein, P., et al.: Concealed hemorrhage due to pelvic fracture. J. Trauma, *4*:832, 1963.
2. Garland, D., Glogovac, S., and Waters, R.: Orthopedic aspects of pedestrian victims of automobile accidents. Orthopedics, *2*:242, 1979.
3. Bucholz, R.: The pathological anatomy of fracture-dislocations (Malgaigne) of the pelvis. J. Bone Joint Surg., *63-A*:400, 1981.
4. Conolly, W., and Hedberg, E.: Observations on fractures of the pelvis. J. Trauma, *9*:104, 1969.
5. Hauser, C., and Perry, J.: Massive hemorrhage from pelvic fractures. Minn. Med., *49*:285, 1966.
6. Holdsworth, F.: Dislocation and fracture-dislocation of the pelvis. J. Bone Joint Surg., *30B*:461, 1948.
7. Peltier, L.: Complications associated with fractures of the pelvis. J. Bone Joint Surg., *47A*:1060, 1965.
8. Dunn, A. W., and Morris, H.: Fractures and dislocations of the pelvis. J. Bone Joint Surg., *50A*:1639, 1968.
9. Hundley, J.: Ununited unstable fractures of the pelvis. J. Bone Joint Surg., *48A*:1025, 1966.
10. Slatis, P., and Huittinen, V.: Double vertical fractures of the pelvis. Acta Chir. Scand., *138*:799, 1972.
11. Judet, R., Judet, J., and Letournel, E.: Fractures of the acetabulum: classification and surgical approaches for open reduction. J. Bone Joint Surg., *46A*:1615, 1964.
12. Kane, W.: Pelvic fractures. *In* Fractures. Edited by Rockwood and Green. Philadelphia, J. B. Lippincott, 1975.
13. Watson-Jones, R.: Dislocations and fracture-dislocations of the pelvis. Br. J. Surg., *25*:773, 1938.
14. Rothenberger, D., et al.: The mortality associated with pelvic fractures. Surgery, *84*:356, 1979.
15. Dommisse, G.: Diametric fractures of the pelvis. J. Bone Joint Surg., *42B*:432, 1960.
16. Pennal, G., Tile, M., Waddell, J., and Garside, H.: Pelvic disruption: assessment and classification. Clin. Orthop., *151*:12, 1980.
17. Rankin, L.: Fractures of the pelvis. Ann. Surg., *106*:266, 1937.
18. Smith-Peterson, M., and Rogers, W.: End-result study of arthrodesis of the sacroiliac joint for arthritis—traumatic and non-traumatic. J. Bone Joint Surg., *8*:118, 1926.
19. Bryan, W., and Tullos, H.: Pediatric pelvic fractures: review of 52 patients. J. Trauma, *19*:799, 1979.
20. Rang, M.: Children's Fractures. Philadelphia, J. B. Lippincott, 1974.
21. Carruthers, F., and Logue, R.: Treatment of fractures of the pelvis and their complications. AAOS Instructional Course Lectures, *10*:50, 1953.
22. Almond, G., and Vernon, E.: Iliac skeletal cross traction—a method of treatment of oyster shell pelvis. J. Bone Joint Surg., *41B*:779, 1959.
23. Grosse, A.: Stabilization of pelvic fractures with Hoffman external fixation: The French experience in external fixation. *In* External Fixation—The Current State of the Art. Edited by Brooker and Edwards. Baltimore, Williams & Wilkins, 1979.
24. Karaharju, E., and Slatis, P.: External fixation of double vertical pelvic fractures with a trapezoid compression frame. Injury, *10*:142, 1978.
25. Riskin, E., et al.: External fixation of unstable pelvic fractures. Acta Orthop. Scand., *50*:362, 1979.
26. Slatis, P., and Karaharju, E.: External fixation of unstable pelvic fractures. Clin. Orthop., *151*:73, 1980.

27. Muller, J., Bachman, B., and Berg, H.: Malgaigne fractures of the pelvis: treatment with percutaneous pin fixation. J. Bone Joint Surg., *60A*:992, 1978.
28. Mears, D.: The management of complex pelvic fractures. *In* External Fixation—The Current State of the Art. Edited by Brooker and Edwards. Baltimore, Williams & Wilkins, 1979.
29. Johnston, R.: Stabilization of pelvic fractures with Hoffman external fixation: The Colorado experience. *In* External Fixation—The Current State of the Art. Edited by Brooker and Edward. Baltimore, Williams & Wilkins, 1979.
30. Gunterberg, B., Goldie, I., and Slatis, P.: Fixation of pelvis fractures and dislocations. Acta Orthop. Scand., *49*:278, 1978.
31. Taylor, R.: Pelvic dislocations. Br. J. Surg., *30*:126, 1942.
32. Jenkins, D., and Young, M.: The operative treatment of sacroiliac subluxation and disruption of the symphysis pubis. Injury, *10*:139, 1978.
33. Letournel, E.: Acetabular fractures: classification and management. Clin. Orthop., *151*:81, 1980.
34. Milch, H.: Ischio-acetabular (Walther's) fracture. Bull. Hosp. Joint Dis., *16*:7, 1955.
35. Pearson, J., and Hargadon, E.: Fractures of the pelvis involving the floor of the acetabulum. J. Bone Joint Surg., *44B*:550, 1962.
36. Tipton, W., D'Ambrosia, R., and Ryle, G.: Non-operative management of central fracture-dislocations of the hip. J. Bone Joint Surg., *57A*:887, 1975.
37. Carnesale, P., Stewart, M., and Barnes, S.: Acetabular disruption and central fracture-dislocation of the hip—a long-term study. J. Bone Joint Surg., *57A*:1054, 1975.
38. Senegas, J., Liorzou, G., and Yates, M.: Complex acetabular fractures: A transtrochanteric lateral surgical approach. Clin. Orthop., *151*:107, 1980.
39. Moyson, F., Duprez, A., Bremer, A., and DeGraef, J.: Evaluation et traiteiment du shock traumatique dans les fractures du Bassin. Acta Chir. Belg., *56*:406, 1957.
40. Batalden, D. J., Wickstrom, P., Ruiz, E., and Gustilo, R.: Value of the G suit in patients with severe pelvic fracture. Arch. Surg., *109*:326, 1974.
41. Flint, L. M., et al.: Definitive control of bleeding from severe pelvic fractures. Ann. Surg., *189*:709, 1979.
42. Ben-Menachem, Y., et al.: Therapeutic arterial embolization in trauma. J. Trauma, *19*:944, 1979.
43. Ring, E., et al.: Arteriographic management of hemorrhage following pelvic fracture. Radiology, *109*:65, 1973.
44. Horton, R., and Hamilton, S.: Ligature of the internal iliac artery form massive hemorrhage complicating fracture of the pelvis. J. Bone Joint Surg., *50B*:376, 1968.
45. Patterson, F., and Morton, K.: The cause of death in fractures of the pelvis. J. Trauma, *13*:849, 1973.
46. Ravitch, M.: Hypogastric artery ligation in acute pelvic trauma. Surgery, *56*:601, 1964.
47. Kane, W.: Complications in treatment of fractures and dislocations of the pelvis. *In* Complications in Orthopedic Surgery. Vol. 2. Edited by C. Epps. Philadelphia, J. B. Lippincott, 1978.
48. Riskin, E., et al.: Operative control of massive hemorrhages in comminuted pelvic fractures. Acta Orthop. Scand., *50*:370, 1979.
49. Hawkins, L., Pomerantz, M., and Eiseman, B.: Laparotomy at the time of pelvic fracture. J. Trauma, *10*:619, 1970.
50. Goodell, C.: Neurological deficits associated with pelvic fractures. J. Neurosurg., *24*:837, 1966.
51. Peters, P., and Bright, T.: Management of trauma to the urinary tract. *In* Advances in Surgery. Vol. 10. Edited by W. Longmire. Chicago, Year Book Medical Publishers, 1976.
52. Rothenberger, D., et al.: Open pelvic fracture: A lethal injury. J. Trauma, *18*:184, 1978.
53. Froman, C., and Stein, A.: Complicated crushing injuries of the pelvis. J. Bone Joint Surg., *49B*:24, 1967.
54. Siegel, R.: Vesico-vaginal fistula and osteomyelitis—A complication of an occult open fracture of the pelvis. J. Bone Joint Surg., *53A*:583, 1971.
55. Lucas, G.: Missile wounds of the bony pelvis. J. Trauma, *10*:624, 1970.

Chapter 18 Concomitant Ipsilateral Fractures of the Hip and Femur

MICHAEL W. CHAPMAN

Fractures of the hip in association with fractures of the femoral shaft are common and are seen at least once or twice per year in a busy trauma practice, even though only 98 cases have been reported in the English literature (Table 18-1). Ipsilateral knee injuries occur in as many as 27% of cases,[1] creating an injury complex that is difficult to treat. Ritchey and associates hypothesize that the mechanism of injury in concomitant fractures of the hip and femoral shaft is a longitudinal compressive force applied to a flexed, abducted femur with the knee flexed.[2]

This combination of fractures tends to occur with high-velocity trauma, such as occurs in motor-vehicle accidents, pedestrians hit by vehicles, or falls from a height. Associated fractures of another long bone, a dislocation of a major joint, or trauma to the chest or abdomen have been reported in as many as 76% of these patients.[1] Therefore, the treatment of these injuries must be looked at in the context of the multiply injured patient.

Diagnosis

The usual hip fracture is an undisplaced transcervical or basilar neck fracture. Subcapital fractures are rare. For this reason, the hip fracture is frequently missed. In only one series have missed hip fractures not been reported,[3] and the overall incidence of delayed diagnosis is 17% (Table 18-1). All complications of nonunion and aseptic necrosis reported in the literature occurred in hips in which the diagnosis was missed initially.[1] A typical case is illustrated in Figure 18-1. A routine anteroposterior roentgenogram of the pelvis is inadequate for detecting the hip fracture because the hip is often in external rotation and not in the center of the film. In all femoral shaft fractures, anteroposterior and cross-table lateral views of the ipsilateral hip with the limb in neutral or internal rotation are recommended. Any patient with a severe knee injury or a femoral shaft fracture who complains of inordinate hip pain at any time in the course of treatment should have repeat roentgenograms taken of the hip to search for an occult fracture.

Extracapsular hip fractures are half as common as the undisplaced transcervical or basilar neck fracture and usually do not present a problem in diagnosis. They are most frequently intertrochanteric, but often are peritrochanteric with a subtrochanteric component, which frequently extends well into the diaphysis. The shaft fractures most commonly occur in the middle third. In Casey and Chapman's series, 14% of such fractures were segmental.[1]

The high incidence of ipsilateral knee injuries mandates roentgenograms of the knee also. The most common associated knee injury is a fracture of the patella with tibial plateau fractures also reported.[1] Soft-tissue injuries occur as well, and

Table 18-1. *Ipsilateral Fractures of the Hip and Femoral Shaft.*

Series	No. of Cases	Type of Hip Fracture: Intra-capsular	Type of Hip Fracture: Extra-capsular	Delayed Diagnoses	Ipsilateral Knee Fractures	Results: Nonunion	Results: Aseptic Necrosis
Delaney and Street (1953)[7]	4	4	0	2	3	0	0
Kimbrough (1961)[4]	5	4	1	4	0	2 (hip)	1
Dencker (1965)[9]	8	3	5	1	2	1 (hip)	0
Schatzker and Barrington (1968)[8]	6	6	0	4	2	2 (hip)	0
MacKenzie (1971)[5]	8	8	0	3	1	0	1
DiStefano, et al. (1972)[11]	1	0	1	*	*	†	0
Fielding, et al. (1974)[12]	1	0	1	*	*	*	*
Bernstein (1974)[6]	15	11	4	1	4	0	0
Wolfgang (1976)[14]	1	0	1	0	1	0	0
Ashby and Anderson (1977)[10]	3	1	2	1	1	0	0
Casey and Chapman (1979)[1]	21	12	9	1	9	0	0
Wright and Becker (1979)[3]	25	*	*	0	*	1 (shaft) 1 (hip)	*
Total	98	49	24	17	23	7	2

*Information not given
†Insufficient followup

the diagnosis of knee ligament instability can be difficult to make in the presence of an unstable femur, particularly if the fracture is in the distal half. If there is any doubt, examination under anesthesia with an assistant stabilizing the femur is indicated. Carefully performed stress roentgenograms or direct fluoroscopic examination may be helpful also. In borderline cases in which the need for surgical repair of the knee ligaments must be ascertained, internal fixation of the femur may be necessary to obtain an accurate diagnosis.

These severely injured limbs must be examined carefully for neurovascular impairment, and any significant deficit may be an indication for femoral arteriography.

Treatment

Institution of traction splinting at the scene of the accident or in the emergency room is important to minimize hemorrhage from the fractures, prevent displacement of an undisplaced hip fracture, and protect neurovascular structures. On rare occasions, an unstable knee may contraindicate traction, and in this circumstance, a distal femoral traction pin can be instituted in the emergency room.

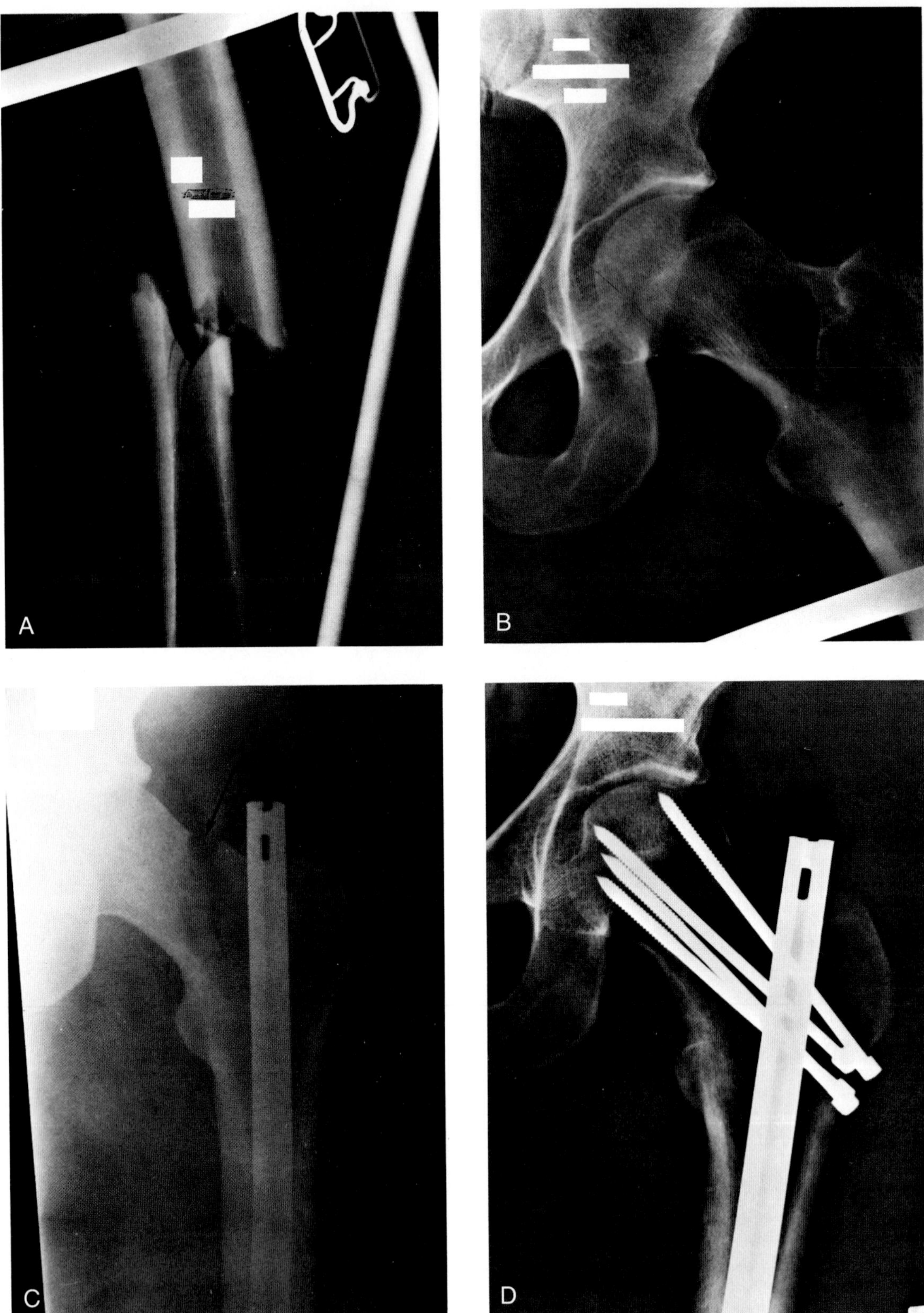
A
B
C
D

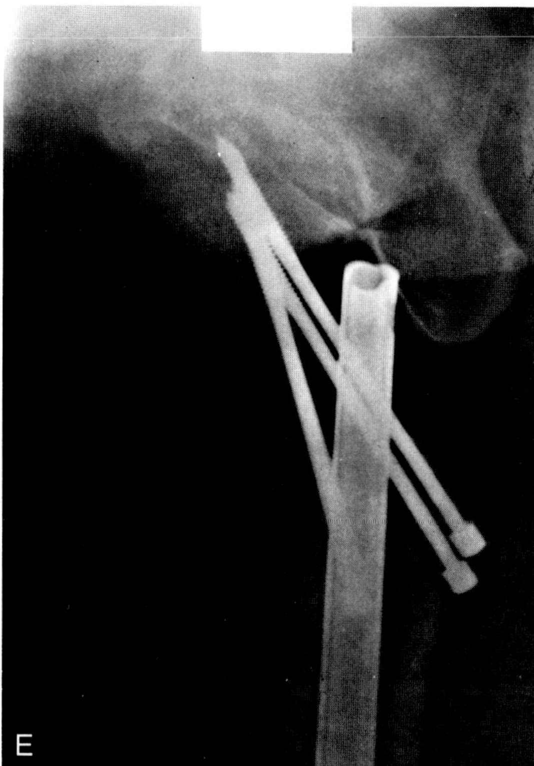

Fig. 18-1. *A*, A 25-year-old man was a passenger in an automobile that was involved in an accident. On admission to the hospital he was found to have a dislocated left first metatarsophalangeal joint, a fractured left ulna, and the closed midshaft fracture of the left femur seen in this anteroposterior roentgenogram. *B*, This anteroposterior roentgenogram of the left hip was interpreted as showing no abnormality. *C*, On the fourth day after injury, the femoral shaft fracture was internally fixed with an intramedullary Küntscher nail inserted by the closed technique under fluoroscopic control. The postoperative roentgenogram seen here revealed a displaced fracture of the femoral neck. Review of the original roentgenogram (Fig. 18-1*B*) revealed a nondisplaced fracture of the neck of the femur. *D* and *E*, The fracture was reduced closed and fixed with four percutaneous Knowles pins as seen on the postoperative anteroposterior and lateral roentgenograms. Both fractures healed, and avascular necrosis did not occur. The rod and pins eventually were removed, and after 44 months of follow-up, the patient had normal function of the hip and knee.

No single method of treatment can be considered standard or even preferable. In polytrauma situations, the surgeon must be flexible, must have many treatment methods available, and must individualize each treatment approach to give the optimal end result with a minimum of risk to the patient.

The treatment in the reported cases includes traction for both fractures followed by a cast,[1,3–5] a spica cast for treatment of the hip and plate fixation of the shaft,[2] a Thornton pin and plate plus traction,[5] traction for the hip and a Küntscher nail for the shaft,[5] a Jewett nail plus traction,[1,6] and Deyerle pins plus traction.[1] When both fractures were fixed internally with independent devices, the combinations reported were: Knowles or Moore pins with a Küntscher intramedullary nail,[1,2,4,7,8] lag screws for the hip and a Küntscher nail,[8] a sliding hip nail or compression hip screw with a separate plate on the shaft,[1,2] a Wainwright splint and an intramedullary nail,[5] Knowles pins plus single or double plates,[1,5] a Smith-Petersen nail with a separate plate,[5] a Neufeld nail and compression plate,[6] Hagie pins plus a compression plate,[5] a Jewett nail with a separate plate,[6] multiple pins with a muscle pedicle graft plus a compression plate,[6] and Nystrom nails plus intramedullary nails.[9] When one device was used to fix both fractures, those employed were a Smith-Petersen nail with a long side plate,[8] a Jewett nail with a long side plate,[6] a Zickel nail,[3,10–12] and Ender pins (augmented in some reports with Knowles pins).[1]

Most authors advocate internal fixation of the intracapsular hip fracture.[1,4–6,8–11] Whether internal fixation is mandatory cannot be proved from the literature. The intracapsular hip fractures treated in traction that had poor results generally were diagnosed late. The results reported were equally good in patients whose hip fracture was treated operatively and nonoperatively.[1] Because isolated intracapsular hip fractures heal better with internal fixation, I believe that the hip fracture should be fixed.

Extracapsular hip fractures can be managed in traction with good results when both fractures are treated with traction. In isolated concomitant ipsilateral fractures of the hip and femoral shaft, the literature shows equally good results with either nonoperative or surgical treatment, as long as the hip fracture is undisplaced and acceptable alignment is achieved in the shaft fracture.

Most authorities, however, advocate internal fixation of both fractures, particularly when the intracapsular hip fracture is displaced, the injury is sustained by a victim of polytrauma, there is an associated ipsilateral knee injury, or the fractures are sustained by an elderly person.

All the respiratory complications in Casey and Chapman's series occurred in patients in skeletal traction.[1] In polytrauma patients who are at risk for the adult respiratory distress syndrome, early internal fixation of both fractures is indicated after initial stabilization. Internal fixation permits immediate mobilization of the patient, which optimizes pulmonary physical therapy. A vertical position can then be achieved by the patient, and drainage and aeration of dependent pulmonary segments can be promoted.

Ipsilateral knee injuries most frequently are responsible for whatever residual disability occurs after these injuries heal.[1] Early, aggressive range-of-motion and muscle-strengthening exercises minimize knee disability, and fixation of both fractures usually is necessary to achieve this end.

Some authors believe that internal fixation of the shaft fracture must be done initially to facilitate reduction and fixation of the hip fracture.[8] My experience has shown that this is not the case; fixation of the hip fracture, when carried out initially, has been uniformly successful.[1] Reduction is achieved by the usual manipulation on a fracture table. The soft tissues provide adequate control of the fracture fragments. Internal fixation of the fracture of the shaft has not been a prerequisite to fixation of the hip fracture. In the San Francisco General Hospital series, all the intracapsular fractures were reduced by closed means and fixed with percutaneous multiple pins.[1]

In multiply injured patients, the surgeon may have to delay operation or do only one operation at the outset. In these circumstances, the fracture of the hip should take precedence over that of the shaft because the shaft usually can be treated in traction or in a cast-brace, whereas conservative care of an intracapsular hip fracture in a multiply injured patient is less likely to be successful.

No one type of internal fixation for both fractures stands out as the best because of the diversity of devices used and the small number of cases reported. Each system offers advantages and disadvantages.

Whichever methods of fixation are chosen, anatomic reduction and stable internal fixation of intracapsular fractures of the hip are mandatory. The fixation of the fracture of the shaft should be sufficiently stable to be free of external immobilization and ideally should permit early ambulation. For most surgeons, in most circumstances, multiple pins, a nail-plate, or a compression hip screw for the fracture of the hip and a separate compression plate for the shaft fracture may be the simplest technical approach. The disadvantage of this approach is that open reduction and internal fixation of both fractures often involve considerable soft-tissue dissection and blood loss. Two surgical exposures or one large incision may be needed. Prolonged operating time may be required.

For this reason, percutaneous fixation techniques are attractive. The shorter operating time, lower blood loss, and minimal infection rate make these methods safer and more applicable to the multiply injured patient who requires immediate fixation.[1,13] The disadvantages are that the patient must be transferred to a fracture table and a fluoroscope is required after other life-salvaging surgery has been performed. If these techniques are to be employed under emergency circumstances, the surgeon must be experienced in the techniques, and excellent nursing and radiologic support must be available.

When suitable, an intramedullary Küntscher or Schneider rod inserted using closed techniques can be used for the shaft fracture, and multiple Knowles or Neufeld pins can be inserted percutaneously for the hip fracture.[1,7] This combination is illustrated in Figure 18-1. This procedure is technically challenging as the intramedullary nail must be placed first without disturbing the fracture of the femoral neck, and the insertion of multiple pins into the femoral neck and head about an intramedullary nail can be difficult.

The Zickel nail requires exposure of the hip region, but can be inserted into suitable fractures of the proximal shaft of the femur without opening the fracture.[10–12,14] Its usefulness is somewhat limited as it is not suitable for intracapsular fractures nor for fractures of the shaft distal to the middle of the femur.

Ender pins have proved useful for these fractures, particularly when combined with percutaneous Knowles pins for an intracapsular hip fracture.[1,12,13] Two cases are illustrated in Figures 18-2 and 18-3. The advantages of Ender pins are that they are biomechanically well designed for subtrochanteric and intertrochantric hip fractures;[11] have proved suitable for shaft fractures;[1,15] can be used for intracapsular fractures when combined with Knowles pins; can be used to fix almost any combination of fractures in the proximal two thirds of the femur; require a small surgical incision causing minimal blood loss; eliminate the need to open the fractures since the nails are inserted by closed technique under fluoroscopic control; are inserted within an operating time for both fractures, including setup time, of usually less than 2 hours; and usually allow early mobilization without external protection. The best stability is achieved when pins are inserted

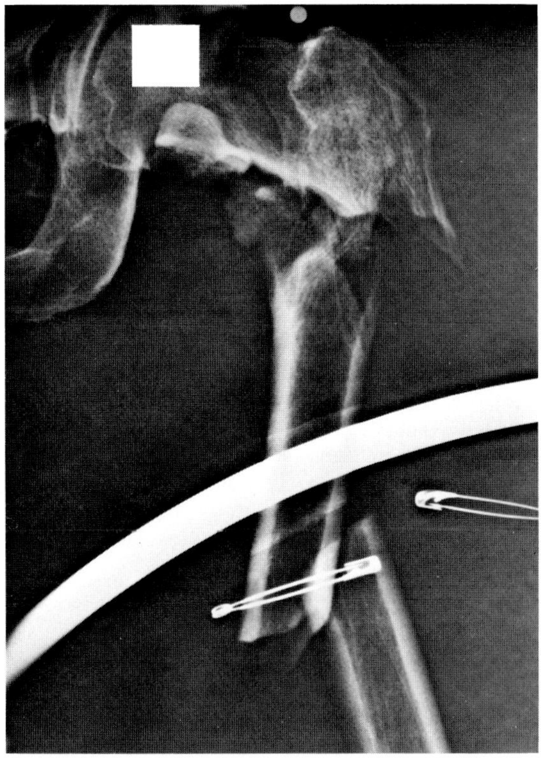

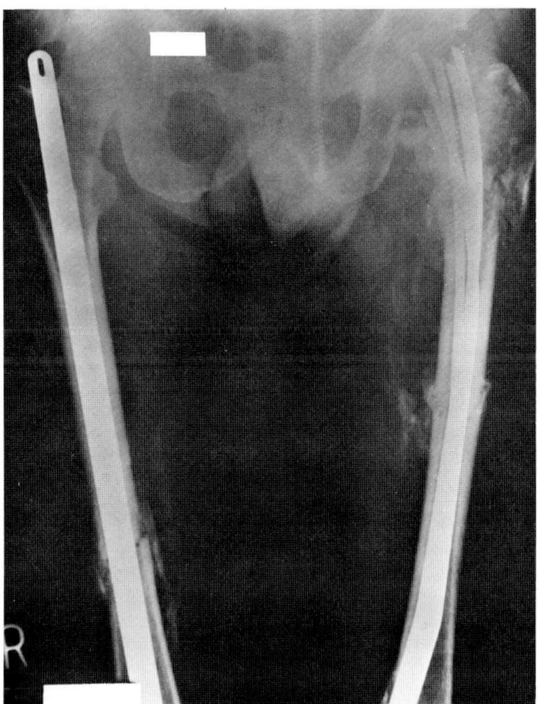

Fig. 18-2. *A*, A 58-year-old man was struck by an automobile and sustained multiple injuries, including fractures of the occiput, ribs, right femur (open), right tibia and fibula (open), left pubic ramus, left tibial plateau (open), and fibula. In addition, he had two fractures of the left femur, one peritrochanteric and one in the midshaft, as seen in this anteroposterior roentgenogram. He also sustained blunt abdominal trauma resulting in a retroperitoneal hematoma. After resuscitation and insertion of a right chest tube, a laparotomy was done and revealed minor mesenteric lacerations. The open fractures were debrided. Both femurs were placed in tibial pin traction, and the tibial fractures were placed in short-leg casts incorporating the tibial pins. *B*, The patient's pulmonary function deteriorated rapidly, and mobilization of the patient to enhance pulmonary care was deemed necessary. To do so, the femoral fractures were fixed on the fourth day after injury by closed intramedullary Sampson nailing on the right femur and Ender pinning on the left femur. A Sarmiento cast was applied on the right tibia and a cast-brace on the left femur. The patient was out of bed the following day. After 3 months, roentgenographic evidence showed healing of all the fractures. The patient was able to walk bearing weight on each lower limb without external support at that time. The fractures healed without incident.

through both femoral epicondyles and into the femoral head and greater trochanter as shown in Figure 18-3B. The disadvantages of Ender pins are that unstable shaft fractures may require protection for 3 to 6 weeks in a cast-brace or intermittent traction; they are insufficient as the sole fixation for transcervical and subcapital hip fractures; and they are contraindicated in most fractures of the distal half of the shaft because of the risk of a fracture extending from the entry hole. Previous experience with Ender pins in routine hip fractures is a necessary prerequisite to undertaking treatment of one of these difficult fractures.

My Preferred Methods

I prefer to fix both fractures internally unless surgery is contraindicated by the patient's general condition, the presence of infection or a highly contaminated open fracture, or the fact that the shaft fracture is so comminuted as to not be amenable to internal fixation. In the latter instance, I treat the intracapsular hip fracture with closed reduction and percutaneous Knowles pin fixation and treat the shaft with a cast-brace using early mobilization with intermittent traction. If surgery is contraindicated and the hip fracture is extracapsular, I treat both fractures with skeletal traction if the patient is capable of withstanding prolonged bed rest. In the polytrauma patient or elderly patient in whom surgery is not possible, I have, on rare occasions, used well-leg traction or a Hoffman external fixation device to facilitate mobilization of the patient.

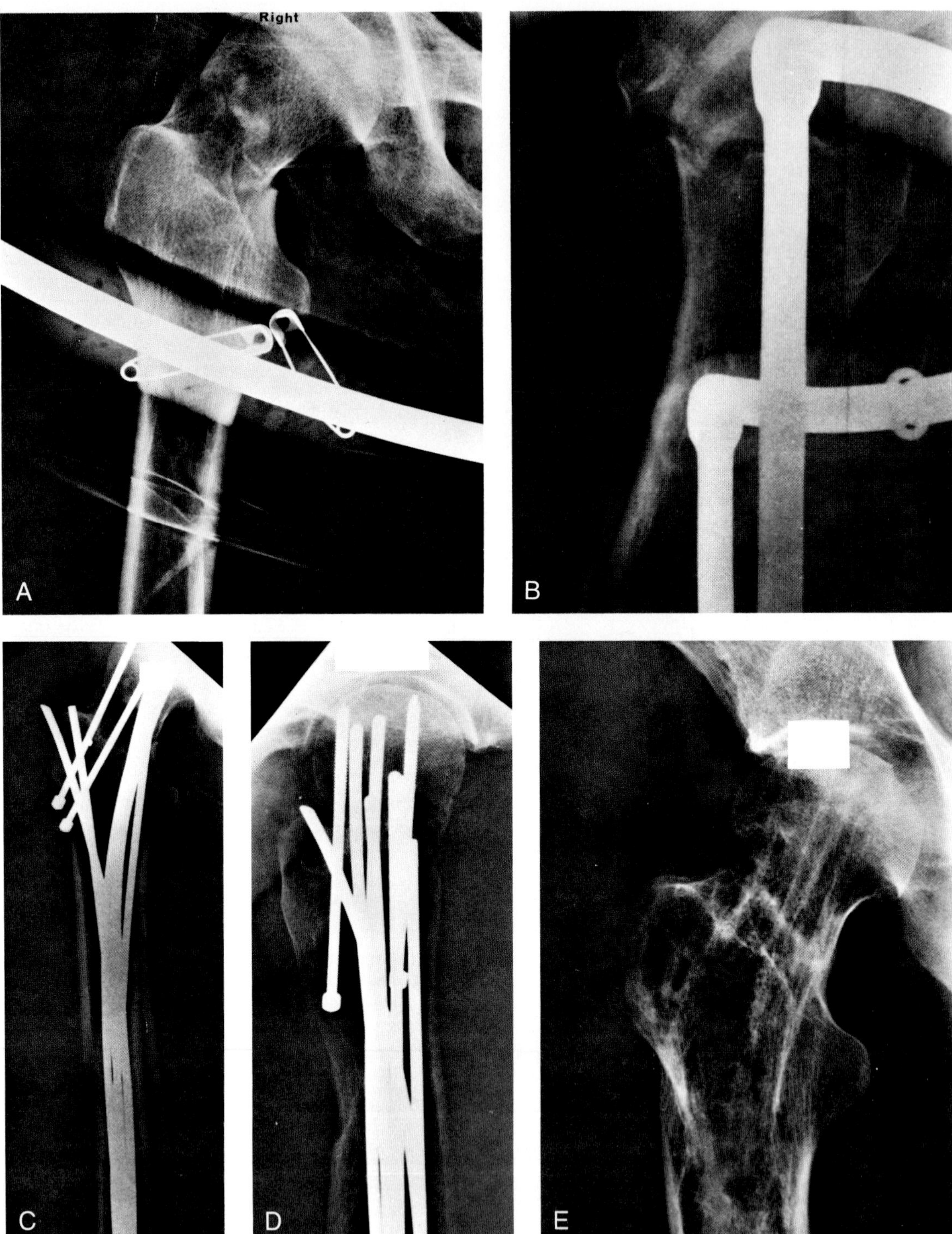

Fig. 18-3. *A* and *B*, This 26-year-old man sustained a comminuted closed fracture of the proximal shaft of the right femur and a displaced (Garden type III) transcervical fracture of the ipsilateral femoral neck when a 90-kg crate fell on him. These anteroposterior and lateral roentgenograms show the hip fracture well, but the shaft fracture extends somewhat more distally. *C* and *D*, These fractures were treated with closed reduction and percutaneous fixation by Knowles pins and Enders pins seen in these anteroposterior and lateral roentgenograms taken 4 months postoperatively. *E*, The fractures healed uneventfully, and aseptic necrosis of the femoral head did not occur. This anteroposterior roentgenogram was taken 11 months after injury (the time of hardware removal).

For most combinations, I prefer to use Ender pins augmented by Knowles pins using percutaneous technique under fluoroscopic control. If the shaft fracture is too distal for Ender pins but suitable for an intramedullary rod (transverse or short oblique and more than 10 cm proximal to the knee joint line) and the hip fracture is intracapsular, I prefer to place a Küntscher intramedullary nail by closed technique followed by percutaneous Knowles pins. If the shaft fracture is not suitable for Enders pins or an intramedullary rod, I internally fix the shaft fracture with a compression plate and fix the hip with either Knowles pins or a compression hip screw. Because all these surgical techniques are standard, they will not be discussed further.

All these options are functionally oriented, and immediate rehabilitation of the patient can begin in the immediate postoperative period. Even patients in traction can begin on isometric exercises of the involved extremity and motion of uninvolved joints.

References

1. Casey, M. J., and Chapman, M. W.: Ipsilateral concomitant fractures of the hip and femoral shaft. J. Bone Joint Surg., *61-A*:503, 1979.
2. Ritchey, S. J., Schonholtz, G. J., and Thompson, M. S.: The dashboard femoral fracture. Pathomechanics, treatment and prevention. J. Bone Joint Surg., *40-A*:1347, 1958.
3. Wright, P. E., and Becker, G. E.: Results of treatment of simultaneous hip and femoral shaft fractures. Orthop. Trans. *3*:43, 1979.
4. Kimbrough, E. E.: Concomitant unilateral hip and femoral-shaft fractures. A too frequently unrecognized syndrome. Report of five cases. J. Bone Joint Surg., *43-A*:443, 1961.
5. MacKenzie, D. B.: Simultaneous ipsilateral fracture of the femoral neck and shaft: report of 8 cases. South Afr. Med. J., *45*:459, 1971.
6. Bernstein, S. M.: Fractures of the femoral shaft and associate ipsilateral fractures of the hip. Orthop. Clin. North Am., *5*:799, 1974.
7. Delaney, W. M., and Strett, D. M.: Fracture of femoral shaft with fracture of neck of same femur. Treatment with medullary nail for shaft and Knowles pins for neck. J. Int. Coll. Surg., *19*:303, 1953.
8. Schatzker, J., and Barrington, T. W.: Fractures of the femoral neck associated with fractures of the same femoral shaft. Can. J. Surg., *11*:297, 1968.
9. Dencker, H.: Femoral shaft fracture and fracture of the neck of the same femur. Acta Chir. Scand., 129:597, 1965.
10. Ashby, M. E., and Anderson, J. C.: Treatment of fractures of the hip and ipsilateral femur with the Zickel device. A report of three cases. Clin. Orthop., *127*:156, 1977.
11. DiStefano, V. J., Nixon, J. E., and Klein, K. S.: Stable fixation of the difficult subtrochanteric fracture. J. Trauma, *12*:1066, 1972.
12. Fielding, J. W., Cochran, G. V. B., and Zickel, R. E.: Biomechanical characteristics and surgical management of subtrochanteric fractures. Orthop. Clin. North Am., *5*:629, 1974.
13. Chapman, M. W., et al.: The use of Ender's pins in extracapsular fractures of the hip. J. Bone Joint Surg., *63-A*:14, 1981.
14. Wolfgang, G. L.: Combined trochanteric and ipsilateral shaft fractures of the femur treated with the Zickel device. A case report. Clin. Orthop., *117*:241, 1976.
15. Pankovich, A. M., Goldflies, M. L., and Pearson, R. L.: Closed Ender nailing of femoral shaft fractures. J. Bone Joint Surg., *61-A*:222, 1979.

Chapter 19 Segmental Fractures of the Lower Extremity and the Floating Knee

ROBERT A. WINQUIST

Segmental femoral fractures, segmental tibial fractures, and ipsilateral femoral and tibial fractures ("floating knee") are complex fractures that require special attention in the multiply injured patient. Although each of these fractures has unique characteristics, all share certain common features. Central injuries, including head, chest, and abdominal injuries, are commonly associated with these fractures. Because central injuries are life threatening, they take priority over the fractures. Segmental fractures and ipsilateral femoral and tibial fractures are often dramatic, but at no time should their presence distract the physician from a total examination of the patient. These fractures in themselves can threaten life by causing adult respiratory distress syndrome in the absence of central lesions, and they can also threaten the viability of the limb.

After major resuscitation of the patient has been carried out and the viability of the limb has been considered, the treatment for the specific injury must be outlined. The major function of the lower extremity, stability in weightbearing, must be considered in defining the ultimate treatment goal and in choosing the treatment. Alignment of the lower extremity, as well as control of length and rotation, is mandatory. Although minor deviations in alignment, length, and rotation are well tolerated, major deviations are unacceptable as an ultimate outcome and may accentuate a persistent nonunion. A further requirement is maintenance of joint motion, which ultimately leads to improved function in an extremity. Early mobilization of the multiply injured patient is also important. Thus, prolonged immobilization in traction and a cast is an inappropriate treatment for most of these fractures. Functional casts with hinges allow joint mobility. Also, any method of internal fixation should allow adequate joint motion.

The treatment plan for the multiply injured patient is quite different from that for patients with an isolated fracture of a femur or a tibia. In the patient with multiple injuries, internal fixation of all fractures should be strongly considered. In addition, when multiple injuries are sustained in a single extremity, stabilization of all fractures should be given even higher priority. Although the treatment must be tailored individually to the patient, the surgeon, and the specific injury, I believe that the tendency should be toward fixation of all fractures in the multiply injured extremity. This treatment will meet the goals of maintaining alignment, providing stability, and allowing motion.

After resuscitation of the patient, the goals of wound healing and bone healing should be given highest priority. Generally, these goals are more difficult to attain in the tibia than in the femur. Open fractures are common with both segmental fractures and floating knees. In all fractures, neurovascular injury must be analyzed routinely and treated immediately. Open wounds require meticulous debridement and careful postoperative management. Localized stripping of the bone leads to delayed healing, and local damage to the muscles and subcutaneous tissue causes late scarring and joint stiffness. The soft-tissue injuries are a reflection of the velocity of the injury and are the best indicator of the eventual outcome of each of these fractures.

The ultimate treatment goals for these complex fractures in the multiply injured patient include soft-tissue healing, bone healing, good alignment, good range of joint motion, minimal complications, and minimal hospital costs. These ultimate goals put our treatments to the ultimate test. These treatments are not always readily attainable; thus, patience is required on the part of both surgeon and patient. Multiple surgeries are often necessary in the more complex cases.

With these general principles in mind, we will investigate the specific fracture patterns and will outline a management plan for the particular problems associated with each.

A review of the literature reveals little discussion specifically on the segmental femoral fracture.[4,5] The integrity of the blood supply, which comes primarily from an endosteal and extraosteal mode, is of primary concern. Rhinelander has shown that reaming of the medullary canal destroys the important endosteal system, but this system is reincorporated in approximately 8 weeks.[6] Stripping of the periosteal system also retards fracture healing, but this system can be restored or can be compensated for by the endosteal system. Danckwardt-Lillieström and Sjögren have demonstrated in animal experiments that the destruction of the endosteal system is an important factor in fracture healing and should not be taken lightly.[7] Küntscher, however, has shown that endosteal reaming does not appear to be detrimental in the femur when intramedullary nailing is performed by a closed method that maintains the periosteal blood supply.[8] Closed intramedullary nailing has proved to be a satisfactory method of fixation that yields a high rate of union, as we have shown in clinical studies.[9]

Segmental Femoral Fractures

This section will deal with double-level fractures of the femur. Included will be fractures below the lesser trochanter that do not involve the knee joint. Fractures with an intact segment will be differentiated from fractures with split segments and comminution. Specifically excluded will be fractures of the femoral neck and intertrochanteric fractures, which have been covered in Chapter 18 and present different problems. Also excluded will be intra-articular supracondylar femoral fractures that require rigid anatomic reconstruction, as these are covered in Chapter 22. In addition, segmental bone loss will not be discussed.

The major problems to be addressed in femoral fractures are mechanical.[1] Injuries to the soft tissues tend to be less severe in femoral fractures than in tibial fractures, and although open fractures are frequent, the problems of major infection and major local vascular compromise are unusual.[2] Therefore, the priorities in treating these fractures are primarily to stabilize the bone to maintain alignment and simultaneously to maintain overall length and rotation while allowing range of motion of the knee. These mechanical goals are frequently difficult to attain in the segmental femoral fracture.[3]

Fracture Types

Segmental femoral fractures must be analyzed carefully and the treatment individualized for each specific fracture type. One must check to see how far the fracture extends proximally and distally. By examining the degree of displacement on initial roentgenograms, one can assess the amount and severity of soft-tissue injury and, thus, better anticipate healing time. Each fracture type presents its own challenges: transverse fractures are easy to align, but rotation may be hard to control; oblique fractures have a tendency toward shortening; comminuted fractures have a great propensity toward both shortening and rotation; open fractures must be debrided.

The timing of surgery is also important. A conflict often arises in determining the appropriate time for surgery. For the multiply injured patient, early stabilization of the fracture, accompanied by mobilization of the patient, is beneficial.[10,11] If the fracture alone is considered, however, delayed surgery stimulates bone healing and allows better preoperative planning, improved operating-room conditions and greater availability of implants.[12,13] If surgery is delayed too long, however, reduction becomes difficult, and a fracture that might have been easy to stabilize early in the course of treatment may become impossible to align. Therefore, I believe that primary stabilization should be used in patients with open fractures and in multiply injured patients with major long-bone fractures. In the more stable patient, however, I believe that delayed surgery offers the possibility of better technique and also is more beneficial to bone healing. Each case, then, must be assessed as to the appropriate time for surgery.

Treatment Alternatives

Nonoperative Treatment. Treatment of a segmental femoral fracture with prolonged traction and a spica cast meets none of the treatment goals of stabilizing the bone, maintaining overall length and rotation, and allowing range of motion of the knee and early mobilization of the patient. I believe that this method should be used only when no other means of treatment is available and, perhaps, then should be used only transiently in the early treatment of these fractures. Roller traction and cast-brace treatment can be considered for these fractures, however. This treatment achieves the goals of early mobilization of the patient and the extremity and results in relatively good ultimate function.[13a] Unfortunately, alignment of segmental femoral fractures in traction and casts is difficult to achieve, and therefore, shortening and varus angulation can be anticipated in a high percentage of cases (Fig. 19-1). Secondary correction of these deformities is difficult to achieve in malunited segmental femoral fractures. In addition, although union is generally not a problem in femoral fractures, the potential for nonunion becomes a consideration in these higher-velocity injuries to the femur with endosteal and periosteal stripping and open wounds. Because treatment of nonunion in a malpositioned fracture is difficult, the use of roller traction and cast-bracing is a less appealing method for handling these challenging fractures.

External Fixation. External fixation is also a less than ideal means of treating segmental femoral fractures. This method provides only a short-term solution, which may make the long-term resolution of the fracture more difficult to attain. Since healing may be a problem in these complex fractures, the distraction produced by an external fixation device becomes a major consideration. A stable frame to the femur is also somewhat difficult to apply without damaging the femoral artery; therefore, half-pin units frequently are necessary. Excellent alignment is difficult to achieve, and loss of position is common (Fig. 19-2). Pin-tract infection and loosening frequently occur at 6 to 8 weeks, particularly if knee range-of-motion exercises have been started. Unfortunately, these fractures rarely heal within the 8-week time period. Thus, shortening, varus angulation, and instability occur with removal of the external fixation device. Bone grafting, plating, and intramedullary nailing become less appealing when a pin-tract infection is present; therefore, treatment following external fixation can be even more difficult to carry out than if the fracture had been treated in traction alone.

I believe that external fixation should be reserved for the severe grade III open injury, and even then, fixation poses difficulties. Although I do not wish to negate this treatment totally for segmental femoral fractures, I do suggest that it be used rarely, and then only as a temporizing treatment.

Plates. The use of plating in femoral fractures has met with little enthusiasm throughout the world. This lack of enthusiasm extends to its use in simple femoral fractures, where its failure has been high. The plate is a load-bearing device that requires prompt healing; otherwise, failure of the plate occurs.[14] If any comminution is present in the fracture, particularly medially, failure is even more common, and bone grafting frequently is required. Atrophy of the bone occurs under the plate, and after plate removal, the patient is at risk for fracture of the bone through the screw holes (Fig. 19-3). Because of the high failure rate with plates in simple femoral fractures, there are only a few advocates of the use of plates in any fracture of the femoral shaft.[15–17]

The problems of plating are compounded in segmental fractures of the femur. Vascular and soft-tissue injury is greater and healing times are longer. Thus, the risk of plate failure is higher. Furthermore, applying the plate is more technically demanding. Comminution and bone defects are common and require bone grafting. Because plates meet the goal of early stabilization of the fracture with excellent alignment and early range of motion of the joint, they may be appealing as an early, and temporizing, solution. However, the large wound and surgical stripping required for plate application greatly increase the risk of infection and nonunion. Therefore, this treatment form is both technically and mechanically unsound; its use is rare in segmental femoral fractures.

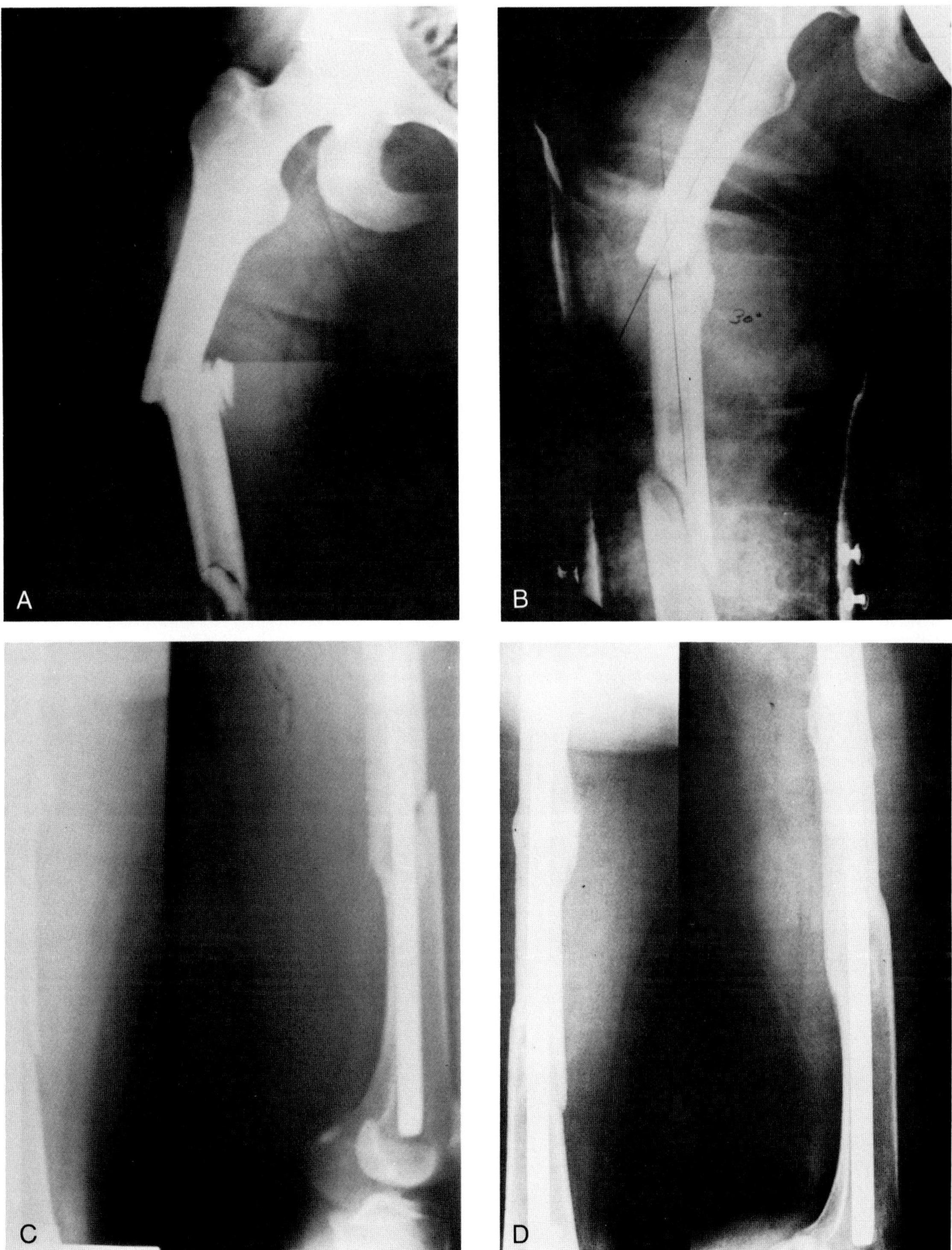

Fig. 19-1. *A*, Roentgenogram of a closed segmental femoral fracture in a 27-year-old woman who was involved in a motor-vehicle accident. *B*, Alignment was achieved with traction, but was subsequently lost; a cast-brace was applied at 2 months. *C*, At 4 months, the cast-brace was removed. The fracture was manipulated to achieve alignment, and closed intramedullary nailing was performed. *D*, Solid union was achieved at 6 months.

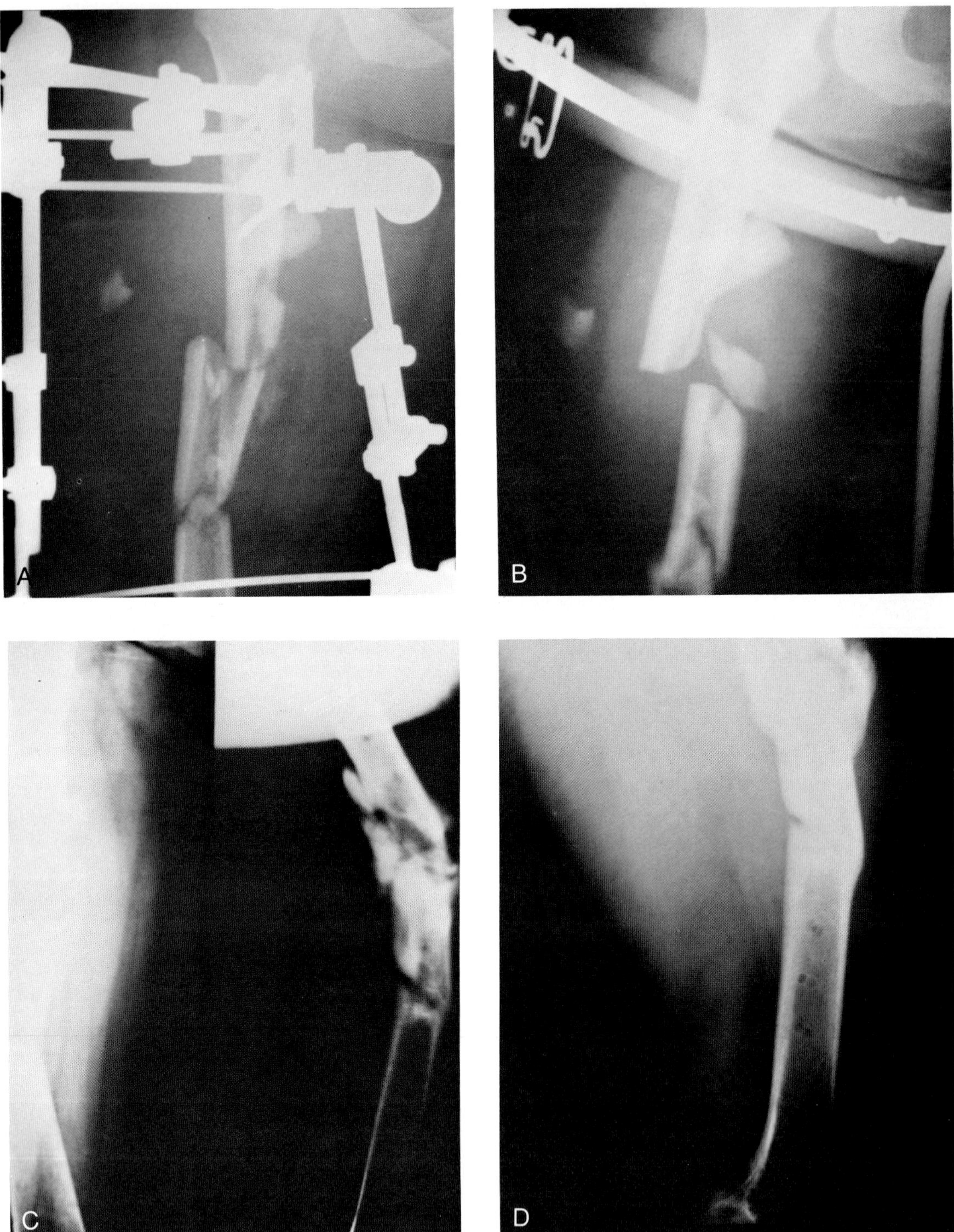

Fig. 19-2. *A*, Roentgenogram demonstrates a segmental femoral fracture with a nondisplaced basilar neck fracture in a 26-year-old woman injured in a motor-vehicle accident. She was treated initially in traction. *B*, A Hoffman external fixation device was applied, and bone grafting was performed to try to stimulate healing. *C*, Progressive angulation occurred, and the bone failed to unite. *D*, One year after injury, the patient had knee stiffness as well as malunion and persistent nonunion at both fracture levels. Her deformity continued to progress.

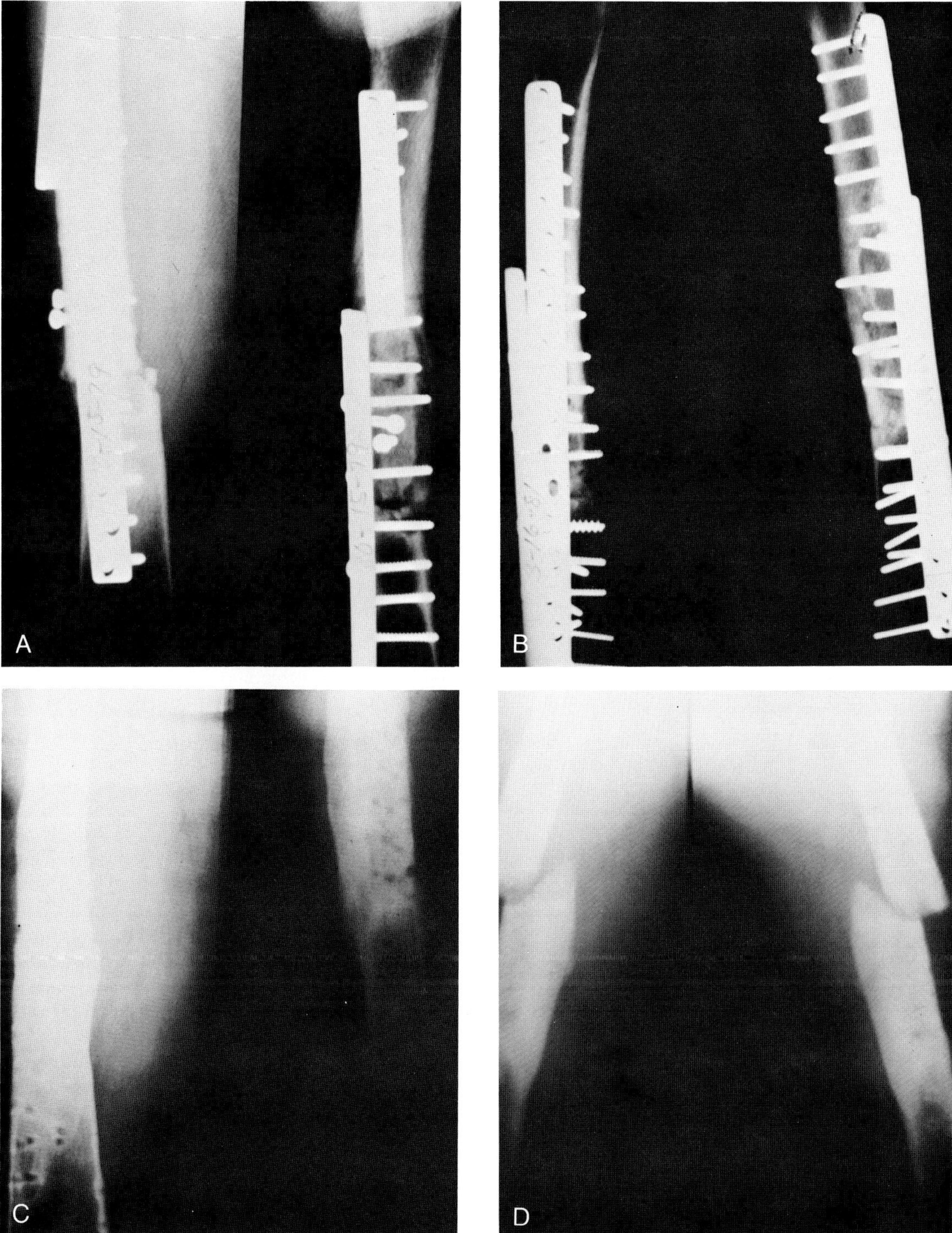

Fig. 19-3. *A*, Roentgenogram taken 5 months after this 26-year-old man was injured in a motor-vehicle accident shows a segmental femur fracture that has been fixed with 2 plates. The distal fracture is unstable. *B*, Because of progressive instability of the distal fracture, both plates were removed and were replaced by longer plates applied at a 90° angle to each other. *C*, Two years after injury the plates were removed. *D*, Three months after plate removal, the patient suffered a refracture at the junction level between the two plates.

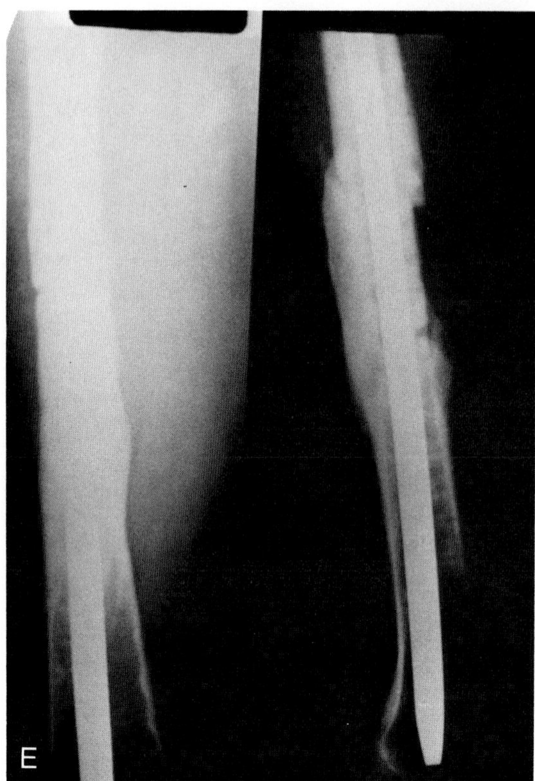

Fig. 19-3 (*continued*). *E*, After little sign of healing in traction, the femur was stabilized with a closed intramedullary nailing.

Intramedullary Nailing. A careful distinction must be made between open and closed intramedullary nailing.[18,19] Closed intramedullary nailing has a reputation for yielding a lower infection rate and a higher union rate than does open intramedullary nailing.[1,9,20–27] This reputation has been borne out in almost all series presented, and although this margin of difference between the two methods may be small in simple fractures, it becomes greater in more complex fractures. With endosteal reaming, as much of the periosteal blood supply as possible must be maintained. Therefore, further stripping to perform an open nailing, particularly a retrograde nailing, should be avoided. In addition, small-diameter intramedullary nails commonly used in open nailings provide inadequate stabilization for these complicated fractures (Fig. 19-4). Further, the rate of infection is increased with the large dissection required for an open nailing. In segmental femoral fractures, the margin of safety is decreased because of the magnitude of the injury; therefore, open nailing in such injuries produces an even higher complication rate than it does in normal simple fractures.

Closed nailing offers the best treatment form available for the segmental femoral fracture (Fig. 19-5). Mechanically, the nail has great advantages. It is an internal splint that bears little load. Therefore, the implant failure common with plates is infrequent with this appliance.[14] Nails with a diameter of at least 13 mm, the usual minimum size for an intramedullary nail, rarely fail. Because the nail provides good alignment and also allows early range of motion of the knee, it approximates the goals of treatment for these complex fractures. Unfortunately, it allows poor management of length and rotary control; thus, these fractures must be observed carefully for shortening and rotation.[27] Also, because periosteal stripping in grade III open fractures may be such that endosteal reaming will impinge too greatly on the blood supply, I am not certain that intramedullary nailing should be considered for this grade of segmental femoral fracture.

Intramedullary nailing in split segmental fractures and comminuted segmental fractures requires even more careful consideration. A simple closed nailing does not maintain adequate length in these fractures, and a combination treatment must therefore be considered.[27] The patient must be kept in traction, either before or after intramedullary nailing is performed, for at least 6 to 8 weeks to maintain bone length. A second treatment option is the use of open cerclage wire (Fig. 19-6); this method generally provides excellent anatomic restoration, but produces a larger operative wound, thus increasing the risk of infection.[27] It also necessitates more periosteal stripping, which increases the risk of nonunion. The use of interlocking nails, which can be inserted by a closed method and maintain length and rotation, is thus an appealing alternative (Fig. 19-7).[9]

Technically, a nailing with interlocking nails is more difficult to perform than is a simple closed nailing. If union is delayed at 3 months, the interlocking screws can be removed to allow impaction of the fracture, thereby decreasing the risk of nonunion. The fracture then is adequately aligned, early motion of the joint is allowed, and

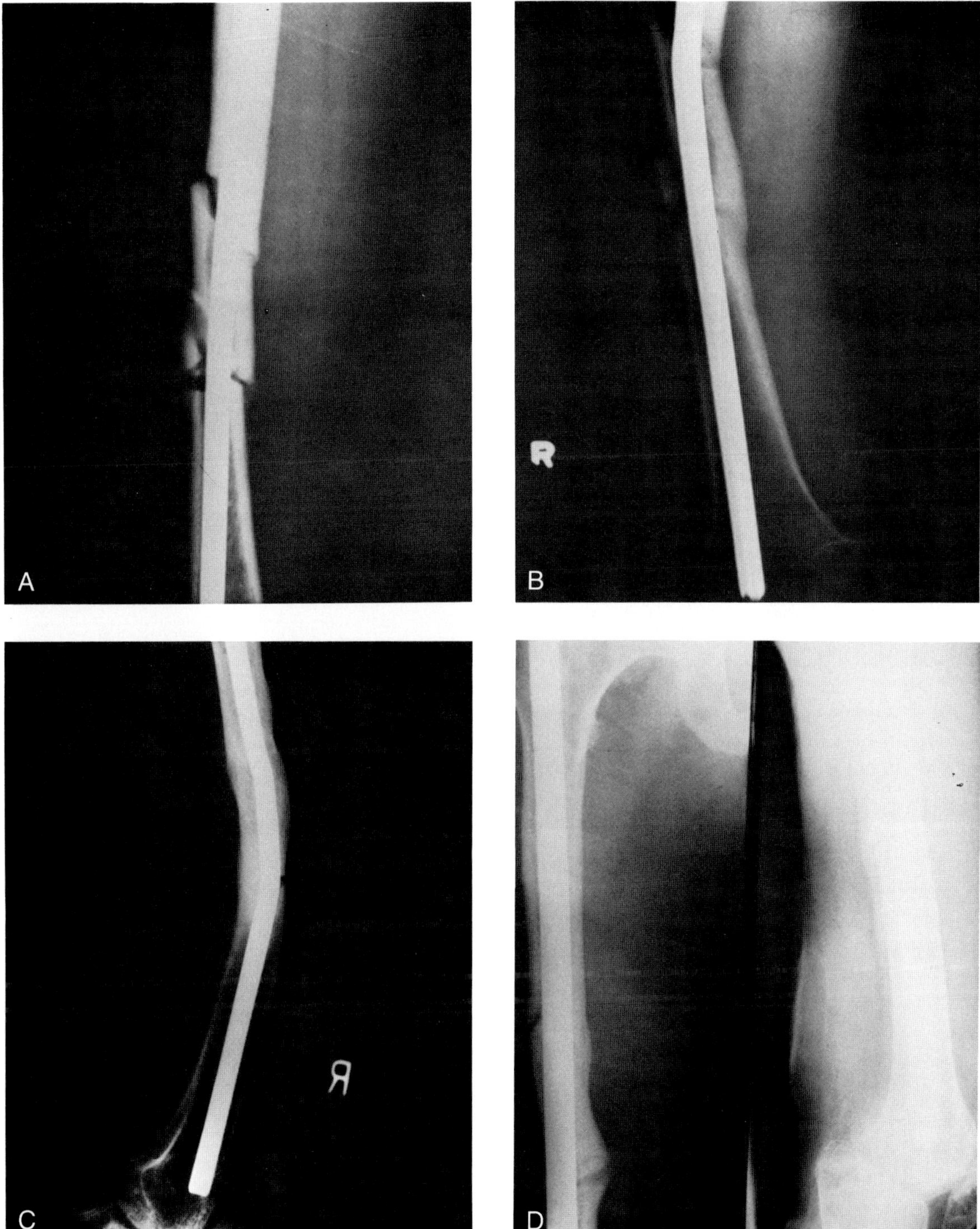

Fig. 19-4. *A*, Roentgenogram of a 26-year-old man who sustained a segmental femur fracture in a motor-vehicle accident. This grade I open fracture was treated with an open retrograde intramedullary nailing. *B*, Brittle bending of the nail at the proximal fracture site is apparent on film taken 3 weeks after the nailing. *C*, The proximal fracture healed, but 6 months after injury, the nail bent at the distal fracture site. The patient continued to experience pain at this site 5 years after injury. *D*, At 5 years, the nail was removed, and with manipulation, the distal fracture was straightened. A second intramedullary nailing was performed, and the bone subsequently united.

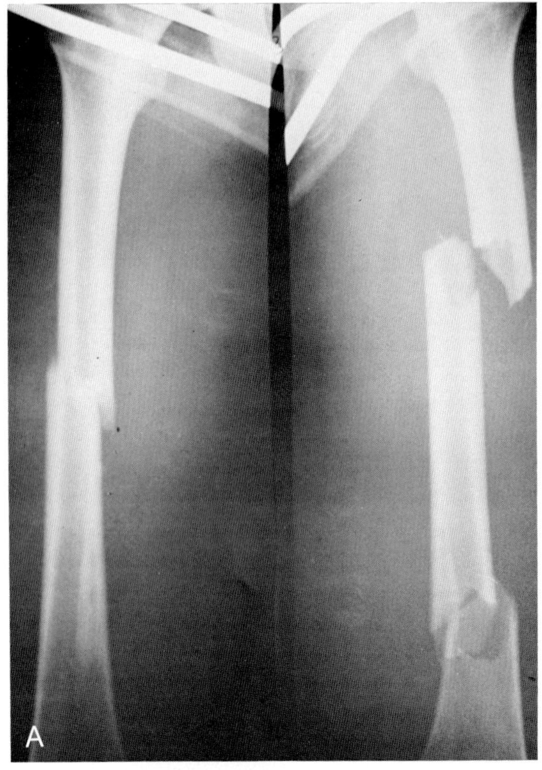

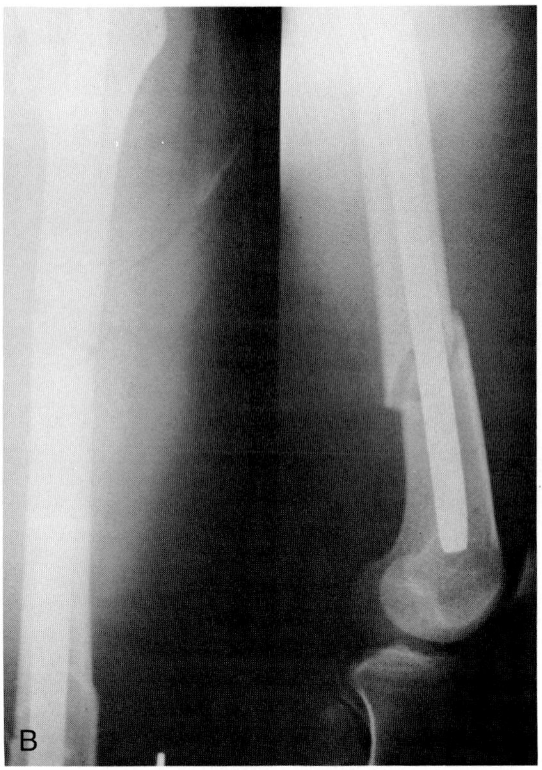

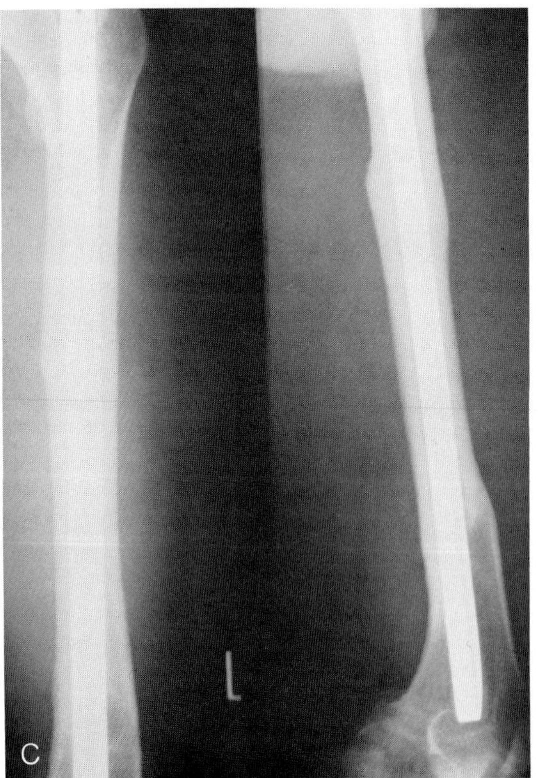

Fig. 19-5. *A*, A 19-year-old man suffered a closed fracture of the right femur and a closed segmental fracture of the left femur in a high-velocity motor-vehicle accident. *B*, A closed intramedullary nailing of both femora was performed 8 days after injury. The patient developed fat embolism following injury, which was treated with pulmonary support prior to nailing. *C*, Solid union of the fracture was achieved 18 months after injury.

length and rotation are maintained in these difficult fractures. Should the bone fail to unite, the treatment is simple in a totally aligned femur: the femur is rereamed and a larger nail is inserted in a closed fashion. Treatment with the interlocking nail has received a great deal of enthusiasm in Germany and should receive further consideration in this country.[28]

In summary, I prefer the following method of treatment for segmental femoral fractures. Segmental fractures of the femur with an intact segment should be treated with closed intramedullary nailing. For comminuted fractures, closed nailing with interlocking nails should be considered. The next option is treatment with a combination of cerclage wiring and intramedullary nailing. This method increases the risk of infection and nonunion but provides excellent anatomic

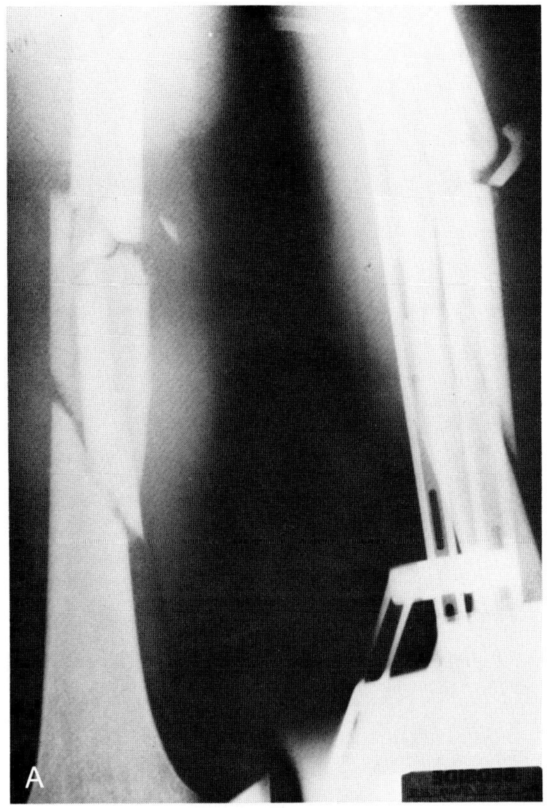

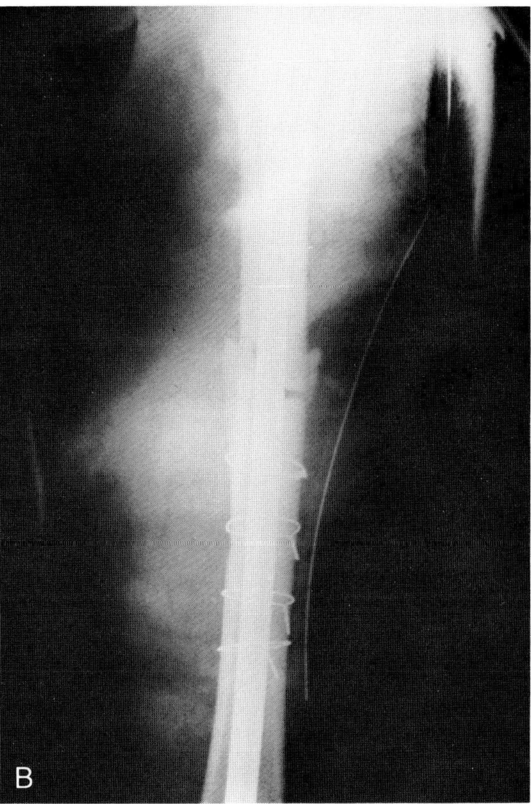

FIG. 19-6. *A*, A 21-year-old man involved in a motor-vehicle accident sustained a closed split segmental fracture of the femur. *B*, Postoperative roentgenogram shows an intramedullary nail and cerclage wiring. Because the patient could not be relied upon to follow a treatment regimen, he was placed in a spica cast for 6 weeks. *C*, Films taken 4 months after injury show the fracture proceeding to union.

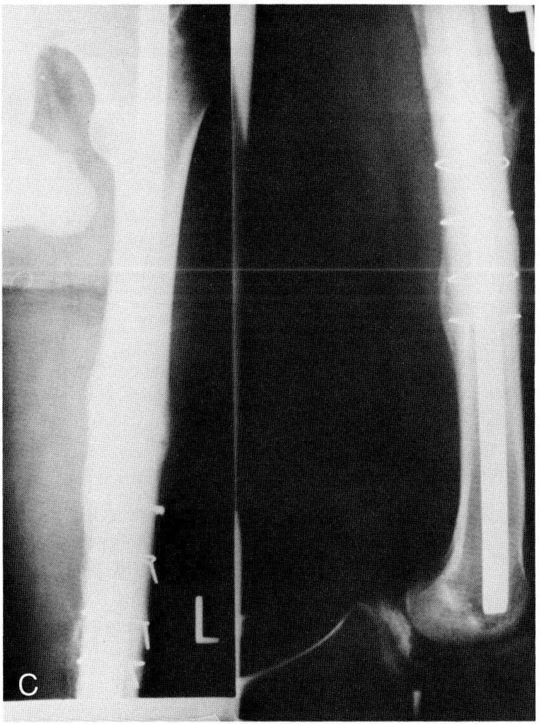

reduction. It also allows relatively early weight-bearing through the nail system and, thus, is ultimately a good treatment system. The mechanical failure rate associated with plating, as well as the large surgical procedure required for plate application, makes this method a poor choice for treatment of the segmental femoral fracture. External fixation has little to offer except in the early management of the severely opened segmental femoral fracture.

Postoperative Management

Postoperative management is important to the overall outcome of the fracture and depends on the specific injury as well as the fixation achieved.[9,29] In determining appropriate postoperative management, the physician must carefully analyze the patient's multiple injuries and

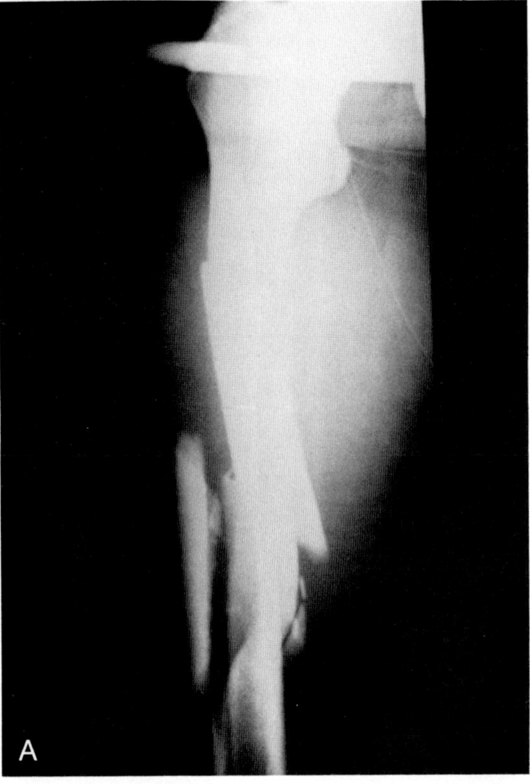

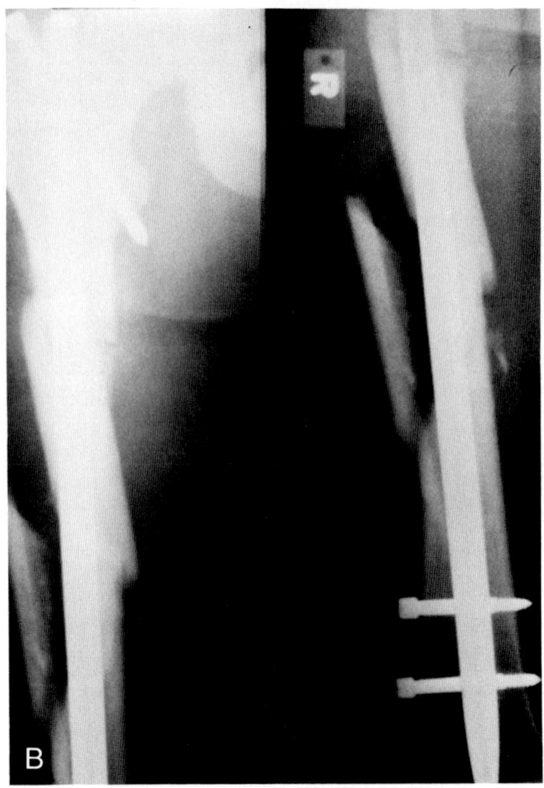

Fig. 19-7. *A*, Roentgenogram demonstrates a comminuted femoral shaft fracture in a 19-year-old man injured in a downhill ski race. *B*, Films taken 2 weeks after operation show overall good alignment with an interlocking nail. *C*, At 14 months, progressive healing has taken place, and the patient has returned to downhill skiing.

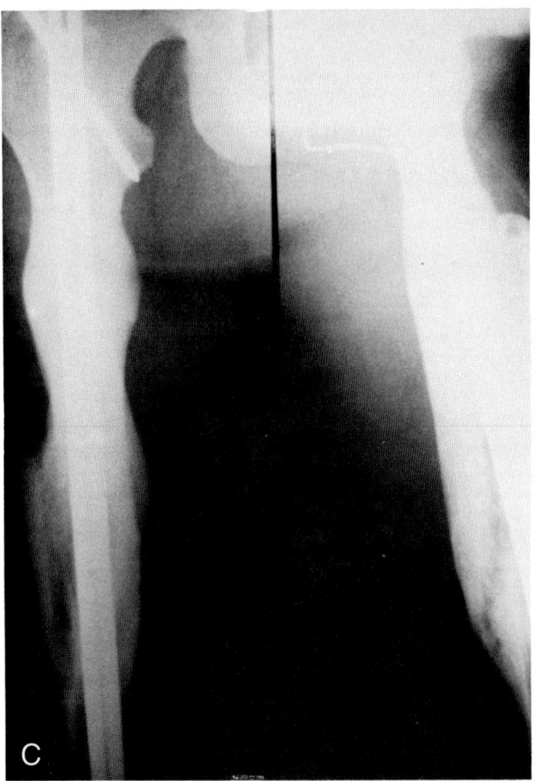

also his personality and ability to cooperate. Early knee motion is desirable, but I have found that as long as the knee is moved within 6 weeks after fracture, final function tends to be quite good. Therefore, unlike the situation with intra-articular supracondylar fractures, early motion for segmental femoral fractures does not mean motion at 5 days but does mean motion within the first few weeks.

Mobilization is important for patients with multiple injuries. In more distal fractures, a cylinder or cast-brace may be required to prevent varus or valgus angulation, particularly if intramedullary nailing is used. This brace can be removed at 4 to 6 weeks. Proximal fractures must be analyzed carefully for rotation, which must be controlled by the use of an antirotation boot, traction or a short-term spica cast. Comminuted fractures must be kept in traction or fixed with an interlocking nail or cerclage wire, and no weight should be borne on the limb for 6 to 8 weeks. The importance of abstaining from weightbearing must be explained to the patient carefully and repeatedly.

The postoperative plan should be determined at the time of the operation and altered only if a good reason for change becomes apparent during the follow-up treatment. The standard postoperative treatment for segmental femoral fractures is early quadriceps rehabilitation, which frees the quadriceps from the fracture scar and allows range of motion of the knee. Range-of-motion exercises for the knee should be started as early as possible, but they should consist of gentle active motion only; vigorous passive motion should be delayed for 8 to 12 weeks. The range of motion achieved must be monitored carefully for a full 3 to 6 months until complete motion is obtained; this is best assessed by having the patient kneel and then sit back on his heels. Rehabilitation of the knee must be followed carefully by the physical therapist, and the strength of the quadriceps muscle should be tested on the Cybex II. Chondromalacia is commonly related not only to the injury, but also to early quadriceps instability and poor tracking of the patella. Because of this potential complication, rehabilitation of the knee is an essential part of treatment of these fractures.[29]

Results

Few papers have appeared on intact segmental femoral fractures and comminuted segmental femoral fractures. My associates and I have experience with 32 cases of intact segmental fractures of the femur with an infection rate of zero and a nonunion rate of zero. In this series, range of motion of the knee averaged 135°, and maximum shortening was 1.5 cm. Maximum rotary malformation was 30°, and maximum valgus angulation measured 11°. All these patients were treated with closed intramedullary nailing. Postoperative treatment was varied and included traction for some comminuted fractures and transient knee cylinders and cast-braces for more distal fractures. The results in this particular series strongly suggest that closed nailing is the best treatment alternative; however, this treatment certainly is not available in all communities.

Results have been reported for several series of comminuted fractures.[30] Cast-brace treatment has produced some good results in several fractures in these series, although no series has addressed itself specifically to the use of this treatment method. Funk, et al.,[5] and Mueller[31] have advised the use of intramedullary nailing with additional internal fixation as the best means for treating the split segmental fracture. We have shown that split segmental fractures and comminuted segmental fractures of the femur have a high incidence of shortening and malrotation when conventional closed nailing is used alone; therefore, traction, cerclage wire, or interlocking nails must be used in combination with intramedullary nailing.[27] Of the 54 cases in our series, 1 infection occurred in a grade I open fracture that was treated with cerclage wire and intramedullary nailing. Two fractures failed to unite. Knee motion averaged 135°. Five patients treated with intramedullary nailing alone had greater than 2 cm of shortening. Malrotation of greater than 20° occurred in 5 patients, and the maximum angulatory deformity was 10°. Although excellent alignment and range of knee motion are being achieved with simple closed intramedullary nailing, the potential for shortening and rotation diminishes the desirability of this treatment and necessitates further means to attain length and rotational control. Major complications of infection and nonunion are rare with this treatment method, however.

Complications

Infection in a fracture represents a major complication and is related primarily to the magnitude of the initial injury and also to poor surgical debridement and poor wound care. When infection occurs, vigorous debridement and draining of the infected area are required. When the tissues are quieted adequately, late sequestrectomy and bone grafting to attain union are necessary.

Nonunion is also a difficult complication to manage. When the fracture is fixed initially with plating or nailing, alignment is excellent. Repeated nailing generally achieves union and also allows weightbearing. Bone grafting may also be necessary. When the initial treatment is administered by nonoperative means, however, alignment of the fracture generally is quite disturbed, and late treatment is difficult. Realignment over an intramedullary nail offers the best mechanical solution, but this is a major procedure and often is most challenging to perform. Because of the great difficulties involved in managing late complications that occur with early nonoperative treatment, I suggest that this treatment generally is not desirable in segmental femoral fractures.

Stiffness of the knee is also a problem with segmental femoral fractures. I have seen this complication only in fractures in which early nonoperative treatment was used, particularly prolonged immobilization in traction and a spica cast. This complication can be resolved with quadricepsplasty, which is generally successful in achieving motion up to 120°. Frequently, this procedure can be performed only in the suprapatellar pouch area, but occasionally, dissection up to the area of the fracture is required. This dissection is done through a lateral incision, elevating the scar tissue circumferentially but leaving a soft-tissue padding over the bone itself. The patient must be treated vigorously with therapy both in the hospital and as an outpatient.

Malrotation with these fractures tends to be asymptomatic unless the arc of internal rotation approaches zero. If even 10 to 15° of internal rotation is maintained, these malunited fractures rarely are symptomatic.[9] When malrotation occurs, it can be corrected easily if the fracture has been aligned surgically. A simple closed intramedullary derotational osteotomy manages this deformity. If the fracture has been initially treated nonoperatively, however, secondary procedures will be difficult to perform.

Angulation with segmental femoral fractures occurs most often when external fixation has traction and cast methods have been used. This complication is rarely seen after primary internal fixation.

Segmental Tibial Fractures

This section will cover segmental fractures, including double- and triple-level fractures, as well as split segmental and comminuted fractures of the tibial shaft. Comminuted fractures of the tibial plateau and comminuted fractures of the distal tibia (pilond fractures) will be excluded, as will fractures with segmental bone loss, which require special attention.

The major problem in treating segmental tibial fractures is management of the soft-tissue injuries. This problem becomes complex in these fractures and requires considerations different from the purely mechanical considerations that apply to the femur. Accurate assessment of the initial soft-tissue injury is essential, as is vigorous treatment of the soft tissues throughout the course of healing. Failure to deal promptly and accurately with the soft-tissue injuries leads to multiple failures. Mechanical considerations are much less important in the tibia than in the femur, and more methods are easily available for treating tibial fractures. The primary emphasis in mechanically stabilizing these fractures is to allow accurate treatment of the soft tissues, which is the major goal.

A review of the literature reveals little information dealing specifically with segmental fractures of the tibia.[32–34] However, information on these fractures is available in many articles on severely comminuted and open tibial fractures.[35–43] The blood supply for the tibia is similar to that for the femur; each is supplied by an endosteal and a periosteal system. Because of the limited soft-tissue envelope, however, the periosteal system is much less abundant in the tibia than in the femur; therefore, vascularity is a problem with any injury to the tibia. The injury disrupts the soft tissues and can cause a great insult to the already limited blood supply. In addition, because the musculature of the tibia is surrounded by tight fascia, compartmental syndromes are a complication to be considered in the tibia—much more so than in the femur.[44]

A severe open fracture with damage to the soft tissues, as well as potential damage to the major neurovascular structures and the possibility of compartmental syndromes, leads to the possibility of amputation with tibial fractures. Amputation is certainly a much more severe consequence of fracture than that which one faces with femoral fractures. Even if the magnitude of the injury is not so severe and these major complications can be avoided, one is still faced with the possibility of infection, nonunion, malunion, and joint stiffness as sequelae of these difficult fractures.[45–48] Conservative treatment of segmental tibial fractures by nonoperative means has led to a nonunion rate of as high as 50%. The only series in the literature that suggest excellent results are those of Lottes,[32] Zucman and Maurer,[34] and Pantazopoulos, et al.,[33] in which all patients were treated with intramedullary nailing. Their series represent some selection of patients, however, since the majority of the fractures treated had either one or two intact segments; thus the authors may not have included the most severe segmental fractures. The specific use of casts, plates, and external fixation devices for segmental femoral fractures will be discussed later in this section.

Definition of the Injury

Segmental tibial fractures occur frequently in the multiply injured patient. As discussed previously, the central injuries demanding immediate attention must be managed appropriately, and the tibial injury then must be defined accurately. The fracture must be analyzed carefully with the use of anteroposterior and lateral roentgenograms. The proximal and distal extent of each fracture must be noted, and the obliquity, as well as the comminution, must be considered at each fracture level. It must be determined whether the fracture is a double- or triple-level segmental fracture and, more importantly, whether the segment is intact. Any comminution may change the treatment alternatives. In addition, any displacement of the fractures noted on initial roentgenograms is a helpful guide in determining later treatment and in anticipating results accurately.

The extent of the soft-tissue injury is the most important criterion for predicting the outcome of a segmental tibial fracture. For defining the soft-tissue injury, the grading system of Tscherne for both closed and open injuries is helpful.[48a] Closed injuries are graded as follows: grade I—minimal swelling and muscle damage with minimal fracture displacement; grade II—moderate swelling and muscle damage with moderate fracture displacement; and grade III—severe soft-tissue injury and swelling with severe fracture displacement and comminution. These grades suggest the velocity of the injury, which is useful in determining the extent of soft-tissue injury. With the use of this grading system, one can anticipate problems with stability and particularly problems with healing. A higher grade signals the physician to watch for further swelling and changes that may affect both the mechanical and soft-tissue management.

Use of a general grading system for open fractures is also essential. These fractures must be graded not only by the size of the skin wound, but also by the estimated bony and soft-tissue injury under the skin. There are four grades of injury for these fractures. A grade I open injury generally is characterized by a puncture wound; soft-tissue stripping and injury beneath the skin are not extensive. A grade II injury has a larger open wound without gross contamination and generally more displacement of the fracture on initial injury. There is a transitional zone in the grading, however, and a patient with a puncture wound to the skin may be found to have a grade II open injury when the soft tissues under the skin are inspected and found to be severely stripped and damaged. A grade III open injury has a large open wound and extensive damage to the skin and soft tissues, as well as extensive displacement of the bone, which causes further tearing of the skin and soft tissues. In these fractures, local blood supply is severely compromised. Grade IV open injuries threaten immediate loss of limb. These injuries include severe fractures to the bone with injuries of the neurovascular system and partial or complete amputations, all of which threaten limb viability.

These grading systems for open and closed fractures are useful. They generally offer the best prognostic tool for determining outcome and also reveal the necessity for vigorous early treatment.[38] Grading is as necessary for closed fractures as for open fractures and helps one to anticipate future problems in the management of these injuries.

Management of the open wound is complex and requires intensive care, generally at a time when operation is not possible. At the accident site, any major debris should simply be removed from the wound and a sterile dressing applied. The limb should be realigned, even in the presence of an open fracture, and a splint should be applied. If debris is pulled into the wound by realignment, this fact should be brought to the attention of the treating physician who will be debriding the wound later. Neurovascular checks at the scene of the accident are important and should be recorded carefully. The patient then can be transported to the emergency room.

In the emergency room, an extensive inspection of the wound is not necessary. Appropriate films should be taken. A swab of the wound should be taken to send to the laboratory, and the patient should be started on antibiotics.[43] My preference is cephalosporin. Tetanus toxoid should be given if appropriate. The wound remains dressed and the limb splinted while the patient awaits transport to the operating room.

In the operating room, careful debridement is necessary. This debridement becomes difficult to perform when tissues are of questionable viability. I believe that any obviously dead tissue should be removed, but that any tissue in question should be left in place; repetitive debridements may be carried out if necessary and offer an advantage over excessive initial debridement. After the major debris and dead tissue have been removed, jet lavage can be helpful in furthering the debridement. When debridement is completed, the leg generally should be prepped again and draped, and the bone should be stabilized at that time. Fasciotomy may be necessary as part of the debridement to prevent compartmental syndromes.[44]

When vascular injury is suspected, a Doppler meter should be used in the emergency room to measure the blood pressure in both legs. If any differences are found in the pressure measurements, an arteriogram should be performed. I generally prefer to perform an arteriogram in the operating room in the following manner: A scout film is taken to ascertain that the x-ray technician is performing the technique correctly and understands which area is to be evaluated. A 50-ml bolus of contrast material then is injected into the femoral artery and three 7- by 17-inch roentgenograms of the extremity are taken as rapidly as possible. With these three films, almost all traumatic injuries can be evaluated accurately if the level of filming has been correct. If an arterial injury is noted, further treatment must be coordinated with the vascular surgeons, and proper timing is necessary. Fasciotomy can be performed as the first part of treatment. The vessels are then localized, and a temporary shunt is applied to allow reinstitution of blood flow to the limb. Debridement then is carried out, followed by stabilization of the bone. The repair of the artery is the final step of the procedure. Timing in such cases is vital, and with early diagnosis, early restoration of blood flow through shunting of the artery, and decompression of the extremity with a fasciotomy, the majority of these limbs can be salvaged.

After wound debridement and stabilization of the bone, the wounds should be dressed and the limb splinted. I believe that a vitally important step in the treatment of these fractures is to place the ankle in a neutral position at the time of the initial debridement and anesthesia, and to keep it in this position throughout the course of treatment. Once the ankle drops into an equinus position, it can be brought up again only with extreme difficulty. Therefore, as part of the first day of treatment of these injuries, appropriate positioning of the ankle is mandatory. Management of the wound is also important. A small wound can be left dressed, and closure can be delayed. In a major wound with severe soft-tissue injury and exposed tendons and bone, however, a method that maintains moisture in the wound may have to be instituted. This goal can be accomplished with the use of plastic wraps or a humidifier system. A slow-drip system or frequent dressing changes with lactated Ringer's solution may be used also. When these major wounds are allowed to dry out totally, further loss of tissue ensues.

Secondary management of the wound is essential to the final outcome of the fracture. No wound should be closed under tension, either during initial debridement or during later treatment. I have found that relaxing incisions generally do not produce excellent results. In most instances, the patient should be returned to the operating room approximately 5 days after injury. The wound should be reinspected and redebrided, if necessary. Delayed primary closure should be carried out only if it can be done without producing a large dead space or requiring a great deal of tension.[46] If there is any question about dead space or tension, a split-thickness skin graft should be applied. Many of these wounds are not ready for closure at 5 days, and repeated debridement or continued dressing changes are necessary.

At present, there is a great deal of emphasis on the use of early flaps. I would caution the orthopaedic surgeon in the use of these flaps. Timing in the application of these flaps is of utmost importance. In a large open wound without severe damage to the surrounding tissues, the application of either a local flap or a vascularized pedicle flap at 5 to 10 days may be possible. However, if there is any threat that the amount of surrounding soft tissue damage cannot be defined accurately, the use of a flap should be delayed. Local flaps applied proximally, using the gastrocnemius or the soleus muscle, give excellent results. At the junction of the middle third and distal third of the tibia, the flexor digitorum communis muscle offers excellent coverage with minimal loss of function. Timing in the application of these flaps, however, is critical; these flaps cannot be used until the wound allows their rapid and thorough healing.

Vascularized pedicle flaps also can be of advantage in soft-tissue healing, but the appropriateness of their use must be assessed carefully. Unfortunately, with these injuries frequently only a single artery remains in the extremity, and this artery potentially can be jeopardized by the application of a vascularized pedicle flap. In addition, when there has been a severe shock injury to the surrounding soft tissues, one may have to proceed to the popliteal fossa to obtain a vascular supply for the flap. Long anastomosis of the artery and, particularly, the vein causes loss of viability of the flap and an undesirable result.

In the initial treatment phase, the application of a vascularized pedicle flap using the latissimus muscle or the gracilis muscle provides excellent muscle and skin coverage, the lack of which is the main problem in most of these fractures. An experienced team is required for its application. I prefer the use of local and vascularized pedicle flaps later in the treatment when the extent of injury can be better defined.

Bone grafting is also part of secondary treatment. This procedure can be performed along with the initial stabilization, at the time of delayed wound closure, or as a tertiary procedure. In the segmental tibial fracture, the emphasis must be on the repair of the soft tissues; treatment of the bone is of secondary importance.

Stabilization of the Fracture

In general, tibial fractures are much easier to stabilize than are femoral fractures. Since many methods are available for stabilization of segmental tibial fractures, there is certainly room for discussion about the proper method of stabilization, as more than one method may be appropriate for each fracture.

Casts. Casts offer an excellent method of external splintage and certainly can be used for stabilization of segmental fractures of the tibia.[49–51] The most appropriate use is in closed injuries in which the soft tissues do not require repeated inspection and debridement. In addition, casts offer the best treatment method for grade I closed injuries in which soft-tissue injury and displacement of the fracture are minimal, and in which the swelling does not change dramatically. These fractures should also have minimal shortening and minimal translation of the bone. Healing should not be a problem in a grade I soft-tissue injury with minimal shortening of the bone, and a cast is the appropriate method of treatment.

Casts can also be used to augment other methods of stabilization. Internal or external fixation of the bone may be performed primarily, and a cast may serve as a supportive splint to neutralize the fracture. The use of a cast is also mandatory for maintaining the ankle in a neutral position from the beginning of fracture treatment.

External Fixation Devices. External fixation offers an alternative form of treatment for segmental tibial fractures.[52] The advantage of this method is that it maintains the position of the fracture with a minimum of soft-tissue stripping, and thus, it does not disturb the endosteal or periosteal system. Unfortunately, it may delay healing because it works as a distraction apparatus. This delay may be an acceptable price to pay for maintaining the position of the fracture, however.

For complicated double- and triple-level segmental fractures, as well as for comminuted tibial fractures, a complex frame may be necessary. One should be able to insert pins in any possible place in the tibia; in addition, one should be able to use a unilateral, triangulated, or quadrilateral frame. It should be possible to make multiplane adjustments, as well as to produce compression and distraction. A frame that can be loosened or tightened during various phases of healing helps to allow more weight to be transmitted through the fracture and thus potentially prevents nonunion. A controversy persists over the appropriate rigidity of the frame. A less rigid frame allows more motion at the fracture site and perhaps allows more natural healing of the fracture. For severely comminuted fractures, as well as for severe soft-tissue injuries, I prefer a more rigid frame that restricts motion, allows revascularization, and permits healing of the soft tissues. If nonunion occurs, this complication can be managed at a later time.

The use of external fixation devices is an excellent method for managing open, comminuted, segmental tibial fractures and may form the primary and most commonly used method of stabilizing these severe injuries (Fig. 19-8). The external fixation systems have become complex and can be applied through a variety of methods. Accurate knowledge of the system selected and its proper application are required for a successful outcome.

Lag screws can be used in combination with external fixation devices. If an oblique fracture is noted during debridement, two lag screws may be inserted to fix the oblique fracture, and an external fixation device may be applied to neutralize the position of the bone fragments. These combination treatment methods can be most useful in segmental tibial fractures.

Plates. Plates provide an additional treatment option for segmental tibial fractures.[42] The general requirements for their use should be that they provide anatomic reduction and excellent stabil-

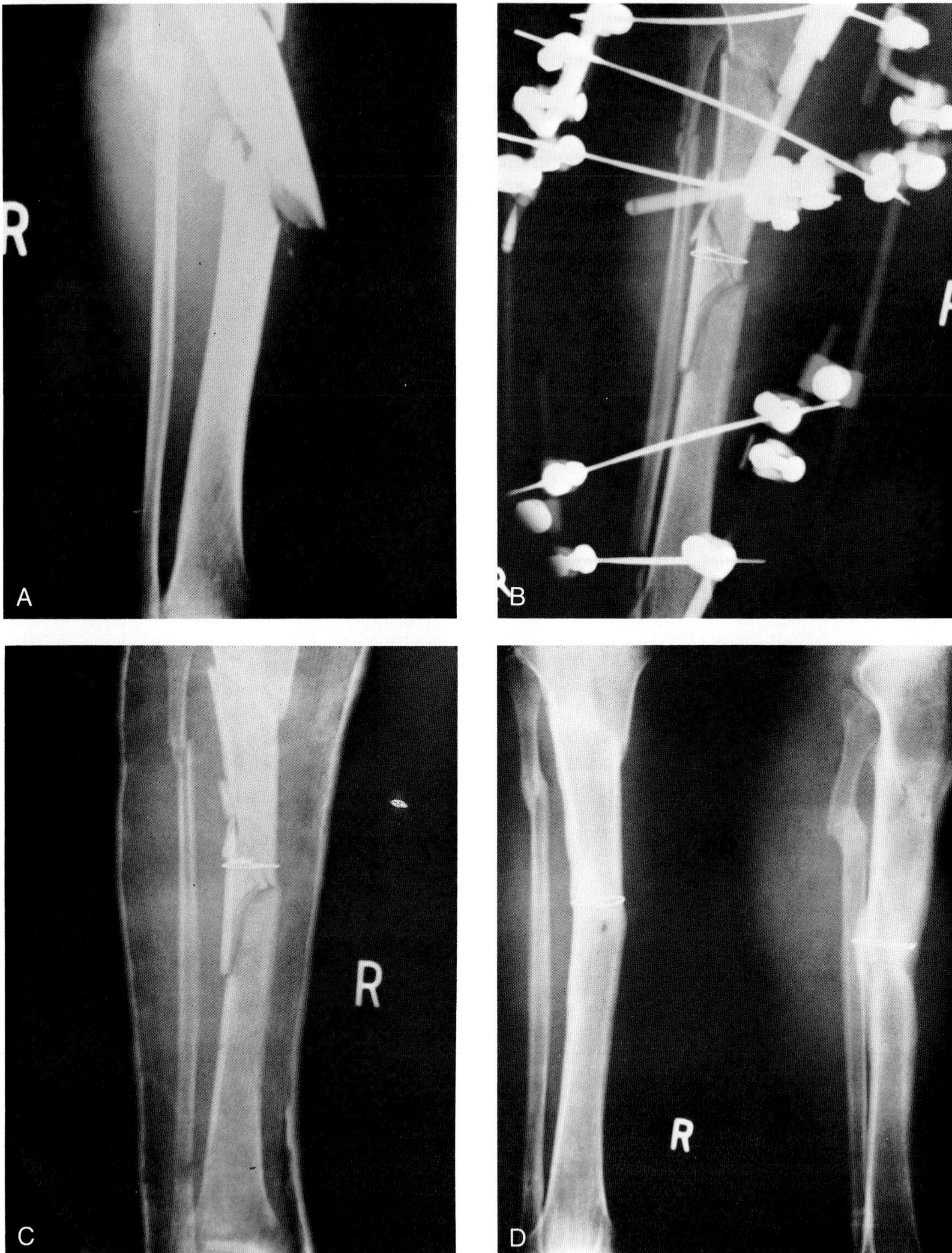

Fig. 19-8. *A*, A 32-year-old man was struck by an automobile and sustained a grade III open segmental fracture of the tibia. *B*, The fracture was aligned partially with a single cerclage wire and supported with an external fixation device. *C*, At 3 weeks, the external fixation device was removed and the patient began walking in a long-leg walking cast. *D*, Roentgenogram taken 2 years later demonstrates solid union without external support. The patient's total time in a cast was 8 months.

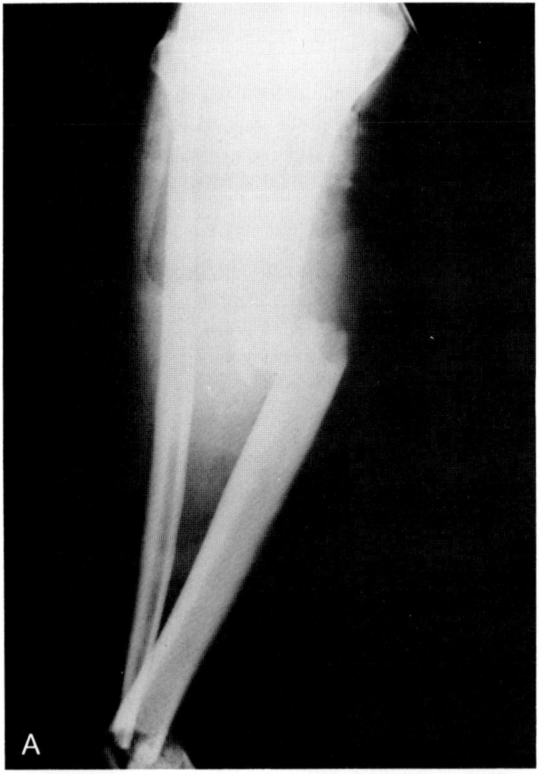

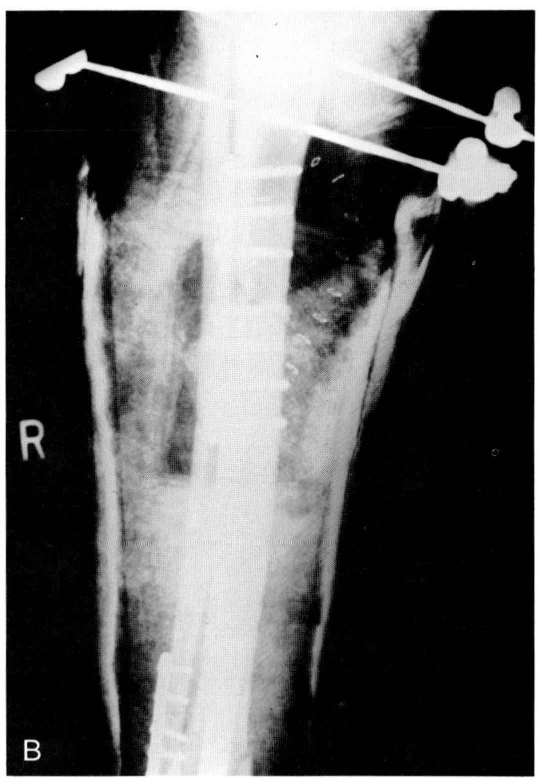

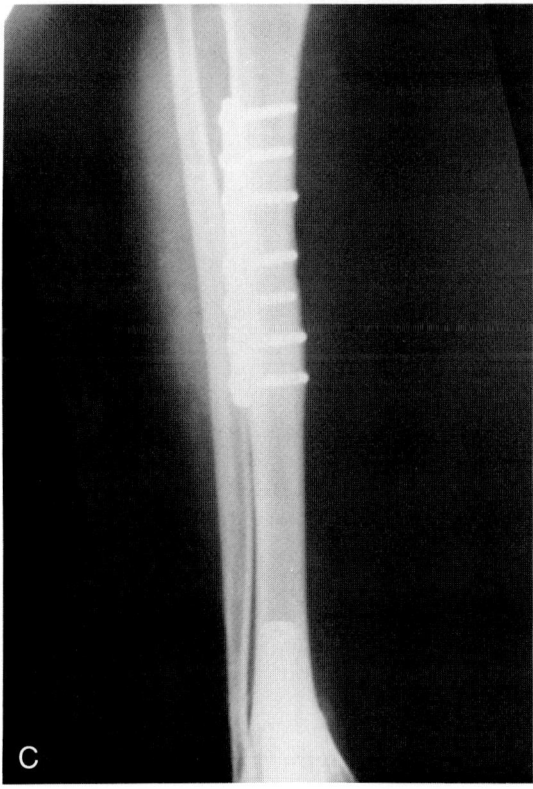

Fig. 19-9. *A*, A motorcycle accident caused a segmental tibial fracture and dislocated knee in this 27-year-old man. *B*, Segmental plates were used to stabilize the tibia, and pins were used to hold the reduction of the dislocated knee following ligament repair. *C*, Seven months later, the tibia had solidly united with good motion of the ankle.

ity. If these goals will not be met, a plate should not be used. In fractures with an intact segment, particularly fractures that are proximal and distal, a plate offers an excellent method of fixation (Fig. 19-9). In segmental tibial fractures, the use of two plates is generally easier than the use of one. If the plates interdigitate, they can be applied at opposite angles on the bone to allow overlapping of the plates and interdigitation of the screws. Contouring the plate to span both fracture levels is complex for a long segmental fracture, and although such contouring is possible, this technique generally is not preferred because of the difficulty in performing it successfully. Unfortunately, plate application leads to further periosteal stripping, and therefore, plates should be used only when excellent stability can be achieved in these segmental fractures.

After plate application in either a closed or open fracture, the wound must be left open if there is any tension on the tissues. In addition, if the bone has a small defect, primary or secondary bone grafting is mandatory. Indications for plate use are specific: if excellent reduction and stabilization of the fracture are not possible, plates should not be used. Technically, plate fixation is the most demanding form of treatment. A great deal of experience in the general use of lag screws and plates is required before their use on a segmental tibial fracture is attempted.

Intramedullary Nails. Intramedullary nailing should be reserved for closed segmental tibial fractures and for grade I open fractures only. We have had limited success with the use of intramedullary nailing in grade II and grade III open fractures of the tibia.

The intramedullary nail is an ideal treatment method for segmental fractures with an intact segment or segments (Fig. 19-10).[33,34] The proximal extent of the fracture must be well below the tibial tubercle, and the distal extent of the fracture can approach the distal tibia as long as the fracture is transverse. As the fracture becomes more oblique, more distal use of the nail is not possible. In comminuted or split segmental tibial fractures, the use of an intramedullary nail is still possible; an interlocking type of tibial nail must be used with screws applied proximally and distally to maintain length. The nail is an excellent treatment choice in closed injuries, particularly grade II and grade III closed injuries. These injuries require stabilization and often involve soft-tissue problems that are difficult to manage; however, one would not desire the problems brought on by a large surgical procedure, such as plating.

Intramedullary nailing causes almost no problems in femoral fractures, and although some vascular compromise is created by endosteal reaming, the extra periosteal blood supply to the femur easily compensates for this loss. Unfortunately, the periosteal blood supply is limited in the tibia, and therefore, endosteal reaming can cause a major compromise of the blood supply, particularly in grade II or grade III open tibial fractures.

Postoperative Management

Postoperative management of the segmental tibial fracture in the multiply injured patient is critical to the patient's outcome and requires a team approach. Cooperation is needed among the patient, the orthopaedist, the nurses, the plastic surgeon, the vascular surgeon, and the nutrition team. For the patient with a severe open tibial fracture with a great deal of soft-tissue injury, nutritional needs should be considered early in the course of treatment to meet the patient's high protein requirements. Management of the wound is complex as well and requires multiple trips to the operating room. On the ward, close attention must be paid to dressing changes. Generally, I try to involve the patients in their own dressing changes as soon as possible, since they have a higher level of interest in the healing of their injuries than does anyone else and thus potentially will be more conscientious in changing their dressings. The reliable patient who is carefully instructed can do an outstanding job of changing dressings.

Patient reliability is an important factor in the choice of postoperative management methods and must be assessed carefully. Reliable patients are able to perform their own dressing changes and follow a prescribed nonweightbearing plan when casts, plates, external fixation devices, and interlocking nails have been used to stabilize the fracture. If a patient is not able to cooperate with this program, prolonged hospitalization or even the application of a spica cast may be necessary to force cooperation. In the management of these complex injuries, the early postoperative phase is critical for a successful outcome. The physician is responsible for assessing the patient's ability to cooperate with the management plan, for instructing the patient in his role in hastening healing of the injury, and for trying to provide the media necessary for the patient's successful care. This task is frequently difficult.

I prefer not to start the patient with a segmental tibial fracture on early range-of-motion exercises. I have found that this exercise program frequently causes the ankle to drift into an equinus position that becomes permanent. This equinus deformity makes later ambulation difficult, since the patient must walk on an unstable platform. In the immediate postoperative phase of treatment, therefore, the ankle should be maintained in a neutral position with careful splinting.

In summary, proper follow-up care is critical to the outcome of the injury. The patient should be seen by the same physician at each visit, since only the treating surgeon understands the complexity of the soft-tissue injury and the insult to the viability of the bone. A postoperative plan must be established at the time of initial treatment and carried through. The fracture must be watched carefully for signs of loosening of an

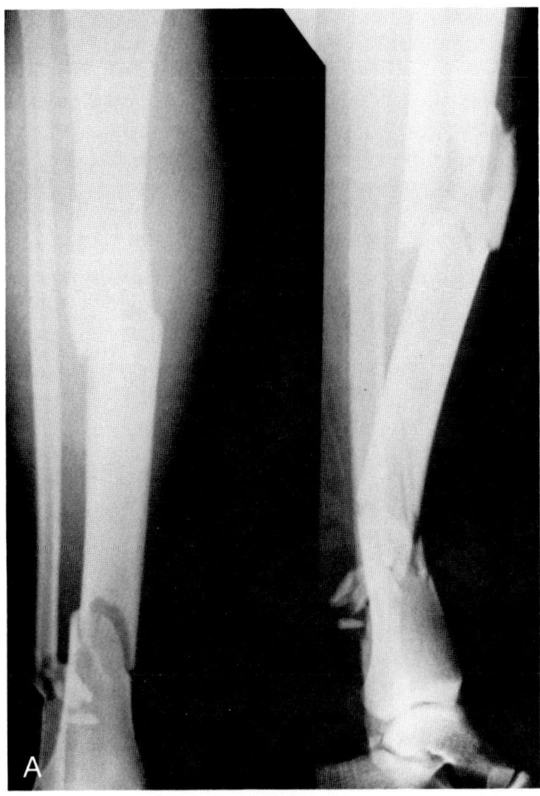

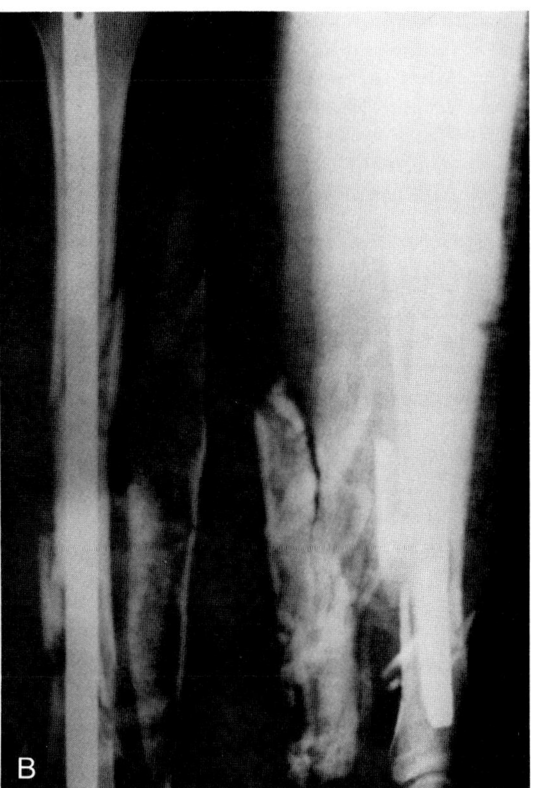

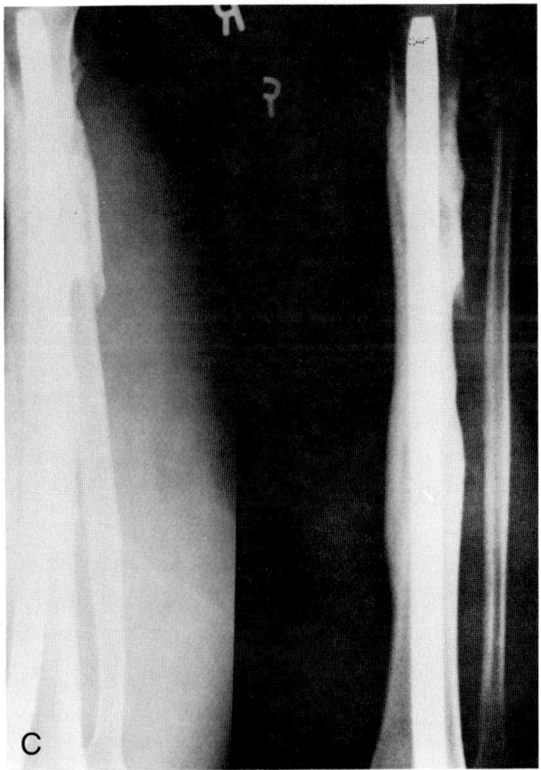

Fig. 19-10. *A*, A 25-year-old man injured in a motorcycle accident suffered a closed segmental tibial fracture with severe swelling. *B*, Within 12 hours, the patient developed a compartmental syndrome with intracompartmental pressures measuring 75 mm Hg. He was treated with four-compartment fasciotomy and intramedullary nailing. *C*, Roentgenogram taken 16 months after surgery demonstrates excellent healing.

implant or implant failure, as well as for failure of bone healing. Multiple procedures frequently are required in the treatment of these complex injuries; one should not hesitate to use multiple bone graftings or to change the method of fixation as required. Healing and return to function generally require from 8 to 18 months. Patients, as well as their families and employers, should be warned of this fact at the beginning of treatment. Time needed for healing is best defined by the velocity of the injury and the grade of the fracture in both closed and open injuries.

Complications

Infection. Infections are common in these complex injuries.[53] By leaving the wounds open, one decreases the risk of a serious infection; since the wound automatically decompresses itself when left open, further destruction of soft tissues by necrosis is prevented. If an infection occurs, the wound should be drained and debrided. Major debridement is generally not necessary. The use of antibiotics preoperatively is helpful, and specific culture should be obtained. Stabilization devices should be left in place if they are providing stability. The wound should be opened and drained, and the patient should be instructed in a program of frequent dressing changes, if he or she can be relied upon to carry out this program. Rapid and total resolution of the infection is not necessary. Prolonged drainage is acceptable if revascularization of the soft tissues and the fracture is taking place. Further surgical debridement should be attempted only if there are systemic signs of infection or if there is increased drainage. Otherwise, time, along with frequent dressing changes, allows revascularization of the area, as well as bony healing, and the infection eventually subsides. If prolonged infection is noted, the emphasis should be toward bone healing and removal of any obvious debris. Final debridement of the infected area and the application of pedicle flaps late in the course of healing generally resolve any persistent infection. In addition, removal of hardware after solid fracture healing has been achieved helps to clear up a chronic area of drainage.

Nonunion. Nonunion is a frequent problem with all tibial fractures, particularly segmental tibial fractures. Two basic approaches to this problem are to restore alignment and restore stability. When these goals have been achieved with the initial treatment, treatment of the nonunion is greatly simplified. An additional, and most important, form of treatment is multiple bone grafting. For fractures in which nonunion is anticipated, multiple bone grafting should be started in the initial treatment phase and repeated at approximately 6 to 8 weeks. When nonunion persists, the procedure should be repeated at approximately 6 months. This treatment encourages healing in some of the more severe fractures. Bone grafting is also an excellent method of treating nonunited fractures that have maintained alignment and stability and simply require further encouragement for bone healing to take place.

In patients with infected nonunited fractures, debridement and drainage are required in combination with one of two forms of bone grafting. The first method is debridement of the local area and application of a cancellous graft after the fracture has been realigned and stabilized. The second method is a bypass graft with a synostosis of the tibia and fibula. The appropriate form of grafting depends on the individual injury. In fractures with persistent nonunion and instability, and in closed nonunited fractures, intramedullary nailing is the procedure of choice, provided that the fracture level is appropriate for this treatment. When intramedullary nailing is performed for treatment of nonunion, the closed technique is used. In fractures in which intramedullary nailing is not appropriate, external fixation or plating may be used to manage nonunion. In each case, the major emphasis should be stimulation of the fracture with bone grafting. Electrical stimulation of the fractured bone is another method used to encourage healing; favorable reports on this treatment form are emerging.[54]

Malunion. Malunion is commonly seen in segmental tibial fractures, particularly when the fracture has been treated nonoperatively. Patients tolerate different degrees of malunion. Usually, 5° of varus angulation and 10° of valgus angulation, as well as 15° of anterior and posterior angulation, are acceptable. External rotation of 15 to 20° and internal rotation of 10° generally cause no symptoms. These figures represent the outer limits of acceptability, however, and may be well tolerated by some patients and not tolerated by others. In addition, deformities in combination tend to accentuate one another. For example, varus angulation and internal rotation accentuate each other, as do valgus angulation and external rotation.

Persistent malunion in a segmental tibial fracture must be corrected. In general, the correction should be made at the level of the malunion. If the area has been infected, however, a more reasonable approach is a distal or proximal osteotomy, clear of the infected area. In this instance, the method of fixation depends on the level of the osteotomy and the experience of the surgeon.

Stiffness. Stiffness of the ankle is a common sequela of segmental tibial fractures. I strongly believe that early range-of-motion exercises do nothing except allow the ankle to drop into equinus angulation and stay in that position. Therefore, I believe that splinting of the ankle at the beginning of treatment is important. Splinting should be done at the time of initial anesthesia. The ankle should be placed in a neutral position that should be maintained carefully throughout the course of healing. When swelling begins to subside at 6 to 8 weeks, motion can be started. I have been most disappointed in cases in which motion was started earlier, as I have found that the ankle drops into equinus and subsequently fails to move. With the ankle in an equinus position, patients find that walking is difficult, since they do not have a stable platform on which to bear weight. Thus, they are walking on a tenuous bone union with a tenuous platform, and this situation prolongs healing and rehabilitation.

Swelling. Swelling is a great problem in these patients. Patients with this complication must remain with the foot elevated for several weeks and should then start to stand or sit for only short periods of time while carefully monitoring the swelling. The swelling generally increases with cast removal. Careful wrapping with elastic wraps or a pressurized stocking is essential, as the ultimate degree of loss of function of the joint seems to be related primarily to the amount of swelling.

Floating Knee

The presence of ipsilateral femoral and tibial fractures, the "floating knee," indicates a multiply injured patient. These fractures pose a potential threat to life from fat embolism, pulmonary embolism, and blood loss. They frequently are accompanied by central injuries to the head, chest, and abdomen and are also commonly associated with other injuries to the extremities. A diagnosis of a floating knee should automatically alert the surgeon to the possibility of major life-threatening complications. Patients with this injury must be carefully managed in the emergency situation and carefully monitored in the emergency room, operating room, and intensive-care unit. Only after all life-threatening, or potentially life-threatening, situations have been treated may the orthopaedist turn his attention to the extremity injuries.

Extremity injuries associated with the floating knee tend to be severe. The bony injury may include damage to the diaphysis of the femur and tibia; one or more of the fractures may extend into the knee, creating supracondylar femoral fractures or fractures of the tibial plateau. Hip fractures or intra-articular distal tibial fractures are excluded from this discussion, since they represent somewhat different problems not associated with problems about the knee.

Complications commonly noted in the extremity with a floating knee are stiffness of the knee, infection, nonunion, malunion, and prolonged loss of function. With floating knee injuries, as many as 70% of the tibial fractures[2] and as many as 22% of the femoral fractures[55] may be open fractures, which require specialized wound management.

The general guideline for treatment of the floating knee is to stabilize the femur and mobilize the knee. Treatment of the tibial fracture is individualized; however, I generally prefer to stabilize the tibia as well as the femur.

Management of the Femoral Fracture

The femoral fracture offers the greatest challenge for mobilizing the patient. Although the soft-tissue injury surrounding the femur tends to be less severe than that around the tibia, the bony instability is greater. The fracture pattern should be analyzed carefully and, on that basis, the potential methods of treatment considered.

Treatment in traction has produced the worst possible results in these combination injuries (Fig. 19-11). This method should be used only as a temporizing means of treatment, or only if other means of treatment are not available. Only rarely is traction indicated for long-range treatment of patients with floating knees. The use of external fixation devices is also seldom indicated. This device is used only in grade III open femoral fractures and has little place in the treatment of the patient with a floating knee.

The two primary treatment forms for the patient with a floating knee are intramedullary nailing and plating. Intramedullary nailing is the treatment of choice; in comminuted fractures, an interlocking nail may have to be used, or the intramedullary nail may have to be supplemented with cerclage wires. Intramedullary nailing of the femur offers a high rate of union and allows early mobilization of the patient and of the knee; also, this method produces a minimum of complications when performed closed (Fig. 19-12). Thus, all treatment goals for the patient with a floating knee are met.

The appropriate timing for intramedullary nailing is more controversial. Riska, et al.,[11] have suggested that primary stabilization of the femur

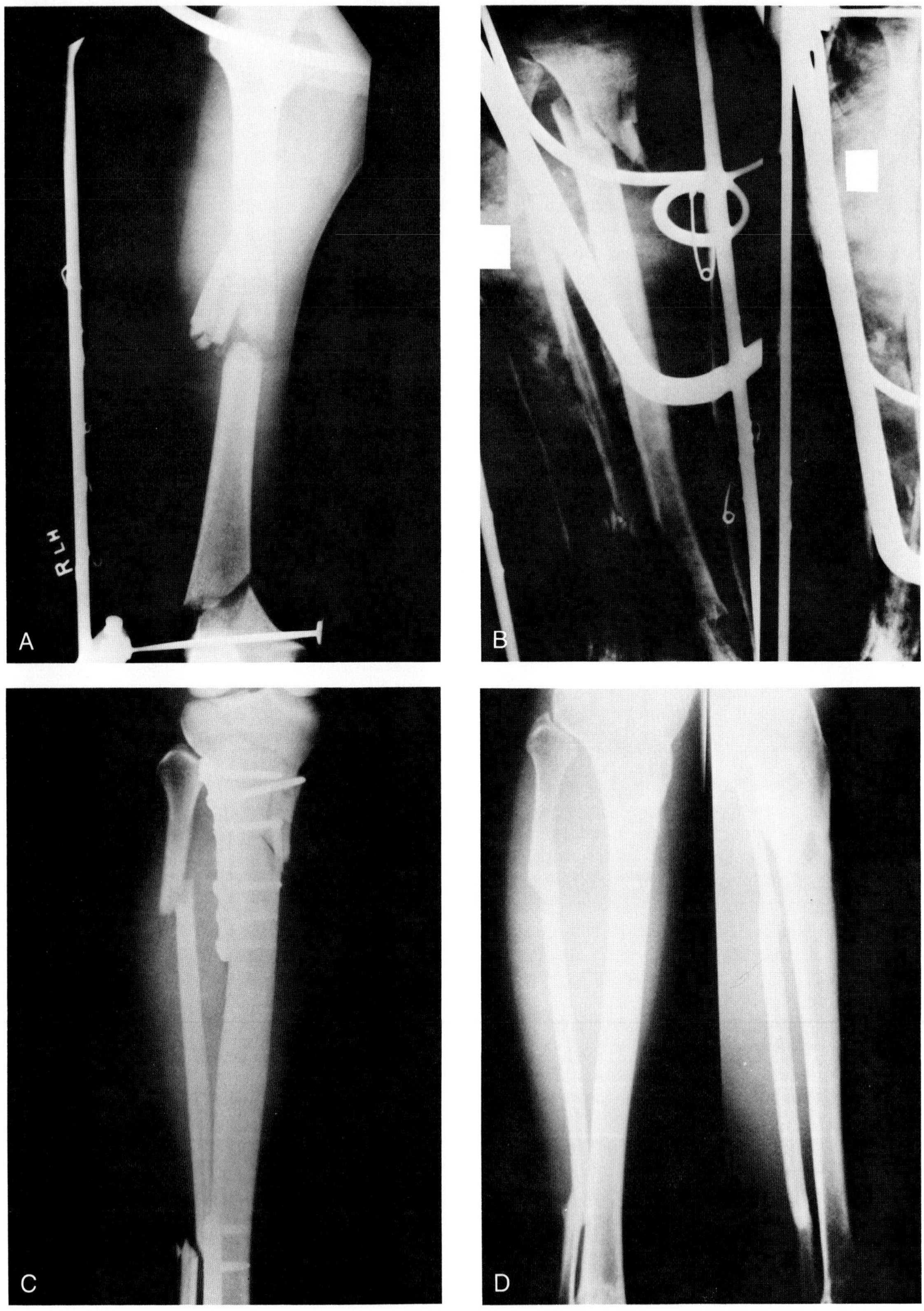
A
B
C
D

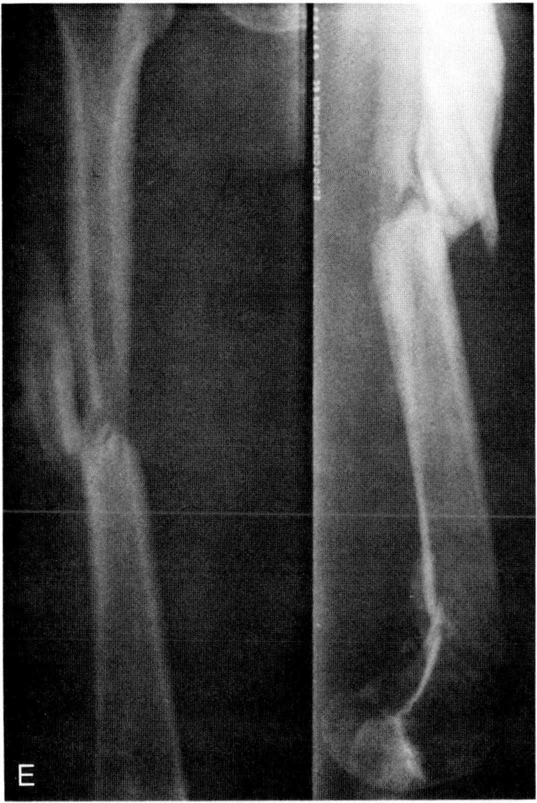

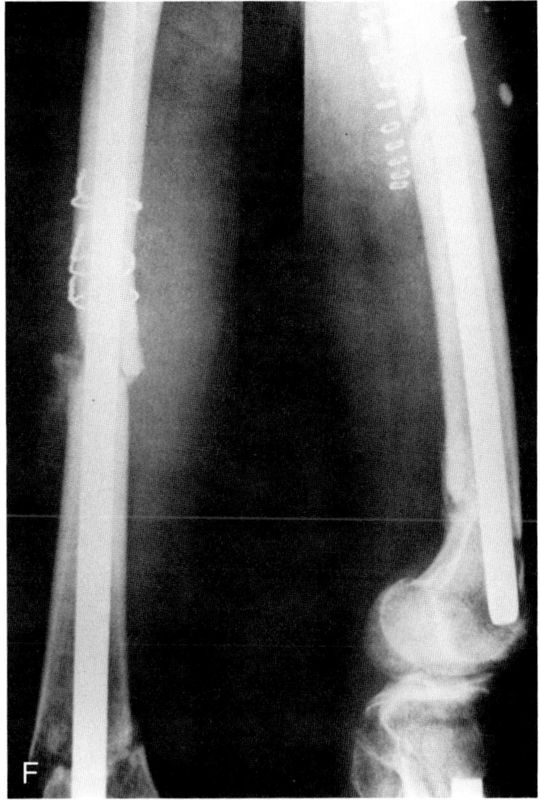

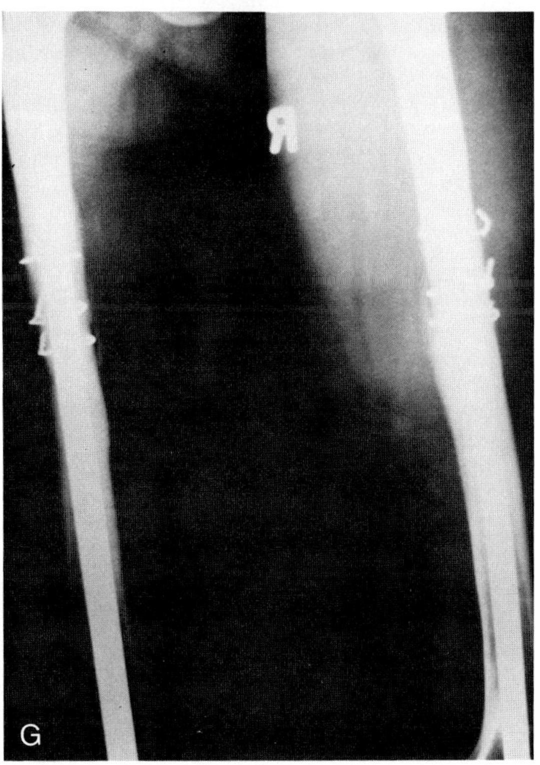

Fig. 19-11. A 26-year-old woman involved in a motor-vehicle accident suffered a grade I open segmental fracture of the right femur (*A*) and an ipsilateral closed segmental fracture of the tibia (*B*). The tibia was partially splinted with proximal and distal plates (*C*) and healed uneventfully (*D*). The femoral fracture was treated with traction and a cast-brace. At 5 months, there was gross motion at the fracture site. Although the patient had worn a cast-brace for 2 months, she had only 5° of knee flexion (*E*). The fracture was treated with realignment, cerclage wiring, intramedullary nailing, and bone grafting (*F*). The femur united, but the patient gained only 20° of knee flexion. After a quadricepsplasty was performed, the patient gained 115° of knee flexion (*G*).

enhances the resuscitation of the patient and decreases the risk of fat embolism. Primary stabilization, which is the preferred method at the University of Washington, Seattle, Washington, requires an organized team of paramedics, emergency room physicians, operating room personnel, and surgeons with the experience to stabilize the fracture in an efficient manner and with accurate techniques, even at inopportune times. The more severe the central or peripheral injury, the higher the indication for primary stabilization.[10] In patients who require mobilization to reduce the risk of complications from chest or

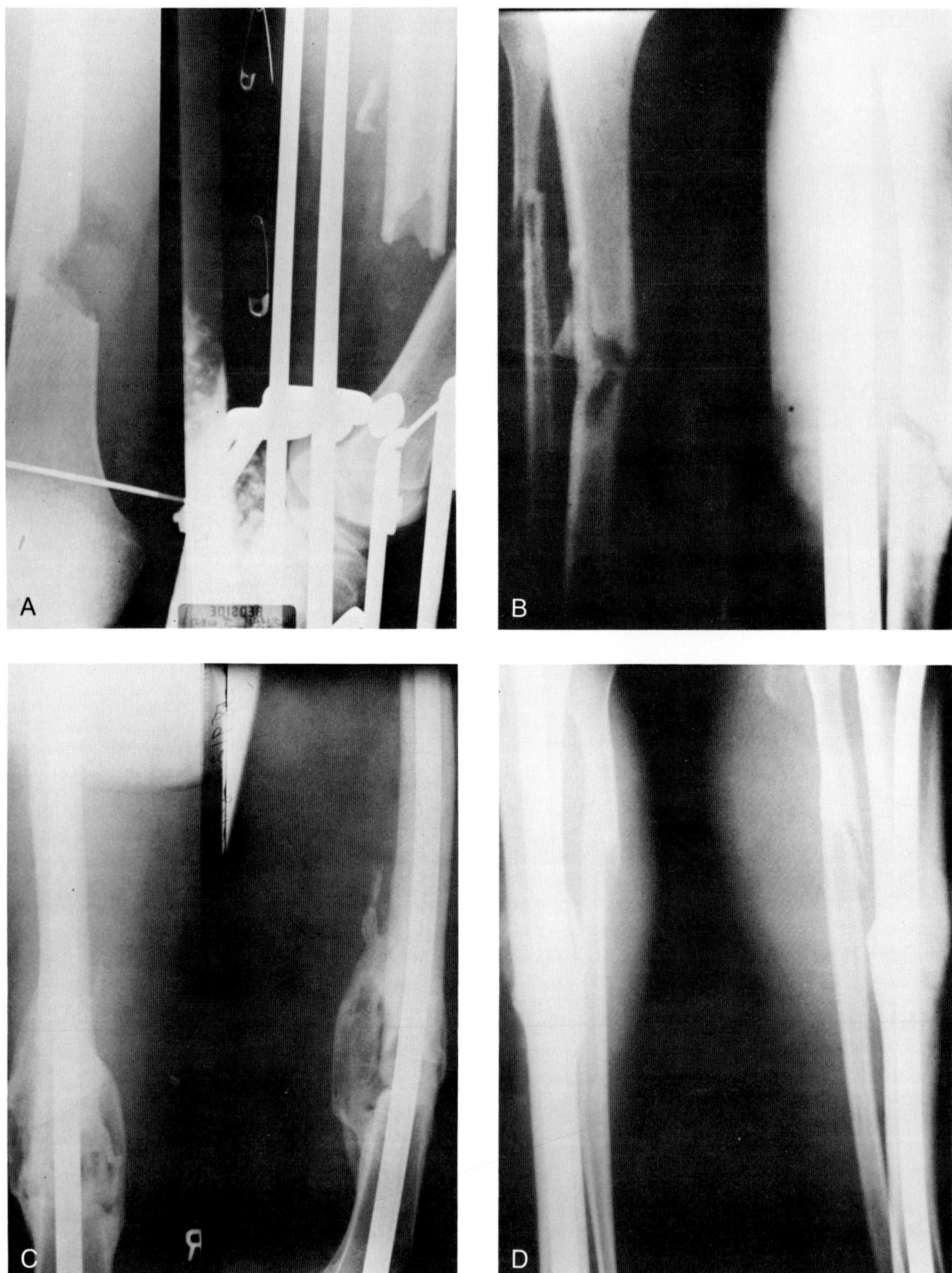

Fig. 19-12. A 15-year-old boy involved in a motorcycle accident sustained a grade I open fracture of the right femur (*A*) and an ipsilateral grade I open tibial fracture (*B*). One year after debridement and primary fixation of both fractures with intramedullary nailing, both the femur (*C*) and the tibia (*D*) had healed without bone grafting. Knee motion was 135°.

abdominal injuries, the preference is to stabilize the femur immediately.

In patients with open femoral fractures, the wound is debrided and the femur stabilized. In patients with open tibial fractures, superficial wound contamination tends to increase in the first 2 weeks after injury. Therefore, we prefer to stabilize the ipsilateral femur immediately to reduce the risk of a femoral infection. The overall management of the patient is much easier once the femur has been stabilized. However, if the hospital or the surgeon is not equipped or prepared to perform primary stabilization, this procedure should be delayed until the appropriate equipment and expertise are available for performance of an excellent procedure. If stabilization is delayed, the patient is placed in longitudinal skeletal traction and observed in the intensive-care unit until the appropriate time for surgery. To make a proper decision about the appropriate time for stabilization, one must carefully assess the working environment. In each institution the decision realistically depends on the experience of the surgeon, the day of the week, the time of day, the attitude of the general surgeons and neurosurgeons, and the availability of the anesthesiologist, nurses, and equipment.

Management of the Tibial Fracture

Although the femoral fracture presents a challenge in terms of mobilizing the patient, the tibial fracture presents a greater overall challenge. As with segmental tibial fractures, the key factor in assessing these fractures is the velocity of the injury. This assessment indicates the severity and the amount of contamination of open injuries and, more importantly, the severity of injury under the skin. The amount of initial angulation and shortening of the bone, if any, gives a good indication of the degree of soft-tissue stripping.

Massive injuries to the soft tissues, even in closed fractures, greatly delay healing. Delayed healing and prolonged immobilization lead to unacceptable results. Therefore, particularly in the floating knee, treatment methods that allow mobilization of the knee must be considered. My preferred method of treatment in patients with this injury is stabilization of both closed and open fractures of the tibia. Controversies rage on this topic, and there is certainly room for a great deal of discussion. The evaluation by Fraser, et al., of 222 patients with floating knee injuries in a multicenter study showed a 30% incidence of osteomyelitis in cases managed by operative treatment of both the femur and tibia.[56] Such statistics would cause one to hesitate to perform tibial stabilization. However, Karlström and Olerud's analysis of a series of patients with floating knee demonstrated the best results in patients in whom both the femur and tibia were stabilized and, thus, strongly supports this method of treatment.[57]

The initial treatment of the tibial fracture should be aimed at the soft-tissue injury. Careful debridement and irrigation are mandatory. Antibiotics are used initially, and the wound is left open. Stabilization of the tibia greatly enhances the treatment of the wound and the overall treatment of the patient. Stabilization can be achieved with external fixation devices, plates, or intramedullary nails. Cerclage wires or lag screws may be combined with these treatment forms. The appropriate method of stabilization is determined by the fracture pattern, the position of the wound, and the degree of stability that can be achieved by treatment. Intramedullary nails are best suited for grade I open fractures. Plates are most appropriate for fractures that can be rigidly stabilized with this treatment (Fig. 19-13). For comminuted fractures and severe open fractures, external fixation appears to be the treatment of choice. With all treatment forms used, management of the wound is the priority and requires multiple debridements and late closure, as was noted for open segmental tibial fractures.

Results

The results of nonoperative treatment of the floating knee generally have been unsatisfactory.[57,58] The concept of stabilizing the femoral fracture is generally accepted.[2,56,57,59] In addition, Karlström and Olerud have strongly advocated the stabilization of both fractures for producing optimum results.[57] However, the findings of Fraser, et al., in a multicenter study showing a complication rate of 26% delayed union and nonunion and a rate of osteomyelitis of 30% cause one to ponder the wisdom of stabilizing both femur and tibia.[56]

Our experience at Harborview Medical Center, reviewed by Veith, et al.,[55] lends support to the concept that stabilization of both fractures offers the best treatment method. Fifty-seven consecutive cases of ipsilateral femoral and tibial fractures, treated between 1968 and 1978, were analyzed. Forty-two patients had diaphyseal fractures of both bones, and fifteen patients had intra-ar-

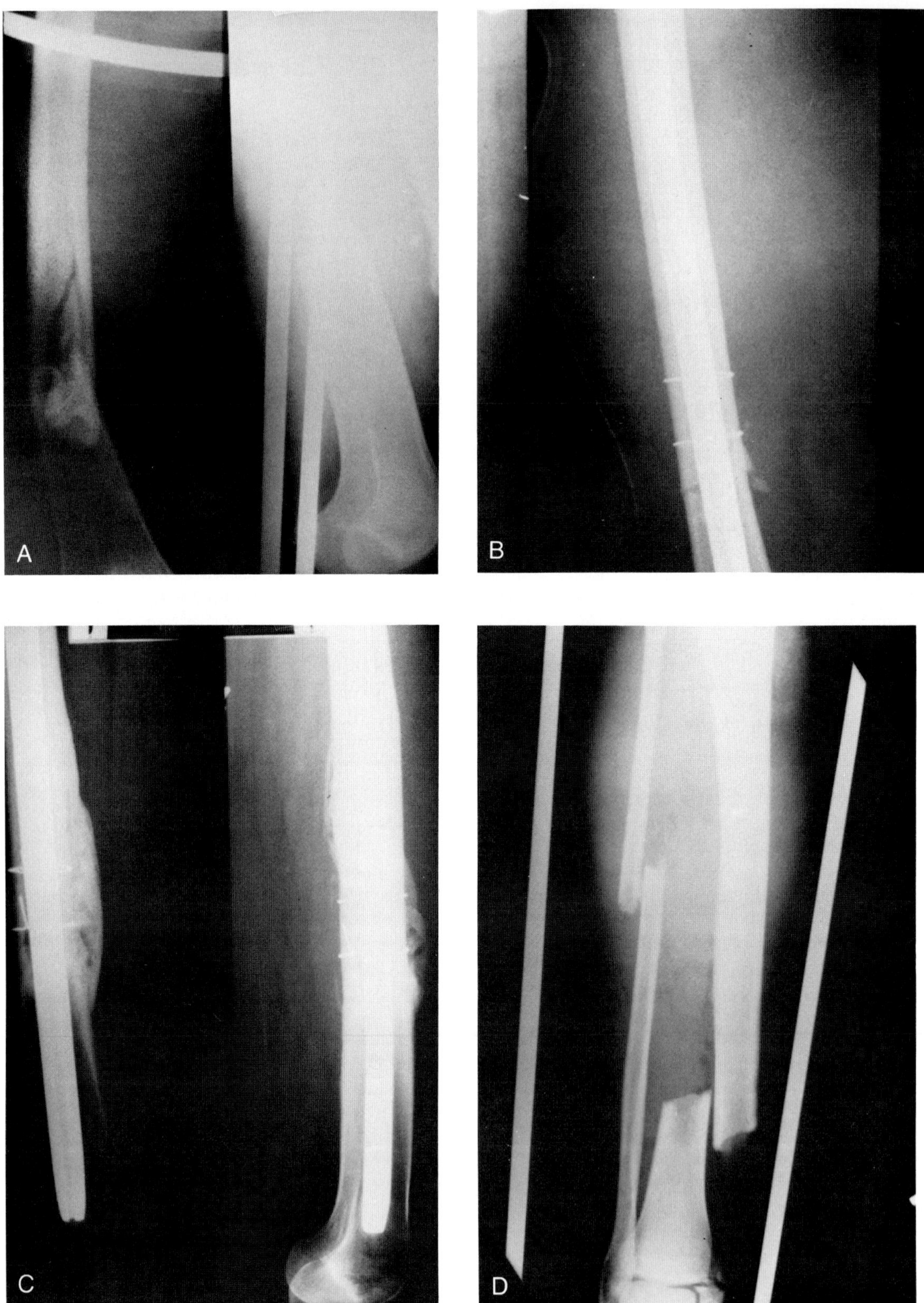
A
B
C
D

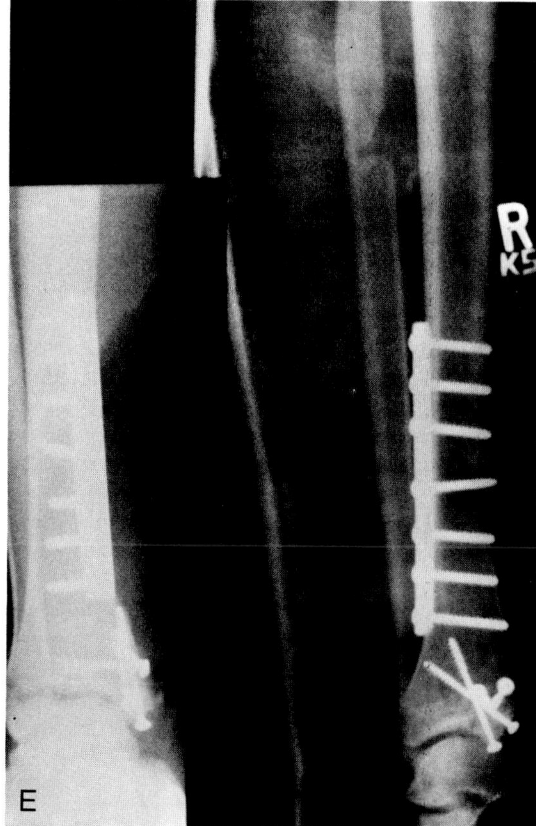

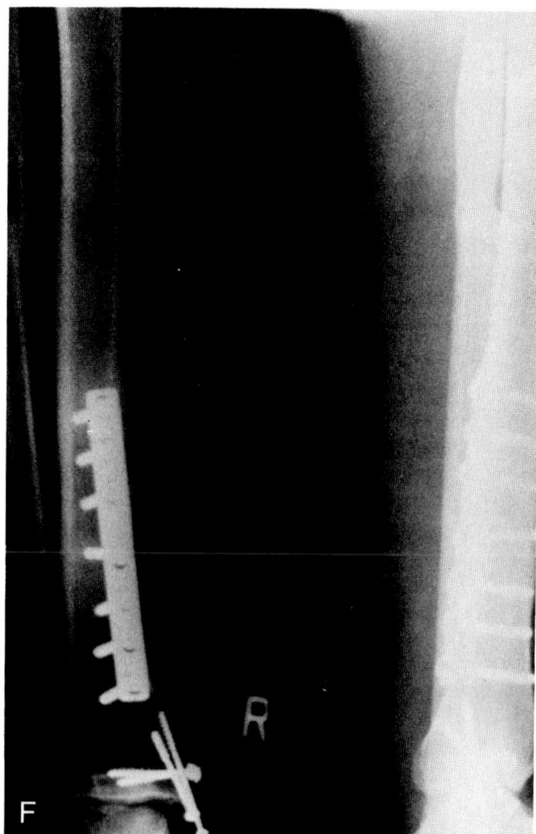

FIG. 19-13. *A*, A motorcycle accident caused this grade I open femoral fracture in a 22-year-old man. *B*, After debridement, primary intramedullary nailing and cerclage wiring were performed. *C*, Films taken 14 months after injury show solid union of the femur. *D*, The patient also sustained an ipsilateral grade II open fracture of the distal tibia with a medial malleolus fracture. *E*, After debridement, both fractures were stabilized primarily by using lag screws for the medial malleolus and a compression plate for the tibia. *F*, At 14 months after injury, solid union of the tibia and medial malleolus was achieved. The patient gained 130° of knee flexion.

ticular injuries of either the supracondylar femur or the tibial plateau. Hip fractures or intra-articular distal tibial fractures were excluded from the series.

In the early years, treatment of these injuries consisted of stabilization of the femur and nonoperative management of the tibia. With time, however, a more aggressive approach to treatment of the tibia evolved, and currently both fractures are stabilized. Twenty-one patients (38.9%) had involvement of the head, chest, or abdomen, and twenty-five patients (46.3%) had additional musculoskeletal injuries to the axial skeleton or to other extremities. Careful analysis of results revealed that the need for stabilization increased as the injury became more severe.

The patients were categorized into two groups. Group 1 included 26 patients treated with internal fixation of the femur and cast on the tibia. Group 2 included 29 patients in whom both the femur and tibia were stabilized. It is interesting that the injuries of patients in group 1 represented a much less severe group of injuries. Multiple trauma occurred in only 30.9% of the patients in this group, and open fractures were present in 38.5% of the patients. By contrast, multiple trauma occurred in 44.8% of group 2 patients, and open fractures were present in 72.4%. In group 2, however, 48.3% were patients with multiple trauma and 72.4% had open fractures. Despite this difference, analysis of both groups showed an improved end result in the patients in group 2, whose injuries had been twice as severe as those of the patients in group 1 but in whom both fractures had been stabilized. The average healing time was 20.7 weeks for group 1 and 18.2 weeks for group 2; hospital time averaged 37 days for group 1 and 35 days for group 2. Good or excellent results were seen in 73.9% of the patients in group 1 and 91.7% of the patients in group 2. Thus, in our series, results appeared to be improved with stabilization of both bones. This treatment is now routinely recommended in open and closed fractures. Cast immobilization is used only in minimally displaced, stable, tibial fractures.

Complications

A number of complications were seen in our series. Fat embolism occurred in 14.8% of the patients; all were treated with pulmonary support. Three patients had pulmonary embolism, and one patient had a hyperosmolar syndrome. Local complications were experienced by one patient with deep-view thrombosis in the calf, one patient who sustained a grade III open tibial fracture with an arterial injury required a below-knee amputation. One patient died 2 months after sustaining a severe head injury.

Of the 114 fractures in the series, 3 became infected. These infections occurred in one open femoral fracture and two open tibial fractures. The femoral fracture had been treated initially with debridement and intramedullary nailing combined with cerclage wiring. When infection developed, debridement and eventual hardware removal, sequestrectomy, external stabilization, and bone grafting were required. The tibia proceeded to union with an excellent result. The two tibial fractures that developed infections were also open fractures. One was a grade I open fracture treated initially with intramedullary nailing. After debridement, with the nail in place, the infection resolved. The second open tibial fracture that became infected had been treated with immediate plating. Debridement, with the plate in position, was required, but the bone failed to unite. Bone grafting was subsequently performed and union was achieved.

Two tibial fractures in the series failed to unite. One was the infected nonunited fracture already described; the other, which had been treated with primary plating, developed a hypertrophic nonunion requiring plate removal and intramedullary nailing.

Nonunion occurred in two femoral fractures. One patient had a segmental bone loss of 5 inches and required nailing with bone grafting; bone union was achieved at 12 months. In the second patient, who had sustained a comminuted intercondylar supracondylar femoral fracture, the plate broke after 11 months; this fracture proceeded to union without further treatment but unfortunately malunited.

Shortening of 2.5 cm and 3.0 cm, respectively, occurred in 2 patients with tibial fractures treated in casts. External rotation of 45°, 45°, and 25°, respectively, was seen in 3 femurs. In one of these patients, a derotational osteotomy was required. In all three cases, rotation was caused by inaccurate positioning of the patient on the fracture table and in the bed postoperatively.

Despite these complications, including the infections, the results in this series still were better in the patients whose fractures were stabilized primarily. Infection and nonunion delayed, but did not change, the ultimate result. This same situation with regard to infected nonunited fractures has been demonstrated by Rittmann, et al.[53]

In our series, chondromalacia was seen in 6.4% of the patients, and ligamentous laxity was noted in 12.8% of the patients at late follow-up. The condition of the ligaments should be evaluated carefully at the time of initial treatment. Stabilization of both bones allows accurate assessment of the knee injury.

Ultimate knee motion averaged 126° in group 1 and 131° in group 2. In group 1, flexion in 5 knees that had been immobilized in plaster for longer than 6 weeks averaged 110°. In group 2, only 2 patients had less than 125° of knee flexion.

Conclusions

Floating knee injuries offer a challenge from the standpoint of both resuscitation of the patient and local care of the fracture. More than 50% of patients with this injury have open fractures. Nonoperative care of these fractures has produced less than ideal results. Early stabilization of both fractures seems to offer the best results, even in the face of such complications as infection and nonunion. Analysis of the Seattle series showed two groups of patients: one treated with femoral stabilization and tibial casting, and the other treated with internal fixation of both the femur and tibia. Despite the increased severity of their injuries, including both central injuries and open fractures, the results were better for patients in the second group. At present, our preferred treatment is stabilization of both fractures along with careful wound management and vigorous treatment of any complications.

References

1. Küntscher, G.: Practice of Intramedullary Nailing. Springfield, Charles C Thomas, 1967.
2. Koostra, G.: Femoral Shaft Fractures in Adults. Femoral Shaft Fracture and Homolateral Lower Leg Fracture. Assen, The Netherlands, Van Gorcum, 1973.
3. Winquist, R. A., and Hansen, S. T.: Segmental fractures of the femur treated by closed intramedullary nailing. J. Bone Joint Surg., *60-A*:934, 1978.
4. Church, J. C. T.: Segmental fractures of femur. *In* Proceedings of the Association of Surgeons of East Africa. J. Bone Joint Surg., *53-B*:355, 1971.
5. Funk, J. F., Jr., Wells, R. E., and Street, D. M.: Supplementary fixation of femoral fractures. Clin. Orthop., *60*:41, 1968.
6. Rhinelander, F. W.: Tibial blood supply in relation to fracture healing. Clin. Orthop., *105*:34, 1974.
7. Danckwardt-Lillieström, G., and Sjögren, S.: Postoperative restoration of muscle strength after intramedullary nailing of fractures of the femoral shaft. Acta Orthop. Scand., *47*:101, 1976.
8. Küntscher, G.: Die Marknagelung von Knochenbrüchen. Arch. Klin. Chir., *200*:443, 1940.
9. Winquist, R. A., Hansen, S. T., and Clawson, D. K.: Closed intramedullary nailing of femoral fractures. Paper presented at the American Academy of Orthopaedic Surgeons Annual Meeting, Las Vegas, NV, 1981.
10. Border, J.: Cardiopulmonary failure. *In* Basic Surgery. Edited by J. A. McCredie. New York, Macmillan, 1977.
11. Riska, E. B., et al.: Prevention of fat embolism by early internal fixation of fractures in patients with multiple injuries. Injury, *8*:110, 1976.
12. Lam, S. J.: The place of delayed internal fixation in the treatment of fractures of the long bones. J. Bone Joint Surg., *46-B*:393, 1964.
13. Smith, J. E. M.: The results of early and delayed internal fixation of fractures of the shaft of the femur. J. Bone Joint Surg., *46-B*:28, 1964

13a. Mooney, V., Nickel, V. L., Harvey, J. P., Jr., and Snelson, R.: Cast-brace treatment for fractures of the distal part of the femur. J. Bone Joint Surg., *52-A*: 1563, 1970.

14. Winquist, R. A., and Frankel, V. H.: Complications of implant use. *In* Complications in Orthopaedic Surgery. Edited by C. H. Epps, Jr. Philadelphia, J. B. Lippincott, 1978.
15. Gant, G. C., Shaftan, G. W., and Herbsman, H.: Experience with the ASIF compression plate in the management of femoral shaft fractures. J. Trauma, *10*:458, 1970.
16. Magerl, F., Wyss, A., Brunner, Ch., and Binder, W.: Plate osteosynthesis of femoral shaft fractures in adults. A follow-up study. Clin. Orthop., *138*:62, 1979.
17. Rüedi, T. P., and Lüscher, J. N.: Results after internal fixation of comminuted fractures of the femoral shaft with DC plates. Clin. Orthop., *138*:74, 1979.
18. Rokkanen, P., Slätis, P., and Vankka, E.: Closed or open intramedullary nailing of femoral shaft fractures? A comparison with conservatively treated cases. J. Bone Joint Surg., *51-B*:313, 1969.
19. Wickstrom, J., and Corban, M. S.: Intramedullary fixation for fractures of the femoral shaft. A study of complications in 298 operations. J. Trauma, *7*:551, 1967.
20. Böhler, J.: Percutaneous internal fixation utilizing the x-ray image amplifier. J. Trauma, *5*:150, 1965.
21. Böhler, J.: Closed intramedullary nailing of the femur. Clin. Orthop., *60*:51, 1968.
22. Christensen, N. O.: Technique, errors and safeguards in modern Küntscher nailing. Clin. Orthop., *115*:182, 1976.
23. Clawson, D. K., Smith, R. F., and Hansen, S. T.: Closed intramedullary nailing of the femur. J. Bone Joint Surg., *53-A*:681, 1971.
24. Gherlingoni, G., Vasceaveo, F., and Murena, P. F.: Closed reduction reaming and nailing in fractures of the femoral shaft. Ital. J. Orthop. Traumatol., *1*:117, 1975.
25. Hansen, S. T., and Winquist, R. A.: Closed intramedullary nailing of fractures of the femoral shaft. Part II: Technical considerations. *In* Instructional Course Lectures, The American Academy of Orthopaedic Surgeons. Vol. 27. St. Louis, C. V. Mosby, 1978.
26. Rasher, J. J., Nahigian, S. H., Macys, J. R., and Brown, J. E.: Closed nailing of femoral-shaft fractures. J. Bone Joint Surg., *54-A*:534, 1972.
27. Winquist, R. A., and Hansen, S. T.: Comminuted fractures of the femoral shaft treated by intramedullary nailing. Orthop. Clin. North Am., *11*:633, 1980.
28. Hempel, D., and Fischer, S.: Marknagelungs-praxis nach Küntscher. Stuttgart, Georg Thieme Verlag, 1980.
29. Nichols, P. J. R.: Rehabilitation after fractures of the shaft of the femur. J. Bone Joint Surg., *45-B*:96, 1963.
30. Connolly, J. F., Dehne, E., and LaFollette, B.: Closed reduction and early cast-brace ambulation in the treatment of femoral fractures. Part II. Results in one hundred and forty-three fractures. J. Bone Joint Surg., *55-A*:1581, 1973.
31. Mueller, K. H.: Intramedullary nailing of comminuted fractures with additional fixation. *In* Instructional Course Lectures, The American Academy of Orthopaedic Surgeons. Vol. 22. St. Louis, C. V. Mosby, 1973.
32. Lottes, J. O.: Medullary nailing of the tibia with the triflange nail. Clin. Orthop., *105*:253, 1974.
33. Pantazopoulos, T., Galanos, P., Agoropoulos, Z., and Hartofilakidis-Garofalidis, G.: Treatment of double tibial fractures by blind intramedullary nailing. Clin. Orthop., *84*:137, 1972.
34. Zucman, J., and Maurer, P.: Two-level fractures of the tibia. Results in thirty-six cases treated by blind nailing. J. Bone Joint Surg., *51-B*:686, 1969.
35. Andersen, M. N., McDonald, K., and Stephens, J. G.: A study of the effect of open and closed treatment on the rate of healing and complications in fractures of the tibial shaft. J. Trauma, *1*:290, 1961.
36. Connolly, J.: Management of fractures associated with arterial injuries. Am. J. Surg., *120*:331, 1970.
37. Gallinaro, P., Crova, M., and Denicolai, F.: Complications in 64 open fractures of the tibia. Injury, *5*:157, 1973.
38. Gustilo, R. B., and Anderson, J. T.: Prevention of infection in the treatment of one thousand and twenty-five open fractures of long bones. J. Bone Joint Surg., *58-A*:453, 1976.
39. Hampton, O. P.: Basic principles in the management of open fractures. J.A.M.A., *159*:417, 1955.
40. Johansson, O.: Viewpoints on primary osteosynthesis in compound fractures. Acta Chir. Scand., *105*:474, 1953.
41. McNeur, J. C.: The management of open skeletal trauma with particular reference to internal fixation. J. Bone Joint Surg., *52-B*:54, 1970.

42. Olerud, S., and Karlström, G.: Tibial fractures treated by A-O compression osteosynthesis. Acta Orthop. Scand. [Suppl.], *140*:3, 1972.
43. Patzakis, M. J., Harvey, J. P., and Ivler, D.: The role of antibiotics in the management of open fractures. J. Bone Joint Surg., *56-A*:532, 1974.
44. Matsen, F. A., Winquist, R. A., and Krugmire, R. B.: Diagnosis and management of compartmental syndromes. J. Bone Joint Surg., *62-A*:286, 1980.
45. Anderson, J. T., and Gustilo, R. B.: Immediate internal fixation in open fractures. Orthop. Clin. North Am., *11*:569, 1980.
46. Chapman, M. W.: The use of immediate internal fixation in open fractures. Orthop. Clin. North Am., *11*:579, 1980.
47. Chapman, M. W., and Mahoney, M.: The role of early internal fixation in the management of open fractures. Clin. Orthop., *138*:120, 1979.
48. Karlström, G., and Olerud, S.: Fractures of the tibial shaft. A critical evaluation of treatment alternatives. Clin. Orthop., *105*:82, 1974.
48a. Tscherne, H.: Personal communication, 1983.
49. Brown, P. W.: The early weight-bearing treatment of tibial shaft fractures. Clin. Orthop., *105*:167, 1974.
50. Dehne, E.: Ambulatory treatment of the fractured tibia. Clin. Orthop., *105*:192, 1974.
51. Sarmiento, A.: Functional bracing of tibial fractures. Clin. Orthop., *105*:202, 1974.
52. Karlström, G., and Olerud, S.: Percutaneous pin fixation of open tibial fractures. Double-frame anchorage using the Vidal-Adrey method. J. Bone Joint Surg., *57-A*:915, 1975.
53. Rittmann, W. W., Schibli, M., Matter, P., and Allgower, M.: Open fractures. Long-term results in 200 consecutive cases. Clin. Orthop., *138*:132, 1979.
54. Bassett, C.A.L., Pilla, A. A., and Pawluk, R. J.: A nonoperative salvage of surgically resistant pseudoarthrosis and nonunions by pulsating electromagnetic fields. Clin. Orthop., *124*:128, 1977.
55. Veith, R. G., Winquist, R. A., and Hansen, S. T.: Ipsilateral fractures of the femur and tibia. Paper presented at the American Academy of Orthopaedic Surgeons Annual Meeting, Atlanta, GA, 1980.
56. Fraser, R. D., Hunter, G. A., and Waddell, J. P.: Ipsilateral fracture of the femur and tibia. J. Bone Joint Surg., *60-B*:510, 1978.
57. Karlström, G., and Olerud, S.: Ipsilateral fracture of the femur and tibia. J. Bone Joint Surg., *59-A*:240, 1977.
58. DeLee, J. C.; Ipsilateral fracture of the femur and tibia treated in a quadrilateral cast-brace. Clin. Orthop., *142*:115, 1979.
59. Hojer, H., Gillquist, J., and Liljedahl, S.-O.: Combined fractures of the femoral and tibial shafts in the same limb. Injury, *8*:206, 1975.

Chapter 20 Major Knee Ligament Injuries and Ipsilateral Fractures

RICHARD E. JONES, III

The knee is the largest and most complex joint of the body. It is the link between the torso and ground contact and moves through flexion, extension, and rotational planes. The static stabilizers of the knee include the contour of the articular surfaces, the menisci, the ligaments, and the capsule. The dynamic stabilizers of the knee are all musculotendinous units that act across the knee. The ligaments of the knee provide proprioceptive feedback into the central nervous system, resistance to abnormal planes of motion, and guides to joint motion.

The recognition and diagnosis of knee ligament injuries in a limb with intact osseous structures depend on demonstration of instability to stress testing. In limbs that are rendered unstable by fractures, the diagnosis of knee ligament injury is difficult to make because of motion at the fracture site. Recognition of knee ligament injuries associated with ipsilateral fractures is complicated further by focusing on the fracture as the major injury to the limb. When the fractured limb is splinted, the knee is not readily accessible for examination. Ligamentous injuries about the knee, therefore, remain occult because of a low index of suspicion. Attention must be focused on the knee and its supporting structures to improve the incidence of recognition of knee ligament damage associated with ipsilateral fractures.

There is general agreement that acute repair of knee ligament injuries gives better and more predictable results than do late repair or supplemental reconstructive procedures. Palmer[1] and O'Donoghue[2] were pioneers in advocating early surgical repair to improve better functional results in knee ligament injuries. The goal of early surgical repair is restoration of the ligaments to preinjury anatomy and tension. Naturally, the differences in injury mechanisms, status of the soft tissues, and blood supply to the ligaments influence the outcome.

The function of the knee joint with impaired ligamentous integrity is compromised. Marshall and Olsson showed that section of the cruciate ligaments in dogs caused significant degenerative changes in the articular surface and osteophyte formation.[3] Jacobsen demonstrated osteoarthritic changes in the knees in a series of 48 patients with cruciate ligament insufficiency.[4]

The functional problems associated with knee ligament insufficiency are magnified by the degree of activity the patient requires. The degree of function necessary for sedentary or walking activity is much less than that required for athletic activities. Functional problems, such as knee "giveway," swelling, and pain, are common in patients with knee damage whose levels of physical activity are high. Therefore, failure to recognize knee ligament damage in a limb with associated fractures causes serious long-term functional disability for the patient.

Knee Ligament Mechanism of Injury and Commonly Associated Fractures

Disruption of the supporting structures of the knee with associated ipsilateral fractures usually is caused by high-energy trauma. Shelton and associates reported on 26 patients with fractures and knee ligament ruptures in the same limb.[5] Of their patients, 22 were involved in pedestrian-auto accidents and 15 of those patients had pelvic fractures and knee ligament injuries. In five patients with pelvic fractures, the foot on the side of the fracture was planted on the ground, and the subsequent stress to the knee caused rupture of the medial ligamentous structures. Both feet were fixed to the ground in eight patients with pelvic fractures. Ipsilateral valgus strain and contralateral varus strain resulted, thereby producing bilateral knee ligament ruptures on the appropriate strained side (Fig. 20-1). In two patients, the extremity on the side of the pelvic fracture was not planted on the ground; consequently, the ipsilateral knee ligaments were spared but the contralateral lateral knee ligaments were ruptured. Shelton and associates speculated that the ligamentous rupture of the knee occurred prior to the stress failure of the bone.

Nagel, et al.,[6] described the most common mechanism of knee ligament damage in automobile accidents. The legs up to the knee were usually situated beneath the dashboard. On impact, the trunk was thrust forward and over with the lower extremities trapped beneath the dashboard. Hyperextension of the knee was produced with various rotational and angulatory stresses causing damage to either the cruciate ligaments or the collateral supporting ligaments (Fig. 20-2). Fractures of the femoral shaft were sustained with essentially the same injury mechanism.

Walling and associates found that 33% of 24 consecutive patients with femoral shaft fractures sustained concomitant ligamentous injury to the ipsilateral knee.[7] The predominant injury mechanisms found in their study resulted from motorcycle accidents in six of ten patients and pedestrian-auto accidents in two of seven patients.

Ipsilateral concomitant fractures of the femur and tibia usually are caused by direct, high-energy trauma. DeLee found 4 of 15 limbs with residual knee instability.[8] Two limbs had anteromedial rotary instability and two limbs had posterior instability.

Fraser and associates reviewed 222 limbs with this injury pattern.[9] Ligamentous injury about the knee was diagnosed within 3 weeks in only 6 patients and after 6 weeks in 11 patients. Of their patients, 99 were traceable, but only 63 were examined. Ligamentous laxity of the knee was present in 39% of those patients seen in follow-up, and in one third of these patients, the laxity

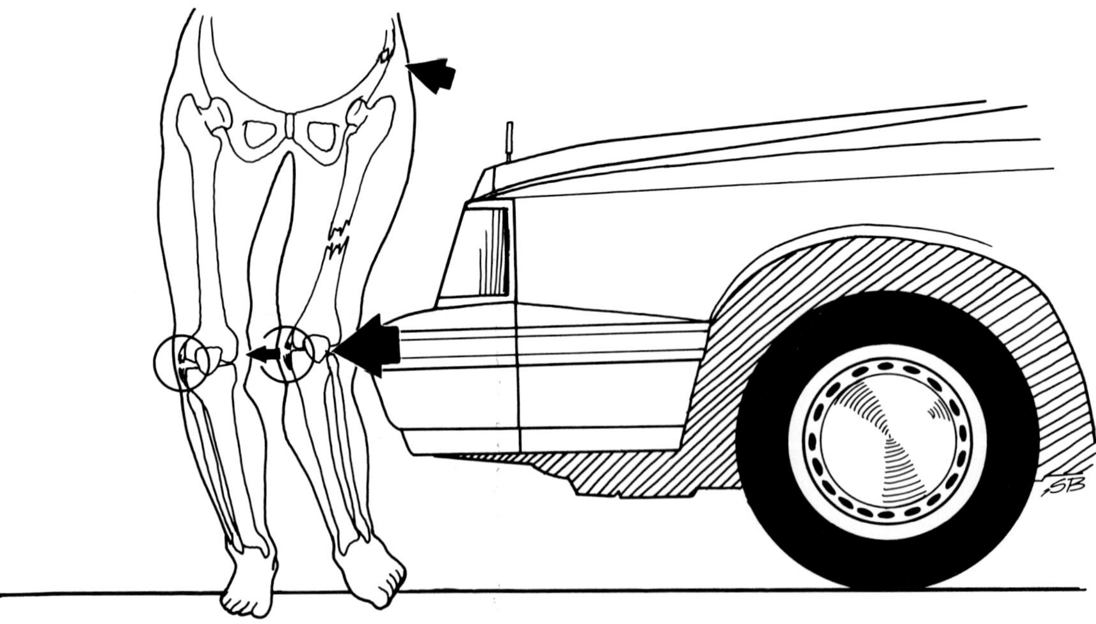

FIG. 20-1. Example of injury mechanism in pedestrian-auto accident.

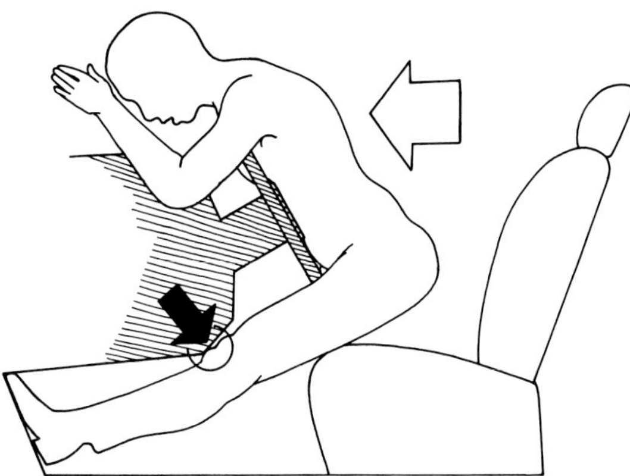

Fig. 20-2. Example of injury mechanism in motor-vehicle accident.

was severe. Thus, the incidence of the ligament injury found at follow-up was five times greater than that discovered during the initial hospitalization. At least two thirds of their patients had multiple-system injury with about one in four patients sustaining craniocerebral injury.

The incidence of knee injury associated with ipsilateral hip injury has been reported variably. Casey and Chapman found 9 limbs with associated ipsilateral knee injuries in 21 limbs with concomitant ipsilateral fractures of the hip and femoral shaft.[10] They did not diagnose any ligamentous injury to the knee, and the knee injuries were largely secondary to direct blows upon the knee. Gillespie retrospectively reviewed 135 posterior dislocations and fracture-dislocations of the hip.[11] He found 25 limbs with knee injuries clearly attributable to a direct blow on the front of the knee, such as fractured patella, traumatic chondromalacia, and fracture of femoral and tibial condyles. There were ten limbs with ligamentous injury of the knee, which were overlooked on initial examination (Fig. 20-3). Medial and anterior instability were present in four patients, medial instability alone in two patients, lateral instability alone in two patients, and anterior instability in two patients. Diagnosis in six of the patients was established at admission, but in the other four patients, diagnosis was late.

Moore has proposed a separate classification of fractures of the proximal tibia that are associated with instability caused by rupture of the soft-tissue supporting structures of the knee.[12] He distinguishes these injuries as fracture-dislocation of the knee in contrast to the typical tibial plateau fracture, which demonstrates knee instability because of loss of support for the opposing femoral condyle. Previous reports of knee ligament damage associated with intra-articular proximal tibial fractures were most likely fracture-dislocations, according to Moore's definition. Stress radiographs are essential for the diagnosis, and Moore recommends operative repair of the soft- and osseous-tissue injuries.

Knee ligament injuries are commonly associated with ipsilateral fractures in situations of high-energy trauma, but prompt recognition of the diagnosis has not been consistent. Furthermore, there is a high degree of associated multiple-system injury. Many patients involved in high-energy trauma incidents sustain craniocerebral injury. The patient with a closed head injury is obtund, frequently for days, and does not complain of pain; consequently, there is no targeting patient complaint that can enhance diagnosis of knee ligament problems.

As Shelton and associates suggested,[5] the knee injury probably occurs before the fracture. It is unlikely that a knee could be loaded and stressed enough to cause ligamentous rupture when the osseous structures are not intact. In such instances, stress would be transmitted to the area of bone disassociation and would not be great enough to cause ligamentous rupture. Of course, if there was secondary entrapment, for instance underneath the automobile or under the driving module, secondary loading of knee ligaments could occur (Fig. 20-4).

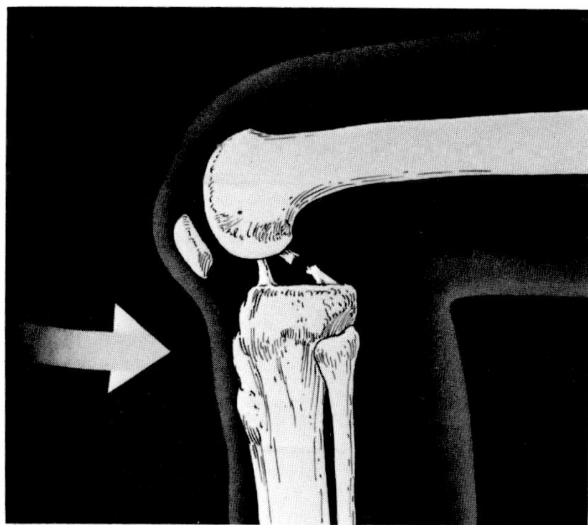

Fig. 20-3. Example of axial loading from automobile accident causing posterior cruciate injury and posterior fracture-dislocation of hip.

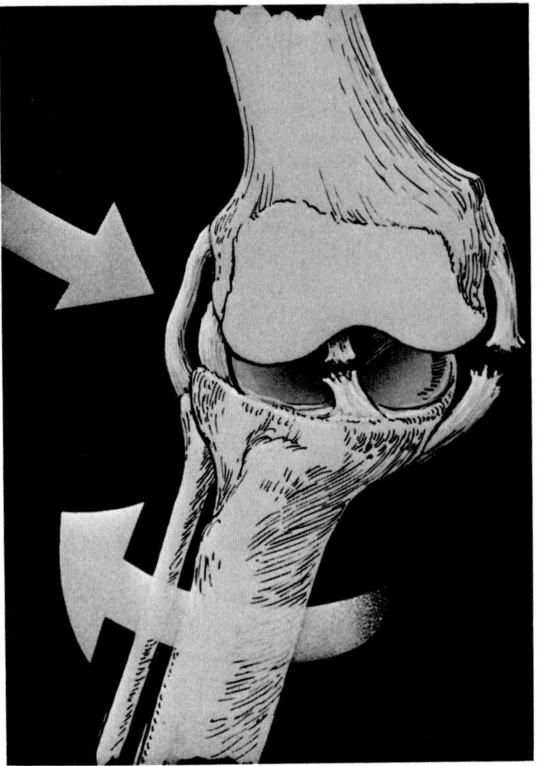

Fig. 20-4. Example of valgus and rotatory stresses causing medial capsular and anterior cruciate injury.

Classification of Knee Ligament Injuries

Ligamentous injuries are graded according to increasing severity and increasing number of fibers disrupted (Fig. 20-5). Grade I injuries show only mild amounts of tearing of the ligamentous fibers, minimal swelling pain, and no significant instability. The integrity of the ligament is largely intact. A grade II injury indicates moderate ligament tearing with increasing physical signs of tenderness and swelling. The end point to stress testing may be soft with grade II injuries, and range of motion may be somewhat limited. Grade III injuries signify complete tearing of the ligament with no functional stability. Limited range of motion, particularly in the extremes of range, significant tenderness, and swelling of the unstable joint are the hallmarks of grade III injuries. Electron microscopic studies show that, although the gross appearance of the ligament may be normal, there may be extensive intimal tearing and attenuation of ligamentous fibers. Therefore, there may be some secondary lengthening and loss of functional capacity even with a grossly intact ligament.

The classification of knee ligament injuries has been somewhat confusing. The Committee on

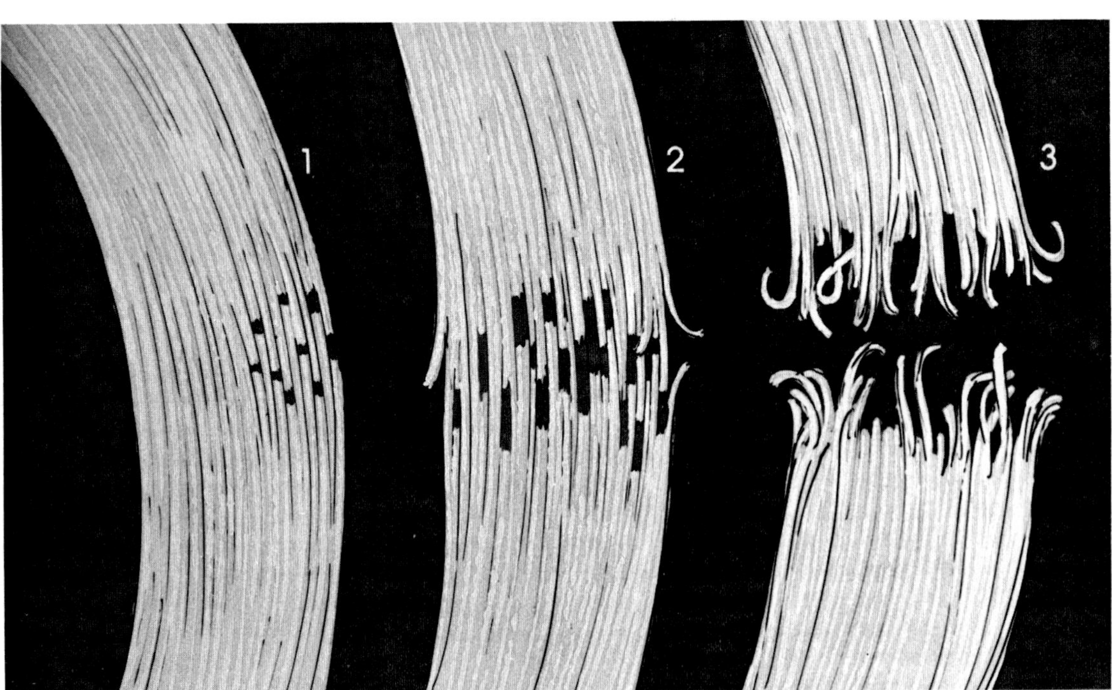

Fig. 20-5. Schematic of grades I, II, and III ligament injury.

Research and Education of the American Orthopedic Society of Sports Medicine has classified knee instability as follows:

I. One-plane instability
  A. One-plane medial
  B. One-plane lateral
  C. One-plane posterior
  D. One-plane anterior
II. Rotary instabilities
  A. Anteromedial
  B. Anterolateral
    1. In flexion
    2. In extension
  C. Posterolateral
  D. Posteromedial
III. Combined instabilities
  A. Anterolateral-posterolateral rotary
  B. Anterolateral-anteromedial rotary
  C. Anteromedial-posteromedial rotary

This classification is based on the direction of displacement of the tibia with relation to the femur. The specific anatomic injuries that produce such displacement to stress testing continue to be the subject of dispute.

Diagnosis of Concomitant Knee Ligament Injuries

History and Physical Examination

A history of high-energy direct trauma with pelvic or lower extremity fractures is strongly suggestive of concomitant knee ligament injuries. Since the initial examination of the patient by emergency medical personnel or by physicians not specializing in trauma to the musculoskeletal system may only target the fracture and its associated deformity, the treating orthopaedist must ascertain the presence or absence of knee ligament injury. Frequently, the leg is splinted by the emergency care team, and consequently, access to the knee for examination is difficult to obtain. Nonetheless, the orthopaedic surgeon must perform a thorough, systematic examination.

Patients who sustain concomitant craniocerebral injury and therefore are unable to give an adequate history should be re-examined carefully when the closed head injury begins to clear, or at 3- to 5-day intervals, to assure that no injuries have been missed. Waddell and Drucker reviewed ten patients involved in pedestrian accidents.[13] Six of those patients had one or more injuries that were not diagnosed at the initial examination. All of those patients sustained craniocerebral injuries, femoropelvic injuries, and knee injuries. The knee injuries included ligamentous rupture and distal femoral or proximal tibial fractures.

If the patient is awake, complaints of pain at the knee or sites of ligamentous attachment can help to target the examination. Extensive ligament disruption, of course, causes diffuse tenderness. Differentiation between meniscal trauma and ligamentous trauma frequently can be made on the basis that compression pain occurs in the compartment with meniscal injury, whereas tension pain caused by stress examination indicates ligamentous injuries. The limbs should be inspected for areas of local abrasion or ecchymosis. Any evidence of a local blow to the knee or of entrapment of the knee should demand a thorough stress examination of the knee.

Effusion of the knee should be considered secondary to knee ligament injury unless proved otherwise. The early development of effusion is the almost pathognomonic of cruciate rupture. Effusion that appears later, particularly while the patient is in traction, should not be attributed to "sympathetic effusion." Rather, it should be considered indicative of knee ligament injury, and definitive diagnostic procedures must be performed.

Ligamentous injury asociated with capsular disruption does not show a significant effusion of the knee. The fluid displaces into fascial planes about the knee because of rupture of the capsule and produces diffuse swelling.

Stress Testing

If ligamentous injury is suspected, stress testing must be performed. As time from the acute injury passes, swelling and muscle spasm make evaluation of the patient difficult. Heavily muscled individuals can guard and stabilize the knee against stress testing. If there is any question of ligamentous laxity, examination under adequate anesthesia should be performed. This examination can be done with local anesthetic infiltration, but is probably best performed under general anesthesia. The patient should be prepared for surgery at that time and told that operative treatment may ensue.

If the contralateral knee is uninjured, it should be tested first to determine the physiologic status of the individual patient. The lateral compartment usually opens to stress testing approximately 25 to 50% more than does the medial compartment. Stress testing of the knee is performed to determine the presence of any of the instabilities previously outlined. However, stress testing is more difficult in the presence of ipsilateral fractures. With femoral fractures in particular, there is no stability in the proximal fragment; therefore, a distal femoral Steinmann's pin should be placed to hold the proximal fragment for evaluation of the ligamentous status. The distal Steinmann's pin should be placed only when ligamentous injury is strongly suspected on the basis of the foregoing type of examination and history.

Fractures of the proximal tibia also preclude stress testing and examination. Transverse fractures should be stabilized with a proximal fragment tibial Steinmann's pin if there is a likelihood of ligament damage. Tibial plateau fractures give the clinical illusion of instability because of depression of the fracture surfaces. Stress radiographs help to make the definitive diagnosis, but occasionally the instability can be determined only after definitive fracture fixation.

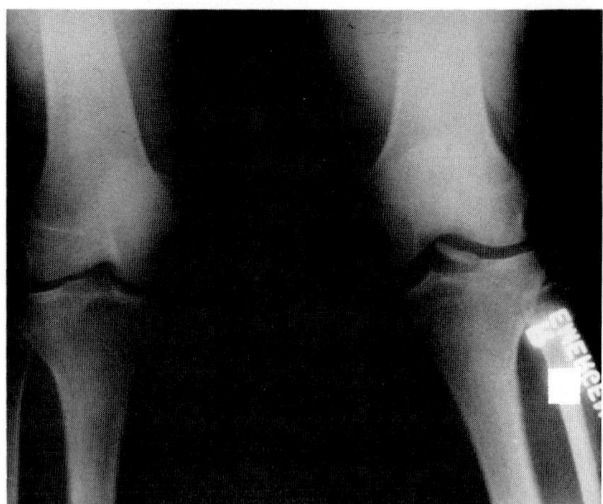

Fig. 20-6. Avulsion fracture of tibial attachment of anterior cruciate ligament.

Radiographic Examination

Radiographs are necessary to completely define the diagnosis of a patient with an injured limb. The plain radiograph should be examined thoroughly for avulsion fractures. Avulsion of the attachments of the ligamentous or capsular structures about the knee renders the knee unstable. Avulsion fractures of the tibial attachments of the cruciate ligaments are much more common than of the femoral attachments (Fig. 20-6). Such cruciate avulsion fractures usually are seen on the lateral radiograph.

On the medial side of the knee, the avulsion fracture more frequently involves the femoral attachment. Late manifestation of trauma to the knee ligament can be seen on the knee radiograph and is termed Pellegrini-Stieda disease. On the lateral side of the knee, the avulsion fracture most commonly seen is from the fibular attachment on the lateral ligaments (Fig. 20-7).

The lateral capsular sign is described as an avulsion fracture of the tibial attachment of the lateral capsule, which usually is found on the plain radiograph and is indicative of significant damage to the lateral side of the knee.

Children with epiphyseal plates still open can sustain ligamentous damage to the knee caused by severe, direct trauma.[14] More frequently, there is an epiphyseal fracture. Careful evaluation of plain radiographs may show the small metaphyseal flake of a Salter II epiphyseal fracture or a more significant epiphyseal damage. Stress radiographs, however, are required to demonstrate the nondisplaced or occult epiphyseal fracture (Fig. 20-8).

All patients involved in high-energy trauma should have roentgenograms taken of the obvious bone with fracture deformity, including the joint above and the joint below. An anteroposterior roentgenogram taken of the pelvis is mandatory since pelvic fractures can also remain occult if the bony landmarks are obscured by surrounding soft tissues.

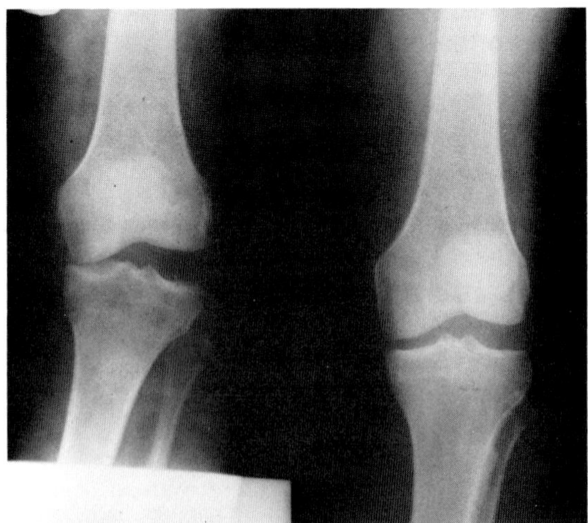

Fig. 20-7. Varus stress test demonstrating injury to lateral supporting structures and avulsion fracture of fibula head.

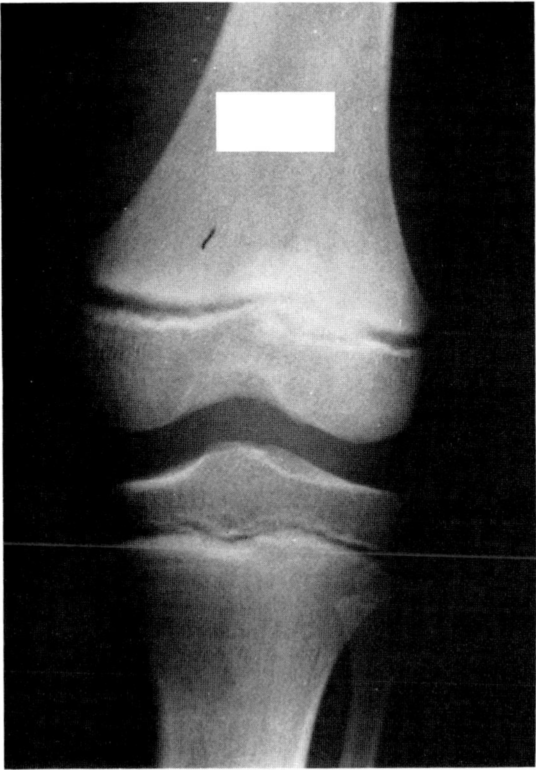

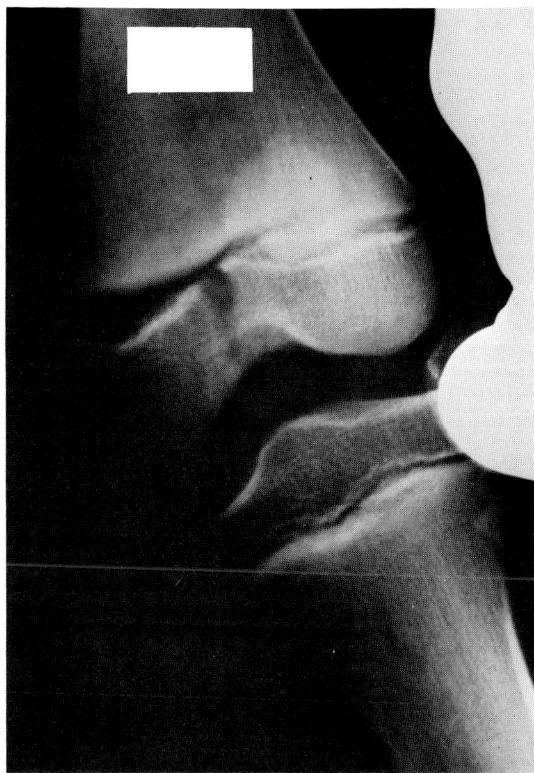

Fig. 20-8. *A*, Plain radiograph of an 11-year-old patient with suspected knee ligament injury. *B*, Valgus stress radiograph demonstrating epiphyseal fracture in an 11-year-old patient with suspected knee ligament injury.

Patients with multiple-system injuries and craniocerebral trauma should be re-examined as their neurologic status clears. If the patient complains of pain, radiographs should be performed to disclose any possible injuries.

Stress Radiographs

Stress testing the knee under radiographic control is particularly important to the diagnosis of knee ligament injuries. A primary indication for stress radiographs is a finding of clinical instability about the knee in a patient with open epiphyseal plates.

Stress radiographs should be performed with varus and valgus stress at 0° and 30° of flexion (Fig. 20-9). At 90° of flexion, the lateral radiographs with anterior and posterior stress application demonstrate damage to the appropriate cruciate ligament (Fig. 20-10). Combined and rotary instability are not always demonstrable by plain stress radiographs. Image intensification of fluoroscopic control can demonstrate combined or rotary instabilities. However, such sophisticated studies rarely can be performed in the presence of associated fractures.

If the associated fractures preclude examination of knee joint stability, some arrangement must be made to perform definitive diagnostic stress radiographs. With femoral fractures, a distal femoral Steinmann's pin must be placed to hold control of the distal femur. In some instances, e.g., tibial plateau fractures, stress radiographs should be performed routinely. Martin states that an increase of 1 cm in the medial clear space of the involved side compared with that of the noninvolved side was indicative of medial ligament rupture in limbs with lateral plateau fractures.[15]

Another form of stress radiograph is the plain film, which can be taken of the knee with the patient in tibial pin traction. Patients with fractured femurs in particular should have anteroposterior and lateral views taken of the knee as well as of the fractured femur in traction. When there is damage to the ligaments of the knee, the constant pull of the traction apparatus shows abnormal bony relationships of the knee on the roentgenogram.

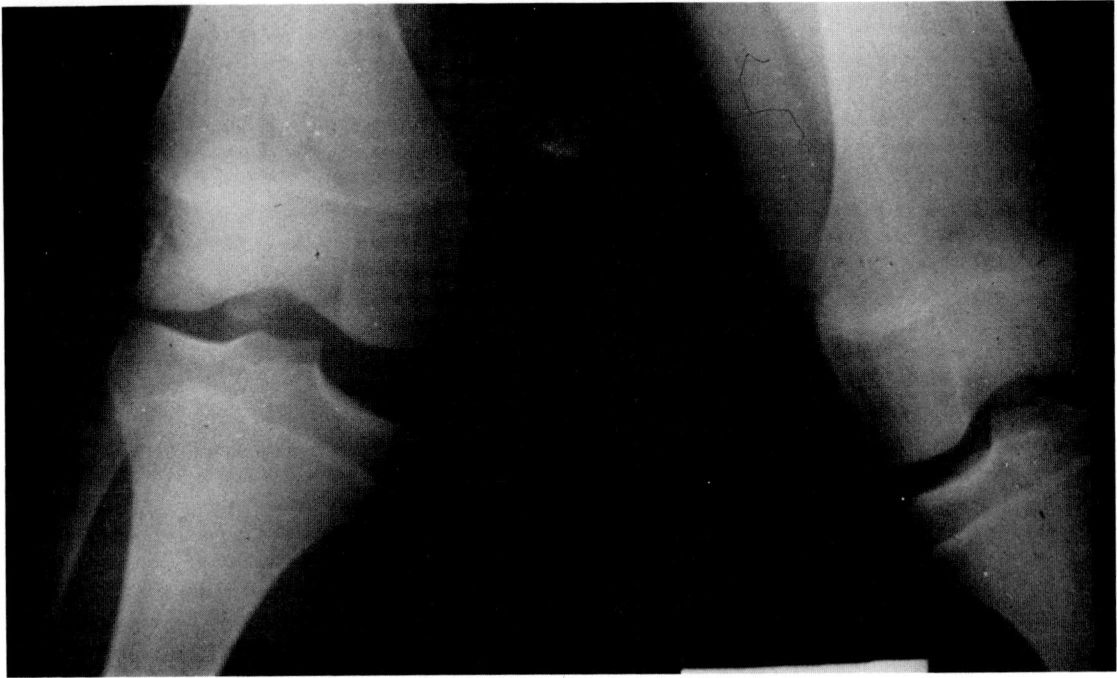

Fig. 20-9. Radiograph of bilateral valgus stress test demonstrating injury to medial supporting structures on the right.

Arthrography

Arthrography can be used in the acute phase to demonstrate knee ligament injuries. Initial aspiration of the knee should be performed and the aspirate examined. When globules appear in the aspirate, an osteochondral fracture usually is present. If the aspiration demonstrates a hemarthrosis, there is good evidence for a ligamentous disruption.

Leakage of contrast material into the periarticular tissues is indicative of grade III ligamentous or capsular damage. If the anterior cruciate can be seen on the lateral view of the acute arthrogram, one can conclude with a high degree of probability that it is intact. Failure to visualize the anterior cruciate ligament usually indicates complete disruption. This is an all-or-none phenomenon in that grade I or grade II injuries to the anterior cruciate ligament would not be picked up in such a study since the fibers remain grossly intact.

Arthroscopic Examination

Just as cardiologists began to make great leaps forward in the diagnosis of heart disease when the electrocardiogram became available to supplement the physical examination, the orthopaedists have been able to make more definitive diagnoses with the help of arthroscopy.[16,17] Diagnosis of ligament injury, delineation of osteochondral fractures, and demonstration of meniscal injuries are possible under direct visualization with the arthroscope.

The patient should be prepared for the operating room, and the surgeon should be ready to undertake definitive treatment if arthroscopy is to be performed. While arthroscopy can be done under local anesthesia, local arthroscopy would be difficult to perform in the patient with ipsilateral fractures. The patient would continue to have pain from the fractures, and manipulation of the knee would only augment that pain and cause muscle guarding and a poor arthroscopic study.

Treatment Options

Nonoperative Management

The treatment of knee ligament injuries by nonoperative means is appropriate for injuries that do not produce instability. Grade I and grade II ligament injuries, particularly of the collateral ligaments, do not require operative repair.

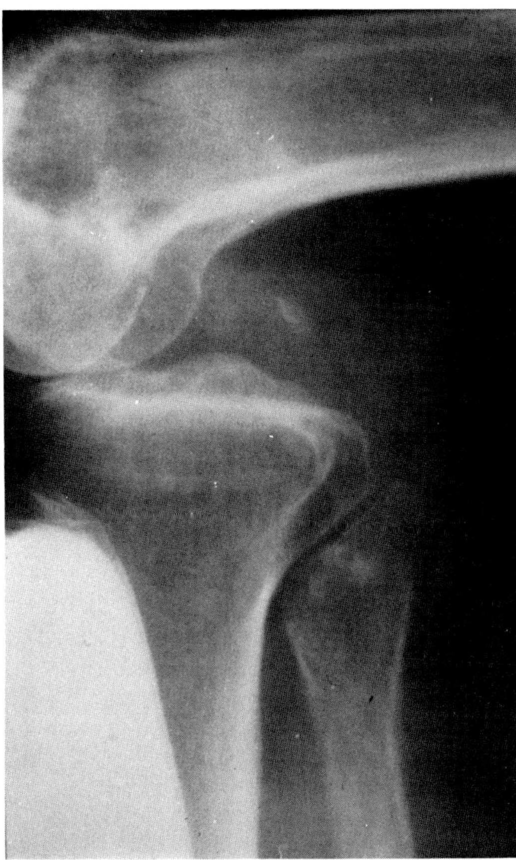

Fig. 20-10. Stress radiograph of posterior drawer test.

Hastings described the use of a controlled-mobilization cast-brace for the treatment of grade III collateral ligament injuries of the knee.[18] He made a particular point that the collateral ligament injury should be isolated and not associated with cruciate ligament tears. Hastings contended that the presence of intact cruciate ligaments implies initial stresses on the knee that are somewhat limited. The diagnosis of isolated collateral ligament tear must be positive and should be confirmed with examination under anesthesia. Hastings suggested initial treatment with a long-leg cast at 90° of flexion and molded to the appropriate rotatory and angulatory alignment that would reverse the injury mechanism and allow healing of the ligament at the shortest relative length. After 2 weeks, the limb is placed in a cast-brace with the same alignment restraints, and controlled mobilization is allowed from 45 to 100°. He described excellent results in his series with the use of historical controls.

Basset and associates[19] also used historical controls to validate controlled mobilization therapy for acute knee ligament injuries treated nonoperatively, e.g., in the case of isolated collateral injury, and operatively, such as combined collateral and cruciate injuries, and for late reconstructive procedures. Satisfactory healing was reported in most of the patients with a carefully applied cast-brace. Again, appropriate reversal of rotation and angulation at the time of injury should be performed.

Cast-brace management of knee ligament injuries requires experience and careful attention to detail in application of the cast-brace. If the rotational or angulatory deforming stresses are not reversed, the ligament will heal in a relatively lengthened state and will cause instability. Treatment of knee ligament injuries in a way that does not immobilize the knee has some major advantages. Immobilization produces significant alterations in connective tissue of the ligament, the articular cartilage, and the biomechanical properties of the bone ligament complex.[20,21] Additionally, since the muscles are functioning actively, atrophy is considerably less than that encountered when the entire limb is immobilized.

My Preferred Treatment

The knee ligament injury associated with ipsilateral fracture is usually the result of high-energy, direct violence. With multiple-system injury, the decision may be made to treat the fractures nonoperatively. In such situations, operative repair of the knee ligament damage is unlikely, and the knee ligament should be managed with a controlled-mobilization cast-brace. When traction is necessary for the fracture, e.g., a diaphyseal femur fracture, modifications of the cast-brace management are necessary. I prefer a modification of Neufeld roller traction using a distal femoral pin for skeletal fixation.[22] The pin is incorporated with the thigh cast. The usual eye bolt hinges are replaced by 30 to 60° or 45 to 90°controlled-mobilization knee hinges (commercially available), which are connected to a short-leg cast. Appropriate angular or rotatory alignment can be obtained by positioning the tibia to allow healing in the shortest functional position (Fig. 20-11).

Dislocation or fracture-dislocation of the hip is another situation in which non-operative management of the skeletal injury may be undertaken. Any associated isolated collateral ligament injury can be treated with controlled mobilization during the time the patient is maintained in traction.

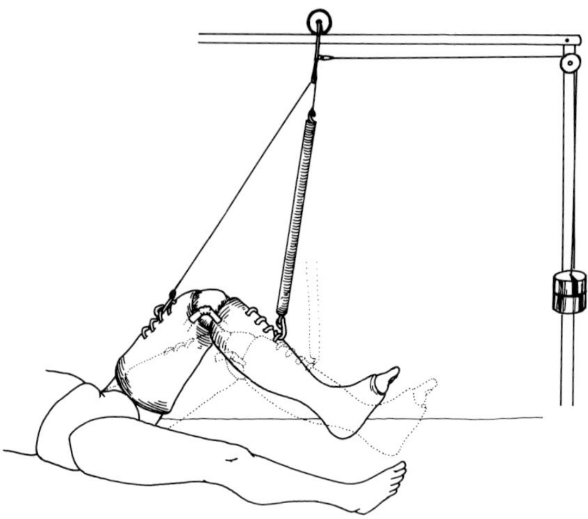

Fig. 20-11. Roller traction setup for treatment of femoral fracture and knee ligament injury.

Because of the violent injury mechanism in these commonly associated complex injuries, there may be open wounds on the limb. The magnitude of soft-tissue loss may also influence decisions on operative management. For instance, knee ligament injury in the presence of ipsilateral, concomitant, open grade II or III femur and tibial fractures may require external fixation to give the best result. Controlled-mobilization knee hinges can be appropriately applied to external-fixation anchoring frames of the tibia or femur or can be attached from a distal femoral pin to an external anchoring frame for the tibia using plaster as the bonding agent.

When a nonoperative approach to the knee ligament injury is elected, I believe that each patient should be placed in a controlled-mobilization cast-brace rather than completely immobilized in the traditional manner. The benefits of functional treatment of the knee ligament injury accrue for the limb components by the increase in mobility allowed for the whole patient. Furthermore, the patient can be initiated early into the concept of responsibility for his own rehabilitation. Rehabilitation exercises with muscle strengthening can be started at the bedside and should be encouraged throughout the convalescent period.

Operative Management

A theme throughout this book is that fracture stabilization allows early mobilization, which is important in the overall management of the patient. Ipsilateral knee ligament injury causing instability is a relative primary indication for operative fracture fixation to allow definitive operative treatment of the knee ligament injury. Such complex injuries are also complex therapeutic problems. Shelton and associates found poor results in their patients with unreduced ipsilateral fractures and unrepaired ligaments.[5] They called the employment of tibial tubercle traction for treatment of femoral and pelvic fractures in the presence of ruptured knee ligaments a ''catastrophe.''

More recently, Walker and Kennedy have also suggested primary rigid internal fixation of femoral fractures when associated with knee ligament injuries.[23] Walling and Spiegel also believed that combined femoral and knee injuries were relative indications for primary rigid fixation of the femur to allow treatment of the knee ligament injury.[7]

The treatment options for fixation of the fractures are thoroughly discussed in the appropriate chapters of this book and need not be repeated. It should be emphasized that early rigid internal fixation is preferable. In the patient with multiple injuries, the best opportunity for complete and definitive treatment of complex knee injuries is frequently in the acute phase. Patients with significant head injuries or with subsequent complicating factors that arise during their hospital stay may be unable to tolerate another operative procedure for a prolonged period of time.

O'Donoghue has championed acute surgical repair of knee ligament injuries.[24] Hughston and Eilers also have emphasized the necessity of early ligamentous repair to a good functional result.[25] Such acute repair is particularly important for the patient who will place high functional demands on the knee.

Repair of Medial Supporting Structures

Ideally, the limb should be positioned in 45° of flexion of the hip with abduction and external rotation and 45° of flexion of the knee; however, this positioning may be compromised by the associated fractures. An anteromedial oblique incision is made beginning distally at the insertion of the pes tendons into the tibia. It extends proximally and posteriorly over the anterior medial triangle of the knee, passes back to the adductor tubercle, and is extended proximally as far as necessary. A medial cutaneous flap then is developed, preserving the neurovascular structures in the subcutaneous tissue and exposing the fascia on the medial aspect of the knee. The medial side of the knee then can be inspected for areas of ecchymosis or gross rupture of the fascia, which can help to target sites of injury. Stress testing should be performed under direct vision. The proximal border of the pes anserinus is observed and palpated, and the deep fascia is incised along that border. Care must be exercised at this juncture to prevent incision of the fibers of the medial collateral ligament that lie just underneath the pes anserinus. The superificial medial collateral ligament can be seen passing beneath the pes anserinus in the mid-medial plane. The pes anserinus should be lifted and the superficial medial collateral ligament inspected along its entire course to define any areas of injury. This can be done with retraction, but frequently one must detach the distal two thirds of the pes tendon from the tibia to allow complete inspection of the superficial medial collateral ligament. The proximal one third of the tendon should always remain attached.

Tears in the medial ligamentous complex that lie deep to the superficial collateral ligament may involve the components of the medial capsular ligament, the anterior third, the medial third, or the posterior third. The most frequently torn areas are the meniscofemoral and meniscotibial portions of the medial third of the medial capsular ligament and the posterior third of the medial capsular ligament.

When the meniscus is not torn through the substance and the coronary attachment to the capsule layer is intact, direct repair can be performed in the arca from which the capsular ligament is torn (either the tibia or the femur). If direct repair is not possible, the capsule should be reattached through drill holes into the bone using heavy synthetic, nonabsorbable suture material.

The meniscus must be retained if at all possible. If there are no substance tears within the meniscus, the meniscus can be reattached to either the meniscofemoral or meniscotibial portions of the ligament. If there are tears within the body of the meniscus, the meniscus should be trimmed to retain as much functioning peripheral meniscus as possible.

The importance of the menisci to knee function cannot be overemphasized. If the meniscus is damanged and, therefore, must be removed, instability of the knee will be more pronounced. Additionally, stress degeneration of the compartment from which the meniscus is removed is the universal outcome. Damage to the meniscus necessitating removal in the presence of anterior cruciate or posterior cruciate injury causes a loss of stability even if ligamentous repair is successful. For this reason, acute anatomic repairs of the medial ligamentous complex and the anterior cruciate ligament occasionally must be supplemented to enhance knee stability. There is no universal agreement on this question. However, in patients with the complex of fracture and knee ligament damage, operative time usually dictates that only acute repair and not supplemental reconstruction can be performed.

Attention then should be directed to the interior of the knee with a median parapatellar incision through the synovium. This incision is not necessary if there is significant disruption of the medial supporting structures. Inspection of all compartments of the knee should be done at this time. The patella femoral compartment should not be forgotten because the injury mechanism with ipsilateral fractures and knee ligament tears frequently includes a direct blow to the knee that causes osteochondral fractures. The lateral meniscus, the medial meniscus, and the cruciate ligaments should be inspected thoroughly. If the cruciates are torn, repair should be instituted with suture placement.

Flexion of the knee to 90° and further development of the posterior medial cutaneous flap readily expose the posterior medial corner of the knee. Delineation and repair of damage to the posterior third of the medial capsular ligament are particularly important. Failure to repair this damage results in anteromedial rotary instability. The posterior third of the medial capsular ligament should be repaired directly, if possible. Nonabsorbable synthetic sutures should be used. If direct suture is not possible, drill holes should be placed in the capsular ligament to anchor the tissue firmly to the bone.

In some instances the posterior medial corner cannot be repaired anatomically. Exposure of the medial aspect of the medial head of the gastrocnemius tendon allows detachment from the posterior femoral condyle. The tendon then should be split distally, leaving the muscular fibers that attach toward the midline of the knee. The tendinous fibers then can be used to supplement the posteromedial corner by penetrating the posterior capsule and directing the fibers medially and anteriorly and reattaching them to the medial femoral condyle, either into available viable soft tissue or through drill holes into the osseous tissue.

An alternative unit available for supplementation is the semimembranosus. Larson has described this procedure in detail.[26] Other alternatives for supplementation include the pes anserinus tendons and the medial one third of the patella tendon.

Positioning of the limb in flexion abduction and external rotation of the hip with 60 to 90° of flexion at the knee allow gravity to take the knee into a varus position. The appropriate rotational correction must be obtained before sutures are snugged down.

Tears of the cruciate ligaments should be sutured before repair of the medial supporting structures is undertaken. However, typing of the cruciate sutures should be performed after the medial structures are repaired.

Repair of Lateral Supporting Structures

Medial complex tears are much more common than lateral complex tears. Operative repair is indicated when varus or lateral rotational instability has been demonstrated by stress testing.

Positioning of the patient begins with a roll under the greater trochanter to provide accessibility to the lateral side of the knee. An anterior lateral oblique incision is made, beginning some 2 or 3 cm distal to the tibial tubercle and extending proximally and posteriorly across the anterior lateral triangle of the knee and on to the lateral epicondyle. The incision can be extended proximally along the line of the iliotibial tract as necessary. The distal limb of the incision may have to be extended somewhat posteriorly to visualize adequately the region of the fibula head. The cutaneous flap is developed posteriorly and laterally to expose the fascia and inspect the lateral side of the knee for ecchymosis. On the lateral side of the knee, the peroneal nerve should be identified and protected throughout the procedure. Stress testing under direct vision helps to determine the injured areas.

Particular attention should be paid to the head of the fibula with inspection for avulsion of the conjoined attachment of biceps and fibula collateral ligament. The lateral capsule attachment to the tibia and the iliotibial tract at Gerdy's tubercle also should be inspected carefully. The posterior lateral capsule and the arcuate ligament also are inspected.

If there is a large lateral capsular rent, anterior lateral synovial incision is not necessary to inspect the joint. If the joint cannot be readily visualized, a synovial incision should be made and a thorough inspection of all the compartments of the knee carried out.

Primary suturing should be undertaken if either of the cruciate ligaments is ruptured, but the sutures should not be tied until lateral repair is completed.

Again, the lateral meniscus must be maintained if possible. Because of the anatomic configuration of the lateral compartment, the lateral meniscus is even more important than the medial meniscus for maintenance of rotational stability.[27]

After inspection and stress testing have identified the lesions, anatomic restoration of the lateral supporting structures should be undertaken. The knee should be flexed 45 to 60° and held in valgus and external rotation to snug up the posterior lateral corner.

Direct suture of the posterior or posterior lateral capsule should be performed. If this is not possible, the posterior capsule should be pulled distally and sutured through drill holes into the tibia with nonabsorbable synthetic suture.

Repair of the lateral collateral ligament in its substance or at its femoral or tibial attachments should be accomplished next. An avulsion of the iliotibial tract should be replaced with barbed staples.

If anatomic restoration of the lateral supporting structures is not possible, supplementation of repair should be performed. Larson suggests the use of advancement of the lateral edge of the arcuate ligament into the posterior capsule, reattachment of the lateral aspect of the lateral head of the gastrocnemius, transplantation of the biceps tendon, or rerouting and transplantation of the iliotibial band for reinforcement of the lateral side of the knee.[26]

Repair of Cruciate Ligaments and Posterior Supporting Structures

Acute repair of anterior cruciate ligament rupture is a controversial subject. There are many advocates of acute repair, including O'Donoghue,[24] Larson,[26] and Marshall and Rubin,[28] who cite late degenerative changes and functional problems in the nonrepaired limb. Such pessimism largely has been documented subjectively through personal experience, and often evaluation has been complicated by inclusion of other major ligament injuries. McDaniel and Damron reported on 53 knees with surgically documented ruptures of the anterior cruciate ligament that were evaluated some 10 years post injury.[29] Although the incidence of anterior and anteromedial rotary instability and meniscal tears was high at follow-up, the radiographic evidence of osteoarthritis was low. Only 10 knees had degeneration of articular cartilage noted at follow-up arthrotomy, and McDaniel and Damron felt this development was more likely related to meniscus injury and changes following menisectomy than to instability of the anterior cruciate ligament. They noted much better results in patients who regained normal thigh circumference than in patients who did not.

It does seem clear that the late development of anterior lateral rotary instability is secondary to chronic anterior cruciate insufficiency.[30] Anterior lateral rotary instability is more functionally disabling than anterior medial rotary instability. The musculotendinous units frequently can compensate for instability in the anteromedial plane, but dynamic stabilization is not as successful with anterior lateral instability.

In the patient without a prospect of high functional demands, anterior cruciate repair may be bypassed. If the menisci are intact, the experience of McDaniel and Damron would seem to indicate that outcomes may not be significantly improved by anterior cruciate repair. If the knee is surgically explored and the anterior cruciate is ruptured, acute repair should be performed, particularly if either meniscus must be removed.

Though injuries demonstrating predominate anterior cruciate instability can occur, such instability usually is associated with other lesions of the ligaments about the knee. Girgi, et al., demonstrated that rupture of the posterior cruciate is possible only after rupture of the anterior cruciate in injuries caused by hyperextension.[31] The posterior cruciate is approximately twice as strong as the anterior cruciate; consequently, rupture of the posterior cruciate is much less common. Rupture of the posterior cruciate is the most disabling of all knee ligament injuries. Though it may occur as an isolated injury (with a posterior directed force on the tibia with the knee in flexion), it is more usually associated with other major knee ligament ruptures.

Accurate repair of the cruciate ligaments depends on restoration of the normal anatomic sites of attachment. The anterior cruciate inserts on the tibia at the junction of the anterior third and posterior two thirds between the tibial spines. The posterior cruciate inserts on the posterior aspect of the tibia, blending in with the posterior capsule. On the femoral side, the anterior cruciate inserts well posterior in the intercondylar notch on the lateral condyle. The attachment of the posterior cruciate to the femur is somewhat more anterior than that of the anterior cruciate, but lies posterior to the midline plane in the notch on the medial condyle.

Tibial detachment of the anterior cruciate is usually at the bone-ligament interface or with an avulsed fragment of bone. Synthetic nonabsorbable suture can be passed readily through drill holes to reattach the anterior cruciate ligament. Such ruptures usually do not interrupt the blood supply of the anterior cruciate entering through the synovial sleeve and fat pad and can be expected to heal with good functional outcome.

Detachment of the anterior cruciate from the femoral side presents several treatment options. The ligament can be reattached to the femur through drill holes that must be tied on the lateral aspect of the lateral femoral condyle. This necessitates a separate incision if exposure is through the anteromedial approach. Several drill guides are available for accurate placement of the drill holes.

My preference for reattachment of the anterior cruciate to the femur is the "over-the-top" method described by McIntosh.[32] The ligament is secured with synthetic nonabsorbable sutures and passed over the posterior aspect of the lateral femoral condyle and firmly secured into the posterior lateral capsule and lateral head of the gastrocnemius muscle. This approach, too, requires making a separate lateral incision to define the plane of the intermuscular septum and then passing a curved clamp through the posterior capsule and into the knee joint to grasp the suture.

Injuries to the substance of the anterior cruciate ligament are difficult to repair. Pulling the proximal fibers distal through tibial drill holes and the distal fibers proximal through femoral drill holes for overlapping of the ligament offers the best of alternatives. The synovium with its blood supply to the cruciate ligament is essential for healing of the ligament. When the synovium is disrupted, incision through the fat pad with plication of the fat pad about the body of the repaired cruciate ligament is reported to facilitate healing.

Detachment of the tibial insertion of the posterior cruciate presents some problems with exposure. The anteromedial incision with the knee flexed at least 90° most often provides adequate visualization of the posterior cruciate after incision of the capsule in the posteromedial "soft spot.'' Occasionally, a formal posterior approach to the knee must be undertaken. An avulsion fracture can be reattached with screws or staples (Figs. 20-12, 20-13). Reattachment of the ligament at the bone-ligament interface usually requires placement of drill holes into the bone. The posterior capsule frequently is torn from the tibia with posterior cruciate injury, and it should be reattached in its anatomic position. Pulling the posterior capsule too far distally limits extension of the knee postoperatively.

Reattachment of the posterior cruciate to the femur should be performed through drill holes extending from the medial femoral condyle. Ruptures of the body of the posterior cruciate should be reapproximated in methods similar to those used with the anterior cruciate ligament.

Supplementation of anterior cruciate repair usually is not indicated in the patient with associated complex fractures. However, the patella tendon, the iliotibial band, the semitendinosus tendons, and the semimembranosus tendons have been described for use as reinforcement or reconstruction of anterior cruciate injuries. Supplementation for the posterior cruciate has utilized the patella tendon, the medial head of the gastrocnemius, and popliteus tendon. If satisfactory anatomic restoration of the posterior cruciate is not accomplished, I prefer immediate supplementation with the tendinous portion of the medial head of the gastrocnemius. The tendon is detached from the femur and placed through the intercondylar notch by drill holes into the medial femoral condyle. The distal portion of the tendon then is split and sutured into the posterior capsule, if available, or by drill holes into the bone. Because the posterior cruciate is the cornerstone ligament of the knee, one must obtain as stable a repair as possible.

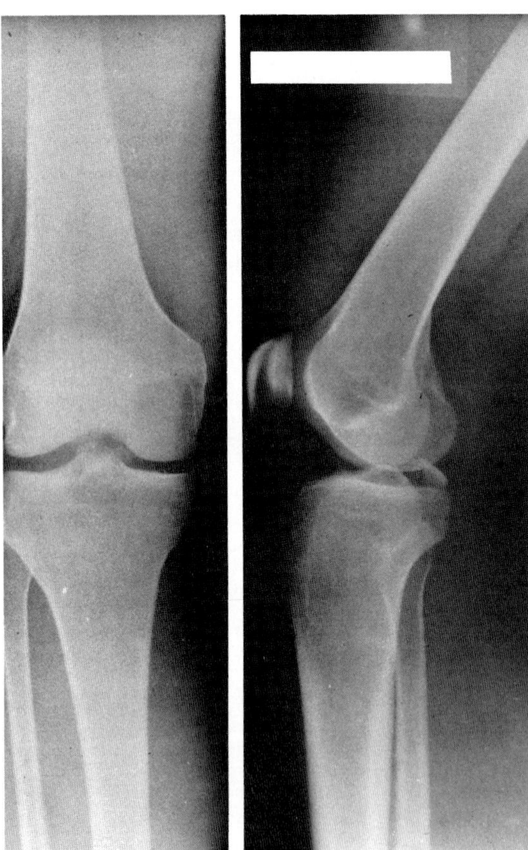

Fig. 20-12. Avulsion fracture of tibial attachment of posterior cruciate ligament.

Operative Closure

After all operative procedures are performed, adequate hemostasis is essential. Good subcutaneous repair, suction drainage, and bulky compressive dressings placed over the flaps help to prevent formation of wound hematoma, particularly with major ligamentous repairs.

Postoperative Care

At the time of final tying of ligamentous sutures, the limb should be positioned appropriately to provide for the least amount of tension on the repair sites. Such positioning is usually at least 45 to 60° of flexion; the greater amount of flexion is used when posterior structures are repaired. Cast immobilization is instituted carefully in the operating room and usually is continued for 5 to 7 days postoperatively. After 5 to 7 days, the cast should be removed and the wounds inspected. At this time, the patient is placed on a controlled-mobilization cast-brace, again with appropriate angulatory and rotatory correction.

Rehabilitation exercises can be performed during the period of external support, which usually is 6 weeks. Naturally, the rehabilitation program is dictated by the associated fractures and their healing course and potential. After the cast is removed, supervised rehabilitation is initiated to include regaining full range of motion and maximum muscular function. The end result is likely to be best when the patient is involved in his own care, is motivated, and is athletically inclined.

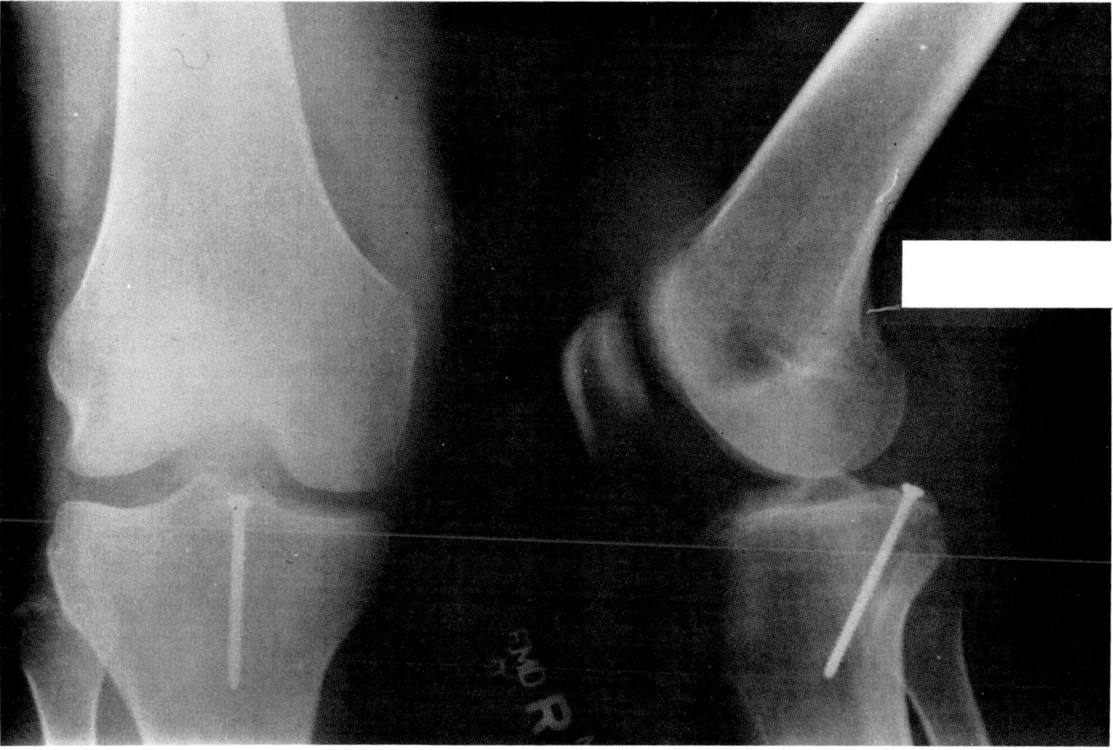

FIG. 20-13. Screw fixation of avulsion fracture of tibial attachment of posterior cruciate ligament.

Summary

Knee ligament injuries associated with ipsilateral fractures are usually the result of direct, high-energy violence. A high index of suspicion is necessary to rule out knee ligament damage. Diagnosis is enhanced by radiographic examination and examination under anesthesia with appropriate stabilization of the osseous structures to allow demonstration of instability by stress radiographs. Aspiration of the knee joint demonstrating hemarthrosis or effusion of the knee in a patient with ipsilateral fractures is good evidence for knee ligament damage. Arthroscopy can aid in the diagnosis of knee ligament injury by direct inspection.

Knee ligament damage is an excellent relative indication for primary stabilization of associated fractures. In most cases, knee ligament repairs should be undertaken on a primary basis as well.

Improved recognition of knee ligament injuries, aggressive management of associated fractures, operative repair of the knee ligament damage, and a rehabilitation program directed at involving the patient in his own care are the keys to functional restoration of patients with these complex injuries.

References

1. Palmer, I.: On the injuries to the ligaments of the knee joint. Acta Chir. (Suppl.) *81*:3, 1938.
2. O'Donoghue, D. H.: Surgical treatment of fresh injuries to the major ligaments of the knee. J. Bone Joint Surg., *32-A*:721, 1950.
3. Marshall, J. L., and Olsson, S.: Instability of the knee. A long-term experimental study in dogs. J. Bone Joint Surg., *53-A*:1561, 1971.
4. Jacobsen, K.: Osteoarthrosis following insufficiency of cruciate ligament in man. Acta Orthop. Scand., *48*:520, 1977.
5. Shelton, M. L., Neer, C. S., and Grantham, F. A.: Occult knee ligament ruptures associated with fractures. J. Trauma, *11*:855, 1971.
6. Nagel, D. A., Burton, D. S., and Manning, J.: The dashboard knee injury. Clin. Orthop., *126*:203, 1977.
7. Walling, A. K., Housang, S., and Spiegel, P. G.: Injuries to the knee ligaments with fractures of the femur. J. Bone Joint Surg., *64-A*:1324, 1982.
8. DeLee, J. C.: Ipsilateral fracture of the femur and tibia treated in the quadrilateral cast-brace. Clin. Orthop., *142*:115, 1979.
9. Fraser, R. D., Hunter, G. A., and Waddell, J. P.: Ipsilateral fracture of the femur and tibia. J. Bone Joint Surg., *60-B*:510, 1978.
10. Casey, M. J., and Chapman. M. W.: Ipsilateral concomitant fractures of hip and femoral shaft. J. Bone Joint Surg., *61-A*:503, 1979.
11. Gillespie, W. J.: The incidence of pattern of knee injury associated with dislocation of the hip. J. Bone Joint Surg., *57-B*:376, 1975.

12. Moore, T. M.: Fracture-dislocations of the knee. Clin. Orthop., *156*:128, 1981.
13. Waddell, J. P., and Drucker, W. R.: Occult injuries or pedestrian accidents. J. Trauma, *11*:844, 1971.
14. Clanton, T. C., et al.: Knee ligament injuries in children. J. Bone Joint Surg., *61-A*:1195, 1979.
15. Martin, A. F.: The pathomechanics of the knee joint. J. Bone Joint Surg., *42-A*:13, 1960.
16. DeHaven, R. E., and Collins, H. R.: Diagnosis of internal derangements of the knee: the role of arthroscopy. J. Bone Joint Surg., *57-A*:802, 1975.
17. Noyes, F. R., et al.: Arthroscopy in acute traumatic hemarthrosis of the knee. J. Bone Joint Surg., *62-A*:687, 1980.
18. Hastings, D. E.: The non-operative management of collateral ligament injuries of the knee joint. Clin. Orthop., *141*:22, 1980.
19. Bassett, F. H., Beck, J. L., and Weiker, G.: The modified cast-brace, its use in non-operative and post-operative management of serious knee ligament injuries. Am. J. Sports Med., *8*:63, 1980.
20. Akeson, W. H., Amiel, D., and Laviolette, D.: Connective tissue reponse to immobility. Clin. Orthop., *51*:183, 1967.
21. Noyes, F. R., et al.: Biomechanics of ligament failure. J. Bone Joint Surg., *56-A*:1406, 1974.
22. Mays, J., and Neufeld, A. J.: Skeletal traction methods. Clin. Orthop., *102*:144, 1974.
23. Walker, D. M., and Kennedy, J. C.: Occult knee ligament injuries associated with femoral shaft fractures. Am. J. Sports Med., *8*:172, 1980.
24. O'Donoghue, D. H.: Treatment of acute ligamentous injuries to the knee. Orthop. Clin. North Am., *4*:617, 1973.
25. Hughston, J. C., and Eilers, A. F.: The role of the posterior oblique ligament in the repair of acute medial (collateral) ligament tears of the knee. J. Bone Joint Surg., *55-A*:923, 1973.
26. Larson, R. L.: Injuries of the ligaments of the knee in fractures. Edited by Rockwood and Green. Philadelphia, J. B. Lippincott, 1975.
27. Yocum, L. A., et al.: Isolated lateral menisectomy. J. Bone Joint Surg., *61-A*:338, 1979.
28. Marshall J. L., and Rubin, R. M.: Knee ligament injuries. Orthop. Clin. North Am., *8*:641, 1977.
29. McDaniel, W. J., and Damron, T. D.: Untreated ruptures of the anterior cruciate ligament. J. Bone Joint Surg., *62-A*:696, 1980.
30. Ellision, A. E.: Distal iliotibial band transfer for anterolateral instability of the knee. J. Bone Joint Surg., *61-A*:330, 1979.
31. Girgis, F. G., et al.: The cruciate ligaments of the knee joint. Clin. Orthop., *106*:213, 1975.
32. McIntosh, D. L.: Acute tears of the anterior cruciate ligament. Presented at the American Academy of Orthopedic Surgeons Annual Meeting, Dallas, TX., 1974.

Chapter 21 Traumatic Dislocation of the Knee

MARVIN H. MEYERS

Traumatic dislocation of the knee is a serious and sometimes devastating injury. Rupture or avulsion of two or more knee ligaments can result in dislocation. Although regarded as an uncommon injury, traumatic dislocation of the knee occurs more frequently than is generally appreciated.

Traditionally, injuries to two or more major knee ligaments have been associated with traumatic dislocation of the knee. Associated fractures are seen in some patients and have not received as much attention as have ligamentous injuries. Recently, fracture-dislocations have been classified and the relation to traditional traumatic dislocation defined.[1]

Although there is disagreement in the literature concerning the mechanism of injury and treatment, all authors concur that vascular complications occur frequently. Early recognition of the extent of damage to the circulation is of paramount importance if the involved limb is to be saved. Knee fractures and peroneal nerve injuries are other common associated complications.

Traumatic knee dislocation is the result of severe direct or indirect violence. The direction of dislocation follows the force. Classification depends on displacement of the tibia in respect to the femur. Thus, the tibia is anterior to the femur in an anterior dislocation, posterior to the femur in a posterior dislocation, lateral to the femur in a lateral dislocation, and medial to the femur in a medial dislocation (Fig 21-1). There also may be rotary components; consequently, a dislocation can be anterior rotary, posterior rotary, lateral rotary, or medial rotary (Fig. 21-2).

Anterior dislocations occur slightly more often than do the other types, and they have a higher incidence of associated complications. The mechanism of injury is usually hyperextension of the knee.[2] The posterior capsule and the cruciate ligaments usually are torn. The medial and lateral knee stabilizers frequently are damaged but may not be disrupted completely. The popliteal artery or its branches and the peroneal nerve are injured frequently.

The incidence of posterior dislocation is slightly lower compared to that of the anterior type of dislocation. Posterior dislocation is caused by a direct force applied to the anterior aspect of the tibia with the knee flexed or by an extreme hyperextension force. The posterior capsule, both cruciates, and either or both collateral ligaments usually are torn. The popliteal artery or its branches are injured in 30% of all posterior dislocations. The peroneal nerve often is injured.

Lateral dislocations are produced by a severe force applied to the lateral aspect of the limb forcing the thigh into adduction while the leg remains in an abducted position. The medial collateral ligament, posterior capsule, and both cruciates usually are ruptured. Vascular injury is least common with this dislocation, occurring in less than 10% of patients. Peroneal nerve injury accompanies lateral dislocation in 15% of the cases.

Medial dislocation is rare. Damage to the lateral structures, both cruciate ligaments, and the peroneal nerve can be anticipated.

Diagnosis depends on usual systematic diag-

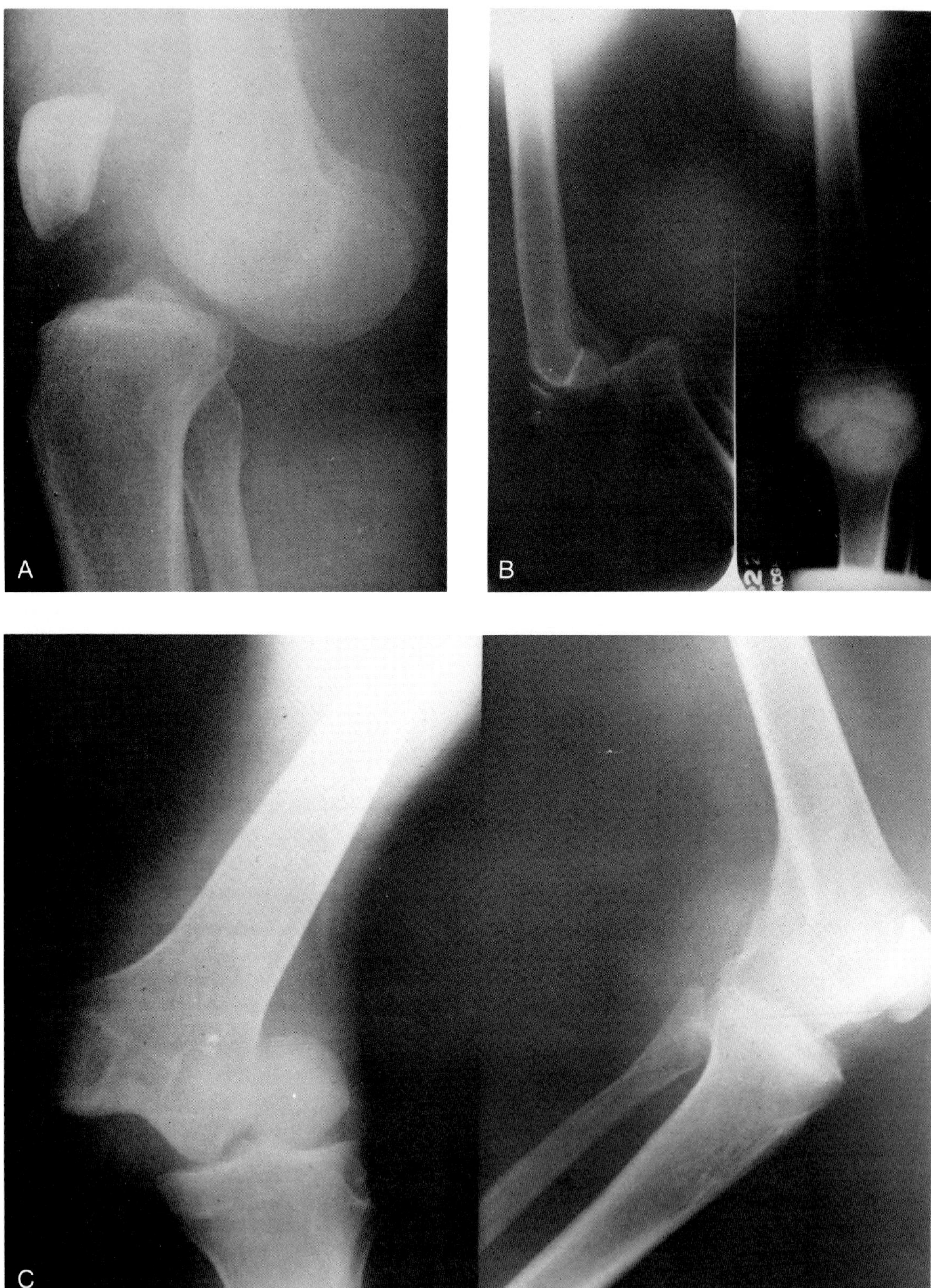

FIG. 21-1. *A*, Anterior dislocation of the knee. *B*, Posterior dislocation of the knee. *C*, Lateral dislocation of the knee.

nostic procedures. A history of the manner of injury, the direction of the forces applied, location of pain, and extent of function are determined. Inspection reveals swelling, the condition of the skin, and location of the deformity, providing that the dislocation has not been reduced (Fig. 21-3). Abrasions, ecchymosis, and hemorrhage are found frequently. Ecchymosis noted in the popliteal area frequently accompanies rupture of the posterior cruciate and posterior capsule of the knee. Palpation reveals tenderness, swelling, defects in the surrounding supporting structures of the knee, and crepitation. Clicking, snapping, and popping may aid in the diagnosis. Manipulation reveals marked instability.

Spontaneous reduction often occurs while the patient is being prepared by paramedical personnel for transportation from the accident scene. Usually, the dislocation can be reduced easily. In some instances, a lateral dislocation may be irreducible, and open reduction then is necessary (Fig. 21-4, *A*).[3] The femoral attachments of the lateral collateral ligament and joint capsule have been detached and drawn into the joint. The soft-tissue structures lie over the tibial tubercle and lateral plateau, thereby preventing relocation (Fig. 21-4, *B*). On occasion, complete relaxation of the patient is required to reduce the dislocation.

Examination under anesthesia is necessary to determine the extent of the ligamentous damage. Surgical repair can be planned only after identification of the damaged tissues.

The roentgenographic examination is important to identify the type of dislocation as well as to identify fractures that may accompany the injury.

Treatment

The treatment plan for traumatic dislocation of the knee follows. An immediate closed reduction is performed in the emergency department. When arterial blockage is present as a result of pressure of dislocated bones on major arteries, restoration of the circulation to the distal extremity follows relief of the pressure. Careful assessment of the vascular status must be made. If there is any doubt concerning vascular impairment, an arteriogram should be made. Prompt vascular repair

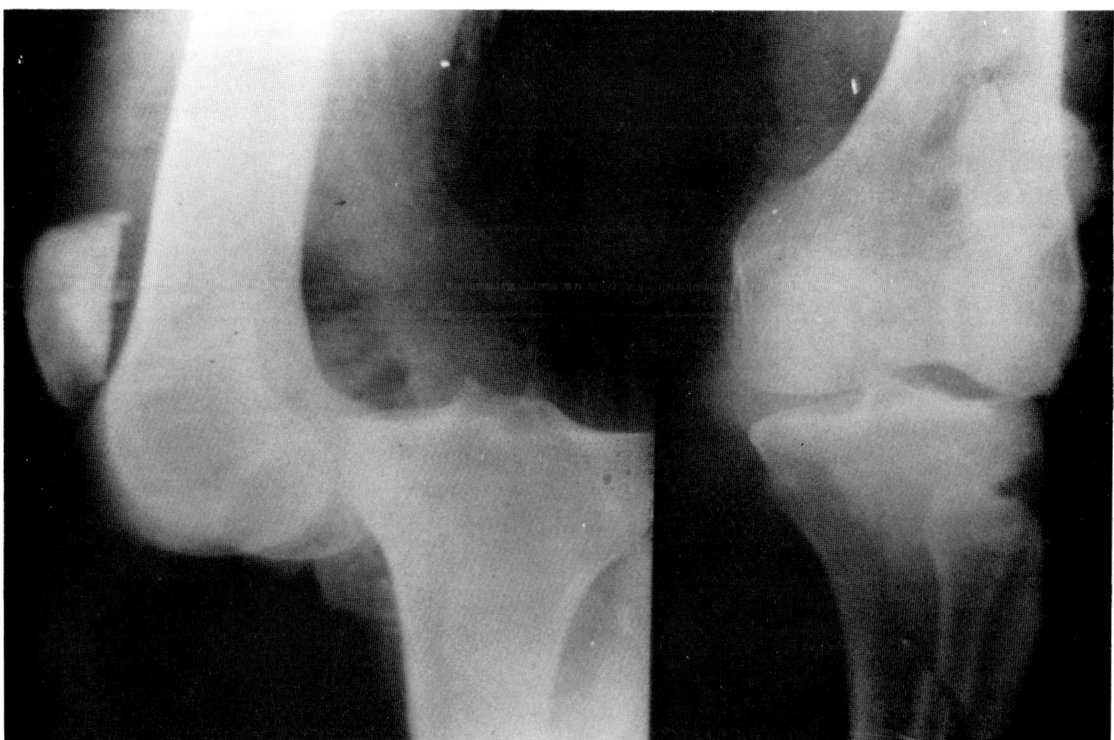

Fig. 21-2. Posterior rotary dislocation of the knee.

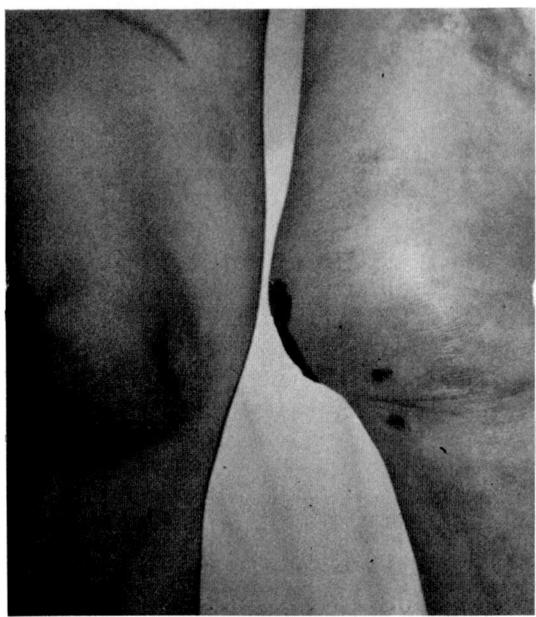

Fig. 21-3. Lateral dislocation of the knee. Note diagnostic features of deformity, ecchymosis, swelling, and skin abrasions.

or thrombectomy must be carried out as soon as possible after injury.

All major knee ligaments that have been torn or avulsed should be repaired. Preoperative evaluation of the integrity of the ligaments is best done under anesthesia. The integrity of the collateral ligaments is determined by stress testing and that of the cruciates by push-pull drawer stability tests. Stress roentgenograms are advised for documentation.

In a large series, both cruciate ligaments were found to be completely torn or avulsed in 85% of all dislocations.[4] Torn cruciates were associated with tears of the medial collateral ligaments in 45% and with lateral collateral ligament tears in 18%. All major knee ligaments were torn in 11% of the cases, and only the cruciates were torn in 11%.

There is a significant difference of opinion in the literature concerning the need for repair of damaged major knee ligaments following traumatic dislocation of the knee.[2,4-7] Animal experiments have demonstrated that ruptures of knee ligaments heal best when approximated with sutures. Most orthopaedic surgeons agree that disrupted knee ligaments require surgical repair shortly after injury to obtain optimal results. When multiple knee ligaments have been torn to the extent that the knee is unstable and dislocated, accurate repair of these ligaments logically would be essential for restoration of knee stability.

Some authors maintain that only prolonged cast immobilization is necessary to ensure a stable knee after traumatic dislocation.[5,7] A personal experience with a large series of patients that have been followed and reviewed adequately

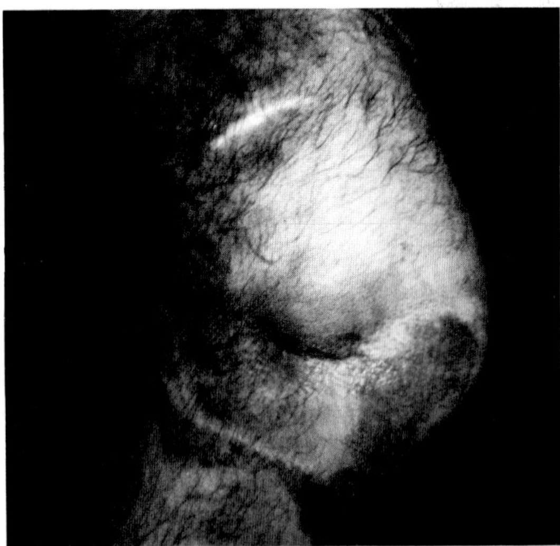

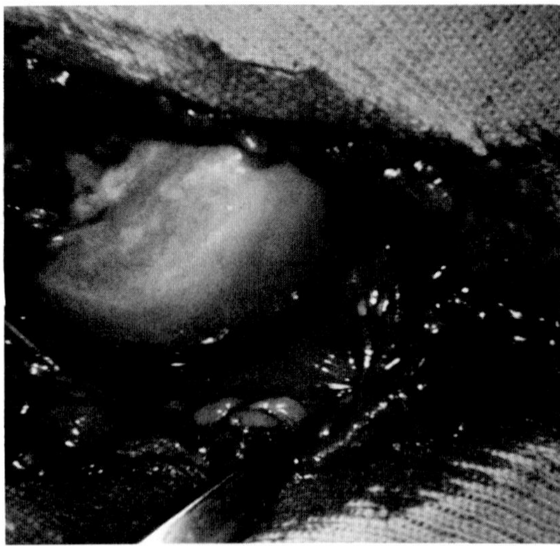

Fig. 21-4. *A*, Irreducible lateral dislocation of the knee. Note puckering of skin over lateral joint line. *B*, Lateral joint capsule and end of lateral collateral ligament trapped in intercondylar notch.

supports the position that surgical repair of all ruptured major knee ligaments after traumatic dislocation results in much better stability than can be obtained by prolonged immobilization alone.[4] When ligaments are not repaired, instability usually can be expected. Patients with unstable knees complain of difficulty when negotiating stairs, walking on tiptoes, running, and dancing. A change of occupation or modification in activities of daily living frequently is necessary.

Repair is best accomplished as soon as conditions permit. If there is a concomitant vascular injury, repair of the damaged major blood vessels takes precedence. Prolonged surgery may preclude treatment of damaged ligaments initially. However, as soon as the vascular status has been secured, repair of the torn ligaments may proceed. Surgical repair of damaged ligaments frequently can be performed along with vascular repair. If surgery can be accomplished within 6 to 8 hours, the ligaments can be sutured and the vascular surgery performed. In some cases, the vascular repair must precede ligament repair. Frequently, a 2- or 3-week waiting period may be required before ligament repair can be undertaken.

Four surgical aproaches can be utilized to repair damaged knee ligaments.[8]

Anteromedial Parapatellar Approach (Langenbeck) (Fig. 21-5)

This approach is undertaken for repair of the anterior cruciate and anterior portion of the posterior cruciate ligament. The incision begins over the medial border of the quadriceps tendon, 10 cm above the patella, and is carried medial to the border of the patella and then laterally below the patella, ending just distal to the center of the tibial tuberosity. The fascia is divided. The quadriceps mechanism is incised and dissected between the vastus medialis muscle and quadriceps tendon. The capsule and synovium then are incised medial to the patellar tendon, the patella, and along the lateral border of the vastus medialis muscle. The patella then can be retracted laterally, exposing the anterior compartment of the knee joint. Flexion of the knee facilitates exposure of the joint. The anterior cruciate ligament and the femoral attachment of the posterior cruciate can be visualized easily.

Medial Approach (Fig. 21-6)

This approach is utilized to repair the medial collateral ligament and either or both of the cruciate ligaments. The exposure obtained through this approach permits repair of the cruciate ligaments whether they are avulsed or torn in their substance.

The incision starts above the superior pole of the patella. It extends downward along the medial border of the patella and then is curved medially over the anteromedial joint line to the posterior border of the tibia, approximately 8 cm distal to the joint. The medial skin flap is reflected backward, exposing the fascia over the medial side of the knee. Palpation and ecchymosis may indicate tears in the medial collateral ligament if the fascia has not been torn already. Division and dissection of the fascia permit examination of the superficial fibers of the ligament.

The incision is developed through the extensor retinaculum along the border of the patella and patellar tendon. Tears in the superficial layer can be identified and the superficial layer reflected proximally to expose the deep portion of the medial collateral ligament.

The synovium is entered longitudinally along the medial border of the patella. Retraction of the collateral ligament permits inspection of the cruciate ligaments. The joint will open widely if the cruciates are torn. Repair of the attachments or the substance of the cruciate ligaments is possible through this approach.

Lateral Approach (Fig. 21-7)

The lateral stabilizers of the knee (lateral collateral ligament, iliotibial band, biceps tendon), as well as the cruciate ligaments, can be repaired through this approach. The incision begins 1 cm lateral to the superior pole of the patella. It proceeds distally at this distance from the patella and patellar tendon to the patella tubercle of the tibia and then swings downward and backward to terminate at the level of the fibular shaft, about 2 cm from its proximal end. The posterior flap is reflected backward to expose the lateral aspect of the knee.

The fibular shaft can be examined and avulsion of the combined attachment of the biceps tendon and fibular collateral ligament can be seen and necessary repairs made. The peroneal nerve can be examined. The iliotibial band frequently is avulsed, and suture is possible.

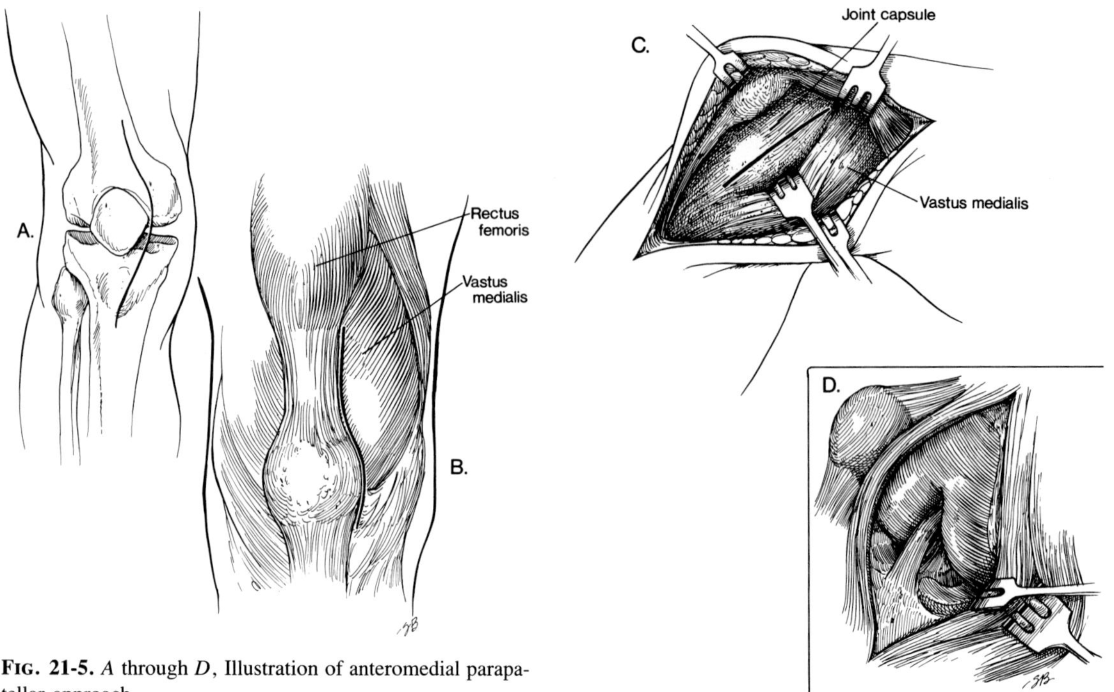

Fig. 21-5. *A* through *D*, Illustration of anteromedial parapatellar approach.

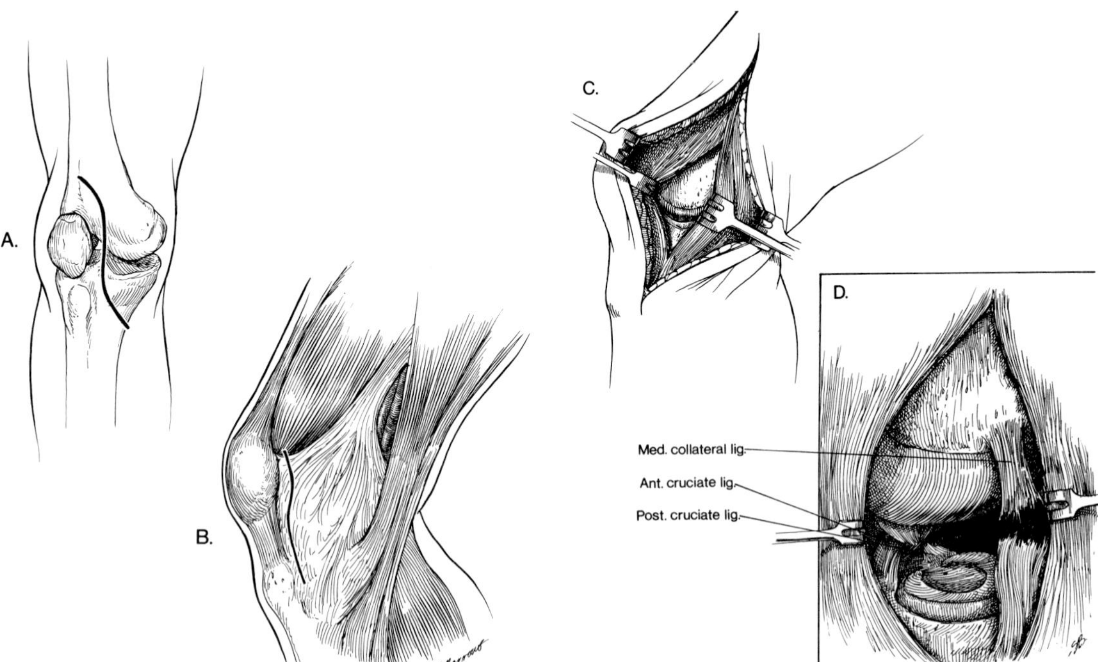

Fig. 21-6. *A* through *D*, Illustration of medial approach.

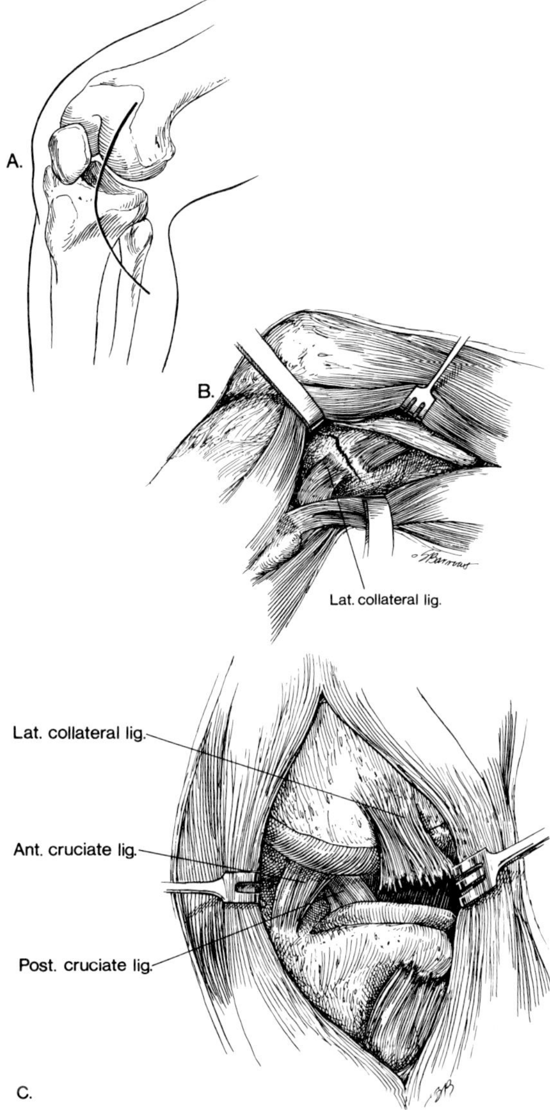

Fig. 21-7. *A* through *C*, Illustration of lateral approach.

The knee can be opened along the line of the skin incision. The cruciate ligaments, as well as the popliteus tendon, may be inspected from this incision and suitable repair carried out.

Posterior Approach (Fig. 21-8)

This approach becomes necessary when only the cruciate ligaments require repair and the posterior cruciate ligament is avulsed from the posterior tibial rim with or without a piece of bone. The anterior cruciate can be sutured through a medial parapatellar approach. Repair of the tibial attachment of the posterior cruciate ligament (with or without a bone fragment) is difficult to accomplish through the medial parapatellar approach. Thus, two incisions are necessary in this situation.

The anesthetized patient is placed in a prone position, and a pneumatic tourniquet is inflated on the thigh. The skin incision begins laterally over the biceps femoris approximately 8 cm above the flexion crease in the popliteal space. It is continued medially over the popliteal fossa in a curvilinear direction, ending 6 cm below the flexion crease on the posterior medial side of the calf. The saphenous vein is identified superficial to the popliteal fascia in the posterolateral aspect of the fossa, and the sural nerve is seen deep to the fascia just medial to the midline. These structures should bc preserved.

The sural nerve is traced proximally to its origin from the tibial nerve. Above this point, the motor branch to the medial head of the gastrocnemius muscle is identified, and the tendinous origin of the medial head is divided proximal to its nerve supply. The muscle is dissected on its medial aspect and retracted laterally, thus protecting the neurovascular bundle, which does not require exposure. The superior medial genicular artery and vein are seen passing medially and should be divided and ligated.

The posterior capsule of the knee joint frequently is torn, exposing the tibial attachment of the posterior cruciate ligament. If the capsule is intact, it is incised and retracted to expose the cruciate ligament.

The ligament can be repaired or reconstructed. When a large bony fragment is avulsed with an intact ligamentous insertion, it can be secured with a cancellous screw. When there is comminution of fragments or when the fragment is too small to accommodate a screw, suture of the ligament and comminuted fragments can be accomplished through two parallel sagittal drill holes in the tibia directed posteroanteriorly. Two sutures are placed and carried through the drill holes and are tied together over the anteromedial aspect of the tibial tubercle in the medial parapatellar wound.

Vascular Complications

Severe arterial injury requiring surgical repair occurs in approximately 20% of all traumatic knee dislocations. Of cases with arterial damage, 50% are found with posterior dislocations, 40%

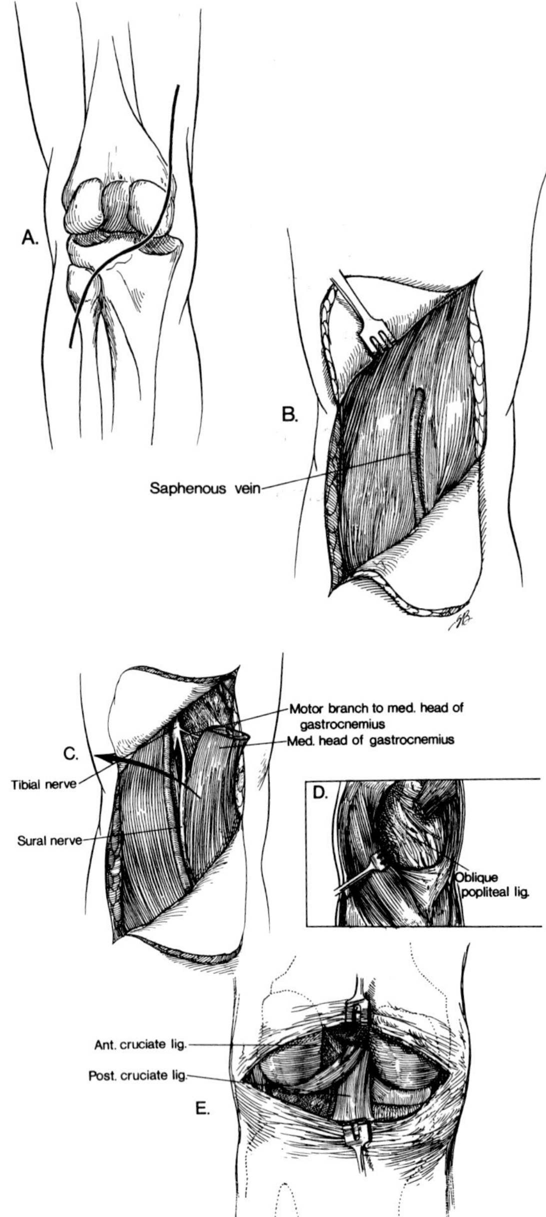

FIG. 21-8. *A* through *E*, Illustration of posterior approach.

with anterior dislocations, and 10% with lateral dislocations.

Procrastination is the foremost error in the management of a patient with vascular insufficiency. Statistically, the golden period for surgical repair is within 8 hours of injury. The incidence of limb loss rises significantly when repair is not accomplished before 8 hours.[4,9-11] The surgeon must be vigilant in monitoring the circulation distal to the injury for several days. An attitude of complacency because of the presence of palpable peripheral arterial pulses may result in failure to recognize the onset of major impairment of peripheral vascular blood supply. A warm distal extremity or evidence of capillary filling after pressure on the skin of the foot and toes does not always indicate that the major arteries are intact. Severe arterial damage frequently is present despite these favorable signs.

The danger signs of vascular injury are the classic five "Ps"—pulselessness, pallor, paresthesia, paralysis, and pain. One or more of these signs should alert the surgeon to the possibility of vascular compromise. If vascular injury is at all suspected, a femoral arteriogram is recommended. Exploration must be carried out when major vascular impairment is discovered. It is important to remember that the optimal time for successful repair of damaged arteries is within 8 hours of injury.

Arterial laceration or complete tears are evident early. Intimal tears followed by thrombosis may be insidious or a late sequela. The hallmarks of excellence in the recognition and treatment of arterial injury in the traumatic dislocated knee are constant vigilance and prompt surgical intervention when indicated.

Fasciotomy of the Leg Compartments

Fasciotomy is necessary after prolonged, severe ischemia and is an important adjunctive procedure for many vascular repairs.[11] This procedure becomes more urgent when both the popliteal artery and vein have been injured. Knee dislocation is caused by a major force resulting in severe soft-tissue damage in many cases and is accompanied by marked swelling and increased intracompartmental pressure that can compromise the vessels, nerves, and muscles in the compartment. Direct measurement of intracompartmental pressures can aid in the decision-making process concerning fasciotomy (see Chap. 8 for pressure measurement and technique of fasciotomy).

Nerve Injuries

Peroneal nerve damage occurs in approximately 25% of all cases of knee dislocation.[4] The injury is usually an axonotmesis; neurapraxia and neurotmesis are uncommon. Peroneal nerve

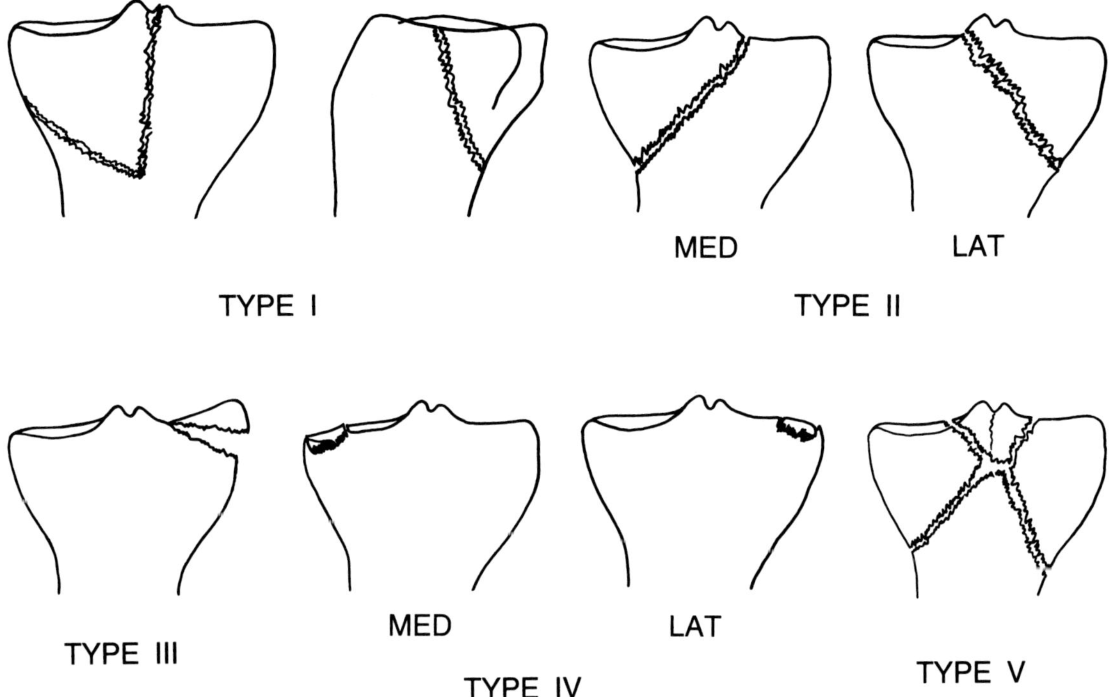

Fig. 21-9. Diagram of types of fracture-dislocations of the knee. (From Meyers, M. H.: Clin. Orthop., *156*:128, 1981.)

function does not return in most instances. Exploration of the peroneal nerve seldom is rewarding when it accompanies a traumatic knee dislocation because the extent of the nerve damage makes repair impossible. The length of nerve involved frequently is too long to permit a satisfactory end-to-end anastomosis or nerve graft.

Fractures

Concomitant ipsilateral fractures of the proximal fibula, intercondylar eminence of the tibia, tibial, tubercle, and tibial plateaus are common in traumatic dislocation of the knee. Fractures of the head and neck of the fibula occur most often. The method of fracture treatment is conventional and should not interfere with ligament repair. When plateau displacement occurs, reduction by manipulation probably cannot be maintained without internal fixation. Avulsion of the intercondylar eminence is, in reality, an avulsion of the tibial attachment of the anterior cruciate ligament and should be repaired surgically. In most instances, avulsion of the tibial attachment of the posterior cruciate ligament requires relocation and fixation.

Fracture-Dislocation of the Knee (Fig. 21-9)

The classification, diagnosis, complications, and treatment of this injury have been described recently in an excellent paper.[1]

Type I is the most frequent and involves only the medial plateau with avulsion of the medial capsule from the fragment. Reduction is accomplished in extension, and the medial plateau fragment is fixed internally to the tibia anatomically. Vascular injury is not seen with this injury.

The diagnosis of a type II injury is made easily because the intercondylar eminence is partially or completely avulsed with the plateau fragment. The medial or lateral plateau may be involved. When the medial plateau is involved, lateral collateral structures may require repair if laxity is demonstrated on stress testing. The opposite is true when the lateral plateau is fractured. Vascular injury and peroneal nerve damage occur in a small percentage of this group.

Open reduction and internal fixation with cancellous screws are the treatment of choice. Ligament tears should be repaired when present.

Type III rim avulsions frequently are accompanied by ligament avulsions or tears. Peroneal nerve injury (10%) and vascular damage (10%) accompany this type of injury. Open reduction and internal fixation of the fracture with screws or pins are the treatment of choice. Repair of all damaged ligaments is advised.

In type IV injuries (rim compression), the ligaments on the side opposite the fracture frequently are torn. Neurovascular injuries are infrequent. All torn ligaments should be repaired in this type of fracture-dislocation.

Type V is characterized by an avulsion of the intercondyloid eminence. Both the peroneal nerve and popliteal artery are injured in 50% of the cases. Open reduction and internal fixation of all fracture fragments, including the fractured eminence, are the treatment of choice.

References

1. Moore, T. M.: Fracture-dislocation of the knee. Clin. Orthop. *156*:128, 1981.
2. Kennedy, J. C.: Complete dislocation of the knee joint. J. Bone Joint Surg., *45A*:889, 1963.
3. Griswold, A. S.: Irreducible dislocations of the knee joint. J. Bone Joint Surg., *33A*:787, 1951.
4. Meyers, M. H., Moore, T. M., and Harvey, J. P.: Traumatic dislocation of the knee joint. J. Bone Joint Surg., *57A*:430, 1975.
5. Conwell, H. F., and Alldredge, R. H.: Complete dislocations of the knee joint: A report of seven cases with end-results. Surg., Gynecol., Obstet., *64*:94, 1937.
6. Myles, J. W.: Seven cases of traumatic dislocation of the knee. Proc. Roy. Soc. Med., *60*:279, 1967.
7. Taylor, A. R., Orden, G. P., and Rainey, H. A.: Traumatic dislocation of the knee: A report of forty-three cases with special reference to conservative treatment. J. Bone Joint Surg., *54B*:96, 1972.
8. Abbott, L. C., and Carpenter, W. F.: Surgical approaches to the knee Joint. J. Bone Joint Surg., *27*:277, 1945.
9. Cole, W. G.: Fractures and dislocations complicated by distal ischaemia. Medical Journal of Australia, *1*:98, 1975.
10. Green, N. E., and Allen, B. L.: Vascular injuries associated with dislocation of the knee. J. Bone Joint Surg., *59A*:236, 1977.
11. Jones, R. E., Smith, E. C., and Bone, G. E.: Vascular and orthopedic complications of knee dislocation. Surg., Gynecol., Obstet., *149*:554, 1979.

Chapter 22 Complex Fractures of the Distal End of the Femur

ROBY D. MIZE

Fractures of the distal femur are frequently complex injuries that are difficult to treat and often leave the patient with significant permanent impairment, particularly if the fracture involves the joint. Although not common injuries, fractures of the distal femur are being seen with increasing frequency because of our modern life-styles and high-velocity means of transportation.

The management of this fracture remains controversial. Over the past 20 years, most studies have compared the results of nonsurgical versus surgical methods. The classic management of displaced fractures of the distal femur has centered on skeletal traction for a variable duration followed by some form of external immobilization. This method is time consuming, carries a high degree of morbidity, and frequently gives poor results. Because of these problems, numerous methods of open reduction and internal fixation have been recommended. Many of these surgical methods have been discarded because of poor results, primarily due to inadequate fixation.

Stewart and associates,[1] in 1966, and Neer and associates,[2] in 1967, reported large series of supracondylar fractures treated by both open and closed methods. Both groups found more favorable results with the nonsurgical method of treatment. Fortunately, significant progress has been made over the past decade in both the nonsurgical as well as the surgical management of this difficult fracture. The ambulatory cast-brace (Fig. 22-1), introduced by Mooney in 1970, has been a significant contribution toward overcoming many of the problems in nonoperative treatment.[3] This nonoperative method requires skeletal traction for a period of 3 to 6 weeks followed by application and use of the cast-brace until the fracture is healed. In 1974, the introduction of roller traction added another dimension to this system (Fig.

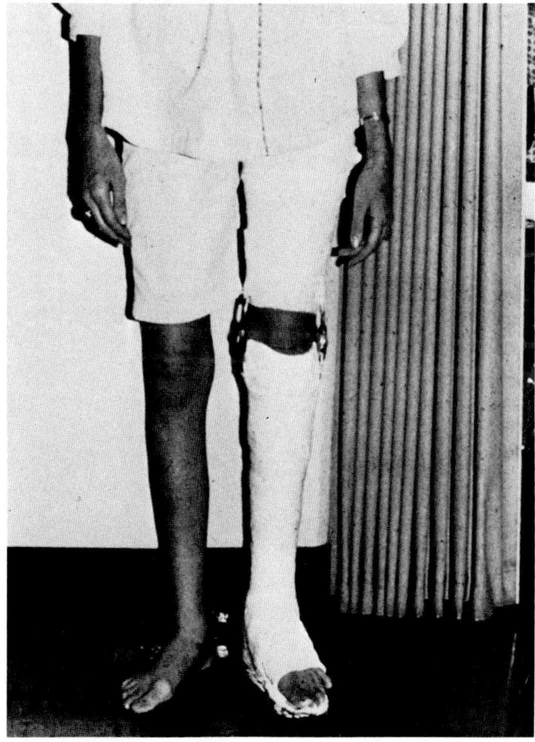

Fig. 22-1. Anterior view of Mooney's ambulatory cast-brace.

22-2).[4] Although these newer conservative methods are safe and better, they are not without complications, and the results are not always gratifying. The primary complication has been malunion with valgus-varus and rotational deformities. Management of fractures with intra-articular extension and displacement is especially difficult.

The surgical treatment of these fractures has been significantly improved through the work of the ASIF (Association for the Study of Internal Fixation) group in Switzerland. Excellent results in the majority of these difficult injuries can be expected by strictly adhering to the technique and principles recommended by the ASIF.

Mechanism of Injury

Fractures of the distal femur occur in all age groups. In young patients, the fracture usually is caused by major trauma occurring in motor-vehicle accidents or by a fall from a height. Motorcycle accidents are a prime cause for this fracture in the younger patient aged 17 to 30 years. Elderly patients may sustain this fracture from trivial trauma such as falling on the flexed knee.

Initial Assessment and Potential Pitfalls in Diagnosis

Fractures of the distal femur usually are not isolated injuries. The patient frequently has been subjected to high-energy forces resulting in multiple-system injuries, which may involve the head, chest, abdomen, and other extremity fractures. These injuries may result in profound shock and may be life threatening. Priority of treatment must be directed toward the life-threatening injury; however, the femoral fracture should not be neglected. Although a distal femoral fracture is ordinarily not life threatening, initial assessment and treatment should proceed simultaneously with the overall resuscitation of the patient.

Physical Findings

A systematic physical inspection of the extremity should be performed. Swelling, painful

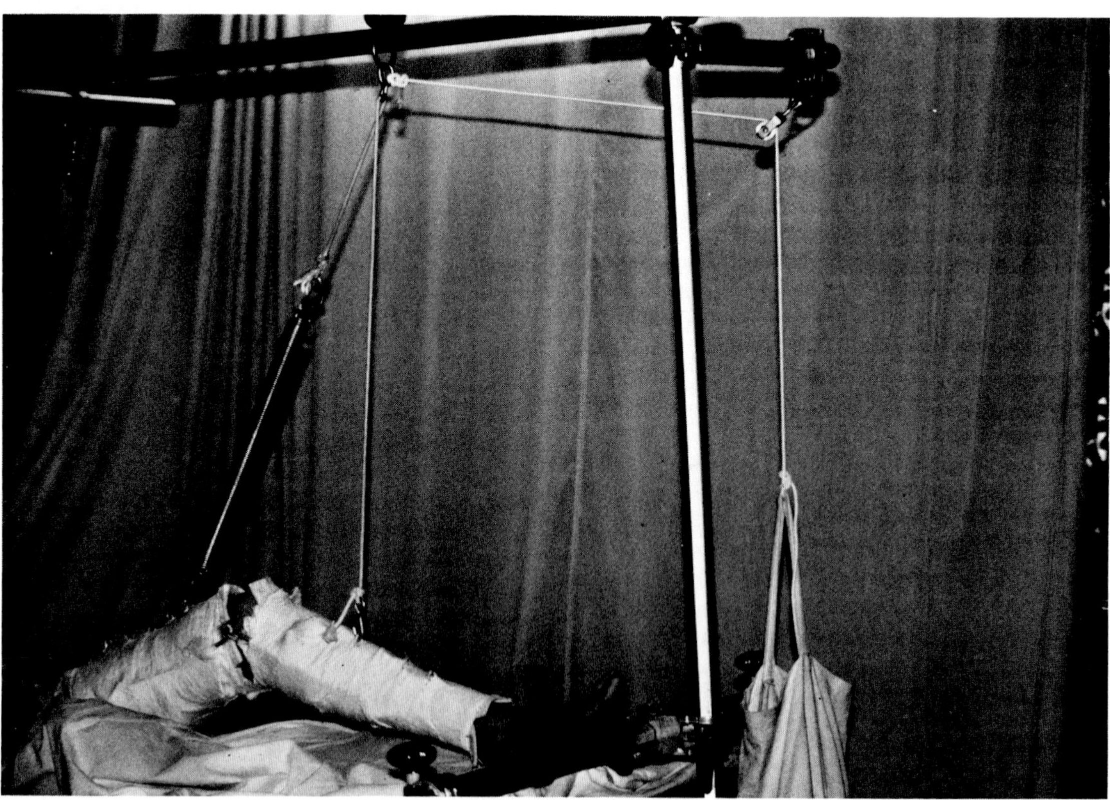

Fig. 22-2. Neufeld's dynamic roller traction system. While the patient is in bed, the hinged cast is attached to an overhead pulley system. The traction can be released to allow the patient to get out of bed.

crepitus with motion, and, perhaps, deformity of the thigh are apparent. The injured limb should be examined for general alignment. One should be gentle when realigning any gross deformity prior to splintage. The condition of the soft tissue must be assessed carefully. A small puncture wound located anteriorly over the suprapatellar pouch area may represent an open fracture.

Neurovascular damage, although unusual with distal femoral fractures, may occur occasionally. A careful motor and sensory examination should be performed distal to the fracture. Circulatory compromise may be detected by coolness, pallor, and diminished pulses in the lower leg or by increased fullness in the popliteal space. This condition is an emergency of the first order and should be dealt with promptly. In cases of suspected vascular damage, arteriography is indicated.

Radiographic Assessment

Good-quality roentgenograms of the entire lower extremity including the pelvis are required for adequate evaluation. Associated fractures or dislocations of the hip, femoral shaft, patella, tibia, and foot should be ruled out. Frequently, these associated injuries are not detected during the initial assessment.

Classification

Fractures of the distal femur occur in such complex and variable patterns that they defy simple classification. Muller and associates have presented an excellent anatomic classification;[5] however, it does not define all pertinent aspects of this injury (Fig. 22-3). In evaluating and categorizing distal femoral fractures, multiple characteristics other than the osseous injury must be considered. A more appropriate assessment should consider the "personality" of the fracture. The "personality" of the distal femoral fracture is determined by:

1. displacement of fragments.
2. degree of comminution.
3. extent and degree of soft-tissue damage.
4. associated neurovascular damage.
5. degree of articular involvement.
6. bone quality (osteoporosis).
7. severity of multiple-system injuries.
8. other fractures.

When one considers all these factors, some distal femoral fractures cannot be classified and thus cause a major problem when attempting to evaluate the results to be expected from open versus closed methods. The fact that so many fractures are not comparable emphasizes the principle that each case must be individualized and all factors considered when formulating a plan of management.

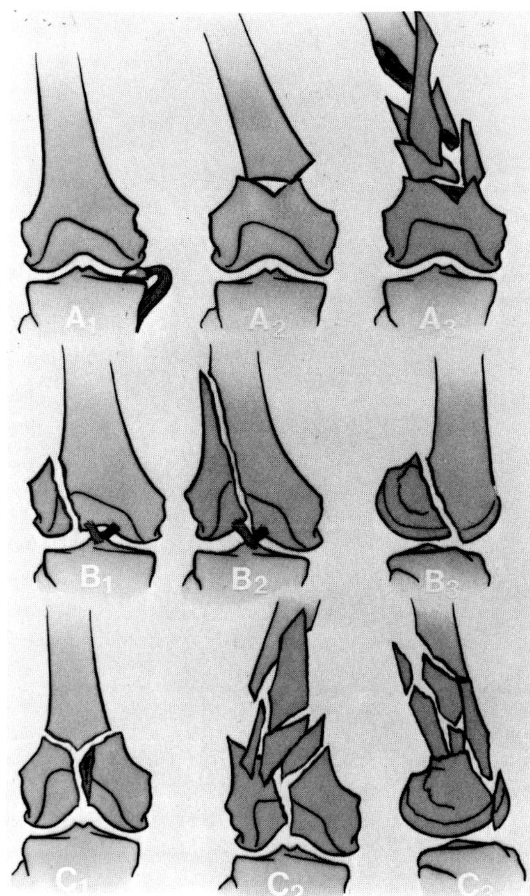

Fig. 22-3. Muller's classification of distal femoral fractures. (Redrawn from Muller, M. E., Allgower, M., Schneider, R., and Willenegger, H.: Manual of Internal Fixation. 2nd Edition. New York, Springer-Verlag, 1979.)

Treatment Options

The primary objectives in treating any fracture are to achieve the best possible anatomic and functional results and to avoid complications in the process. Whether one favors open or closed methods, achieving good results with a distal femoral fracture is not an easy task. Allgower has reminded us that "no surgeon can refrain completely from internal fixation as well as no one would operate on all fractures."[6] The final decision must be made by the surgeon.

Closed Treatment

Some surgeons advocate closed treatment for all fractures of the distal femur, including the intra-articular type. Others believe a trial of closed treatment should be instituted when there are no absolute indications for surgery. Treatment is initiated by inserting a skeletal traction pin through the proximal tibia at the level of the tibial tuberosity. The limb is supported in a well-padded, balanced splint with the knee flexed about 15 to 20° and the lower leg parallel with the mattress. Fifteen to twenty pounds of traction weight, depending on the size of the patient, are attached to the proximal tibial pin, thereby resulting in a force vector in line with the femoral shaft.

The position and alignment of the fracture fragments are determined with biplane roentgenograms. If reduction is unacceptable, a closed manipulation under general anesthesia is performed. The manipulation should be gentle so that damage to the neurovascular bundle, which is in close proximity to the fracture, does not occur. The distal fragment usually is angulated posteriorly because of the deforming muscle forces. If this angulation is not corrected by manipulation, a second Steinmann's pin may be inserted in the distal femoral fragment for vertical pull. Daily inspection of the traction system is required, and sequential roentgenograms are needed to assure acceptable position and alignment of the fracture fragments.

Skeletal traction is maintained for 3 to 6 weeks. A physical therapy program is started to maintain muscle tone and to obtain joint motion. Following traction, the limb is placed in the hinged cast-brace, and the patient begins gait training. The patient must be followed closely with roentgenograms to determine alignment and stage of healing. Union usually is complete in about 12 weeks, at which time the cast-brace is removed.

Roller traction is similar to a cast-brace, is applied shortly after admission to the hospital, and allows the patient to be out of bed within 2 to 5 days following injury. Early results with this method are encouraging; it affords early ambulation, early hospital discharge, and clinical union. There is minimal morbidity compared to that of other closed methods of treatment.[7]

Complications of closed management include the well-known hazards of prolonged bed rest, malunions, shortening, limitation of motion, articular surface incongruity, and residual traumatic arthritis. Delayed unions and nonunions occur, but are less frequent with cast-brace treatment. Although the closed treatment method has distinct limitations, every orthopaedist should be familiar with this form of management.

The closed method of treatment requires meticulous attention to detail to achieve good results. A high degree of tolerance is required by both the physician and the patient during the prolonged bed-rest phase.

Internal Fixation

The objectives of surgical treatment of distal femoral fractures are anatomic restoration and stable fixation. Numerous studies support the use of internal fixation for this difficult fracture.[8–13] Excellent results can be obtained in the majority of patients if the basic objectives are achieved.

Enthusiasm for a system is not a substitute for good judgment. Stable internal fixation gives excellent results; however, this procedure frequently is difficult and sometimes impossible to achieve. Successful use of this method requires adequate instrumentation, knowledge, and application of the principles of internal fixation. The lack of adequate facilities and sufficient experience with open treatment of supracondylar femoral fractures are contraindications to the use of this method. The patient is better served by closed methods of treatment or prompt referral in such situations.

In 1979, Schatzker and Lambert reported a series of supracondylar fractures of the femur that were treated by open methods using the implants and instruments developed by the Swiss ASIF group.[14] This series was analyzed and divided into two groups. In one group, the basic principles of accurate reduction and rigid fixation were followed strictly. The other group was treated with the same equipment; however, the basic objectives were not achieved. The results were striking. In the group in which principles had been followed, 71% showed good to excellent results, whereas in the other group, only 21% achieved these results. This study reveals that good results can be obtained in the majority of patients when accurate reduction and stable fixation are achieved. Furthermore, the study should serve as a warning that the surgical treatment of supracondylar fractures is difficult, and good results are not assured simply by using ASIF equipment alone. The principles are equally important.

Indications

Assuming the surgeon and his institution meet the proper criteria, the following are considered indications for internal fixation.

1. The fracture in which reduction cannot be obtained or maintained should be fixed internally. Criteria for acceptable reduction vary considerably among surgeons.
2. Displaced intra-articular fractures, especially in major weight-bearing joints, should almost always be reduced anatomically and stabilized internally to allow early motion (Fig. 22-4).
3. Multiple fractures:
   a. The distal femoral fracture combined with ipsilateral or contralateral fractures should be fixed to begin early mobilization of the knee and to facilitate control of the limb.
   b. Bilateral femoral fractures should be fixed internally to facilitate general care (Fig. 22-5). Bilateral skeletal traction is not tolerated well.
4. The severely injured patient with multiple-system involvement, such as head, chest, and abdomen, should be stabilized surgically as soon as reasonably possible. Patients with head injuries sometimes are impossible to control in traction. Early stabilization may be a life-saving procedure in patients with chest and abdominal injuries who cannot tolerate prolonged bed rest.
5. Extremely obese patients are best managed by internal fixation because of the difficulty in treating them with skeletal traction or a cast-brace.
6. Vascular damage associated with a distal femoral fracture should have internal stabilization to protect the vascular repair.

Relative Indications

1. The management of elderly patients has to be individualized. It would be preferable to fix these fractures surgically to avoid the hazards of prolonged bed rest; however, obtaining stable fixation is difficult and sometimes impossible because of osteoporosis. Adjunctive methyl methacrylate may be needed to gain stability, and frequently, a cast-brace must be used post-operatively. Roller traction may be an alternate method in selected patients. The advanced age of a patient should not, in itself, be a contraindication to internal fixation. Mize and associates obtained good to excellent results in 8 of 11 patients who were 70 years or older at the time of surgical fixation.[13]
2. The treatment of open fractures is controversial. Each patient must be individualized and calls for considerable judgment by the treating physician. The soft tissues should be in sufficiently good condition to withstand major surgery. These patients usually have severe associated injuries, and early stabilization is desirable to facilitate early mobilization of the patient and care of the soft tissues. The cornerstone of open-fracture treatment remains thorough wound debridement.
3. The patient who prefers not to be treated with prolonged bed rest and in whom a satisfactory stabilization can be obtained should be considered for surgical fixation.

Contraindications

In general, surgery is not advised for patients with severe osteoporosis or massive severe comminution. Surgical fixation may also be contraindicated in patients with an infection or severely contaminated soft tissues that cannot be debrided adequately. Rarely, internal fixation may be indicated in the massively traumatized extremity as a limb-saving procedure.

My Preferred Method

In most instances, I treat complex fractures of the distal femur by open methods. With this approach, good anatomic and functional results can be achieved in the majority of patients with this injury. Unless there is an indication for immediate surgery, the injured limb initially is placed in balanced suspension with about 15 pounds of skeletal traction applied through a proximal tibial pin placed about 4 cm distal to the tibial tuberosity. The injury, treatment options, and potential surgical hazards are reviewed with the patient and, if possible, with the patient's family.

I prefer the Swiss ASIF instrumentation and strictly adhere to their recommended operative principles.[5] Success with the Swiss method can be expected only by combined use of their instruments and principles. In most instances, the 95° condylar angled blade plate is used (Fig. 22-6, *A*); however, for selective cases, the heavy clo-

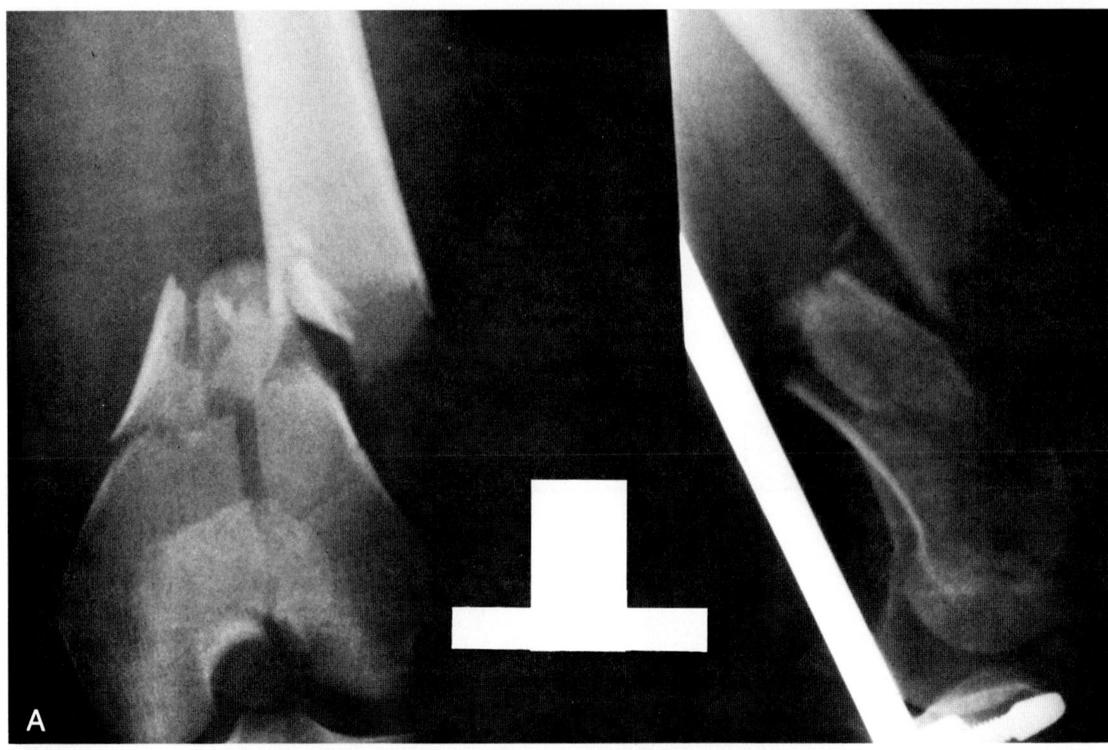

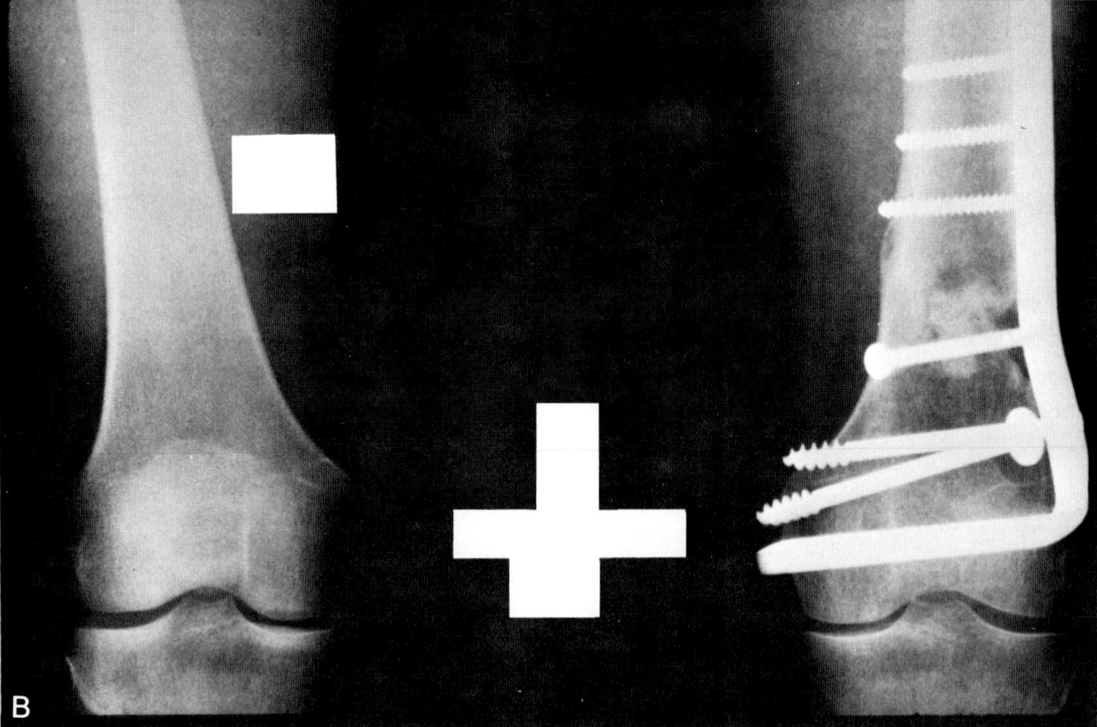

FIG. 22-4. *A*, Severely comminuted intra-articular fracture in a 19-year-old woman. In addition to the intercondylar split in the sagittal plane, there is also a displaced split of the medial condyle in the coronal plane. *B*, All fractures are well healed 1 year following internal fixation. Note the inappropriately long blade that was a source of pain over the medial soft tissues.

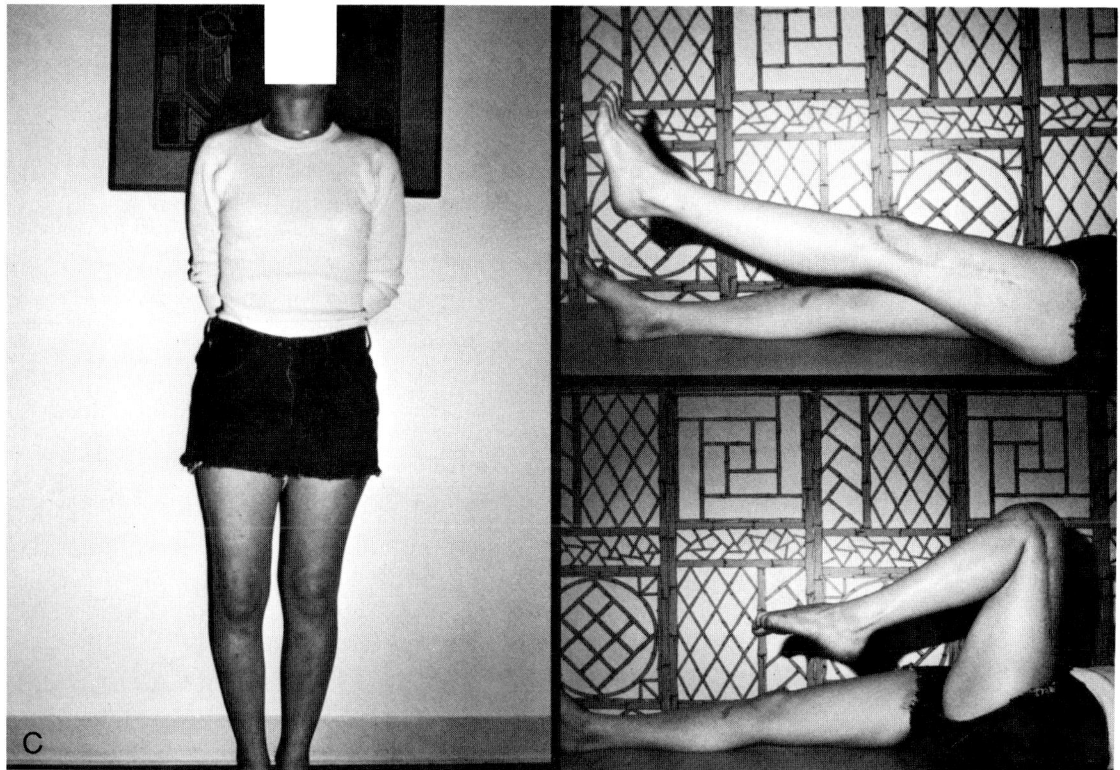

FIG. 22-4 (*continued*). *C*, One year after surgery, patient shows good anatomic alignment and function.

verleaf buttress plate designed for the distal femur can be used (Fig. 22-6, *B*). Surgical assistants and operating-room nurses who understand this equipment and the surgical procedure are required.

Preoperative Planning

In periarticular fractures of the distal femur, it is helpful to obtain roentgenograms of the opposite normal femur. One must have accurate anteroposterior and lateral roentgenograms centered on the joint. The outlines of the normal femur and fracture lines are drawn on the roentgenogram. The plate and proposed position of the screws are drawn on the roentgenogram with the aid of a plastic template. All necessary instruments and implants should be available prior to surgery. It is important to review and discuss the procedure with the assistant surgeon. Although internal fixation of these fractures is performed preferably within 1 to 2 days following injury, all the previously mentioned conditions should be met before surgery.

Operative Technique

The T or Y condylar fracture with split condyles has been chosen for purposes of demonstration. The patient is positioned supine with a pillow or bolster under the knee to allow 90° of flexion. The lower extremity is prepared and draped in the usual manner for bone surgery. The anterior iliac crest or greater trochanteric area should be prepared and draped in the event a bone graft is needed.

The fracture is exposed through a lateral incision to the level of the knee joint, extending distally and medially as far as the tibial tuberosity. Care must be taken to remain anterior to the lateral collateral ligament (Fig. 22-7). The fascia lata is split in line with its fibers and extended down to the condylar area by splitting the iliotibial tract where its fibers diverge. The synovial covering is entered and the lateral superior geniculate artery is identified and controlled. The vastus lateralis muscle is elevated off the intermuscular septum and lifted anteriorly and medi-

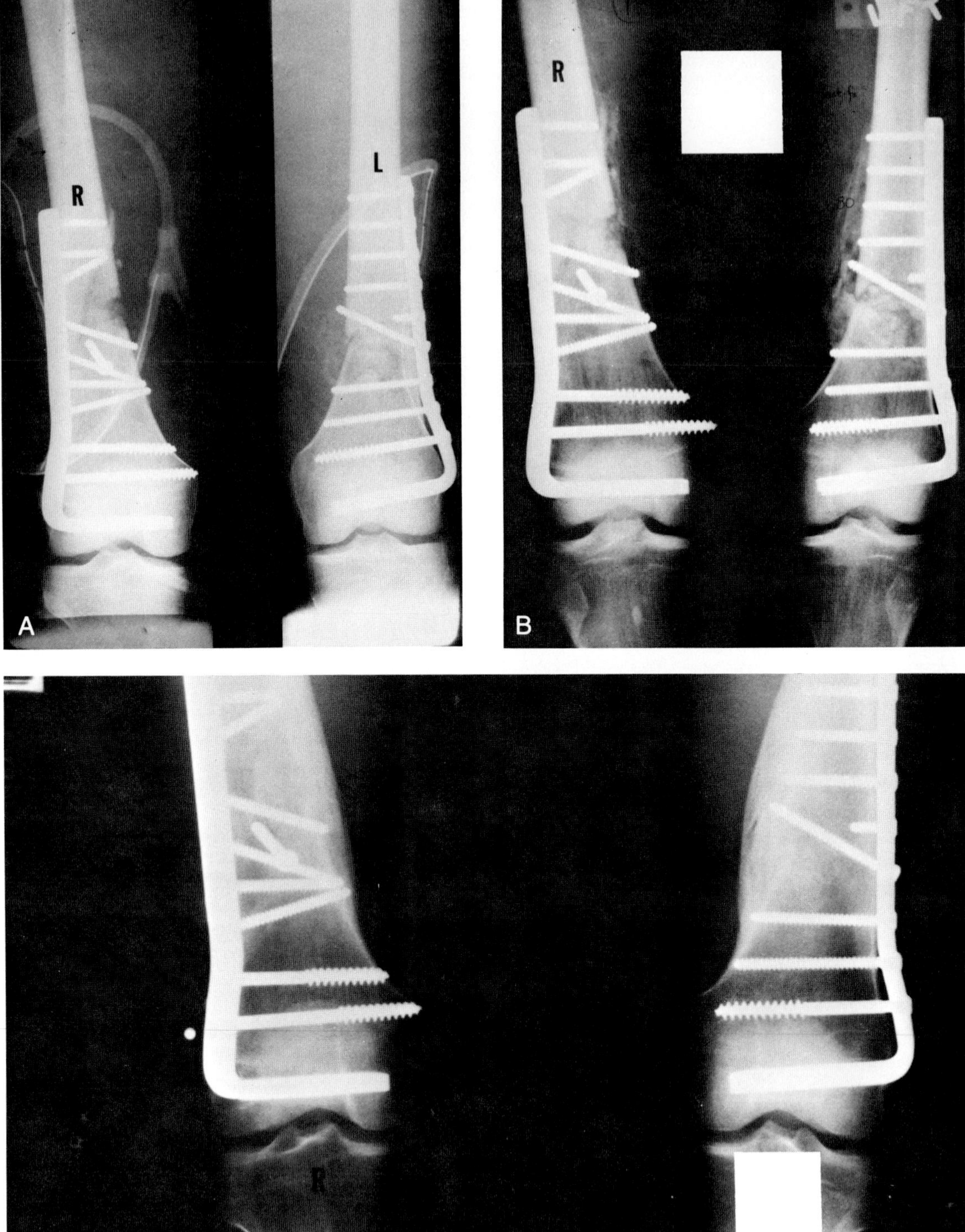

Fig. 22-5. *A*, Bilateral supracondylar fractures in a 21-year-old man on day of surgery. Note the comminution resulting in defects on the medial aspect of both fractures. Cancellous bone grafts were used to fill these defects. *B*, At 6 weeks post-surgery, the bone grafts are beginning to consolidate. *C*, At 1 year following surgery, both fractures are united solidly.

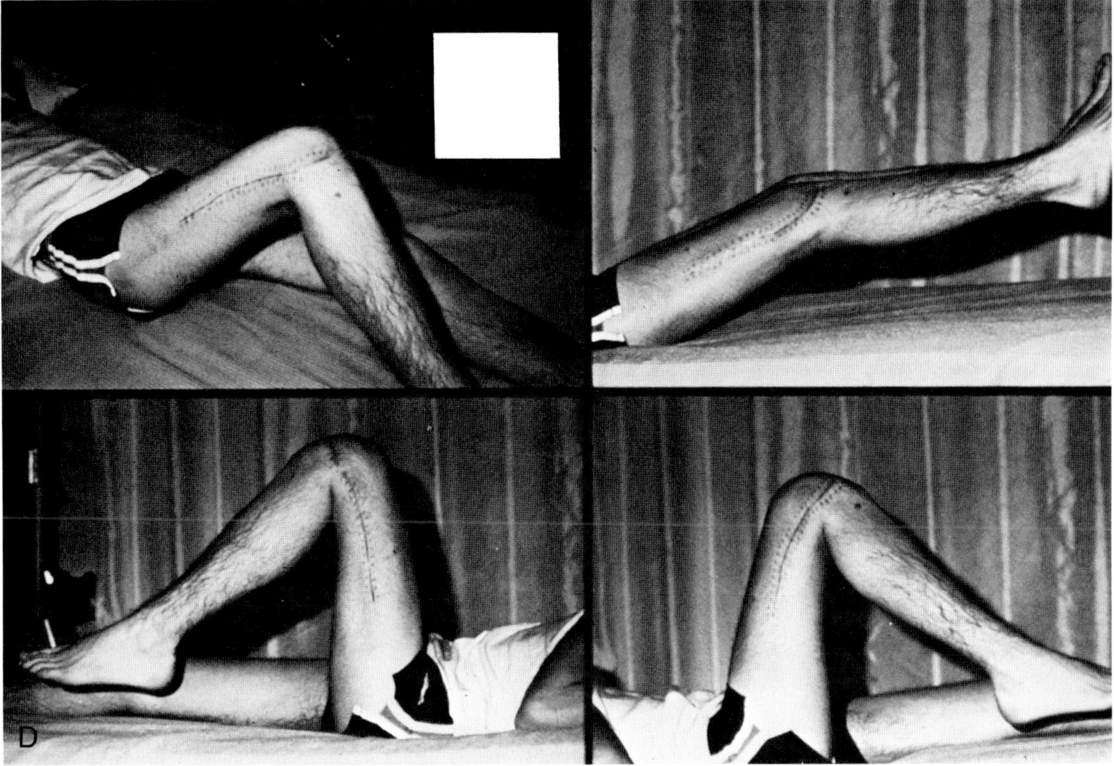

Fig. 22-5 (*continued*). *D*, At 1 year, the patient has an excellent functional result.

ally (Fig. 22-7, *C*). The perforators are ligated to minimize blood loss. The transmuscular approach should be avoided because it leads to scarring and binding down of the quadriceps. The joint is entered anteriorly to the lateral collateral ligament, and adequate exposure of the articular surfaces is accomplished (Fig. 22-7, *C*).

Early in our experience with fractures that had extensive articular involvement and displacement, it was occasionally necessary to reflect the quadriceps mechanism and infrapatellar tendon with a block of bone from the tibial tuberosity to gain sufficient exposure (Fig. 22-8).[13] With repeated experience, one can conceive the anatomy and will rarely have to use this exposure. The technique is good and can be done safely if exercised with caution and attention to detail.

The condyles are reduced with the knee flexed to 90°, and restoration of the articular surface and patellofemoral groove is obtained. Temporary fixation of the condyles is accomplished with a few crossed Kirschner wires. The condyles then are stabilized with two 6.5-mm cancellous screws with washers (Fig. 22-9). Care must be taken to avoid obstruction of the proposed site of entry of the special seating chisel; the threads should not cross the fracture line. These threads should be inserted slightly proximal to the proposed site of entry of the blade and should be either posterior or anterior to the middle of the shaft, far from the projected path of the plate. These screws do not have to be parallel. Washers should be used to prevent sinking of the screw heads into the lateral cortex (Fig. 22-9). The temporary Kirschner wires are removed.

After the condyles are fixed, one of two methods may be used.

1. The blade plate may be inserted into the distal fragment and the supracondylar component of the fracture can be reduced and placed under axial compression. This method should be used when the comminution in the metaphyseal area would not support the reduction without the protective strut of the plate.

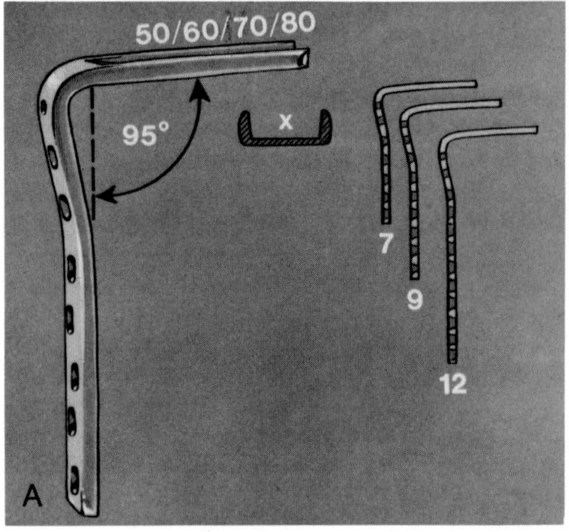

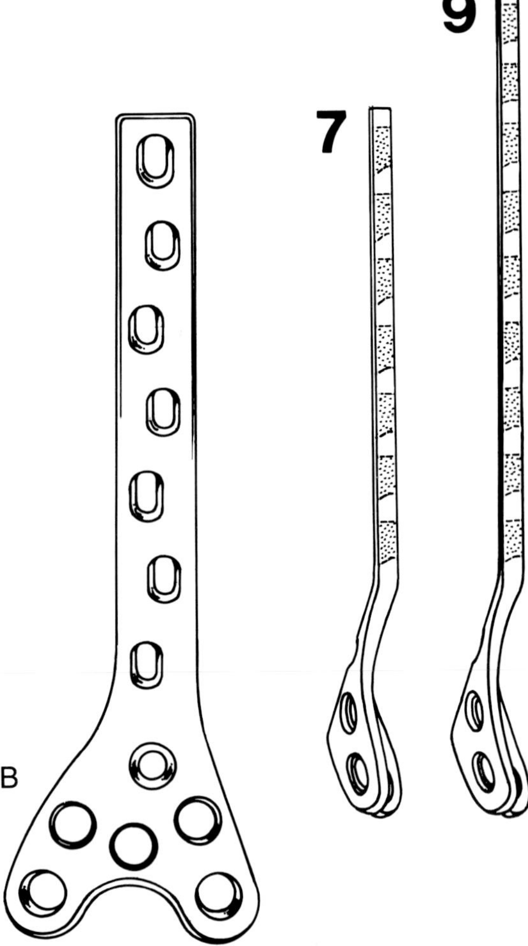

Fig. 22-6. *A*, The ASIF 95° condylar angled blade plate. *B*, The ASIF heavy condylar plate designed to fit the lateral side of the distal femur.

2. The stabilized condylar fragment can be reduced to the proximal fragment and temporarily fixed with multiple crossed Kirschner wires prior to inserting the condylar plate (Fig. 22-9, *B*). Frequently, the major fragments can be stabilized with one or two 4.5-mm cortical lag screws prior to the application of the blade plate.

Three Kirschner wires are used to determine the position of the blade plate (Fig. 22-10). This part of the procedure is most exacting, and one must pay close attention to the placement of these wires. The knee is bent to 90°, and the first wire is inserted transversely through the knee joint, parallel to the joint axis. The second Kirschner wire is inserted between the patella and the anterior surface of the lateral and medial condyles. This second wire serves as a guide to the inclination of the patellofemoral joint. These two wires indicate the desired direction of the blade. The distal femur is a rhomboid, and this second guide wire slopes downward from lateral to medial (Fig. 22-10, *A*). A third wire now is driven through the middle of the condyle, about 1 cm above the joint and in line with the long axis of the femur. This third wire should be parallel with the first and second wires and serves as the definitive guide for the seating of the chisel. The alignment of the third wire should be checked with the condylar positioning guide; all wires should be parallel (Fig. 22-10, *B*). The condylar positioning guide is a mirror image of the side-plate portion of the blade plate.

The point of entry for the blade should be about 1.5 cm from the knee joint and in line with or slightly anterior to the middle of the femoral shaft (Fig. 22-10, *C*). The blade never should be placed posterior to the lateral midline. The point of entry is prepared by drilling 3 holes with the 4.5-mm drill tip (Fig. 22-11, *A*). The 7-mm router is used to enlarge the 3 holes and to convert them to a slot (Fig. 22-11, *B*). The proximal side of the slot is beveled for a few millimeters with an osteotome to receive the shoulder of the angled blade plate and to prevent shattering of the lateral cortex (Fig. 22-11, *C*).

The U-profile of the seating chisel is identical to the profile of the blade plate. The seating chisel is attached to its guide, making sure the U-profile is toward the knee joint. The chisel is driven into the distal fragment by using light blows with the mallet. The flap of the chisel guide must be parallel to the long axis of the femoral shaft, and the seating chisel must be parallel to the third directional Kirschner wire (Fig.

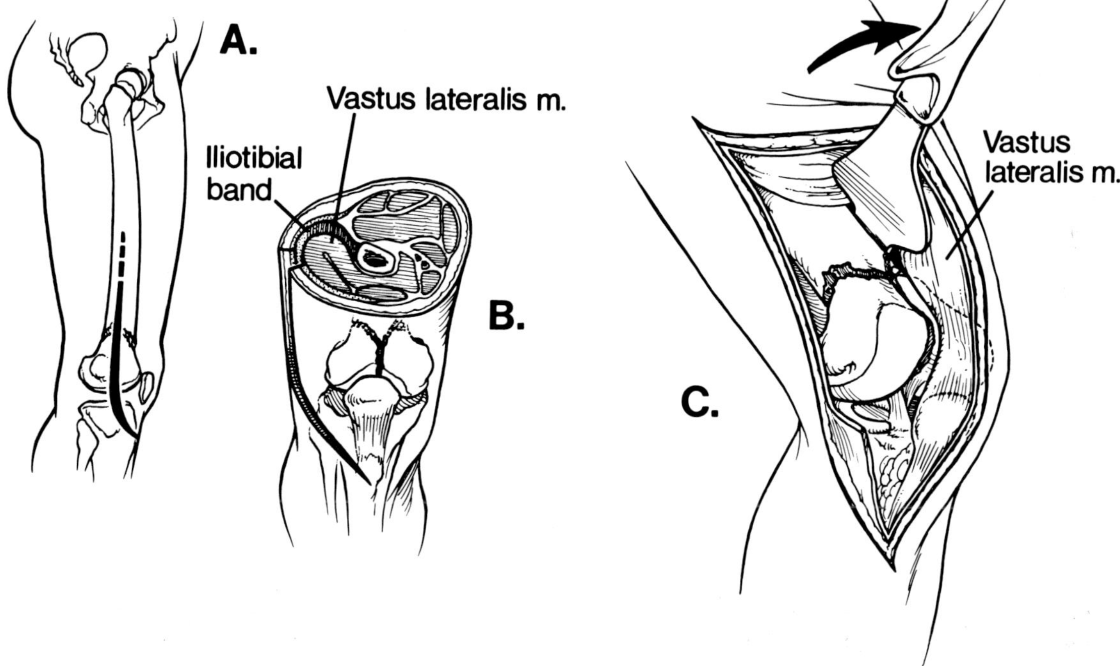

Fig. 22-7. Lateral surgical approach to the distal femur. The incision is anterior to the lateral collateral ligament. The iliotibial band is opened in line with the skin incision. The distal femur is exposed by lifting the entire vastus lateralis muscle from the intermuscular septum and retracting anteriorly and medially. (Modified from Muller, M. E., Allgower, M., Schneider, R., and Willenegger, H.: Manual of Internal Fixation. 2nd Edition. New York, Springer-Verlag, 1979.)

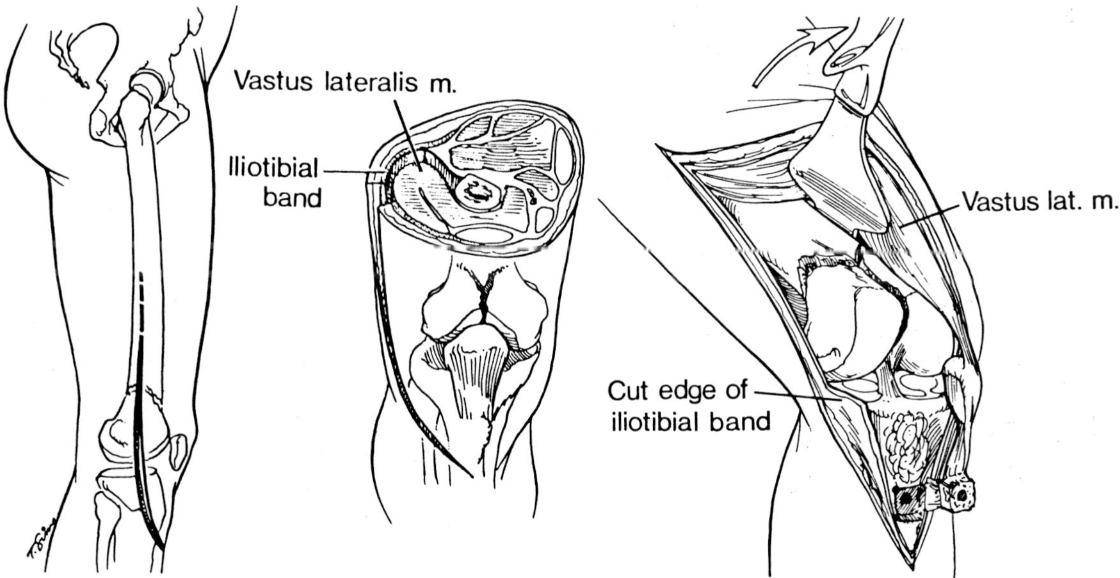

Fig. 22-8. The skin incision for the modified extensile approach extends down to a point fifteen millimeters distal to the tibial tuberosity but has no medial arm. Proximally the dissection is carried down to the femur posterior to the vastus lateralis muscle and anterior to the intermuscular septum. After the tibial tuberosity is elevated, a good exposure of all components of the fracture is achieved, but it is less extensive than that obtained by the extensile exposure. Redrawn from Mize and Associates, JBJS 64-A page 878. July, 1982.

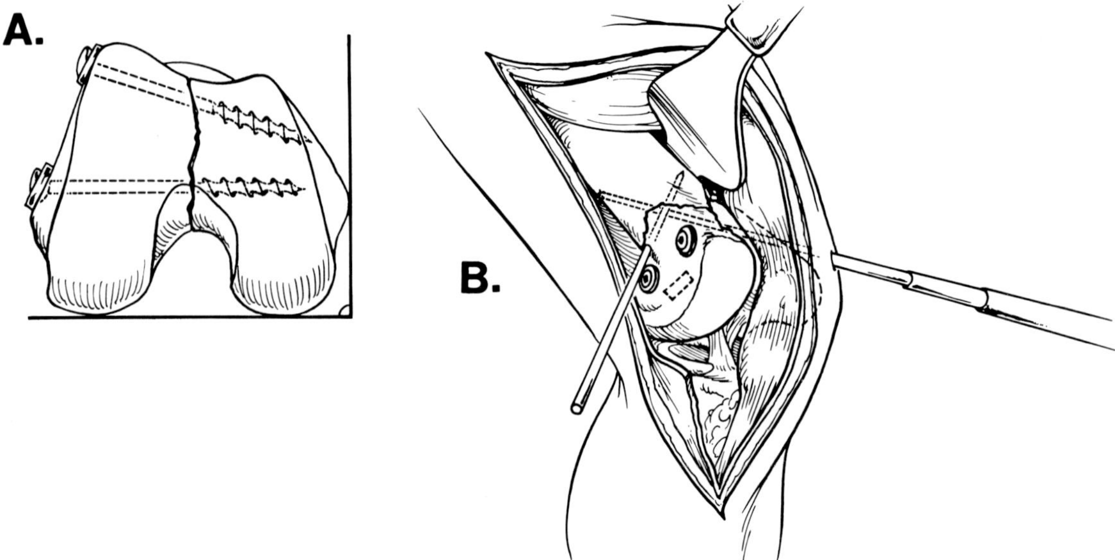

Fig. 22-9. The articular surface and split condyles have been restored and fixed with two 6.5-mm cancellous screws with washers that have been placed away from the proposed site of entry of the blade. (Modified from Muller, M. E., Allgower, M., Schneider, R., and Willenegger, H.: Manual of Internal Fixation. 2nd Edition. New York, Springer-Verlag, 1979.)

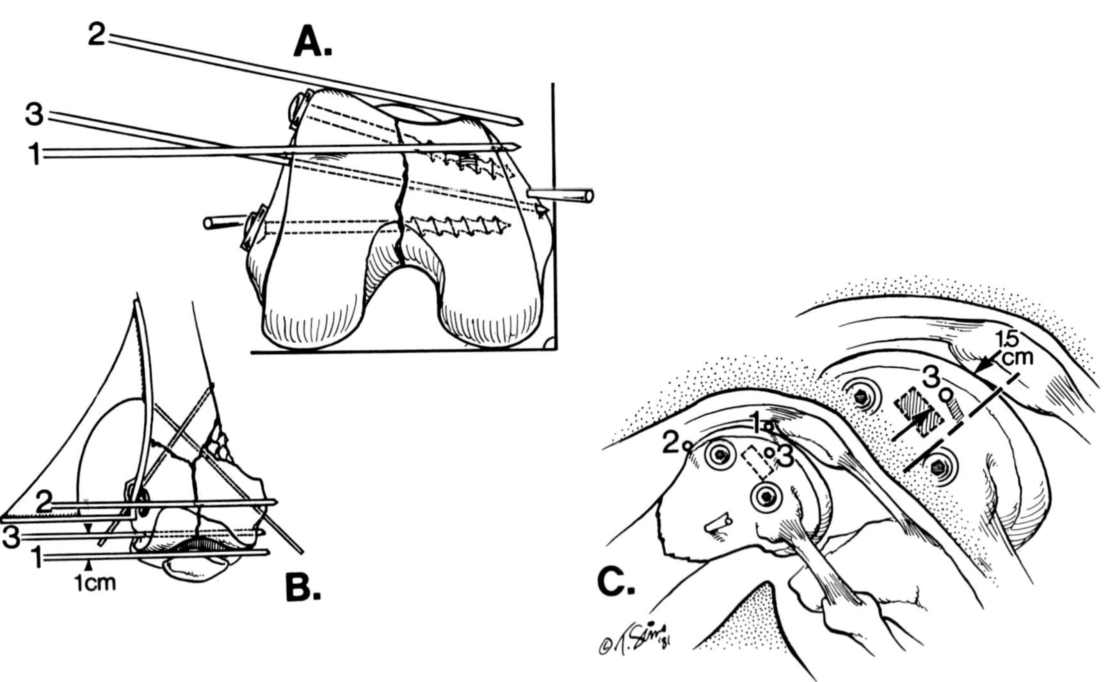

Fig. 22-10. Placement of the three directional guide wires. The first wire is parallel to the joint axis. The second wire shows the inclination of the patellofemoral joints and slopes down from lateral to medial. The third wire is parallel to both the first and second wires and serves as the definitive guide for the seating chisel. The point of entry of the blade should be about 1.5 cm from the joint and in line with the femoral shaft. (Modified from Muller, M. E., Allgower, M., Schneider, R., and Willenegger, H.: Manual of Internal Fixation. 2nd Edition. New York, Springer-Verlag, 1979.)

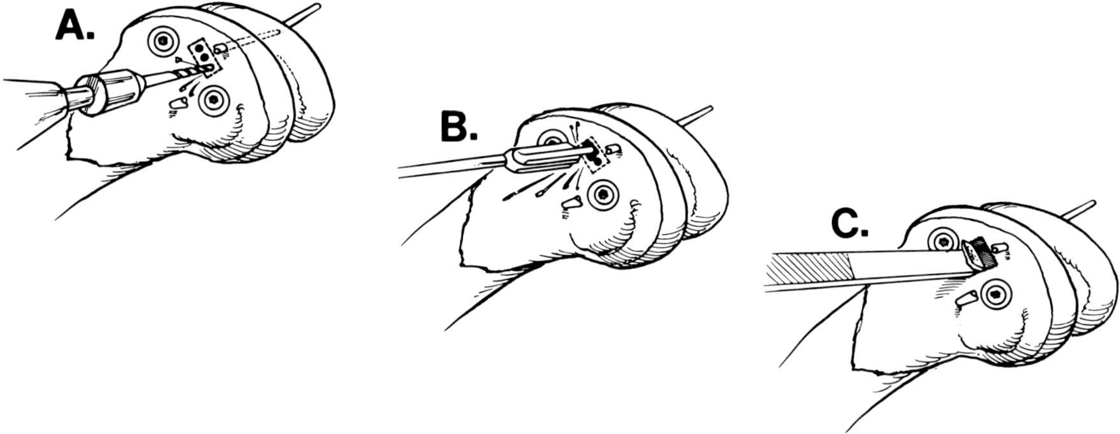

Fig. 22-11. *A*, Three 4.5-mm holes drilled at proposed site of entry. *B*, The 7-mm router used to convert the 3 holes to a slot. *C*, The slot is beveled proximally to receive the shoulder of the angled plate. (Modified from Muller, M. E., Allgower, M., Schneider, R., and Willenegger, H.: Manual of Internal Fixation. 2nd Edition. New York, Springer-Verlag, 1979.)

22-12). The slotted hammer is used to control the alignment and direction of the seating chisel (Fig. 22-12, *A*), thereby ensuring that the precut channel allows placement of the blade parallel to the knee joint and allows correct alignment of the plate in both sagittal and coronal planes.

The assistant must apply firm counterpressure against the medial condyle as the seating chisel is driven in to prevent disruption of the fixation of the condyles. The length of the blade is determined by the depth to which the seating chisel has been driven into the bone and can be checked by noting the gradations marked on the seating chisel (Fig. 22-12). This measurement can be compared to the predetermined length on the preoperative drawing. Keep in mind that the distal femur is a rhomboid and that the medial wall is sloped at about a 25° angle (Fig. 22-12, *B*). Thus, a blade that appears to be the correct length on an anteroposterior roentgenogram is in fact too long. A 50-mm blade usually is appropriate in a small patient. In a large patient, the surgeon rarely uses larger than a 70-mm blade. If the tip of the blade penetrates the medial cortex, it will irritate the medial soft tissues and cause pain. The slotted hammer is used to remove the seating chisel.

The selected condylar plate is attached to the plate holder. The plate holder is used for the insertion and removal of plates. The plate should be attached in such a way that the long handle is in line with or parallel with the blade of the condylar plate (Fig. 22-13, *A*). Rotation and alignment of the plate are controlled with the slotted hammer. The blade is driven in with light blows and should easily follow the previously cut channel. Check frequently to ensure that the plate is lining up exactly with the middle of the shaft. Remove the plate holder and use the impactor to drive the last 5 to 7 mm of the blade into the bone. Supplement the fixation of the blade to the distal fragment by inserting one or two 6.5-mm cancellous screws through the plate into the distal fragment immediately above the blade (Fig. 22-13, *B*). Check to ensure that the proximal component of the fracture is well reduced. To achieve axial compression, the surgeon should use the removable tension device even if the plate has the dynamic compression holes. Place the plate under tension and check the reduction and stability of the fixation; if both are satisfactory, the plate should be screwed home to the femoral shaft.

Attention is directed to the medial buttress. If this area is defective because of comminution, autologous cancellous bone grafting should be performed to fill the defects (Fig. 22-5, *A*, *B*, and *C* and Fig. 22-12, *B*). The medial side of the fracture is under compressive forces. If a medial gap is present, it will collapse under axial loading and create bending forces on the plate exactly opposite the medial defect. The plate eventually breaks with the cyclic loading. The bone graft is used to fill and buttress the medial gap. Failure to

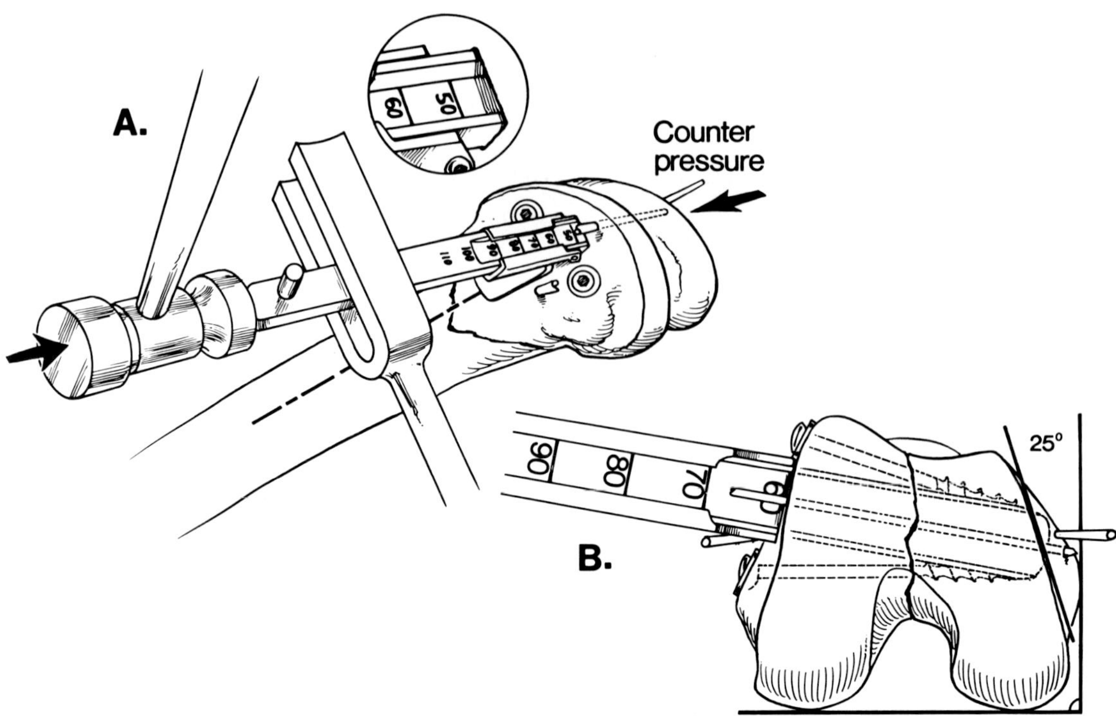

Fig. 22-12. The seating chisel is driven into the condyles. The slotted hammer is used to control the direction of the chisel in all three planes. The chisel cuts a channel that is parallel to the third directional wire. Note the rhomboid configuration of the distal femur. (Modified from Muller, M. E., Allgower, M., Schneider, R., and Willenegger, H.: Manual of Internal Fixation. 2nd Edition. New York, Springer-Verlag, 1979.)

graft these defects portends subsequent implant failure, loss of reduction, and delayed union or nonunion. The graft can be taken from the inner table of the anterior iliac crest or the ipsilateral trochanteric area. The graft should not be taken from the greater trochanter of the side opposite the fracture. The greater trochanter is on the tensile side of the proximal femur and, with full weightbearing, may act to increase stress to the point that a fracture can occur through the donor site. I therefore prefer the anterior iliac crest as a source for most bone grafts.

The wound is closed carefully. The vastus lateralis muscle is not sutured to the intermuscular septum because doing so causes slow recovery of full knee motion postoperatively. Carefully sewn mattress sutures are used to approximate the skin. Tight strangulating sutures have no place in fracture surgery.

Postoperative Management

The limb is placed on a frame with the hip and knee flexed to 90° (Fig. 22-13). This position prevents quadriceps shortening, makes postoperative range-of-motion exercises easier, and decreases the amount of swelling. Suction drainage is used to prevent hematoma formation. These drains are removed 24 to 48 hours after the operation. The 90°–90° position is maintained for about 4 days. While the limb is on the frame, the physical therapist begins gentle active assisted range of motion exercises. The patient is reminded about the "race between fracture healing and plate breakage." The potential danger of premature full weight-bearing is stressed to both the patient and the patient's family.

On about the fifth postoperative day, the patient is allowed to sit on the side of the bed and dangle his legs. Gait training proceeds from parallel bars to the use of a walker or crutches. If the fracture has been fixed rigidly, the patient may begin immediate partial weight-bearing of about 10 kg (20 lbs). The patient who remains completely nonweight-bearing with the hip and knee flexed may develop circulatory stasis and rapid disuse osteoporosis. A functional cast-brace occasionally is applied for the elderly patient with tenuous fixation, for the patient with marked comminution, or for the unreliable patient. As a

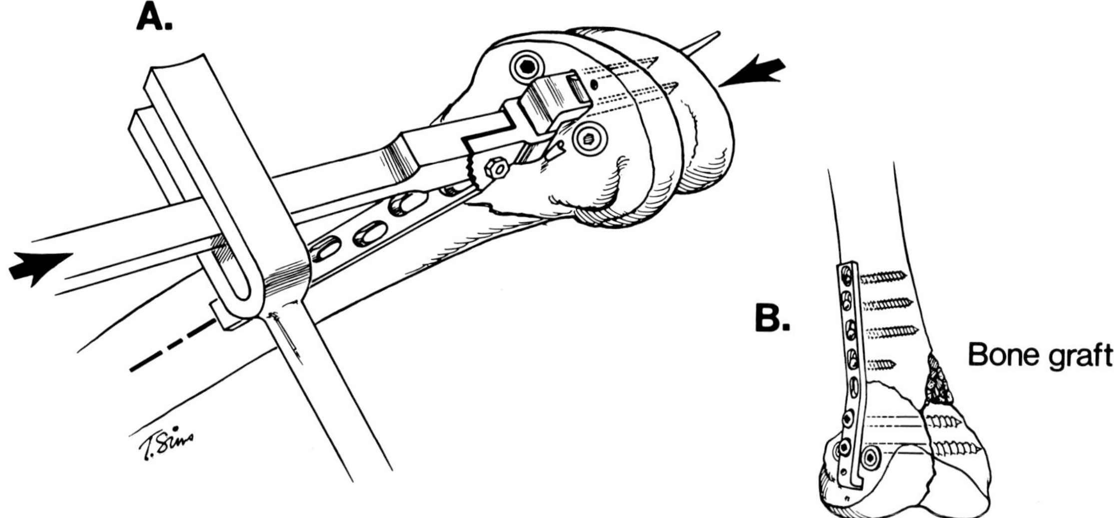

Fig. 22-13. *A*, The plate holder is used to insert the angled blade plate into the previously cut channel. Alignment and rotation are controlled with the slotted hammer. *B*, Fixation of the condyles is augmented by placing two 6.5-mm cancellous screws through the round holes directly above the blade. The side plate is secured to the shaft. The medial defect has been filled with cancellous bone graft. (Modified from Muller, M. E., Allgower, M., Schneider, R., and Willenegger, H.: Manual of Internal Fixation. 2nd Edition. New York, Springer-Verlag, 1979.)

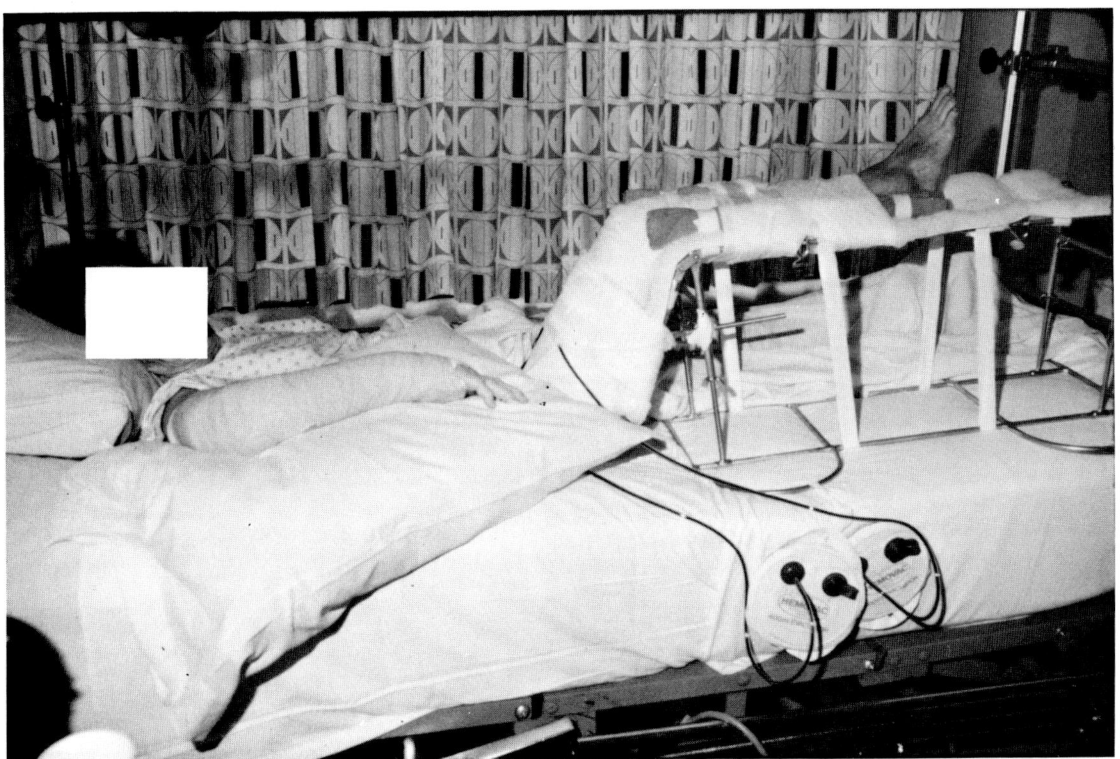

Fig. 22-14. Seventy-one-year-old woman with multiple fractures one day following surgery. Note the 90°-90° position of the limb and suction drainage of both the thigh and iliac crest donor site.

rule, the patient uses 2 crutches for about 2 to 3 months. If there is radiographic evidence of sufficient bone healing at the end of this period, the patient may progress to 1 crutch, which is used on the side of the fracture for an additional 1 to 2 months. Full weight-bearing is allowed with a healed fracture at about 4 months.

Complications

The surgical management of supracondylar and intercondylar fractures of the distal femur is fraught with a wide range of potential complications. All reported series of these injuries mentioned delayed union or nonunion, malunion, delayed wound healing, infection, joint contracture, loosening or breaking of the fixation device, post-traumatic arthritis, and refracture after removal of the implant.

The patient with a relatively simple, two-fragment, supracondylar fracture is vulnerable to any of these complications. A patient with a more complex fracture of the distal femur or with multiple injuries presents an even greater challenge to the treating physician. Therefore, the physician must not increase the risk of these complications by committing technical errors in management.

All these complications can be minimized if the surgeon exercises respect for the soft tissues by using gentle, smooth, operative technique, using tissue planes, minimizing periosteal stripping, and avoiding long operating times. Accurate anatomic reduction and stable internal fixation must be obtained. Satisfaction with "getting the fractures generally aligned" only invites complications. Cancellous bone grafting should be routine in cases of marked comminution with bone loss and defects. This procedure enhances healing and helps to prevent implant failure.

References

1. Stewart, M., Sisk, T. D., and Wallace, S.: Fractures of the distal third of the femur—a comparison of methods of treatment. J. Bone Joint Surg., *48-A*:784, 1966.
2. Neer, C., Grantham, S. A., and Shelton, M.: Supracondylar fracture of the adult femur—a study of 110 cases. J. Bone Joint Surg., *49-A*:591, 1967.
3. Mooney, V., Nickel, V., Harvey, J., and Snelson, R.: Cast-brace treatment for fractures of the distal part of the femur. J. Bone Joint Surg., *52-A*:1563, 1970.
4. Mays, J., and Neufeld, A. J.: Skeletal traction methods. Clin. Orthop., *102*:144, 1974.
5. Muller, M. E., Allgower, M., Schneider, R., and Willenegger, H.: Manual of Internal Fixation. 2nd Edition. New York, Springer-Verlag, 1979.
6. Allgower, M.: Cinderella of surgery—fractures? Surg. Clin. North Am., *58*:1071, 1978.
7. Montgomery, S., and Mooney, V.: Femur fractures—treatment with roller traction and early ambulation. Personal communication, 1980.
8. Slatis, P., Ryoppy, S., and Huittinen, V.: AOI osteosynthesis of fractures of the distal third of the femur. Acta Orthop. Scand., *42*:162, 1971.
9. Olerud, S.: Operative treatment of supracondylar-condylar fractures of the femur. J. Bone Joint Surg., *54-A*:1015, 1972.
10. Chiron, H. S., Tremoulet, J., Casey, P., and Muller, M.: Fractures of the distal third of the femur treated by internal fixation. Clin. Orthop., *100*:160, 1974.
11. Shelton, M., Grantham, S., Neer, C., and Singh, R.: A new fixation device for supracondylar and low femoral shaft fractures. J. Trauma, *14*:821, 1974.
12. Schatzker, J., Horne, G., and Waddell, J.: The Toronto experience with the supracondylar fracture of the femur, 1966–1972. Injury, *6*:113, 1974.
13. Mize, R. D., Bucholz, R. W., and Grogan, D. P.: Surgical treatment of displaced comminuted fractures of the distal end of the femur. An extensile approach. J. Bone Joint Surg., *64A*:871, 1982.
14. Schatzker, J., and Lambert, D.: Supracondylar fractures of the femur. Clin. Orthop., *138*:77, 1979.

Chapter 23 Complex Ankle Fractures

JEFFREY W. MAST
PHILLIP G. SPIEGEL

In the evaluation and treatment of the multiply injured patient, fractures of the ankle can be missed or their treatment delayed because of more urgent associated injuries. Nevertheless, prompt diagnosis and initial treatment, preliminary or definitive, that re-establishes the joint axis and preserves a congruent articular surface, optimally set the stage for recovery of full ankle function. A reduction is accomplished more easily during this acute period than at any other time. Methods of treatment are varied and should be selected to fit the demands of the individual situation. Many patients, particularly those with head injuries, may have a guarded prognosis for weeks. Correction of poorly conceived early or delayed treatment is frequently impossible when the patient begins to recover at a later date.

In this chapter, complex ankle fractures are discussed. Although comminution of bone makes management of fracture patterns complicated, the term "complex" is used in this chapter to describe fractures that combine peripheral instability of the joint complex with axial shortening caused by displacement of the tibial shaft or impaction of bone of the distal tibia (Fig. 23-1).

"Simple" malleolar fractures can lead to various degrees of talar dislocations because of fractures of the tibial malleoli or rupture of their ligamentous functional equivalents. The discussion of pathomechanics, classification, and treatment, both closed and open, of these fractures is well covered in many other sources and will not be repeated here.[1-8]

A few malleolar fractures are complex because, in addition to the usual rotational forces responsible for the fracture pattern, significant axial loading is present at the moment of impact, thus producing large fracture fragments of the tibial plafond. These fractures are sometimes as-

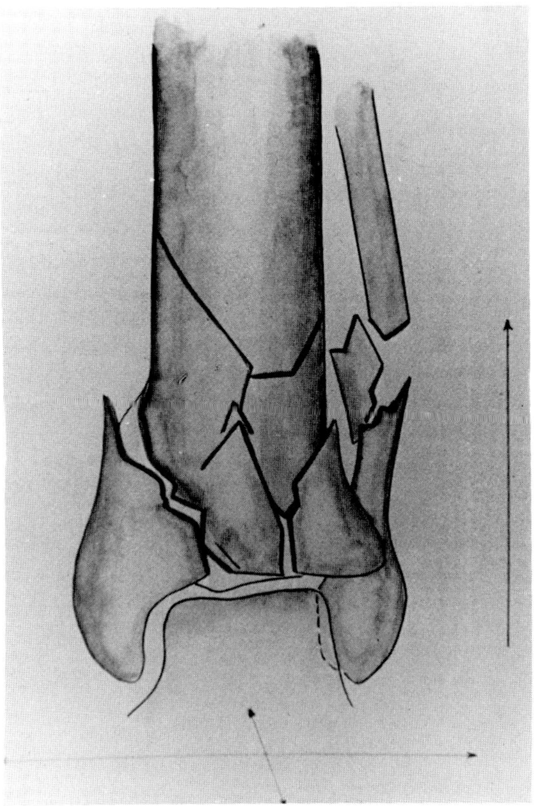

Fig. 23-1. Complex ankle fractures combine peripheral instability of the joint with loss of tibial length.

sociated with compression of subchondral cancellous bone, leading to the problems of shortening, articular incongruity, and instability of the talus.[9]

The following fracture types will be discussed in this chapter: (1) Lauge-Hansen pronation dorsiflexion type of fractures; (2) variants of malleolar fractures as described by Lauge-Hansen with vertical loading as an additional component; and (3) compression and spiral extension types of pilon fractures.

The discussion of these fractures is pertinent to a volume devoted to the polytrauma patient as many authors have shown that these types of injuries are seen frequently in patients who are subjected to violent trauma and who usually have concomitant serious injuries.

Mechanism and Incidence of Injury

Vertical compression forces are the common denominator of fractures that affect significant areas of the ceiling of the ankle mortise, or the plafond. These forces may act singularly on the distal tibia, with the particular area of destruction determined by the position of the foot at the time of impact,[10,11] or may represent a component of more complex forces, including rotation.[12]

The most common causes of these fractures are jumps or falls from a height, motor-vehicle accidents, skiing accidents, or falls forward with the foot trapped under a heavy object; but, any mechanism that produces significant vertically directed force may be responsible.[13]

These complex ankle fractures represent from 1 to 10% of fractures of the lower leg.[12,14] These figures may be misleading, however, as there is no agreement as to which fractures should be included in the classification. Because of the common etiologic factor of vertical compression, other fractures, such as contralateral os calcis, tibial plateau, acetabular, and compression fractures of the vertebral column, especially the first lumbar vertebra, are seen commonly in conjunction with complex ankle fractures.

Classification

Lauge-Hansen's classification brought order to the confusion that existed in the understanding of the commonly repeated patterns of malleolar fractures.[4] Also, he described a pronation dorsiflexion mechanism to explain the highly comminuted fracture of the distal tibia affecting the roof of the ankle joint.[15]

In this pronation dorsiflexion injury, which is frequently produced by a jump or a fall from a height, the first event is a fracture of the medial malleolus at its base, followed by the crushing of the anterior lip of the tibia. A supramalleolar fracture of the fibula follows, and finally, a transverse fracture of the posterior portion of the tibia occurs. The end result is a comminuted intra-articular fracture of the distal tibia and fibula (Fig. 23-2).

Lauge-Hansen fractures of the supination external rotation type and the pronation external rotation type with axial loading also may produce fractures of the tibial plafond and qualify as complex ankle fractures. (Fig. 23-3).[12]

Jahna and associates,[13] Rüedi and Allgoewer,[10,11] and Weber[16] have noted that the pilon fracture patterns are affected by the position of the foot at the time of impact. If the foot is in neutral position, the talus is driven directly upward into the distal tibial metaphysis, thus producing a Y-shaped explosion fracture of the joint. If the foot is dorsiflexed, an anterior marginal fracture of the distal tibia is produced. If the foot is plantarflexed, a posterior triangular fracture fragment results (Fig. 23-4).

Rüedi and Allgoewer,[11,17] who encouraged a more optimistic outlook on the results obtainable from surgical stabilization of these pilon fractures, havc proposed a classification based on the degree of comminution and displacement. Type A consists of a cleavage fracture without major dislocation of the articular surface. Type B consists of significant fracture and dislocation of the joint surface without comminution. Type C denotes impaction and comminution of the distal tibia (Fig. 23-5).

If necessary, further subdivision can be done based on the position of the foot at the time of injury and the major articular fragments produced. Although these subdivisions are useful for documentation of results, they do not change treatment plans.

Maale and Seligson add an additional classification to the previously described fracture patterns—a distal extension of spiral fractures of the tibia into the intra-articular portion of the tibial plafond (Fig. 23-6).[12]

In summary, we favor a classification system of complex ankle fractures that separates the fractures of the tibial plafond caused by combined

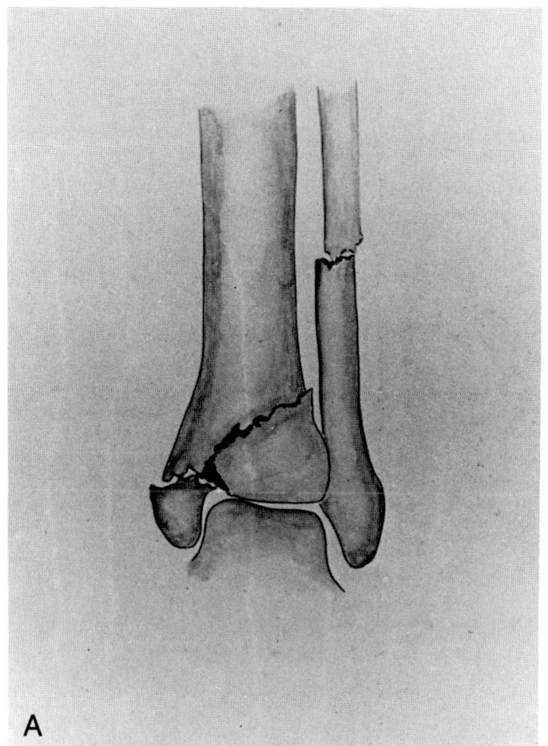

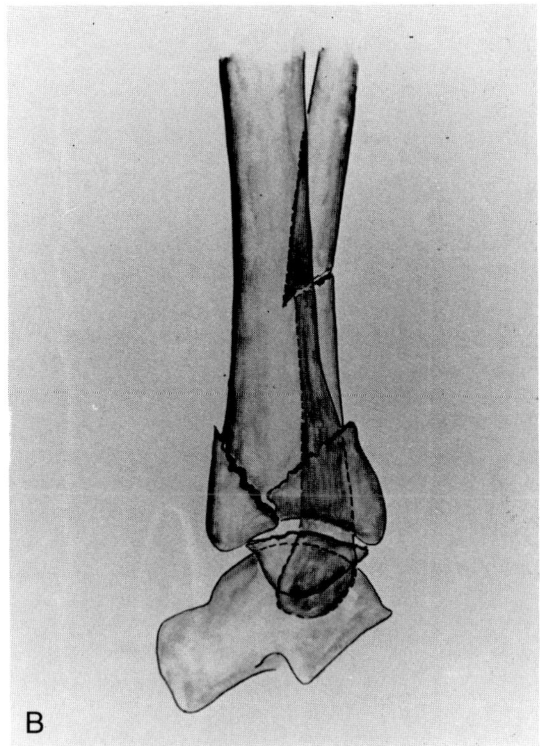

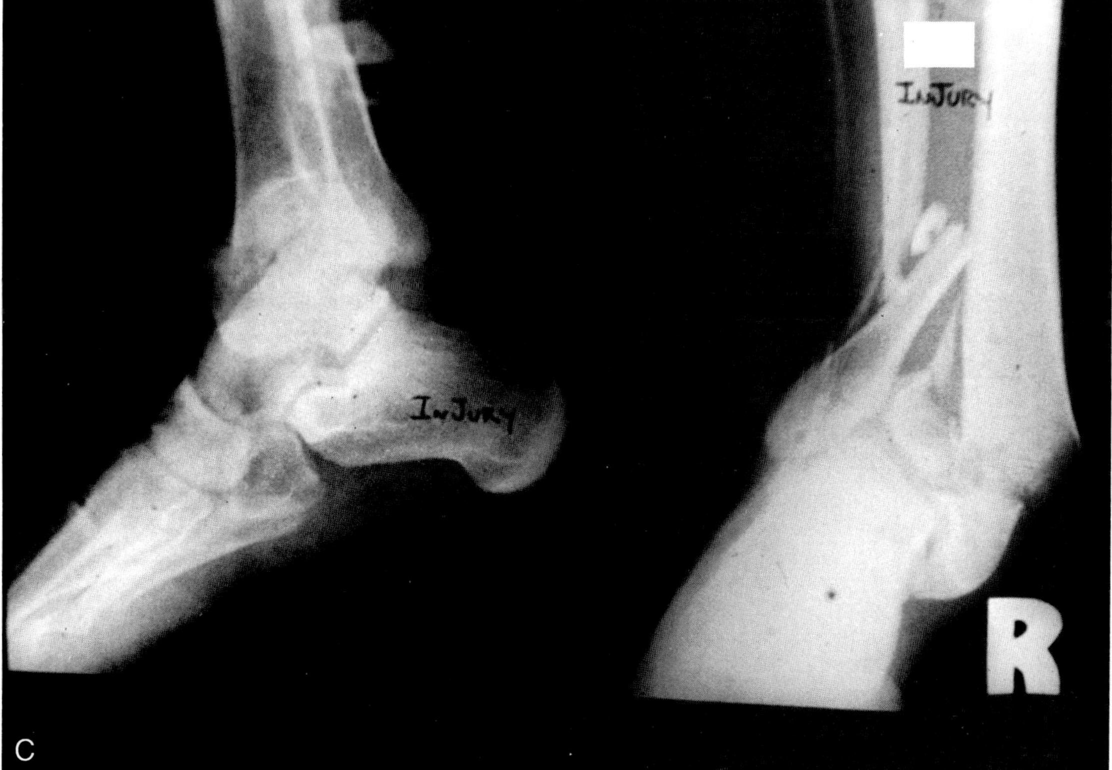

FIG. 23-2. *A* and *B*, Anteroposterior and lateral views of a Lauge-Hansen pronation dorsiflexion injury of the tibia and fibula. *C*, A 25-year-old man sustained a Lauge-Hansen pronation dorsiflexion injury after falling 25 feet (type IIIC fracture tibial plafond). Immediate open reduction and internal fixation were performed without use of a medial buttress plate (earlier case in series).

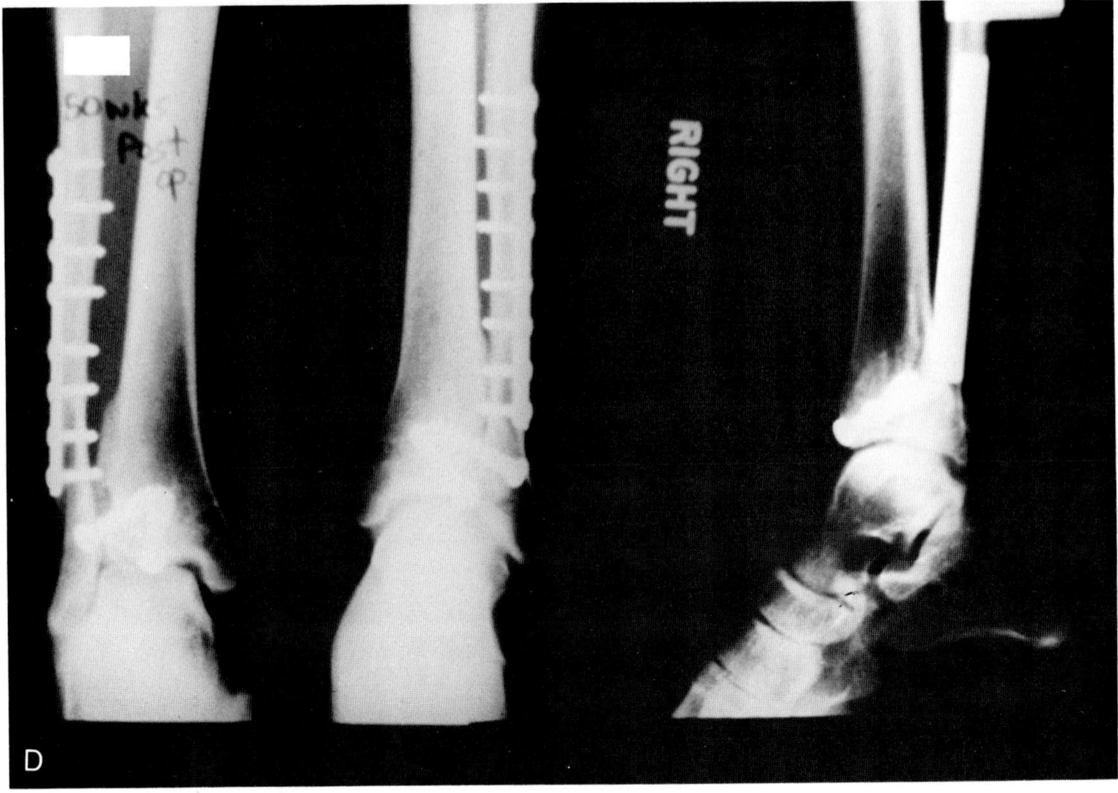

Fig. 23-2 (*continued*). *D*, Result at 50 weeks. The patient experienced full range of motion with no pain and was fully employed at previous job. (Case courtesy of George W. Prutzman, Jr., M.D.)

axial and rotatory stress from those caused by more purely compressive forces. As most surgeons realize, the latter group produces almost irreversible destructive fragmentation and impaction of the distal tibia.

In this chapter, we will refer to the following types of ankle fractures:

Type I—malleolar fractures with posterocranial talar luxation due to large posterior plafond fragments, i.e., Lauge-Hansen Ser IV and Per IV (see Fig. 23-3).

Type II—spiral fractures of the tibia with extension into the plafond, i.e., Maale-Seligson (see Fig. 23-6).

Type III—compressive fractures with pure impaction of the talus into the distal tibia with or without fibular fractures. This type includes Lauge-Hansen's pronation dorsiflexion ankle fracture (see Fig. 23-2). These pilon fractures are then subdivided according to Rüedi and Allgoewer into subgroup A (cleavage fractures of the distal tibia without major dislocation of the articular surface), B (significant fracture-dislocation of the joint surface without comminution), and C (impaction and comminution of the distal tibia) (see Fig. 23-5).

Diagnosis

The history of a jumping injury or an accident associated with axial compression forces should alert the surgeon to the possible presence of the complex ankle fracture.

Since this type of injury produces lesions requiring anesthesia for treatment, questions regarding pre-existing medical conditions, allergies, sensitivity to anesthetic agents, or bleeding disorders should be asked when taking the initial history. A history of previous trauma to the musculoskeletal system is best obtained at the outset, particularly if the traumatized extremity has been injured previously.

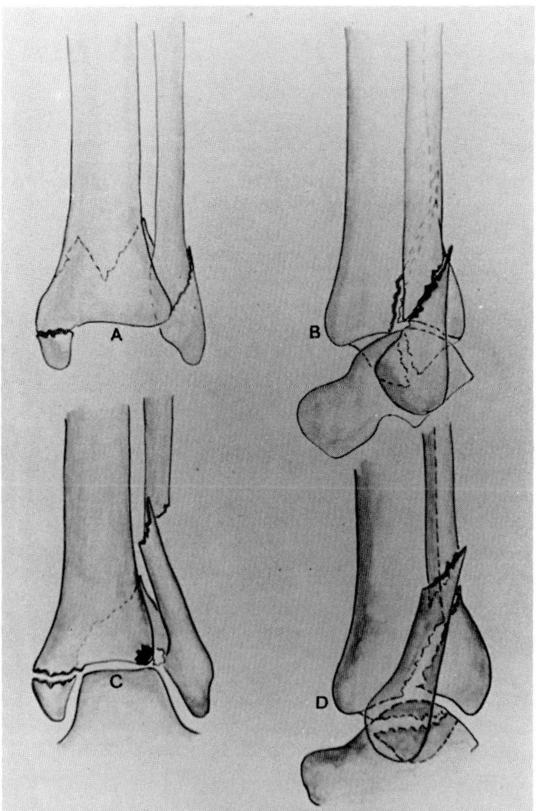

A careful physical examination should disclose the presence or absence of associated injuries. On examination of the affected ankle, a search for proximal tenderness of the fibula or tibia should be included, and a careful evaluation of the neurologic and vascular status and of the general condition of the skin must be made.

Routine roentgenograms usually disclose the nature of the fracture; however, special studies and/or roentgenograms of the contralateral side may be useful. In patients who appear to have an intact fibula in the distal third, roentgenograms of the affected leg should include the entire tibia and fibula because the presence of a proximal fibular fracture may be discovered.

Special roentgenograms should include oblique views, and occasionally, anteroposterior and lateral tomography is necessary. By utilizing these roentgenograms, one can best determine the true degree of comminution, as well as the degree of displacement and the presence of key fragments.

Roentgenograms of the normal side can serve as a template for making a preoperative drawing with the use of tracing paper. If the fracture cannot be drawn in a satisfactorily reduced and stabilized position preoperatively, the surgical end result probably will not be gratifying. Silhouettes

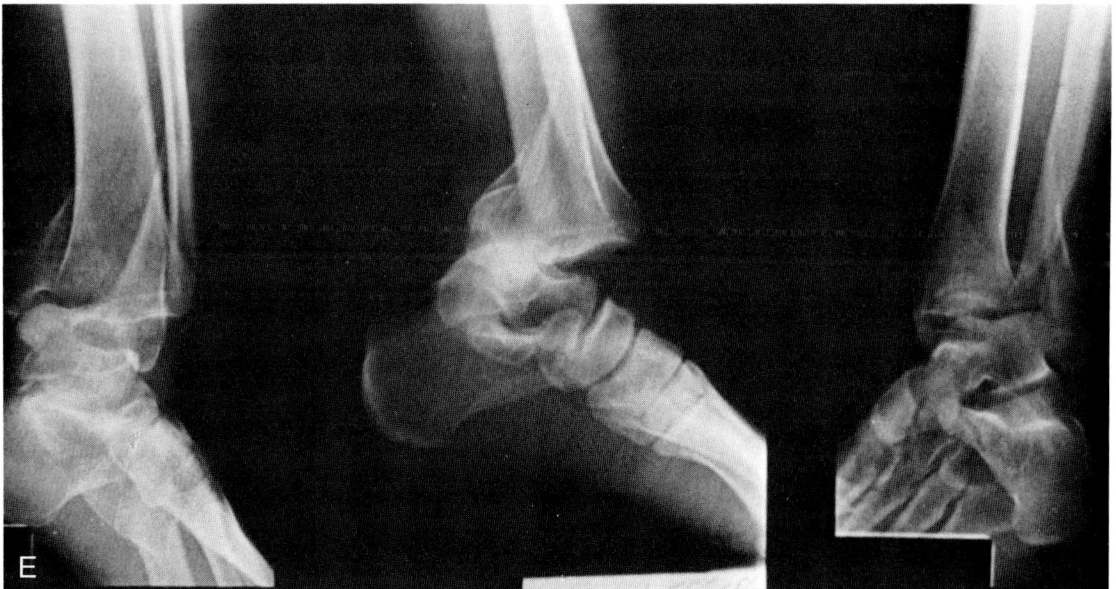

Fig. 23-3. *A* and *B*, Anteroposterior and lateral views of supination external rotation—stage IV injury. *C* and *D*, Anteroposterior and lateral views of pronation external rotation—stage IV injury. Both of these injuries are a result of substantial vertical loading at the time of injury and produce a significant posterior tibial fragment. (These injuries represent type I complex ankle fractures.) *E*, A 30-year-old male skydiver with improper landing technique sustained supination external rotation (stage IV) injury with vertical loading. Immediate open reduction and internal fixation were performed.

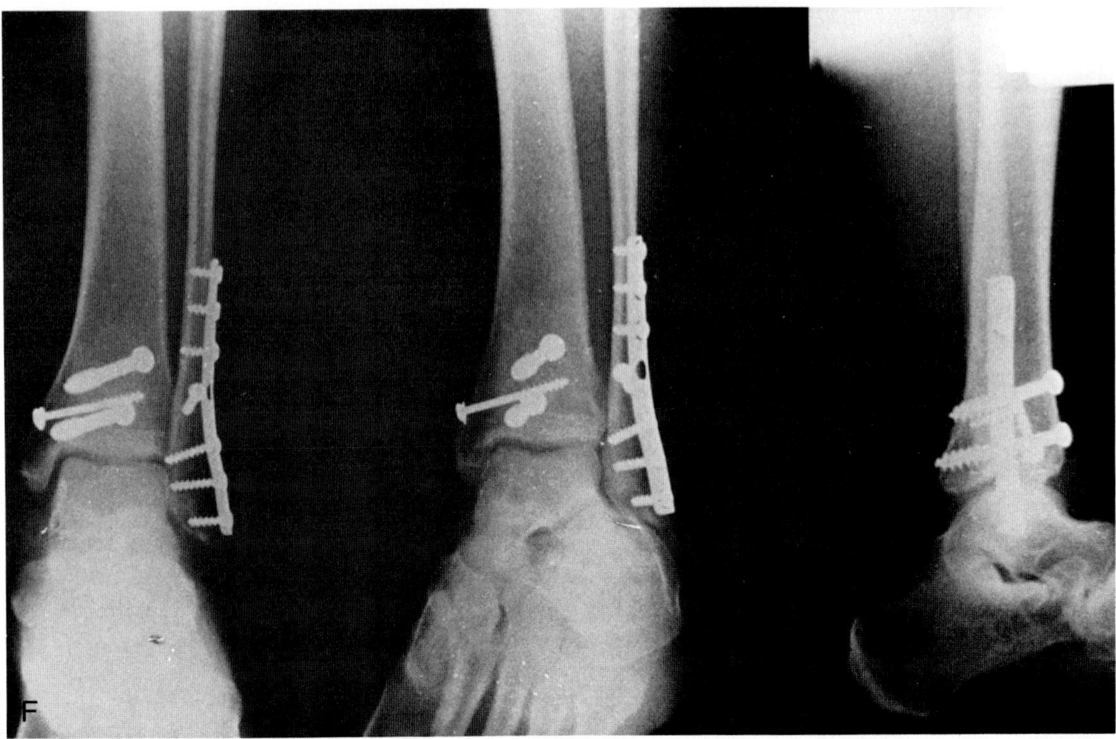

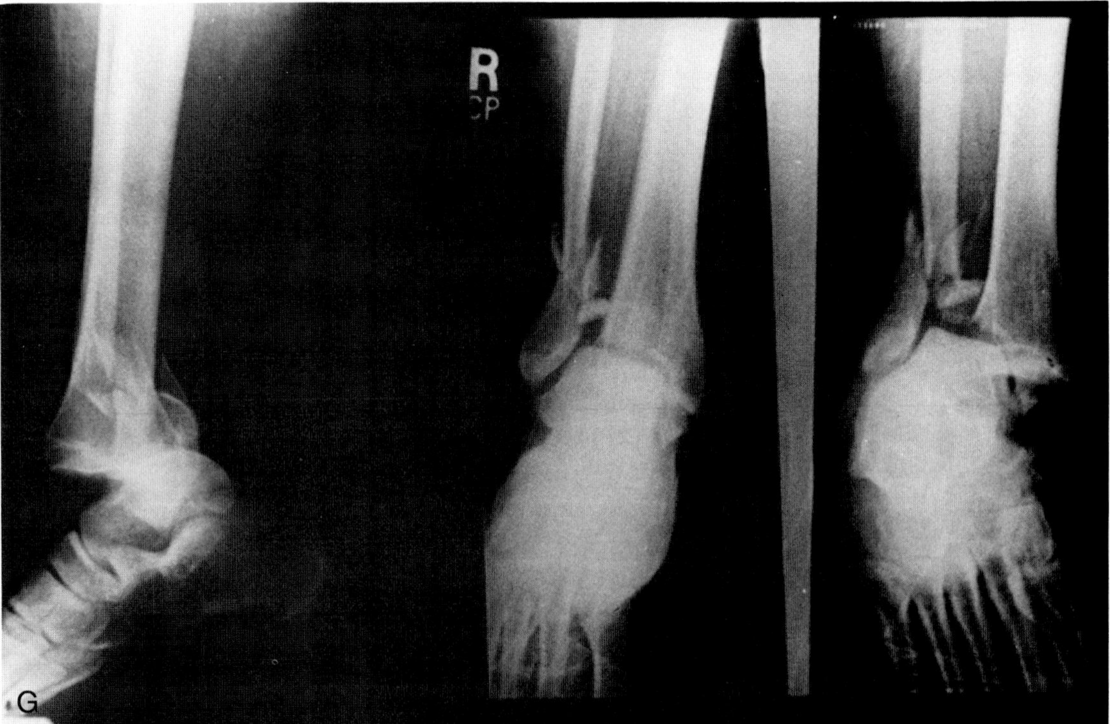

Fig. 23-3 (*continued*). *F*, Result at 6 months. The patient experienced full range of motion with no pain and returned to playing racquetball. *G*, A 28-year-old woman who fell from a height sustained pronation external rotation (stage IV) injury with vertical compression. Immediate open reduction and internal fixation were performed.

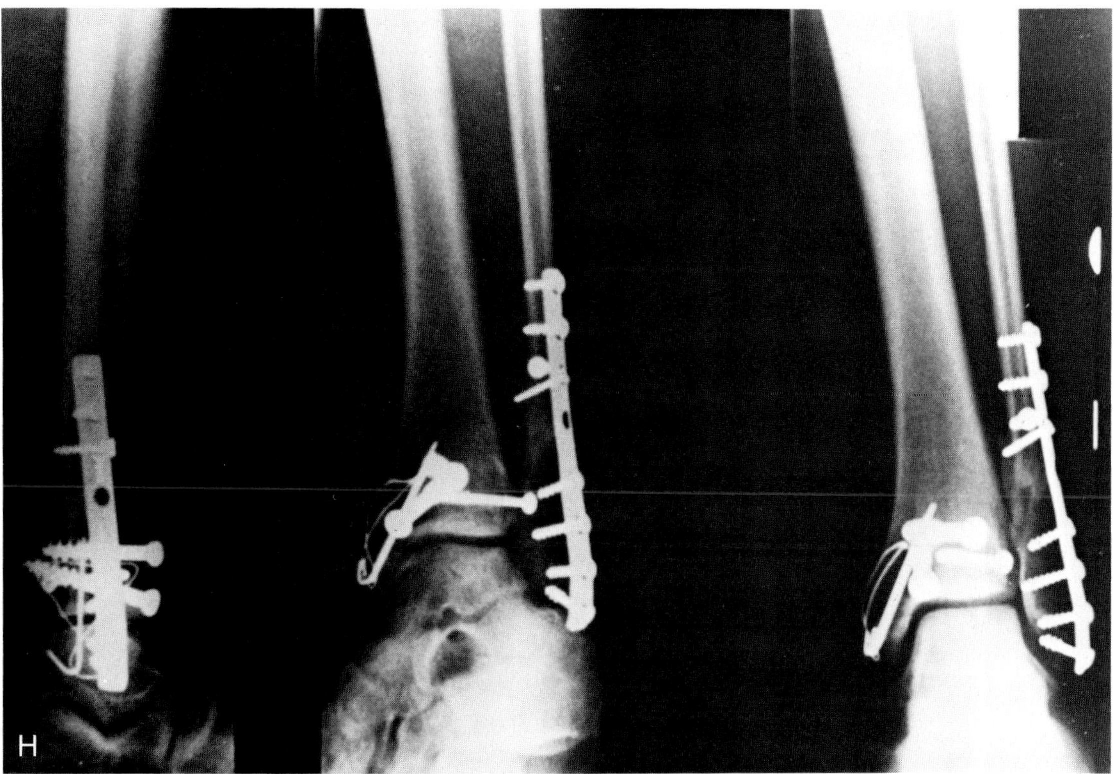

Fig. 23-3 (*continued*). *H*, Result at 8 months. The patient returned to full activity, including her role as ice-skating instructor.

of most implants to be used can be drawn on transparent sheets.

In these fractures, we do not feel that stress films or arthrography are of particular value. Given the present state of the art, we feel that computerized axial tomography scanning is not of any greater value than standard tomography.

Methods of Treatment

The treatment of these difficult fractures depends on several factors, e.g., "the personality" of the fracture (classification), the patient's general condition, and the experience and expertise of the surgeon.

Plaster of Paris

Plaster of paris remains a viable method of treatment; its greatest limitation is the difficulty of holding fracture length. Because complex fractures, as defined, have instability plus shortening, maintaining distraction is a major consideration. (There is not total agreement on this point. Jahna, et al.,[13] make the point that when comminuted type III C fractures of the tibia and fibula are treated closed, the surgeon should aim for 5 to 10 mm of shortening. An attempt at anatomic reduction of the fibula should not be planned because such attempts aggravate the instability caused by the impaction defect of the distal tibial metaphysis.) In types I and II fractures, initial reduction may be possible, and the ease of plaster application is appealing. If time is crucial and soft-tissue problems are not severe, plaster may serve well as a temporizing measure. Unfortunately, physiologic motion beneficial to joint injuries is not possible in plaster, and with time, reductions of these unstable fractures are difficult to maintain. Because of these disadvantages, plaster is not recommended as a definitive treatment.

Kirschner Wires and Steinmann Pins

The proper application of pins and wires may serve as a means of maintaining length by inserting the pin into the os calcis and using traction via a Böhler-Braun frame. The pin's insertion is not time consuming, soft-tissue lesions are visible and can be treated, and some "early motion" can be instituted. However, the disadvantages of applying pins are significant in the polytrauma patient. The technique "immobilizes the patient, not the fracture."[17] This consideration is of paramount importance when one remembers the pulmonary complications in the multiply injured patient. Even though this form of treatment may require a relatively short time period (2 to 3 weeks), it occurs during the crucial period for pulmonary complications in a patient who is in an enforced supine position. Additionally, pin-tract infections, particularly in the os calcis, can occur and are difficult to eradicate. The quality of the reduction with this method may be acceptable, but is not anatomic if central intra-articular fragments are present. Traction application must be well done technically and watched carefully.

In rare instances, e.g., for limb salvage or because of circumstances that compromise the time available for surgery, temporary alignment may be maintained by vertical transarticular pin fixation, as described by Childress.[18] The fact that the entry point of the pin is far from a future operative site is advantageous if this technique is selected for temporary stabilization.

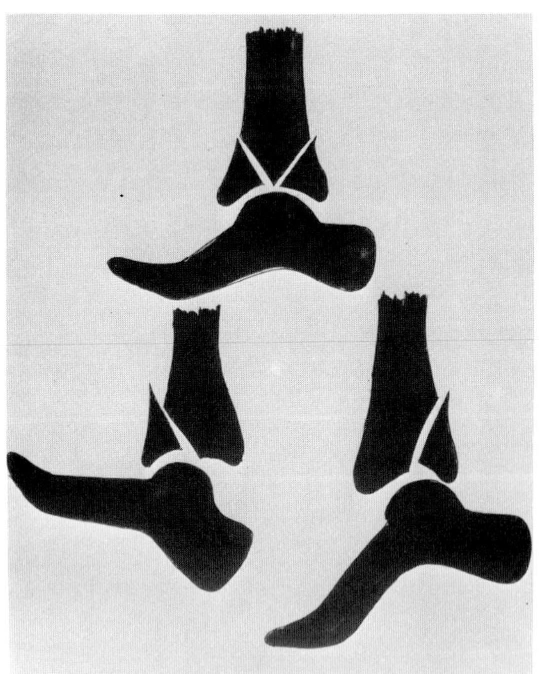

Fig. 23-4. Mechanism of injury in pilon fractures. (Redrawn from Rüedi according to Weber).

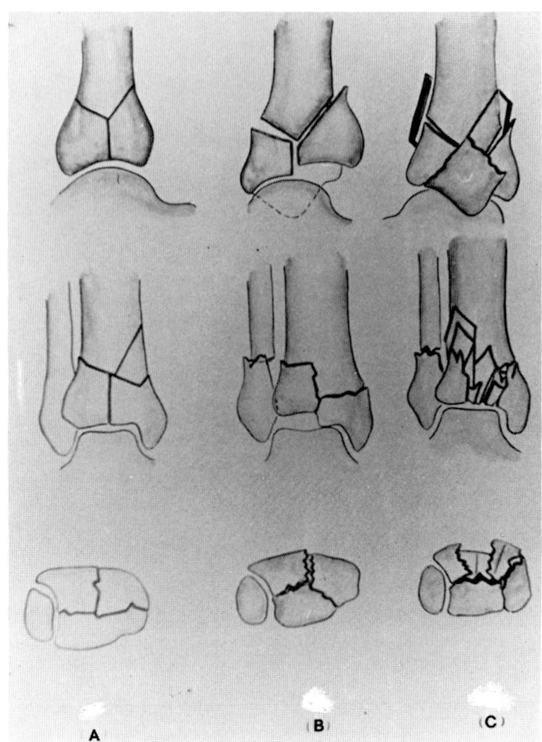

Fig. 23-5. Grading of pilon fractures based on severity of injury (type III complex ankle fractures). *A*, Simple cleavage fractures without intra-articular involvement. *B*, Intra-articular displacement with little comminution. *C*, Intra-articular displacement with marked comminution. (Rüedi & Allgoewer)

This technique seems adequate to hold the talus reduced in type I fractures that have major marginal fractures or in type III fractures in which compression of only the anterior or posterior pillars is present. Otherwise, this method is an unsatisfactory way of maintaining length.

Dual pins also have been used to control more completely the vectors influencing reduction.[13,19] This technique has been successful in experienced hands, but again shares essentially the same disadvantages as the other techniques with pins.

If reduction is satisfactory and the status of soft tissue is not a problem, dual pins may be incorporated in a cast at an early date and length maintained. The major disadvantages of dual pins are the difficulty in obtaining an anatomic reduction and the limited opportunity to introduce early motion. In addition, a calcaneal pin is sometimes incriminated in the subsequent loss of subtalar motion.

The logical extension of the dual-pin method is the use of an external fixation device, either ini-

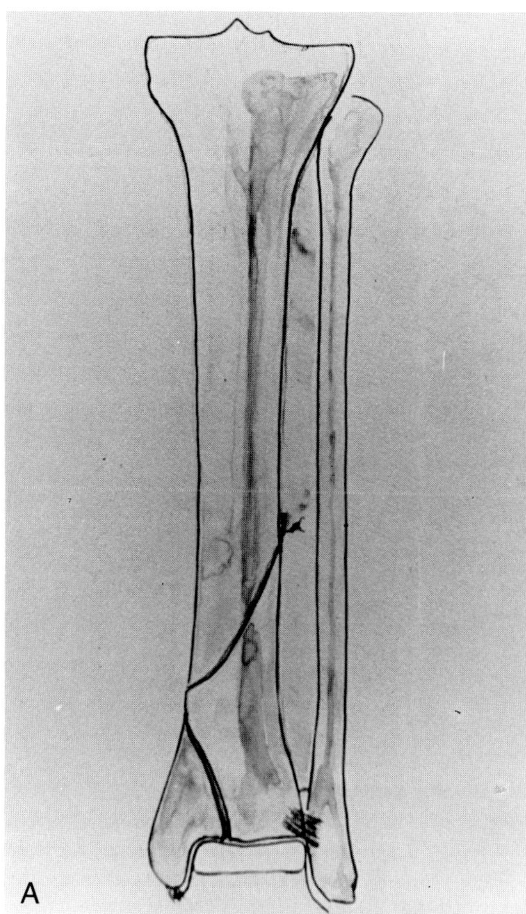

tially or later.[20] A description of the various frames and configurations is beyond the scope of this chapter. In certain situations, the technique certainly has advantages that may outweigh the disadvantages of the possible complications of pin-tract infections, joint immobilization, and poor patient acceptance.

Screws

Screw fixation and percutaneous pin fixation are advocated by Scheck[21] and Jahna and associates,[13] particularly when a key fragment is identified and can be stabilized. This technique is used as a limited open reduction and is applied in combination with dual-pin traction.

Screw fixation of the tibial articular surface is definitely applicable to type I fractures (see Fig. 23-3, *E* through *H*) and usually is associated with plate fixation of the fibula to restore length.[5,6] In this type of fracture, the plafond fragments usually are large and confined to the posterior surface. The corresponding opposite cortex is intact, and good interfragmentary compression can be obtained, which, in association with the reduced fracture anatomy, produces the desired stability. The advantages of direct vision afforded by a good surgical exposure and the ability to obtain an anatomic reduction are balanced by the opening of a closed fracture and an associated infection rate.

Early motion may be instituted with this fixa-

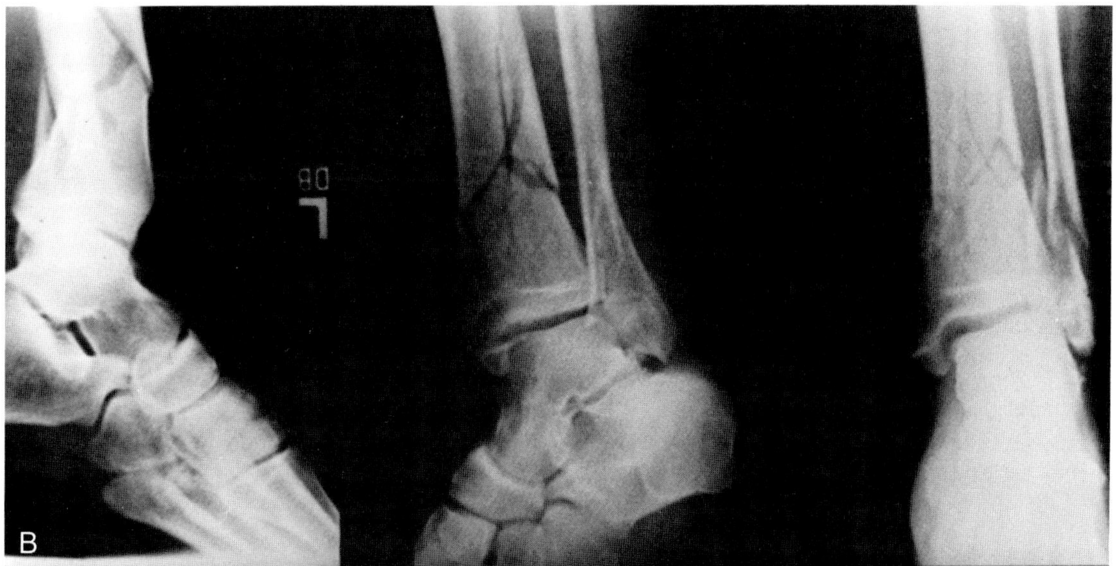

Fig. 23-6. *A*, Spiral extension type of complex ankle fracture. The spiral tibial fracture extends into the articular portion of the plafond (type II complex ankle fractures). *B*, A 54-year-old man fell off a bicycle and sustained a spiral extension fracture. Immediate open reduction and internal fixation with spoon plate and bone graft were performed.

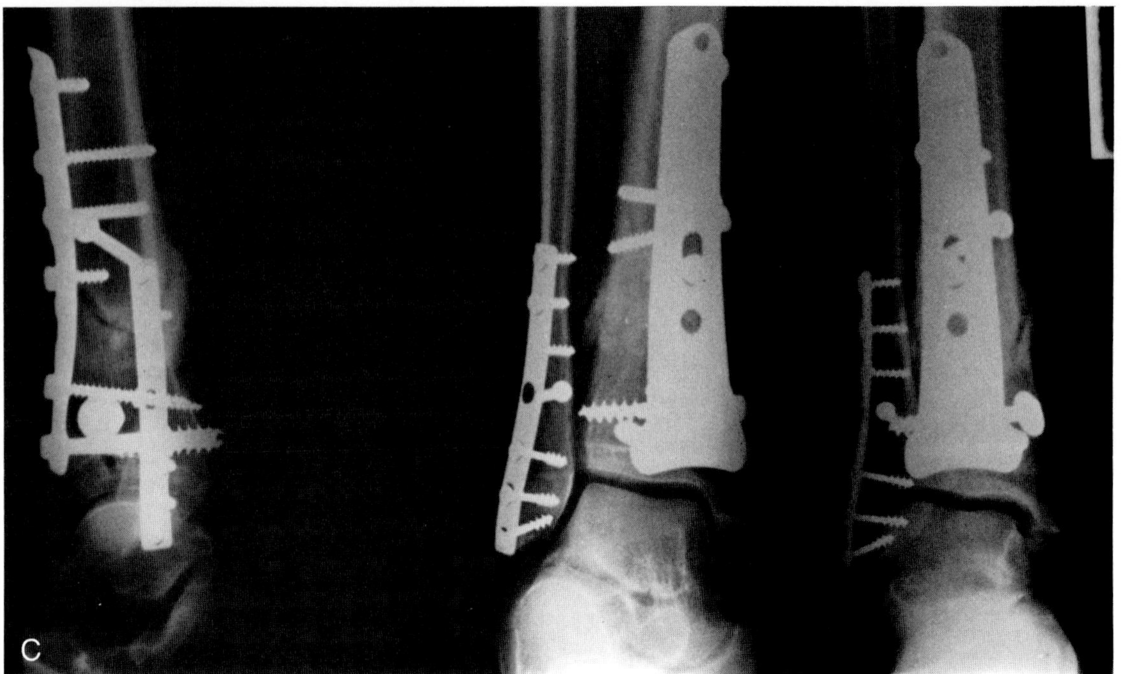

Fig. 23-6 (*continued*). *C*, Result at 5 months. The patient experienced full range of motion with no pain and was back at work as a cab driver.

tion. Screws may be designed as lag screws, in which case they must be selected with regard to proper thread length. The thread must not cross the fracture line. Standard screws also may be made to lag by proper overdrilling of the near cortex of the fracture so that the threads grasp only on the far cortex. Tightening of the screws causes the fracture fragments to compress against each other. Screw fixation alone has been shown to be precarious in types II and III fractures because a late axial deformity can occur.

Plates

Plates in combination with screws offer the most complete solution for types II and III, A, B, and C fractures. However, the sizes and shapes of plates that are used for this anatomic location are varied, and the surgeon must be familiar with the advantages and disadvantages of each plate. Thorough knowledge of normal osseous anatomy is crucial because the plates frequently must be altered by cutting or contoured by twisting and bending.

Plates Used Laterally

The one-third tubular plate is used most frequently for fixation of the fibular fracture. The longest one-third tubular plate available has 8 holes, and occasionally, a longer plate is needed in a badly comminuted fibular fracture. In this instance, two 8-hole plates can be overlapped at their terminal 2 holes, thereby increasing plate length to the equivalent of a 14-hole plate.

Leach[22] and Rouff and Snider[19] have reported that they have successfully treated patients with type III fractures with fixation of the fibula alone. Essentially, this approach represents the first principle of the ASIF/AO approach to the internal fixation of this fracture type.[6] The advantages of this method are obvious in that one need not deal with the more complex and time-consuming tibial part of the procedure, while still being able to restore the length of the comminuted distal tibia. However, this approach requires postoperative cast immobilization, thus sacrificing early motion. Additionally, an early or late varus deformity is a likely occurrence when the fibula is fixed at length without concomitant buttressing of the tibia. Also, this method seems to be at odds with Jahna and associates,[13] who favor the Böhler principle of allowing approximately ½ cm of shortening to occur to increase stability and to decrease the size of the metaphyseal defect.

Plates Used Medially

In the formula for the proper internal fixation of pilon fractures proposed by the ASIF/AO,[6] a medial buttress plate is needed to prevent anticipated late varus deformity. The plates available and ordinarily used for this purpose are the standard narrow 4.5-mm DC plate, the "T" plate, and the cloverleaf plate. Because the narrow DC plate is bulky, medial wound closure is sometimes compromised and postoperative complaints can occur as a result of the plate's location immediately beneath the skin.

The thinner "T" plate, originally designed for the medial tibial plateau, is useful in this location as well. However, when a low transverse fracture of the medial malleolus is present, the "T" plate, which demands a supramalleolar positioning, is awkward. Additionally, the "T" plate utilizes only 4.5- and 6.5-mm screws, which can make the "T" plate a bulky implant for the medial side of the distal tibia.

The cloverleaf plate has a shape suggested by its name. Its inferior flange adapts nicely to the medial malleolus, and in addition, the plate utilizes 3.5- or 4-mm screws. Frequently, one of the "leaf" extensions of the plate must be cut off to facilitate its optimal placement. Cutting the plate sometimes is a technical problem at the time of operation and should be anticipated by having a bolt or pin cutter available.

Plates Used Anteriorly

The spoon plate is exceptionally well suited for fractures of the anterior plafond or for fractures in which the posterior cortex of the distal tibia is not highly comminuted. Meticulous application of the plate to the anterior surface of the distal tibia is necessary to align the inferior contour of the plate with the plafond itself. Such alignment ensures a proper postoperative joint axis because the V-shaped contour of the plate rests accomodatingly on the progressing anterior crest of the distal tibia controlling varus/valgus angulation. The plate is well covered by the soft tissue on the anterior surface of the ankle and, although it uses standard screws, is well tolerated postoperatively.

Plate fixation in general implies a significant operative time because it is preceded by reduction and preliminary fixation with Kirschner wires. Bone grafting increases the time of the operative procedure, but is necessary in fracture types III, B and C. Again, preoperative planning is necessary to explore the possibility of a successful surgical intervention.

The possibility of infection, skin slough, and other musculoskeletal postoperative complications must be considered more likely as a procedure becomes longer and soft-tissue exposure becomes more extensive.

Other Instruments

Other helpful instruments are Hohman retractors of varying sizes, reliable power tools, and an external fixation device, femoral distractor, or articulating tension/distraction device. These devices may be invaluable in achieving successful surgical intervention with minimal devitalization of bone.

The femoral distractor or external fixation device is used to maintain length temporarily while definitive internal fixation is carried out.[23] The distractor or similar fixation device is used medially. Two pins are placed perpendicular to the anatomic axis and, therefore, parallel with the joint axis of the ankle, one in the proximal tibia and the other distal into the talus. Distraction is then carried out until length is regained (Fig. 23-7). Length usually can be judged by the reduction of contiguous fragments at one or more locations in the fracture zone. At this point, temporary fixation of the reconstructed articular surfaces is carried out with Kirschner wires, and roentgenograms should be obtained. The additional steps of fixation are no different from the basic steps outlined by Rüedi[17] and discussed later in this chapter.

This technique is particularly useful when the fibula is intact, or is so comminuted that it is useless as an aid in regaining length of the tibia. In patients in whom the fibula is fractured and can be used to regain length, external distraction usually is not needed.

The articulating tension device also is useful. With proper application of the plate to the distal fragment, in this case the reconstructed articular surface, this instrument may be used as a distraction device to gain the extra centimeter or so of length of the medial cortex of the tibia. This increased length is often advantageous as the comminuted metaphyseal area can be reduced indirectly without disrupting the blood supply to the comminuted fragments in that area. In addition, after the comminuted metaphyseal defect is grafted, the distal hook of the tension device may be turned into a compression mode for the frac-

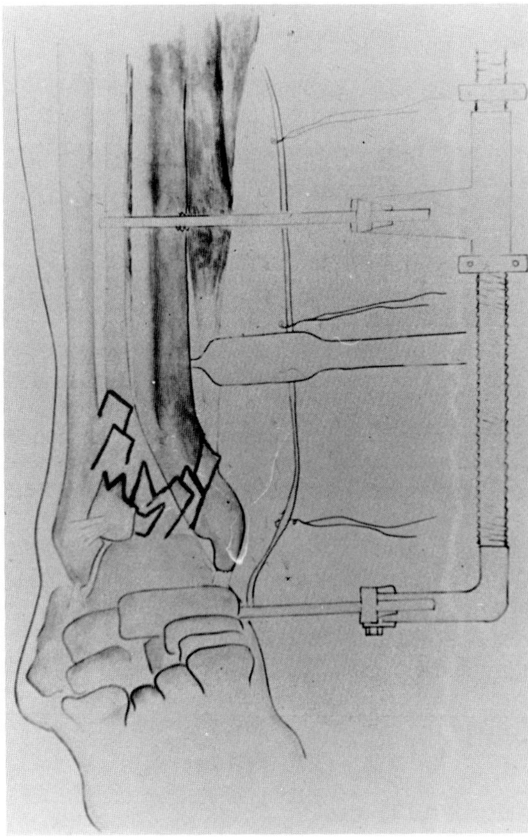

Fig. 23-7. The use of an ASIF/AO femoral distractor in the fixation of a comminuted type IIIC fracture. The intact fibula alerts the surgeon to the anticipated problem of regaining tibial length.

ture and a tensioner for the plate. A correct amount of plate tension compresses the cancellous graft and lends increased stability to the fixation (Fig. 23-8).

Preferred Treatment

Type I Fractures

Type I fractures are essentially malleolar fractures with large plafond fragments (see Fig. 23-3). These fragments are usually posterior. The posteroinferior tibiofibular ligament and the deep transverse ligament usually are attached to the fragments.

A fresh fracture is best operated on during the first 12 hours after injury, before swelling becomes a major problem. If the period of operative time available is limited for some reason, e.g., other major fractures or vital injuries, a closed reduction and cast can be used as a temporizing measure. Axial pin fixation, described earlier, may also be of value. The definitive surgery then may be carried out under more controlled circumstances after soft-tissue swelling has been resolved.

The operative treatment of the fracture consists of a posterior longitudinal approach to the fibula with fixation of the fibular fracture by a lag screw and neutralization plate.[6] Because of the ligamentous attachment of the posterior Volkmann's fragment, length usually is restored by open reduction and internal fixation of the fibula.[5] The tibia is approached by a long anteromedial incision from just anterior to the medial malleolus proximally and 1 cm lateral to the anterior crest

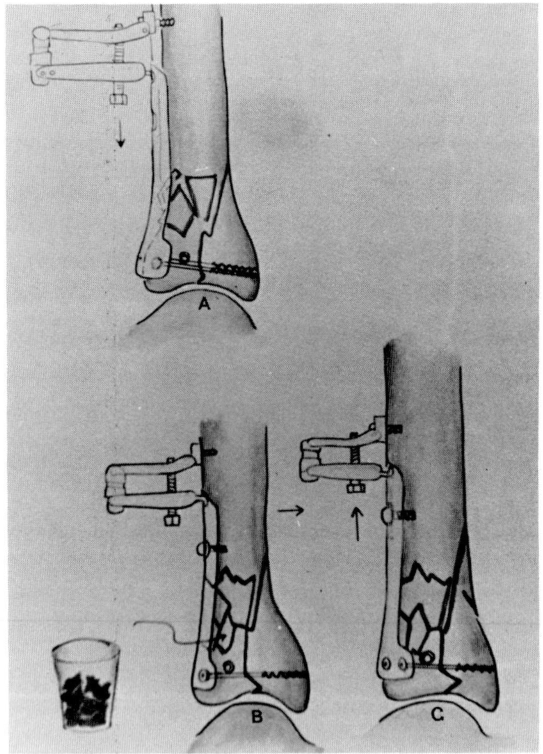

Fig. 23-8. The use of the ASIF/AO articulated tension device in a type IIIC fracture. *A*, The plate and tensioner are applied, and distraction is carried out. *B*, Bone graft is used to fill the residual metaphyseal defect while the tension device remains in place. *C*, The device then is applied into a compression mode, compressing the metaphyseal bone graft and placing the plate under tension, thereby stabilizing the fracture.

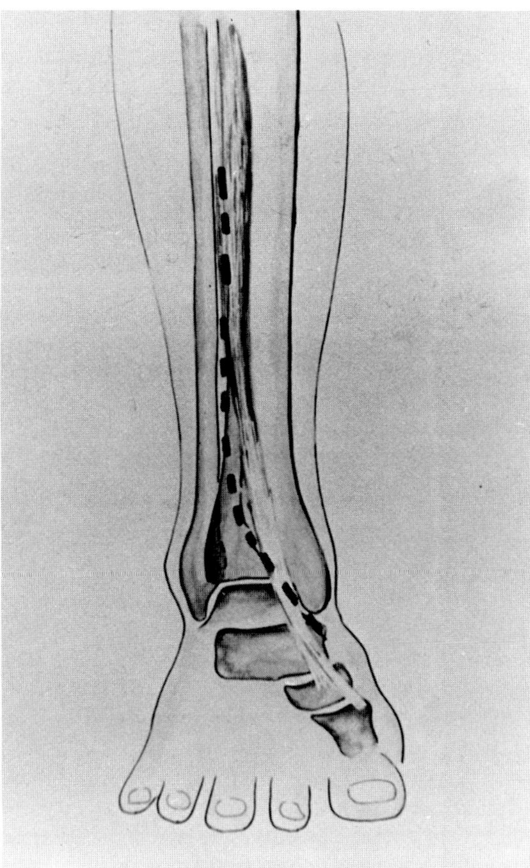

FIG. 23-9. Standard anteromedial approach as advocated by the ASIF/AO. This incision is useful in almost all fractures involving the distal tibial metaphysis.

of the tibia longitudinally (Fig. 23-9). If the medial malleolar and the posterior fragment are large (one third to one half of the articular surface), they can be viewed from this exposure by continuing the subperiosteal dissection around the posteromedial corner of the distal tibia. The fracture reduction then can be "fine tuned," and the posterior fragment can be fixed from anteriorly to posteriorly with appropriate lag screw(s). Next, the medial malleolar fragment is reduced and fixed by lag screws or tension-band fixation. The joint itself must be inspected for loose bodies, which should be removed prior to final reduction.

Type II Fractures

Type II fractures are spiral extension types of fractures (Fig. 23-6). The fracture extends distally from a spiral fracture of the tibia into the ankle joint.

An anterior incision from 1 cm lateral to the anterior tibial crest to the medial malleolus provides excellent exposure.[6] The principles of stable fixation must be observed carefully, and fracture fragments should be exposed delicately. Fixation of the shaft fractures after reduction usually precedes the reconstruction of the articular surfaces. These shaft fragments are stabilized by lag screws. The articular fragments may be temporarily reduced with Kirschner wires. An appropriate narrow DC plate then may be twisted and contoured to fit the medial aspect of the tibia and used to neutralize the comminuted area. Definitive screw fixation of the plafond fragments then may be carried out utilizing at least one or two screws through the plate.

Occasionally, the femoral distractor may be used to bridge the comminuted fracture area and to regain length, thereby greatly facilitating the reduction and preserving most of the soft-tissue attachments to the fragments in the area of comminution.

Type III Fractures

The principles of the operative treatment of this type of fracture are: (1) reduction and stable fixation of the fibula, (2) reconstruction of the tibial articular surface, (3) cancellous autograft of the metaphyseal defect, and (4) application of a medial buttress plate.[6,17,19,24,25]

The surgical approach is a straight posterolateral incision parallel to the posterior border of the fibula and an anteromedial incision extending from the leading edge of the medial malleolus and curving anteriorly and slightly lateral to extend proximally and longitudinally 1 cm lateral to the anterior crest of the tibia. The periosteum just medial to the tibialis anticus tendon is incised, and medial and lateral subperiosteal dissection is carried out. With this approach, one can reach laterally to the anterolateral tubercle of Chaput and posteromedially to the middle one third of the posterior tibia. The distance between the two incisions should be at least 7.5 cm to prevent skin slough.

Preoperative drawings should be made as described earlier. Critical dimensions may be noted on the drawing to localize the exact position of the plate and lag screws.

A bone graft usually is needed to fill in the metaphyseal defect, and proper consent for this part of the procedure should be obtained preoperatively.

The timing of surgery is important. Ideally, these fractures are best corrected as soon as possible after injury, before post-traumatic edema becomes a factor. Soft-tissue management must be meticulous as, even in the best of hands, some degree of skin slough can occur.

If the surgery is not done immediately in closed fractures, a waiting period of 7 to 10 days is necessary until the skin edema has been resolved. After debridement, open fractures are treated operatively like closed fractures; however, the skin incision is best left open and a delayed primary closure is performed at 3 to 5 days.

In a relatively small percentage of type III fractures, the fibula is not broken or may be too comminuted to allow stable fixation at length. This situation should alert the surgeon to possible problems.

When the fibula is fractured in such a way that it can be reduced and fixed stably, the problem of gaining length is largely overcome by initially proceeding with this step. When the fibula cannot be treated in this manner, the tibia must be approached as the first step. If the tibia is also highly comminuted, both in its anterior and posterior column, as in type III C fractures, screw fixation occasionally will be impossible. Such fractures become apparent when an attempt is made at preoperative drawing. When this fracture is recognized preoperatively, rigid internal fixation is doomed to failure. In these cases, stabilization is probably best approached indirectly by utilizing traction or an external fixation device. If the fracture is already open and has been thoroughly irrigated and debrided, a primary arthrodesis may be anticipated after cutting off the cartilaginous surfaces of the dome of the talus and the shattered tibial roof. Proper alignment then may be obtained with properly placed pins incorporated into a traction or fixation device (Fig. 23-10). When the fragments are large, as in fracture type III B, internal fixation should be possible. Again, the use of a distraction device, such as the femoral distractor or an external fixation device, may allow the surgeon more control while fitting the jigsaw puzzle back together (the condition of the fibula does not allow one to use it as an aid in regaining the length and proper axis of the tibia). This technique is valuable as a substitute for regaining "fibular length" while introducing axial stability so that comminuted fragments may be pieced together more easily.

The surgical technique we use is presented in detail in *The Manual of Internal Fixation*.[6] In the usual situation not complicated by the conditions previously described, the initial step in our procedure consists of plating the fibula. This step is followed by reduction of the fragmented articular surface by using the talus as the template for the distal tibial joint surface. Temporary fixation then is carried out using Kirschner wires.

Two possibilities exist at this point. If there is some metaphyseal comminution, the first alternative is to use a bone graft to fill the metaphyseal defect caused by impaction. In the next step, a plate, usually a "T" or cloverleaf, is contoured to fit the medial aspect of the distal tibia. The plate is attached proximally buttressing the reconstructed tibial pilon (Fig. 23-11). Occasionally, the fracture is better suited to the use of an anterior "spoon plate," particularly when there is an unfractured or minimally fractured posterior pilon (Fig. 23-12). Following plate application proximally, the definitive interfragmentary screws are placed and the Kirschner wires are removed.

An alternative is well advised in the presence of a larger metaphyseal defect. It is a technique used occasionally by R. Ganz and M.E. Mueller. After reconstruction of the articular surface with Kirschner wires, definitive lag-screw fixation of the joint surface is carried out. At this point, a small amount of cancellous autograft may have to be added to the central position of the epiphysis to support the subchondral fractures. The plate then is precontoured according to the usual turn of the medial distal tibia. The plate is applied distally and the articulated tension device is applied proximally to the edge of the plate. The hinged hook on the device then is reversed, and the plate and joint surface are distracted together to the proper amount. Cancellous bone graft then is impacted into the resulting defect. The tensioner then is reversed, and the cancellous graft is compressed by adding a careful amount of tension to the plate. This technique is particularly gratifying when an anterior spoon plate is used.

Suction drainage is placed before the skin is closed. Since one of the postoperative complications is skin slough along the anterior medial skin flap, it is wise in selected patients to close only the subcutaneous tissue over the hardware. After between 5 and 7 days have passed, treatment should continue with the performance of a delayed primary closure or of a skin graft of split thickness.

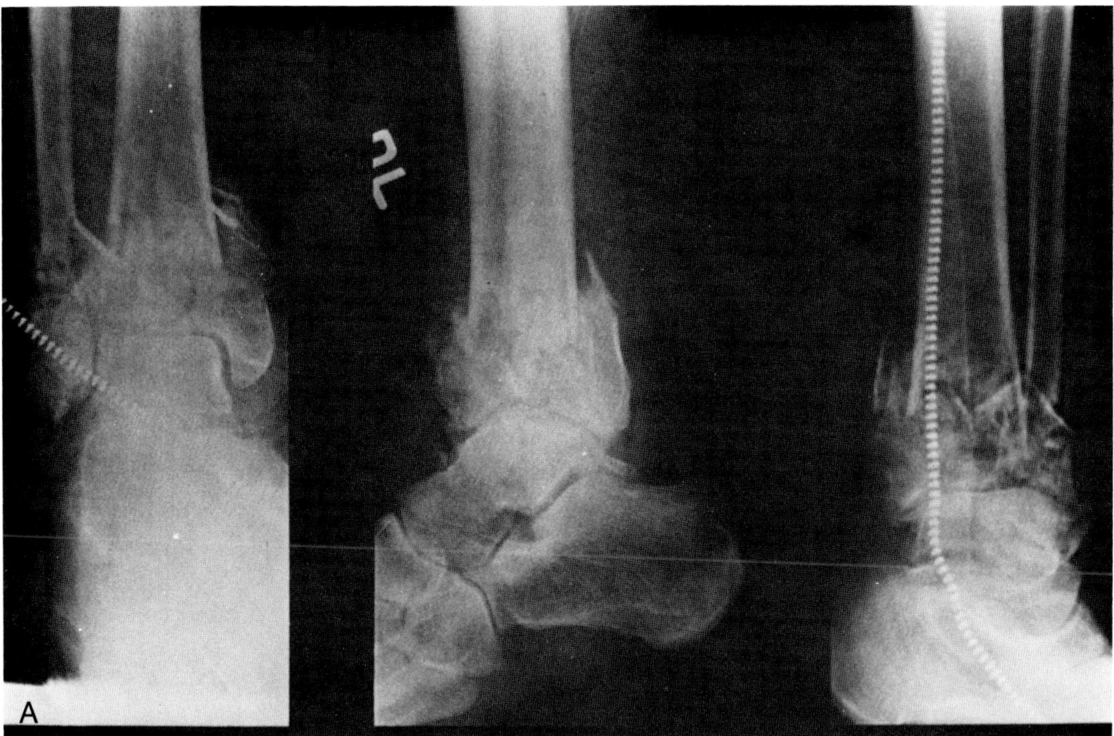

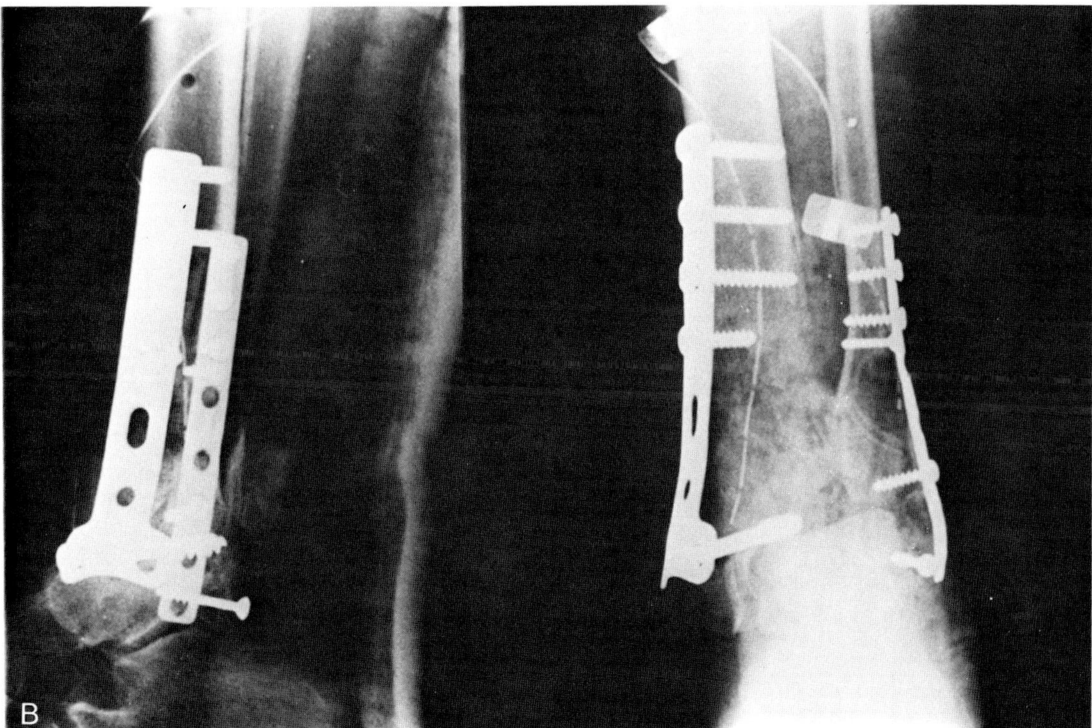

FIG. 23-10. *A*, A 55-year-old man MVA. Grade I open type IIIC fracture of distal tibia. *B*, Open reduction and internal fixation were attempted immediately. Preoperative drawings should have shown that internal fixation would have been unsatisfactory.

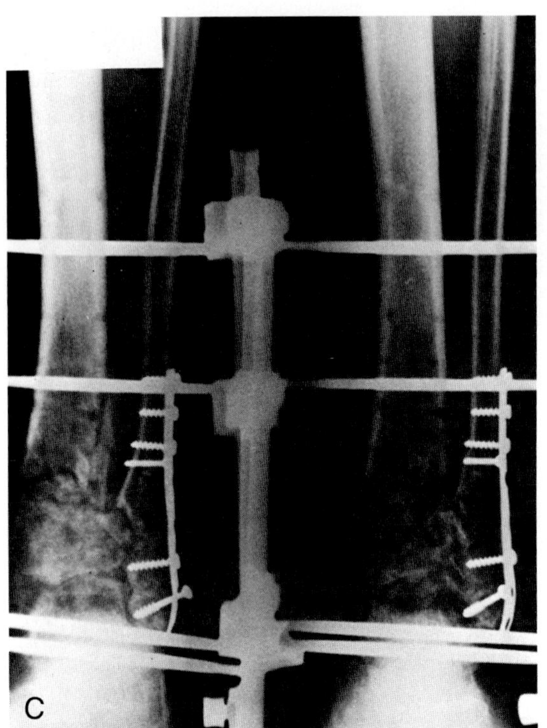

Postoperative Regimen

A well-planned and well-executed operative procedure best satisfies the requirements of optimal treatment of intra-articular fractures, i.e., anatomic reduction of the fracture and stable fixation to allow early motion. The extremity is placed in a U splint on the medial and lateral sides of the leg with the ankle at 90° or neutral allowing dorsiflexion postoperatively.

This splint is maintained for 10 days to 2 weeks, and nonweightbearing walking with crutches is allowed. The sutures then are removed, and the reliable patient is fitted with an elastic stocking and allowed 20 pounds of weightbearing with crutches. Casts are generally not used unless the patient cannot be trusted to follow instructions. At 6 to 12 weeks, guided by the radiographic evidence of fracture healing, the patient is allowed to begin full weightbearing without external support. Metal removal usually is deferred for 12 months.

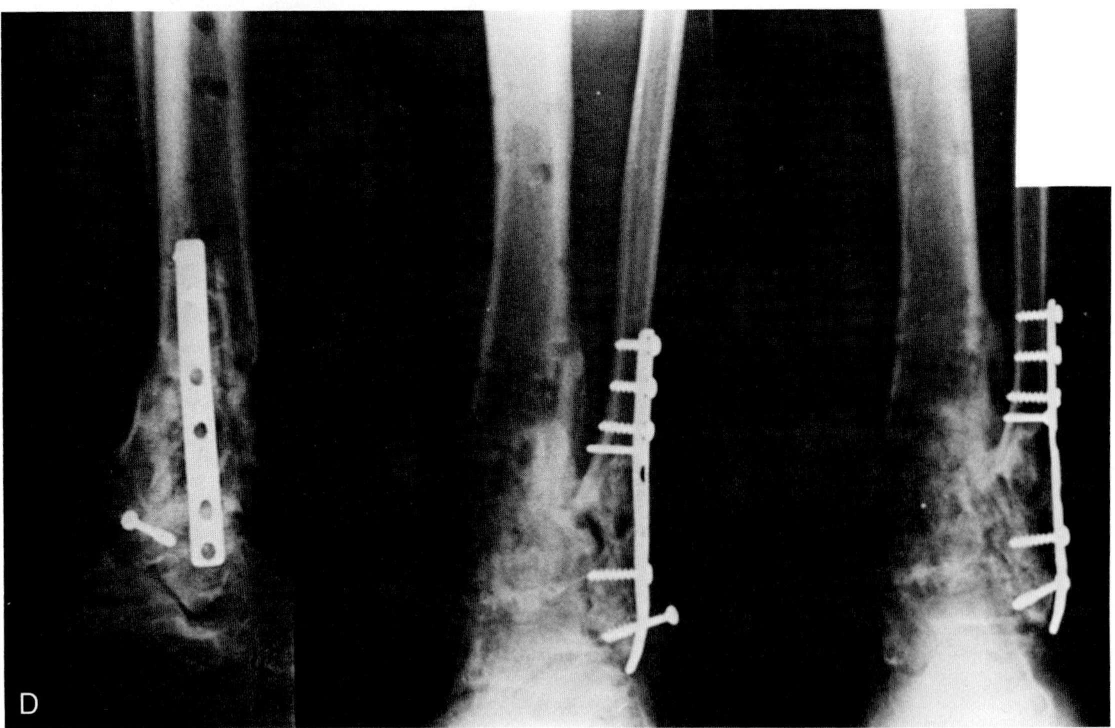

Fig. 23-10 (*continued*). *C*, At 12 hours after initial surgery, the patient was operated on again to remove the tibial plate, add additional bone graft, and resect the articular surfaces of the ankle. The foot was held in the desired position by an external fixation device. *D*, Follow-up at 6 months. Primary tibiotalar arthrodesis has been obtained. The patient walks with a limp that is lessening continually.

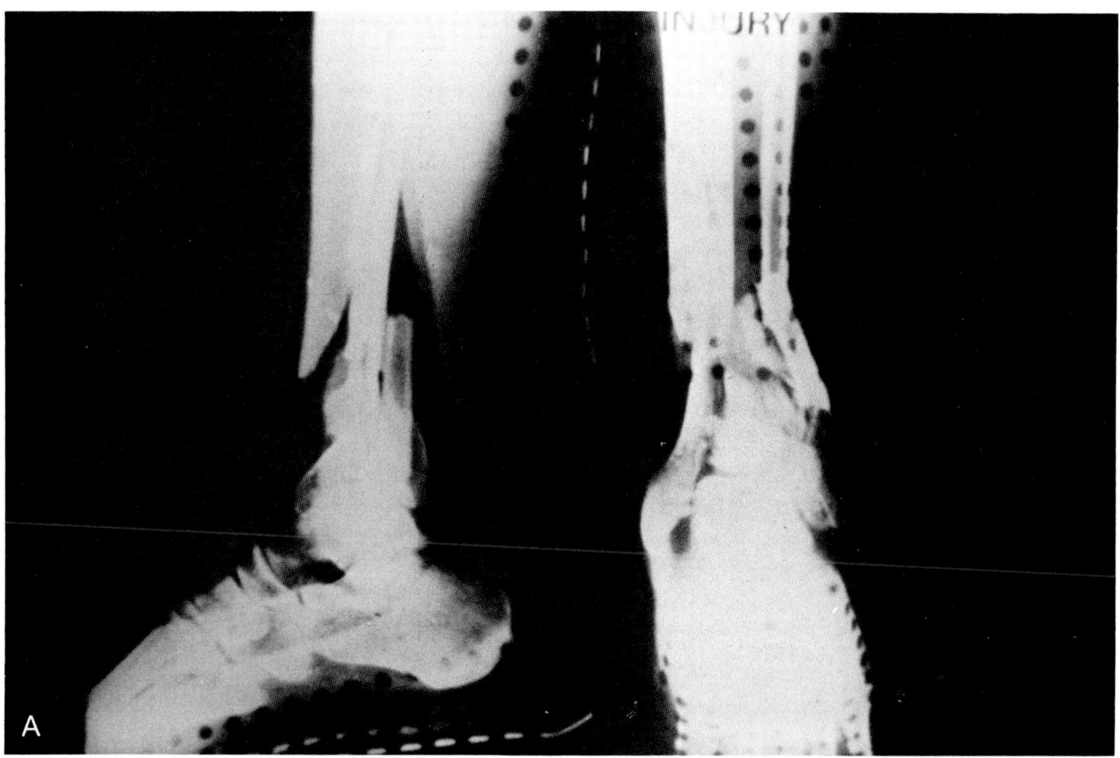

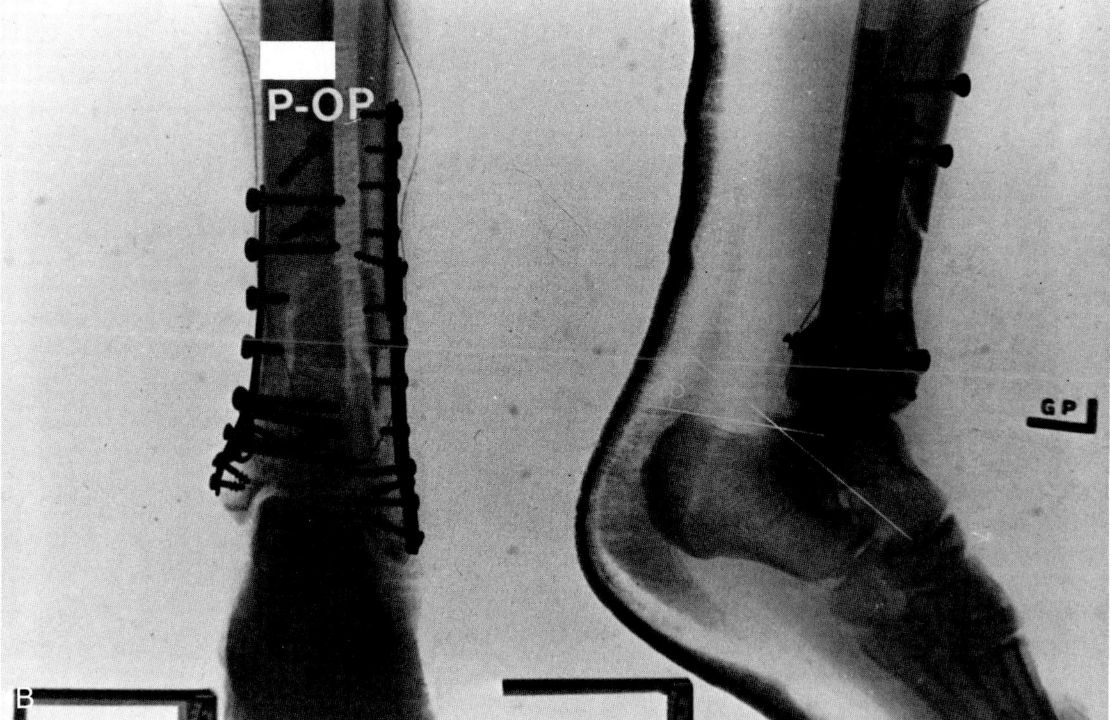

FIG. 23-11. *A*, A 42-year-old man, who was forced to jump off an 18-foot water tower, sustained a grade I open type IIIC fracture of the distal tibia. *B*, Postoperative films show use of cloverleaf plate on tibia and overlapped one-third tubular plates on fibula.

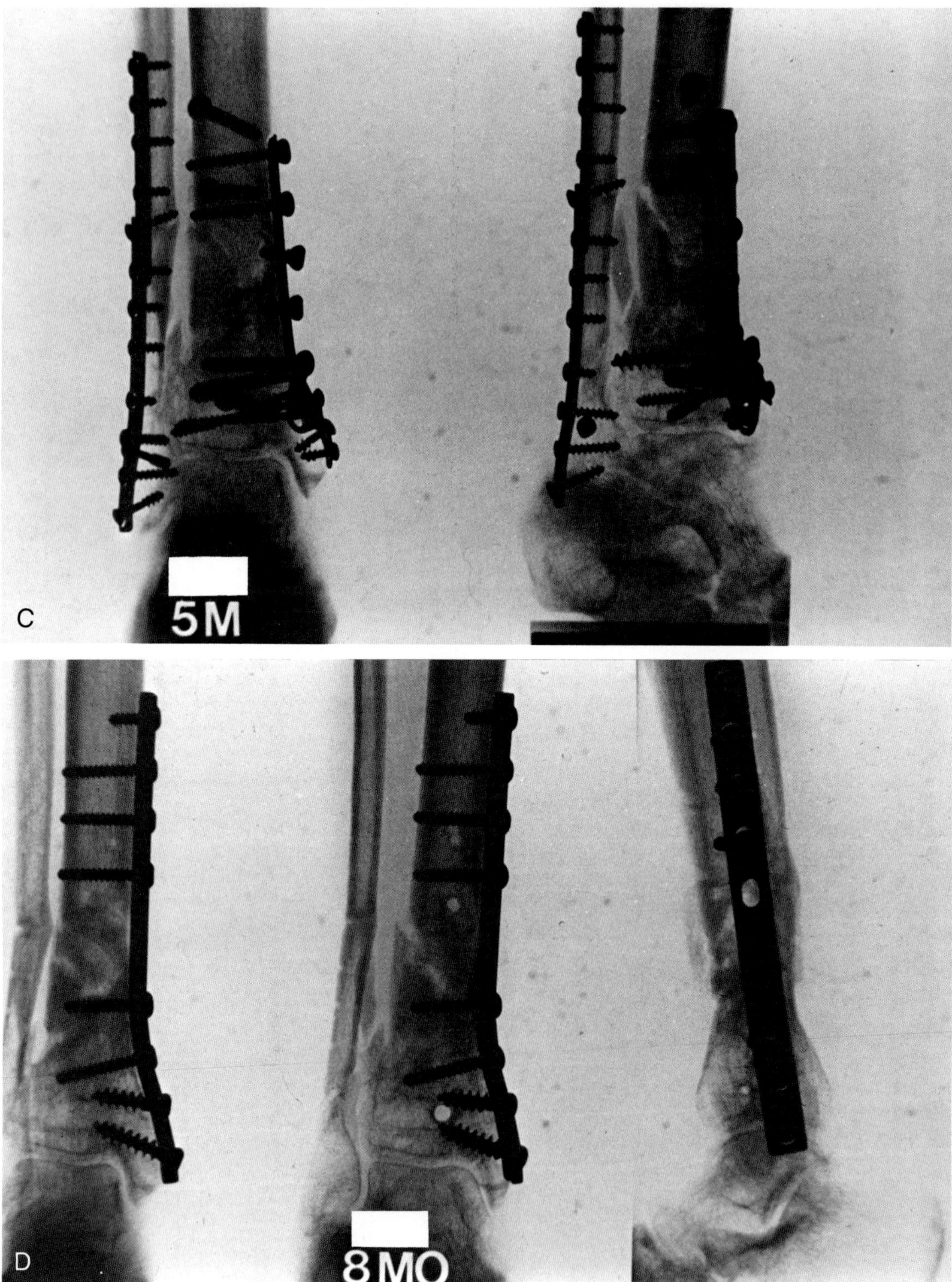

Fig. 23-11 (*continued*). *C*, At 5 months after injury, tibial nonunion is present, as evidenced by loosened screw (third from top of plate). *D*, At 8 months after injury, healing is present after repair of nonunion. The patient went back to his previous job at 1 year with full range of motion and no pain.

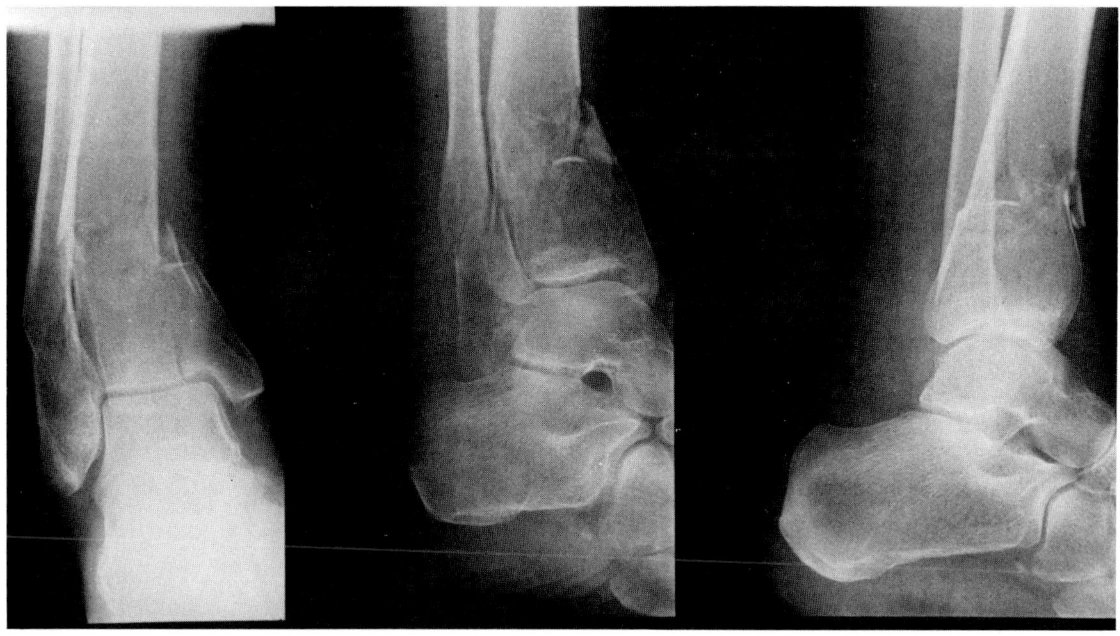

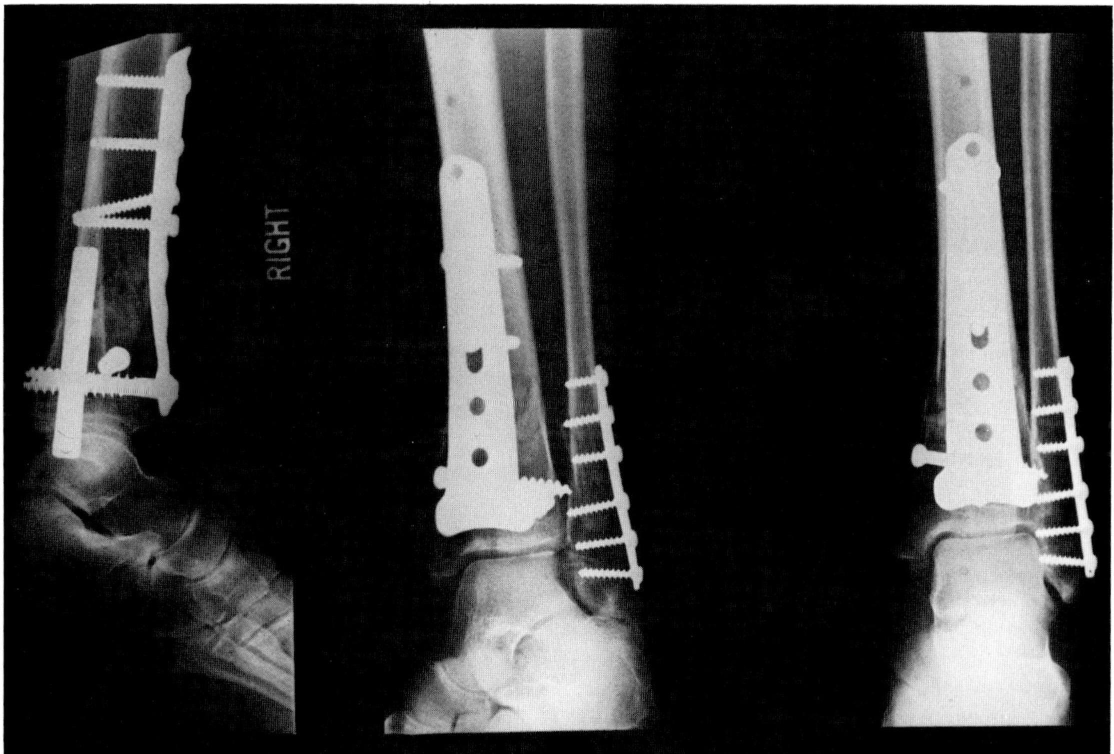

FIG. 23-12. *A*, A 36-year-old woman fell while jumping the wake during waterskiing. Type IIIA distal tibial fracture is evident. Immediate open reduction and internal fixation using anterior spoon plate and bone graft were performed. *B*, At 3-month follow-up, the patient showed full range of motion with no pain and returned to full activities, including sports.

In types III B and C fractures, or others that require bone graft to fill defects produced by impaction of cancellous bone, the same protocol is followed, except weightbearing is deferred for 12 weeks. During this time, however, active motion is encouraged.

Complications

Complications can be divided according to the time of their onset, i.e., intraoperative (technical) complications as well as early and late postoperative complications.

Intraoperative complications include screws entering the joint, malreduction in varus or valgus or inadequate reconstitution of the articular surface, failure to use a bone graft or medial buttress plate, and failure to achieve proper length of the fibula or tibia. These errors can be avoided by careful preoperative planning and by taking intraoperative roentgenograms and viewing them prior to any wound closure so that necessary changes can be made.

Common early complications are skin slough, especially of the anteromedial flap, superficial and deep wound infections, hematoma accumulation, and thrombophlebitis. Although these problems cannot be avoided completely, their incidence certainly can be reduced by meticulous surgical soft-tissue technique with the skin handled as little as possible. When necessary, retraction is obtained via small sutures in the subcutaneous tissue rather than by self-retaining retractors or "rakes." Hohman retractors can be used, but should be "relaxed" whenever the surgeon's attention is directed elsewhere. Judicious use of secondary skin closure when indicated prevents many sloughs. When primary closure can be accomplished without tension, only the skin itself is closed, preferably by the Allgoewer-Donati suture technique. Suction wound drains are always used.

Late postoperative complications include nonunion, malunion, and traumatic arthrosis. Because of the comminution seen in these fractures and the tenuous vascularity of the distal tibial metaphyseal area, a significant incidence of nonunion may be encountered even with the best technique. A second procedure necessary to treat the nonunion is often easier to perform than is the initial procedure since usually all but one fracture line will have consolidated (Fig. 23-11). Throughout this postoperative period, full motion should be encouraged; as a result, "fracture disease" will not be a problem.

Of paramount importance in preventing an increased rate of nonunion are the avoidance of any unnecessary stripping of soft tissue from the fracture fragments, the use of cancellous bone graft in all defects, and well-planned rigid internal fixation. By these means and those discussed earlier, malunions also can be avoided.

The problem of traumatic arthrosis is more enigmatic. As Rüedi and Allgoewer[10] have pointed out and Kellam and Waddell[23] have also shown, the initial degree of displacement and comminution of the fracture are not prognostic indicators as to whether arthrosis will develop, and thus primary arthrodesis rarely is indicated. Rather, the accuracy of anatomic reconstruction of the articular surface correlates with the incidence of arthrosis. A poor reconstruction heralds a poor late result. In addition, these authors also point out that the patients who eventually developed osteoarthritis had onset of their symptoms within 1 year following injury. The reason for this phenomenon is only speculative, but one could presume that it is related to the degree of initial articular damage to both the talus and the tibial roof on a gross and microscopic basis. In addition, Kellam and Waddell believe that avascular necrosis of some subchondral bone fragments leads to collapse of the mortise and rapid development of incongruity of the articular surface and resultant arthritic change.[23]

In any event, anatomic reconstruction with rigid internal fixation allows early motion, avoids most stiffness, and minimizes the incidence of arthrosis of the ankle joint. Rüedi and Allgoewer[11] have pointed out that a good result at 1 year tends to remain a good result and that the ankles in which anatomic reconstruction was achieved seemed to improve with time.

Results

The results of treatment of these disastrous injuries are varied depending on the form of treatment employed and the experience of the surgeons caring for the specific problems.

Best results have been obtained by Heim and Näser (90%),[24] Rüedi and Allgoewer (80%),[10,11] and Hackensbruch (80%),[26] all Swiss surgeons who utilize the approach of stable internal fixation.

In North America, experience with this approach is largely unpublished at present, although the results of a potpourri of operative tactics have been moderately successful.[12,21,22,27-29]

Some criticism of the Swiss results exists because of the high proportion of ski fractures represented in the reported series. This criticism seems valid when one considers the high-energy violence that produces this type of fracture in urban or industrial communities.

Since 1974, the Reno Orthopaedic Clinic has preferred operative reduction and internal fixation as treatment of fractures of the ankle. During the past 6 years, 37 patients have been treated, of which 25 had Type III B and C complex ankle fractures. Overall, we have obtained 78% good to excellent results with the methods of stable internal fixation discussed earlier. These patients have nearly a full range of motion, minimal, if any, pain and swelling, and are back to athletics or are working in the employment that they had pursued prior to their accidents.

Of this group, one patient developed infection and three patients had skin slough, one of whom required secondary skin grafting. Four patients have radiographic changes of arthrosis. Two subsequent arthrodeses and one total ankle arthroplasty have been performed. Additionally, one patient had a primary arthrodesis (Fig. 23-10).

Summary

Complex ankle fractures constitute a unique group of anatomically definable disruptions of the tibiotalar joint. The operative management of these injuries allows for the best results obtainable. From the timing and planning of the operation, through the procedure itself and onto the functional aftercare, the surgeon is the conductor of a carefully orchestrated biologic continuum. The success of the final result is in direct proportion to the wisdom, skill, and experience of this operator.

References

1. Ashurst, A. P. C., and Bromer, R. S.: Classification and mechanisms of fractures of leg bones involving the ankle. Arch. Surg., *4*:51, 1922.
2. Burwell, H. N., and Charnley, A. D.: The treatment of displaced fractures at the ankle by rigid internal fixation and early joint movement. J. Bone Joint Surg., *47*:634, 1965.
3. Dabezies, E., D'Ambrosia, R., and Shoji, H.: Classification and treatment of ankle fractures. Orthopedics, *1*: 365, 1978.
4. Lauge-Hansen, N.: Fractures of the ankle IV—clinical use of genetic roentgen diagnosis and genetic reduction. Arch. Surg., *64*:488, 1952.
5. Mast, J. W., and Teipner, W. A.: A reproducible approach to the internal fixation of adult ankle fractures: rationale, technique and early results. Orthop. Clin. North Am., *11*:661, 1980.
6. Mueller, M. E., Allgoewer, M., Schneider, R., and Willenegger, H.: Manual of Internal Fixation. 2nd Edition. Heidelberg, Springer Verlag, 1979.
7. Pankovich, A. M.: Adult ankle fractures. J. Cont. Med. Educat. Orthop., *3*:17, 1979.
8. Wilson, F. D.: Fractures and dislocations of the ankle. *In* Fractures. Vol. 2. Edited by Rockwood, C. A., Jr., and Green, D. D. Philadelphia, J. B. Lippincott, 1975.
9. Coonrad, R. W.: Fracture-dislocations of the ankle joint with impaction injury of the lateral weight bearing surface of the tibia. J. Bone Joint Surg., *52*:1337, 1970.
10. Rüedi, T., and Allgoewer, M.: The operative treatment of intra-articular fractures of the lower end of the tibia. CORR, *138*:105, 1979.
11. Rüedi, T., and Allgoewer, M.: Fractures of the lower end of the tibia into the ankle joint. Injury, *1*:92, 1969.
12. Maale, G., and Seligson, D.: Fractures through the weightbearing surface of the distal tibia. Orthopedics, *3*:517, 1980.
13. Jahna, H., Wittich, H., and Hartenstein, H.: Der Distale Stauchungsbruch Der Tibia (Supplement). Unfallheilkunde, *137*:1, 1980.
14. Rüedi, T.: Fractures of the lower end of the tibia into the ankle joint, results nine years after open reduction and internal fixation. Injury, *5*:130, 1973.
15. Lauge-Hansen, N.: Fractures of the ankle V pronation-dorsiflexion fracture. Arch. Surg., *67*:813, 1953.
16. Weber, B. G.: Die Verletzungen des Oberen Sprunggelenkes. Stuttgart, Verlag Hans Huber, 1972.
17. Rüedi, T., and Allgoewer, M.: Spätresultate nach operativer Behandling der Genlenkbruche am distalen Tibiaende. (SOG Pilon-Frakturen). Unfallheilkunde, *81*:319, 1978 (English abstract).

17a. Border, J.: Cardiopulmonary failure. *In* Basic Surgery. Edited by J. A. McCredie. New York, Macmillan, 1977.

18. Childress, H. M.: Vertical transarticular pin fixation for unstable ankle fractures. CORR, *120*:164, 1976.
19. Rouff, A. C., III, and Snider, R. K.: Explosion fracture of the distal tibia with major articular involvement. J. Trauma, *11*:866, 1971.
20. Brooker, A. F., and Edwards, C. C.. External fixation—the current state of the art. Baltimore, Williams & Wilkins, 1979.
21. Scheck, M.: Treatment of comminuted distal tibial fractures by combined dual pin fixation and limited open reduction. J. Bone Joint Surg., *47A*:1537, 1965.
22. Leach, R. E.: A means of stabilizing comminuted distal tibial fractures. J. Trauma, *4*:722, 1964.
23. Kellam, J. F., and Waddell, J. P.: Fractures of the distal tibial metaphysis with intra-articular extension—the distal tibial explosion fracture. J. Trauma, *19*:593, 1979.
24. Heim, V., and Näser, M.: Die Operative Behandlung Der Pilon Tibial-Fraktur. Technik Der Osteosynthese Und Der Resultate Bei 128 Patienten. Arch. Orthop. Unfallchirurg., *86*:341, 1976 (English abstract).
25. Heim, V., and Pfeiffer, K. M.: Small Fragment Set Manual. Heidelberg, Springer Verlag, 1974.

26. Hackensbruch, W.: Die Pilon—Fraktur des ski Fahrers. Fortschr. Med., *95*:219, 1977 (English abstract).
27. Nelson, M. C., and Jensen, N. K.: The treatment of trimalleolar fractures of the ankle. Surg. Gynecol. Obstet., *71*:509, 1940.
28. Pierce, R. O., Jr., and Heinrich, J. H.: Comminuted intra-articular fractures of the distal tibia. J. Trauma, *19*:828, 1979.
29. Wheelhouse, W. W., and Rosenthal, R. E.: Unstable ankle fractures: comparison of closed versus open treatment. South. Med. J., *73*:45, 1980.

Chapter 24 Complex Fractures of the Foot

SIGVARD T. HANSEN, JR.

The foot is the end organ of the lower extremity and is a highly specialized anatomic unit. When functioning normally, the foot adapts to numerous surfaces and types of footwear and to a tremendous variety of stresses and activities. To witness the ultimate potential of the human foot, one need only watch such events as an Olympic gymnastics competition or a track-and-field meet.

To appreciate the anatomy and biomechanical adaptations and principles involved in the workings of the foot, one should read the many works by Inman and co-workers.[1-3] The complex interaction of various bones, joints, ligaments, and muscles must be thoroughly understood before minor or major injuries can be dealt with properly. The complex gait mechanics wherein external and internal rotation of the leg during the stance phase first cushions weight acceptance and then stiffens the foot for toe-off are an example of sophisticated normal function of the foot. This function depends on a normal subtalar joint complex, including the talocalcaneal, talonavicular, and calcaneocuboid joints. These joints are vulnerable to a variety of injuries but are particularly susceptible to damage by fractures of the talus, os calcis, and navicular. A significant portion of the surfaces of the talus and navicular bones is devoted to articulation; therefore, fractures of these bones are commonly intra-articular and have the potential for post-traumatic arthritic change. The talus is also susceptible to avascular necrosis, which can result in much more severe damage to both subtalar and ankle joints.

Although motion between the joints is less important in the midfoot than in the subtalar and ankle joints, the position of the midfoot bones is important to the general shape and arch of the foot. Fractures in the cuneiforms and tarsometatarsal joints do not cause serious or disabling arthritic change because the joints simply can be fused. On the other hand, dislocation or misalignment must be well corrected, if for nothing more than to facilitate shoe fitting.

In the forefoot, any injury that disrupts the weightbearing balance across the metatarsal heads or that causes stiffness at the metatarsophalangeal joints is of functional significance. The metatarsals must be restored as closely as possible to normal length and inclination, and for normal gait, there must be at least 25 to 30° of free passive dorsiflexion at the metatarsophalangeal joints.

These considerations noted for each area of the foot are of great significance in choosing methods for treating complex fractures of the foot.

Diagnosis, Priorities, and Pitfalls

Diagnosis of complex foot fractures is not difficult because soft-tissue coverings are not thick and simple physical examination is quite revealing and accurate. Careful neurologic examination, both motor and sensory, is important, as is vascular assessment. Examination of function reveals tendon or muscle deficits, and passive stressing reveals instability from ligamentous injury. Films should be taken in at least the anteroposterior and lateral projections; if questions are unresolved, lateral oblique views of the foot and anteroposterior views of the heel should be added. As with the ankle, suspected sprains, particularly of Lisfranc's joint, should be evaluated with stress films. Open fractures, dislocations causing stress on soft tissues and vascular compromise, and fractures causing vascular disruption or compartmental syndromes demand immediate attention.

Diagnostic pitfalls include occult fractures that are undisplaced; these fractures are most commonly noted in the talus. Other confusing symptoms may be caused by partial nerve lesions, such as the partial tear of the sural nerve occasionally seen with inversion injuries. Partial vascular lesions that leave an intact but diminished blood supply may lead to unreasonable late expectations. For example, if a significant proportion of the vascular supply is lost at the time of injury, a foot may have enough vascularity to heal, but may not be able to tolerate cold weather.

Among the many possible treatment pitfalls are poorly planned incisions and excessive undermining or retraction of incisions, which leads to skin necrosis. When skin incisions are planned poorly, the creation of neuromas by the transection of various nerves may occasionally cause significant painful foci. Susceptible nerves include the sural nerve, the medial plantar calcaneal nerve, and the dorsal foot branches of the peroneal nerve.

Placing permanent, heavy suture knots in areas of thin soft-tissue coverage over bony prominences may cause painful suture granulomas or pressure areas. As in other areas of the body, sutures in the skin of the foot should never be placed too tightly. In areas of concave skin surface, such as behind the malleoli, one should use everting sutures to bring the live areas of skin together and prevent inversion of the heavy, dead skin surfaces, which cause delayed healing. The thick plantar skin, especially, should be carefully sutured so as not to cause inversion and delayed healing.

Soft-Tissue Problems and Considerations

The skin on the dorsum of the foot is thin and covers a rather superficial complex of veins, tendons, and nerves. These structures are vulnerable to crushing injury, misguided surgical approaches, and excessive retraction. In general, incisions should be made in line with the underlying structures, not transverse to them. A common exception is the lateral transverse sinus tarsi approach, but the incision is safe if one simply protects the tendons. The incision generally should go straight through the soft tissues, leaving subcutaneous tissue attached to the skin. Intermittent and gentle retraction should be done with sharp hooks. Forcible retraction, as well as the use of fixed retractors or blunt or crushing clamps, may cause skin necrosis. There is little extra laxity in the skin of the foot, and little skin is available for flaps if necrosis does occur.

The skin on the sole of the foot is highly specialized with thick fibrofatty subcutaneous tissue for tolerating weightbearing. Although this tissue must be preserved carefully, well-placed surgical incisions on the sole are well tolerated, contrary to prevailing opinion. In most patients, these incisions heal with an almost imperceptible and nontender scar. If there is an acute traumatic laceration of the sole, if the sole is contaminated, or if there are open fractures, the skin should not be sutured primarily. The wound should be well cleaned and the skin merely dressed closed. The sole heals safely and completely with this treatment. When the viability of skin flaps is in doubt after trauma, skin viability may be accurately assessed by the use of the fluorescein dye injection technique. For example, if the plantar skin of the heel has been avulsed, the use of this technique may show that the skin is nonvascular, and early amputation of the foot may be required, especially if there are other significant local injuries.

Finally, crushing fractures of the os calcis or midfoot may be associated with compartmental syndromes of the plantar region. If there is massive tight swelling, compartmental pressures should be monitored mechanically or at least carefully examined clinically by palpation and skin sensation. If surgical intervention is required, the sole can be decompressed by a long linear incision over the abductor hallucis muscle and by a blunt opening of the deeper layers with dissecting scissors. After decompression, the foot can be immobilized in a splint or padded cast for 5 to 7 days, and a delayed primary closure of the wound can be performed. Our experience indicates that this treatment preserves the plantar intrinsic muscles and specialized weightbearing tissues for later rehabilitation.

The foot may be affected severely by compartmental syndromes of the deep posterior or other compartments in the leg. These compartmental syndromes may occur in conjunction with blunt crushing injuries, tibial fractures, vascular injury proximal to the leg, and even fractures around the ankle, including the talus. The deep posterior compartmental syndrome, which is probably the most commonly missed, leaves the foot with stiffness in some variation of equinus, varus, and cavus, and with clawing of the toes. Associated contractures of structures in the sole of the foot may also be present. The deformity may be corrected by excising the tendons from the deep compartment at the ankle; frequently, the sole of the foot may also need to be explored and scarring contracted tissues excised or divided. Correction is difficult, however, and is unnecessary if compartmental syndromes are recognized and treated acutely and prophylactically.

Treatment Options: Indications and Contraindications

The primary goal of treatment of intra-articular fractures is anatomic restoration of the bone. Ideally, the fracture must be stable enough so that early motion also can be carried out. Fractures of the talus, calcaneus, and navicular ideally should be treated by stable internal fixation. Theoretically, the best treatment should be open anatomic reduction and lag-screw fixation, and the second best should be open or closed reduction and fixation by Kirschner wires. Although the second method offers a decreased risk, it is a less secure and less accurate method.

Treatment by closed reduction and casting is an acceptable method for fixation of some intra-articular fractures, but does not fulfill the ideal requirement for these fractures, which is stable anatomic fixation that allows early motion. There are obvious contraindications to open reduction and internal fixation, however; these include fractures that are too comminuted to be fixed successfully, and fractures in which the operator's skill and experience in internal fixation leave question as to whether the attempt may lead to more potential harm than clear improvement. Some physicians believe that open fractures are a contraindication to open reduction and internal fixation, but we believe the opposite is true. The need for stable internal fixation is increased with open fractures, especially if fixation can be done with lag screws alone. Stable internal fixation decreases edema and pain and helps to protect soft tissues, allowing them to ward off infection more successfully.

In summary, the primary indication for open reduction and internal fixation is a fracture in the hindfoot that can be stably fixed and anatomically restored. In practice, talus fractures most often are of this type, navicular fractures frequently are, and fractures of the os calcis occasionally are. Debate about the efficacy of internal fixation of calcaneal fractures continues, and some surgeons clearly have developed the skills to perform this internal fixation successfully,[4,5] particularly in the younger patient with normal bone. However, most physicians have better results in treating these fractures with closed reduction and brief immobilization, followed by early motion and prolonged protected weightbearing.

In navicular fractures that are quite comminuted, attempted anatomic restoration of the talar joint surface might be combined with primary fusion to the first cuneiform. Although the talonavicular joint is important for maintaining motion, the comminuted fracture may gain more benefit from this stabilization to the distal row. The relatively small size and lunar shape of the navicular make more pure intrinsic fixation difficult.

For fractures of the midtarsal bones and the tarsometatarsal joint area, the same treatment options are available: open reduction with lag-screw fixation, open or closed reduction with Kirschner wires or fixation with Steinmann's pins, and closed reduction and casting (Figs. 24-1 through 24-6). Here again, the open reductions are slightly more risky in terms of potential added injury and/or postoperative infection but offer the benefit of a more anatomically correct restoration. In these fractures, the aim of treatment is not so much joint preservation as it is overall preservation of the shape and alignment of the bones and proper distribution of load during weightbearing. This treatment approach may offer as beneficial an outcome as would treatment aimed specifically at joint preservation. In certain fractures, e.g., in badly dislocated Lisfranc's joint fractures or dislocations, one might frequently consider primary fusion at the first and second tarsometatarsal joint areas.

In the forefoot, intra-articular fractures and fractures of the metatarsal shaft have the most potential for causing disabling residuals. Treatment options for the metatarsals include open reduction with plate fixation, occasionally screw fixation alone in oblique fractures, and open or closed reduction with either crossed Kirschner wires or intramedullary Kirschner wires. If ade-

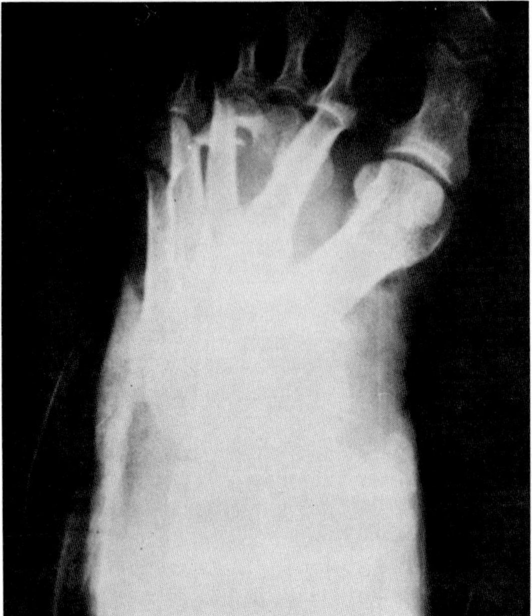

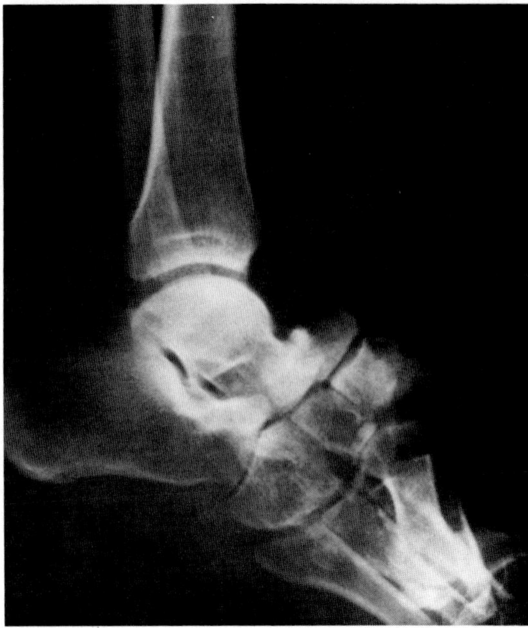

Fig. 24-1. *A* and *B*, Immediate postinjury films of the foot of a 50-year-old longshoreman who sustained a severe longitudinal compression injury when a hatchcover dropped on the back of his foot as he was kneeling on the deck of a ship. The patient had a grade II open injury over the midtarsal area, with rather marked comminution of the tarsonavicular and marked disruption of the midfoot as well as the metatarsal heads. He was taken immediately to the operating room, where initial cleansing of the open wounds and limited debridement were carried out, followed by internal fixation.

quate closed reduction is possible, closed reduction with cast immobilization is acceptable and frequently is quite successful. As always, closed reduction has a lower risk in terms of added injury, but the reduction is less accurate. One must remember that the tolerance for malunion in some patients is small in the forefoot. A 3- to 5-mm change in length may affect the weightbearing surfaces enough to produce painful keratoma formations under the adjacent metatarsal heads as these structures increase their share of the load. The reverse may also be true: a slightly plantarflexed metatarsal may be accompanied by excessive weightbearing and keratoma development.

Intra-articular fractures at the metatarsophalangeal joint should be treated as they are treated in the hand. Treatment options are similar to those previously described; open reduction and Kirschner-wire fixation are the most practical and effective methods.

My Preferred Method of Treatment

Talus Fractures

For treatment of fractures of the talus, all arguments fall on the side of stable anatomic fixation, which is best accomplished by open reduction and lag-screw compression fixation.[6] Anatomic fixation of the joint surfaces on all sides of the talus is necessary for normal joint motion in the future. Compression screws can provide adequately secure fixation to allow early motion and, occasionally, even partial or full weightbearing. In larger young adults with simple fractures, often one or two 6.5-mm cancellous screws can provide secure fixation. In smaller bones, the use of 4.5-mm lag screws may be more realistic, and occasionally malleolar screws may be used.

Because anatomic reduction of talar fractures is important, adequate exposure during reduction is mandatory. Medial and lateral linear incisions may be required for fractures in the head or neck of the talus. For more posterior neck or medial body fractures, the transmalleolar approach, as described by Deyerle and associates, may be used.[7] Lateral body fractures may be exposed best by the use of a slightly posterior Ollier type of skin-crease incision. For a frontal plane fracture through the midbody, the screw also might be inserted from the posterior direction through a posterior medial vertical incision or a posterior transverse incision. The fracture is best held in reduction by large "towel clip" bone-holding

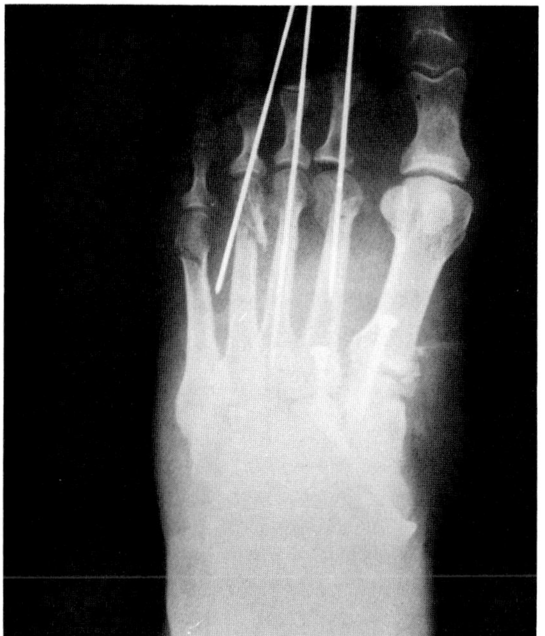

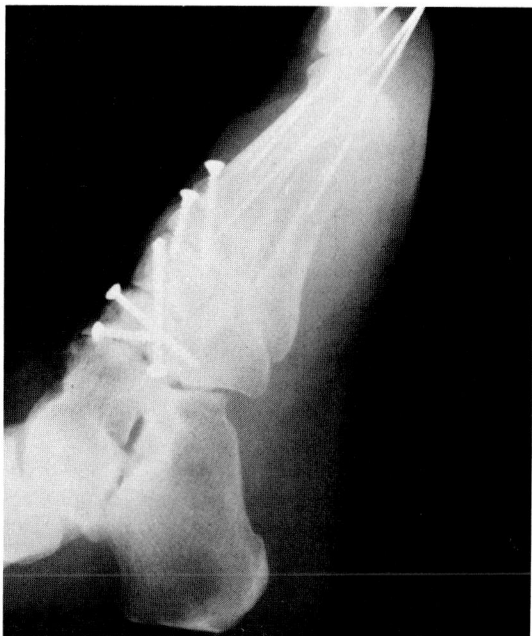

Fig. 24-2. *A* and *B*, Immediate postoperative films show internal fixation with screws in the tarsal area and with Kirschner wires in the metatarsal neck area. The three portions of the tarsonavicular were fixed with three different lag screws, one using the middle cuneiform to help to obtain purchase. The first and second tarsometatarsal joints were reduced under direct vision and fixed with screws; this fixation is our preference as the best method to hold these joints in an anatomically correct position. Goals of this method are to try to maintain the talonavicular joint as a workable joint, to maintain the length and inclination of the metatarsal shafts by stable fixation of the tarsometatarsal joints, and to gain stability in this region and in the metatarsal head and neck area to allow the even distribution of weight across the metatarsal heads.

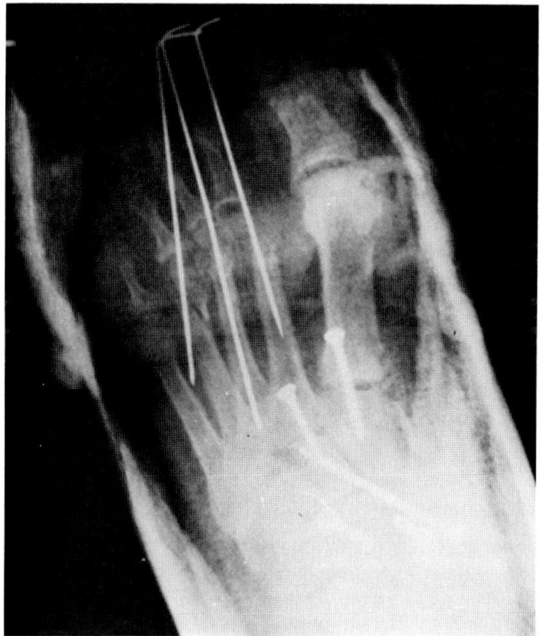

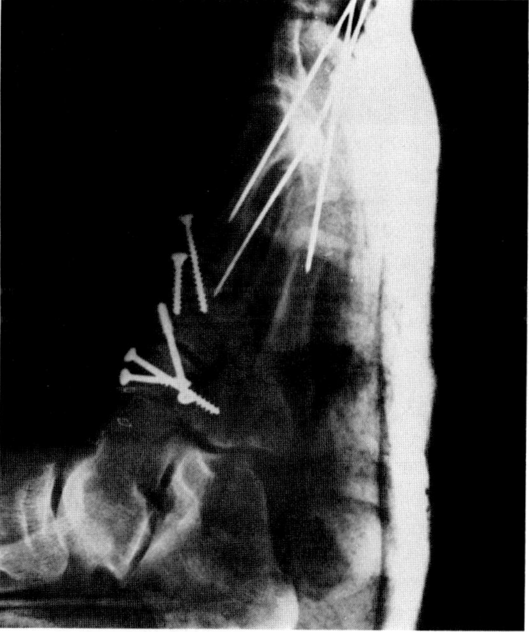

Fig. 24-3. *A* and *B*, Films taken 1 week postoperatively show the foot in a cast after the patient had delayed primary closure of open wounds on the dorsum of his foot. The fixation devices are shown in place. Reduction in the tarsal area is quite anatomic, and reasonable alignment of the metatarsal heads has been achieved.

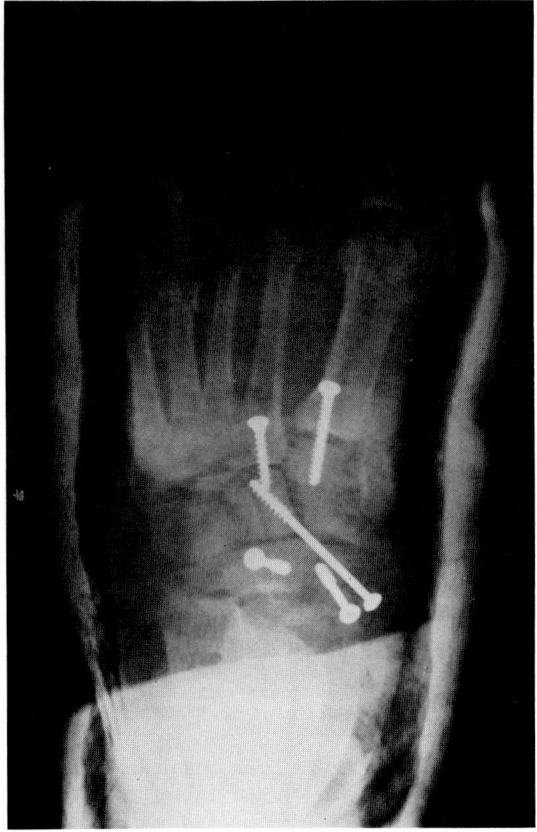

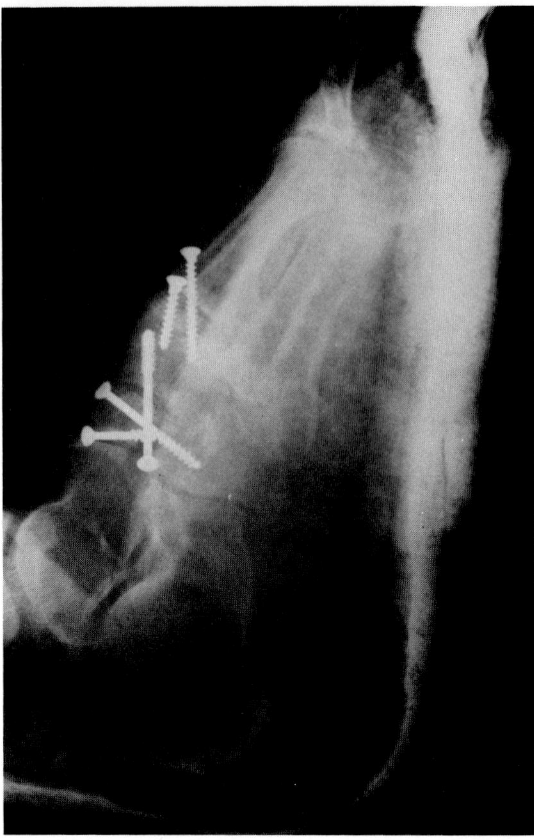

Fig. 24-4. *A* and *B*, Anteroposterior and lateral views, with the foot still in plaster, show removal of the intramedullary Kirschner wires in the metatarsals. We routinely perform this removal at 4 to 6 weeks postoperatively because the wires tend to penetrate the skin and, to some degree, violate the metatarsophalangeal joints. At this point, we take the Kirschner wires out and try to mobilize gently the metatarsophalangeal joints. The tarsal fixation remains in place until the patient is ready to bear full weight without a cast, which may be 4 to 6 months in this case.

forceps, which are kind to soft tissues. The screws are placed perpendicular to the fracture line after appropriate drilling and tapping and careful measuring so that no threads cross the fracture line and good compression is obtained. The probable final benefit of this treatment is the maintenance of existing vascularization and enhanced revascularization, which reduce significant avascular necrosis.[7] For whatever theoretic reasons, we have seen a low incidence of avascular necrosis in the talus since we initiated this approach to talar fractures more than 5 years ago.

Postoperatively, we use a short-leg cast with elevation for about a week, then gradually allow the patient to proceed to touch-down weightbearing for 2½ to 3 weeks. The leg then is fitted with a snug supportive cast, and the patient is started on progressive weightbearing, depending on the security of the fixation and the presence of other injuries. At about 8 weeks, full weightbearing in a short-leg walking cast usually is tolerated. Depending on our findings on the films, the cast usually can be removed at 12 to 16 weeks.

Os Calcis Fractures

Os calcis fractures often show a prime contraindication to open reduction and internal fixation; that is, there is marked comminution and, thus, little chance that operation will anatomically restore the joint surface and provide enough stability to permit early motion. Therefore, the risks of open reduction and internal fixation would not be justified in these fractures, as the exposures are difficult and wound healing is frequently slow or imperfect. Palmer,[8] LeTournel,[4] McReynolds,[5] and others, however, point out that hesitancy in treating these fractures operatively comes from failure to understand the fractures and that operative restoration produces an improved result.

In an open os calcis fracture that can be improved by internal fixation, we would certainly use compression screws or perhaps Kirschner wires. In nonarticular fractures—or even articular fractures with only two to four major fragments and good bone character—that look as if they could be anatomically and stably fixed, or at least significantly improved, we might also use compression screws. Although we occasionally utilize the technique of packing markedly displaced joint surfaces back into place with iliac bone graft, we are not yet facile enough with that technique to discuss it well.[8] For most closed, comminuted intra-articular fractures without gross misalignment, our treatment is closed reduction or reduction with temporary pins for leverage. We then elevate the leg for several days. We have the patient move the foot for another week, being especially gentle in the subtalar joint motions. The leg then is placed in a short-leg walking cast in a slightly equinus position, and touch-down weightbearing is initiated for an additional 4 to 6 weeks. After this time, the ankle is casted in a more neutral position, and walking is increased to full weightbearing for 4 to 6 more weeks. The leg then is taken out of the cast and put into a Jobst stocking and shoe with a slight heel elevation; the patient is progressed gradually to weightbearing with constant activity to allow joint motion to be regained. We expect that optimum recovery may require 18 months or more. For fractures requiring operation, our postoperative management is essentially the same, although with good bone and adequate fixation, weightbearing can be accelerated significantly.

Navicular Fractures

Our protocol for navicular fractures is similar to that for talus fractures. Some of these navicular fractures are completed stress fractures, which usually occur in the sagittal plane near the midline and are minimally displaced. In such cases, we make a linear incision lateral to the navicular

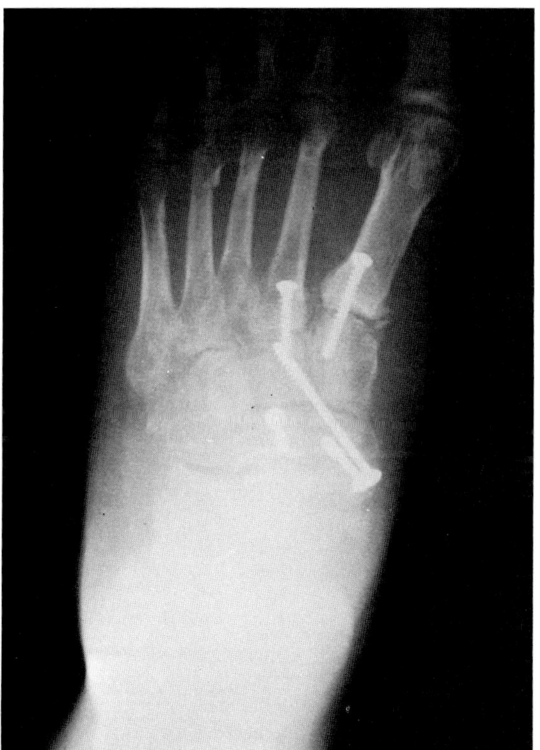

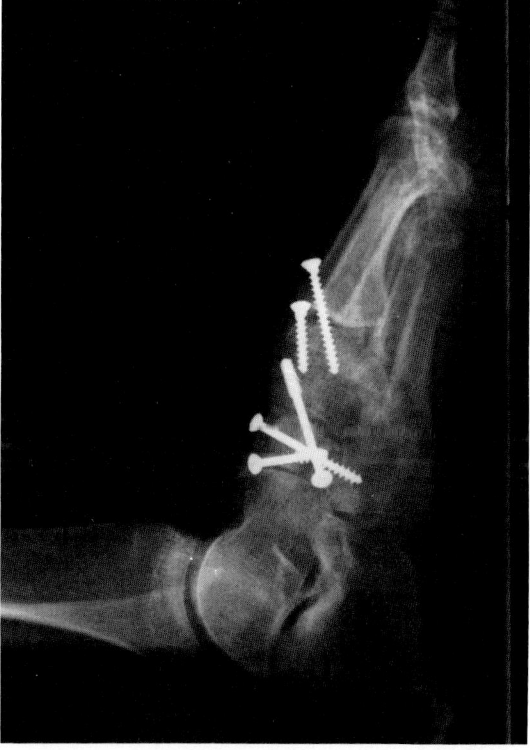

Fig. 24-5. *A* and *B*, Anteroposterior and lateral views 3 months after operation. The patient now is free of the cast and has begun mobilization (limited to touch-down weightbearing with crutches). One small, soft-tissue wound on the dorsum of the foot is healing slowly, but does not seem to communicate with bone or other significant tissues; its slow healing most likely is related to vascular damage.

and strip little soft tissue so as not to damage the blood supply. A stab wound is made over the medial tubercle, and a large "towel clip" forceps is used to reduce and fix the fracture. Two or more 4-mm cancellous lag screws are placed perpendicular to the fracture line; an image intensifier is used for control if necessary. If the fracture is indeed a stress fracture, we use a small drill to further drill across the fracture line, thereby enhancing the blood supply.

In traumatic fractures, apparently often caused by violent compression, there is usually mild to moderate comminution and some dorsal extrusion of the fragments. We approach these fractures through a dorsal medial incision, protecting the anterior tibial tendon but exposing the navicular, the head of the talus, and the talonavicular joint. The incision also is extended distally to isolate the navicular cuneiform joint and the first cuneiform. We then attach a small distracting device, such as a Roger Anderson distractor. This device spans from the medial malleolus to the base of the first metatarsal, and the area is distracted gently until the navicular is reduced by ligamentotaxis. Then, if possible, we fix the navicular to itself with lag screws placed perpendicular to the fracture line or lines. If necessary, we curette the naviculocuneiform joint cartilage sharply and carefully and extend screws across to the first and second cuneiforms. Extending the screws to these bones gives better stability to the fixation and creates a primary fusion to the first cuneiform; all attempts are made, however, to preserve a good talonavicular joint surface. This method also may help to maintain the blood supply and to avoid avascular necrosis, which seems to occur (at least partially) in displaced fractures of the navicular as well as of the talus.

If the talonavicular joint becomes markedly arthritic and/or painful in spite of the fusion to the first cuneiform, a triple arthrodesis is necessary, but salvaging and spacing by repairing the navicular and saving its bone stock produces a better ultimate result.

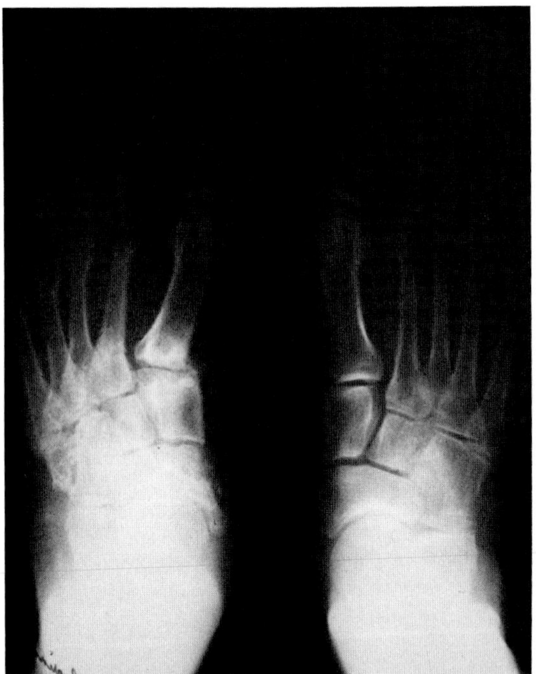

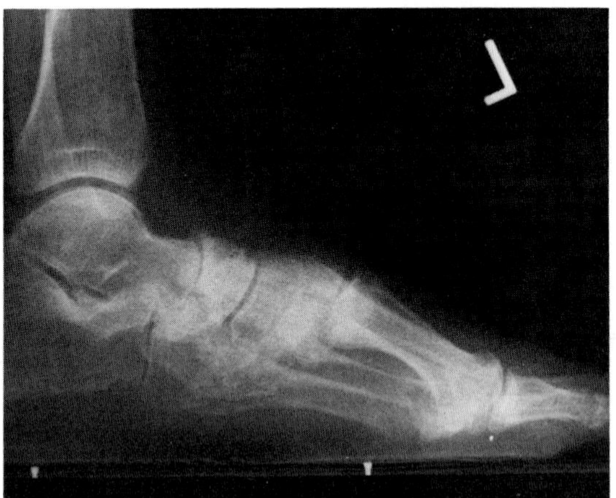

Fig. 24-6. *A* and *B*, Anteroposterior views taken 2 years after injury show a comparison with the opposite foot. A standing lateral view also is shown. The overall shape of the affected foot is similar to that of the normal foot, and mineralization through the forefoot is similar. Of course, there is sclerosis in the midfoot of the affected limb. The lateral film reveals that the first tarsometatarsal joint is not at its ideal position; there is also some secondary arthritis in the talonavicular joint. The overall shape of the foot, however, is quite serviceable, as shown by the fact that the patient is back at work, although restricted from his original heavy work as a longshoreman. He walks with only a trace of a limp and wears standard shoes on both feet. Although fusion at the talonavicular joint and possibly the first tarsometatarsal joint may eventually become necessary, the overall shape and function of the foot are excellent considering the severity of the initial crushing injury.

The postoperative course for navicular fractures is similar to that for other foot fractures; nonweightbearing is maintained for perhaps a little longer, and then, weightbearing is resumed gradually according to roentgenographic signs of union and the amount of stability gained through the original fixation.

Tarsometatarsal (Fracture) Dislocation

For this potentially disabling and deforming injury, we have changed from our previous protocol of closed reduction and occasional open reduction with percutaneous Kirschner wires or fixation with Steinmann's pins to open anatomic reduction and transfixion of the joints with countersunk compression screws. The entry point for these screws is 1.5 to 2 cm distal to the joint in the metaphyseal portion of the first and second metatarsals through a small triangular divot made in the bone with either a rongeur or a small oscillating saw. The screw is aimed from this point across the center of the appropriate tarsometatarsal joint after the fracture has been carefully and anatomically reduced. Although we generally use malleolar screws, we occasionally use a 6.5-mm lag screw in the first tarsometatarsal joint in a larger bone; occasionally we use a 4.0-mm lag screw in the second tarsometatarsal joint or in smaller bones.

Unstable fractures of the more lateral joints also might be treated with screw fixation, although one might use percutaneous Kirschner wires in these fractures. If screws are used, a single linear incision between the third and fourth metatarsals may allow fixation of both of these bones. This incision is similar to the single linear incision made between the first and second tarsometatarsal joints to repair these joints. In cases of gross instability without fracture, immediate fusion of the tarsometatarsal joints may be advisable, at least at the first and second metatarsal level; again, fixation would be done by compression screws. This anatomic fixation seems to prevent late complications of instability, swelling, deformity, and disability. Healing is more secure when the bone is fractured, and less protection is needed in fractures than in pure dislocations. Although 5 years of follow-up in our patients have shown good results, late degeneration of the joints may yet prove to be a problem.

Postoperative care of tarsometatarsal fractures and dislocations requires 3 to 5 days of elevation and then only touch-down weightbearing with the leg in a padded cast for 2 to 6 weeks. After the first 6 weeks, if the screws have provided good stability, we allow the patient to progress to full weightbearing over a total of 10 to 12 weeks with the leg in a cast—guided by our findings on film. The cast then is removed, and a supportive shoe with an orthotic device is worn for at least 6 months. Return to function is graded from walking to gentle running, occasionally to heel-toe figure-eight running, and then to sporting activity if the patient desires.

Hardware generally is removed at about 3 months, or before unrestricted activity is allowed. A screw must be removed where it crosses an unfused joint; when not removed, the screw soon breaks when the patient resumes activity.

Metatarsal Shaft Fractures

In metatarsal shaft fractures, we settle only for essentially anatomic reduction so as to maintain normal distribution of load among the metatarsal heads during weightbearing. If possible, we treat the fracture with closed reduction and casting, but we use intrafragmental screws, one-third tubular plates and screws, or large intramedullary Kirschner wires as needed. Especially in open or complex fractures, we use rigid intrafragmental screw fixation or screw and plate fixation. For fractures of the first metatarsal, we commonly use either screws and a plate or screws alone.

For open wounds in the foot, we always delay closure for 5 days after initial rigid anatomic fixation of the fracture has been achieved. Postoperative care for metatarsal shaft fractures is similar to that for other fractures of the foot, but these fractures may heal more quickly. If intramedullary wires have been used, we remove them at 4 to 6 weeks to minimize damage to the metatarsophalangeal joint.

Intra-articular Fractures of the Metatarsophalangeal Joints

These fractures are fixed anatomically with Kirschner wires if possible, and the lower leg is immobilized in a cast for about 6 weeks. After this time, the Kirschner wires are removed and motion is begun.

Complications

Wound-edge necrosis occasionally occurs for a variety of reasons ranging from severe initial injury to excessive retraction during reduction. Fracture of hardware is common, especially if 4.0-mm cancellous screws inserted across joints, as in tarsometatarsal joint fixation, are left in place. Because these screws break when the patient resumes activity, the solution is either to remove them before full activity is resumed or to use a larger screw. Malleolar screws, for example, may be less susceptible to breakage. The broken screws cause slight pain, but only the available broken part with the head needs to be removed and the symptoms resolve in virtually all cases.

Results

Our results in treating these varieties of foot fractures in the manner described have been gratifying. Infection related to internal fixation is not an apparent problem, as we have seen a low incidence of infection. A careful study of 42 open ankle fractures that we treated with immediate internal fixation and delayed primary closure revealed no permanent infections and no deep infections at any time.[9] We believe that rigid stabilization routinely reduces pain and edema, causes earlier healing of skin and other soft tissues, and protects the bone and soft tissues from infection rather than predisposing them to infection. In general, bone healing has been excellent, as has overall functional restoration of the foot, whenever good anatomic restoration of bones and/or joints has been achieved and early motion begun. In almost all cases, except in the os calcis, adequate reduction and stabilization have been achieved. Although early motion is desirable with intra-articular fractures, the most common mistake made in treating many foot problems is premature removal of the foot from the cast. We feel that anatomic restoration of the bone is the most important objective of treatment and that early motion is the second most important objective. In fractures that have been internally fixed, we try to be sure that union has occurred before we begin the patient on aggressive motion or weightbearing. In intra-articular fractures treated by motion without stable internal fixation, motion is initiated much earlier (e.g., at 1–2 weeks).

In summary, one must bear in mind that the foot is the functional end organ of the lower extremity. For this reason, if full rehabilitation is to be obtained in the multiply injured patient, fractures of the foot must not be regarded as a low priority but must be treated as aggressively and as accurately as are all other fractures in the lower extremity and with equal expertise.

References

1. Inman, V. T.: The Joints of the Ankle. Baltimore, Williams & Wilkins, 1976.
2. Inman, V. T., and Mann, R. A.: Biomechanics of the foot and ankle. *In* DuVries' Surgery of the Foot. 4th Edition. Edited by R. A. Mann. St. Louis, C. V. Mosby, 1978.
3. Inman, V. T., Ralston, H. J., and Todd, F.: Human Walking. Baltimore, Williams & Wilkins, 1981.
4. LeTournel, E.: Personal communication, 1982.
5. McReynolds, I. S.: The case for operative treatment of fractures of the os calcis. *In* Controversies in Orthopaedic Surgery. Edited by R. E. Leach, F. T. Hoaglund, and E. J. Riseborough. Philadelphia, W. B. Saunders, 1982.
6. Peterson, L.: Fracture of the neck of the talus. A clinical study. Acta Orthop. Scand., *48*:696, 1977.
7. Deyerle, W. M., Burkhardt, B., Comfort, T., and Giles, W.: Displaced fractures of the talus—an aggressive approach. Association of Bone and Joint Surgeons Thirty-third Annual Meeting, Lexington, KY, April 8–12, 1981. Orthop. Trans., *5*:465, 1981.
8. Palmer, I.: The mechanism and treatment of fractures of the calcaneus. Open reduction with the use of cancellous grafts. J. Bone Joint Surg., *30-A*:2, 1948.
9. Franklin, J., Johnson, K., and Hansen, S. T., Jr.: Open ankle fractures treated by immediate internal fixation. Presented at the American Academy of Orthopedic Surgeons Annual Meeting, Anaheim, CA, 1983.

Chapter 25 Complex Fractures and Dislocations of the Shoulder

MELVIN POST

The shoulder is a complex articulation; its integrity is essential for normal function. Trauma that impairs the normal anatomy of this region hinders the function of the whole upper extremity. Fortunately, most shoulder injuries are easily treated if the injury is well understood and correctly managed. A relatively small number of injuries are difficult to manage under the best of circumstances and may be termed complex. In essence, most complex shoulder injuries are made much less troublesome when a correct diagnosis is established initially, the mechanism of injury and anatomy comprehended, and the principles of fracture care scrupulously followed. This chapter will describe complex injuries that need special treatment for the shoulder to function effectively.

Fractures of the Clavicle

The clavicle is the supporting strut that connects the upper extremity to the axial skeleton. It provides stability for the shoulder. In the child, longitudinal growth occurs from a single medial epiphysis. The bone is injured easily because it lies subcutaneously in its entire length. The outer portion is flattened, whereas the middle portion is composed of tubular cortical bone. Moreover, its close anatomic relationship to the first rib and major neurovascular structures may cause serious problems following injury.

Mechanism of Injury

The clavicle is one of the most frequently broken bones, especially in children. A force directed against the outer end of the clavicle may cause a shearing fracture in its midportion; however, the bone also may be fractured by a fall from a height or by a fall on the outstretched hand, elbow, or shoulder. In these situations, the shoulder is pushed forcefully inward toward the chest wall. Fractures may result from direct violence, as occurs with a sport injury when force on the point of the shoulder may cause fracture of the lateral clavicle.

Allman classified clavicle fractures into three groups.[1] Group I is comprised of fractures of the middle third of the bone where the bone is unsupported by ligaments. The region of greatest frequency of fracture is just medial to the attachment of the coracoclavicular ligament. In older patients, the bone tends to comminute when fractured. The medial fragment is often elevated by the sternocleidomastoid muscle.

Group II fractures involve the outer end of the clavicle lateral to the coracoclavicular ligament and comprise 10% of clavicular fractures. Such fractures are caused by direct violence. Neer divided these injuries into two types.[2] Type I injuries include fractures wherein the coracoclavicular ligament is intact and has little tendency to displace; type II fractures usually are associated with displacement of the clavicle because rupture of the coracoclavicular ligament makes reduction difficult. There is little or no displacement if the costoclavicular ligament is intact.

Group III fractures occur in the medial end of the clavicle and rarely are caused by direct violence. When the costoclavicular ligament is intact, there is little displacement.

Associated Injuries

Occasionally, combined injuries of the clavicle and the upper ribs may occur.[3] The scalenus anticus muscle attaches to a tubercle on the first rib. The subclavian vein lies in front and the subclavian artery behind the scalene anticus muscle. Other muscles attach to the ribs. The scalene medius also attaches to the first rib behind the subclavian artery. Both scalene muscles elevate the first rib during inspiration. The serratus anterior arises from the upper eight ribs and fixes the rib posteriorly during inspiration. Upper rib fractures may occur through three mechanisms: (1) an indirect force transmitted via the manubrium, (2) avulsion fracture at the weakest portion of the rib produced by the scalene anticus, and (3) injuries to the muscle that transmit an indirect force to the costal cartilage and anterior aspect of the first rib and fracture the posterior portion of the first rib. Thus, when severe acromioclavicular injuries and type II fractures of the lateral clavicle are present, the surgeon should look for fractures of the upper ribs.

Treatment

The chief goal of therapy, regardless of the location of the fracture, is to restore a healed strut in an anatomic position that is as near normal as possible. In most instances, good alignment and a good result are simple to attain by conservative means since the blood supply to the clavicle is so abundant. The age of the patient in large measure determines the treatment.

In the newborn, a fracture of the clavicle merely requires gentle care and quiet to avoid pain for approximately 2 weeks. Overriding and displacement of the fracture ends usually remodel to normal in time.

In the child, the clavicle heals when a figure-of-eight splint is used for immobilization. Weekly visits at least are required to ensure that the splint is tightened. The splint should not be replaced each visit as such changes make alignment of the shoulder blade difficult to maintain. In older, cooperative children with an incomplete fracture, a sling may be used in lieu of the figure-of-eight splint.

The younger the child, the less time is needed for immobilization. Healing usually occurs in 3 to 4 weeks in a 3-year-old child and in 6 to 8 weeks in a ten-year-old child. In teenagers with a displaced fracture of the middle third of the clavicle (group I), alignment of the bones ends may be difficult to maintain after reduction. If the patient is known to be cooperative, a figure-of-eight splint may be used, but otherwise, a plaster-of-paris cast should be employed. A plaster of paris yoke tends to be inadequate.

In the adult, the healing process is longer and presents additional problems. Clavicular fractures in the adult tend to displace easily, which may impede healing. In these patients, the best treatment is a plaster-of-paris spica cast with immobilization maintained for at least 6 to 8 weeks.[4] During application of the plaster-of-paris cast, the patient should be supine on a smooth narrow plate suspended between two tables. Gravity draws the shoulders backward. Following cast application, the metal plate is withdrawn.

Operative treatment is rarely indicated for group I fractures, especially for children and only slightly less so for the young adult and mature patient. There are two valid criteria for open reduction of the clavicle: (1) when there is soft-tissue interposition, and (2) when there is true neurovascular deficit resulting from the fracture.[5–7] The incidence of these circumstances is not high in group I fractures.

Open reduction is not an innocuous procedure. It requires two procedures—one to insert the internal fixation device, whether it be a plate or intramedullary Steinmann pin, and another to remove the device when the fracture is healed. Risks relating to nonunion,[8,9] anesthesia, and infection are increased as a result of the procedure, and the resulting scar and sometimes deformity may be more unsightly than those that occur when closed reduction methods are used. In an extensive comminution, a larger incision than originally intended and more stripping of soft tissues from the bone than anticipated may be needed. Studies indicate that open reduction may be a major factor in nonunion.[8] When marked deformity from a malunion occasionally occurs and is unacceptable, an osteotomy and realignment of the clavicle can be performed. In these rare instances, internal fixation with a plate or intramedullary Steinmann pin with the addition of an iliac bone graft is recommended.[10] The patient should be informed that nonunion can result and that there will be a scar.

In a type I fracture, the distal clavicle may be treated with a figure-of-eight bandage. Type II acute fractures should be treated with open methods in most adults because external immobilization is often ineffective in maintaining the position of the fracture fragments. Open treatment methods include insertion of one or two $^{3}/_{32}$-inch pins across the acromion and bone fragment of the lateral clavicle into the reduced fragment of the medial clavicle. External support is utilized for 8 weeks postoperatively.[11,12] Blind pinning is never justified. The lateral cut ends of the pins should be bent beneath the skin to prevent migration. In acute or old cases of unreduced displaced fracture of the lateral clavicle, internal fixation of the medial fragment to the coracoid with synthetic polyester tape and autogenous bone grafting is worthwhile. In the rare event when the surgeon is confronted with a previously excised short fragment of the lateral clavicle and a superiorly dislocated medial clavicle fragment resulting from rupture of the coracoclavicular ligament, transfer of the coracoid with its active short biceps to the clavicle can be performed as in the treatment for a chronic acromioclavicular dislocation. In the elderly or poor-risk patient, a state of nonunion is compatible with good function, and acceptance of this complication may be prudent.

If a compression of the subclavian vessels or brachial plexus occurs and causes symptoms, whether from injury, exuberant callus, or malunion, the pressure phenomena should be removed.[5,7,13] Regardless of the method employed to relieve pressure, removal of the clavicle is not an entirely harmless procedure as the clavicle does stabilize the shoulder.[14]

Fractures of the Scapula

The scapula is a large, irregular flat bone; its main functions are to provide the shallow glenoid for articulation with the humeral head and to give leverage for the attachment of muscles, such as the deltoid, that move the arm and shoulder. The scapula is well covered by a relatively large number of muscles that cushion the bone and serve to protect it from injury. Unless there are extensive associated injuries, injury of the scapula is not difficult to detect. These fractures have been well described.[15–19]

Most patients sustain fractures of the scapula by severe force, either direct or indirect. Automobile and motorcycle accidents account for a large percentage of the total number of such fractures seen. Imatani showed a mean patient age of 28 years with a range of 17 to 56 years in 1 study of fractures of the scapula.[20] Associated injuries are caused by high-velocity impact and take precedence over the fractured scapula itself. In one study, 88% of 121 patients with scapular fracture had associated injuries, which often led to delayed diagnosis and treatment of the scapular fracture.[21] These associated injuries were often multiple and included a 44% incidence of rib fracture and a 26% occurrence of clavicular fracture. Unusual scapular injuries have been reported, including an intrathoracic dislocation of the inferior angle.[22] A greater preponderance of fractures occurs in men than in women.

When the patient is conscious and carefully examined, discovery of a scapular fracture is easy. The patient tends to splint the arm at the side or to keep the extremity slightly abducted avoiding all movement, especially when there is extensive comminution of the body and spine of the scapula. Moreover, the patient with fractures of the body and spine usually lies tilted away from the injured side of the scapula. Tenderness, ecchymosis, hematoma, and abrasions often are found at the site of fracture. The patient may complain of increased pain during deep inspiration. In the acute phase of injury, muscle power about the shoulder girdle often is impossible to test because of muscle spasm and local hemorrhage.

Whenever fractures of the scapula are suspected, roentgenograms should be taken in the anteroposterior, neutral, tangential, and axillary positions with the arm gently abducted if possible. The axillary film is especially useful for demonstrating the glenoid and any displaced fragments at the axillary border. Accessory ossification centers occur at the proximal and distal parts of the coracoid process and should not be interpreted as a fracture.[23]

Fractures of the spine and body of the scapula require only symptomatic treatment. The patient should be evaluated thoroughly for other injuries to the rib cage, lungs, neurovascular system, and vertebral column.[21] Anatomic reduction of these fractures is not necessary nor are the means to accomplish reduction justified.

Treatment

The vast majority of fractures of the scapula can be treated conservatively. Immobilization in a sling or in Velpeau position is useful. After 10 to 14 days, or longer (when much of the pain has subsided), gentle motion exercises may be started and increased until normal shoulder function is achieved. Complications usually are not encountered, and operative treatment of scapular fractures is considered rarely. However, if the acromion is fractured and displaced downward as a result of a severe blow on the acromial process, the fractured acromion may rotate downward and narrow the space between the superior aspect of the humeral head and undersurface of the acromion. In this event, abduction motion may be diminished. If this complication is suspected early, open reduction and internal fixation with Steinmann pins can be considered. If an ununited acromial epiphysis is suspected, contralateral roentgenograms of the shoulder should be taken for comparison to rule out a fracture.[24] An acromial fracture occasionally may be associated with anteroinferior dislocation of the glenohumeral joint, and in this event, the fracture fragments can be stabilized with Steinmann pin internal fixation to prevent malalignment, thus obviating a chronic anteroinferior shoulder dislocation. Bone union results when the fragments are well aligned.[19] Since conservative treatment of fractures of the glenoid have given satisfactory results in my experience, open reduction of displaced fragments of the glenoid should be considered only in rare situations.

Fractures of the glenoid and neck of the scapula may be undisplaced, displaced, or burst injuries. If the glenoid rim is avulsed in traumatic shoulder dislocations, the small fragment may be observed on the axillary view and anteroposterior films. In any event, this injury may account for recurring shoulder dislocations.[15] Large glenoid fractures are more likely to lead to chronic dislocation.[25] In general, scapular neck and glenoid fractures do not require open treatment for a satisfactory result. Only Velpeau immobilization for 3 to 4 weeks for undisplaced fractures and a plaster shoulder spica cast for 6 to 8 weeks for highly comminuted or displaced fractures are needed.

Finally, fractures of the coracoid are uncommon and may result from a severe blow to the shoulders. The bone is avulsed by the sudden forceful traction of the muscles that attach to it or by the impact of the dislocated humeral head.[26,27] Fractures of the coracoid can be caused by repeated stress.[28] In most instances, treatment should be conservative, immobilizing the extremity for 2 to 3 weeks until there is significant pain relief. Open treatment may be indicated for the acute case in which neurologic deficit results from brachial plexus injury. All markedly displaced symptomatic fractures may be treated with open methods by excising the fragment and reattaching the conjoint tendon after the acute phase. If the acromioclavicular joint is dislocated, the dislocation and coracoid fracture may be treated by open reduction and internal fixation. Recognition of a coracoid fracture is especially important when the surgeon plans to hold a dislocated lateral clavicle to the coracoid either by synthetic polyester tape or a Bosworth screw.[29]

Fractures of the Proximal Humerus

Fractures of the upper humerus constitute a considerable percentage of upper extremity fractures. The abundant cancellous trabecular network in the proximal humerus helps to cushion the humeral head from serious injury in the young. The elderly person does not have this advantage because of advancing osteoporosis where the bone is weakened. Even with minimal force, there is a higher incidence of fracture of the upper humerus in older individuals.

Blood Supply

The much larger posterior humeral circumflex artery arising from the third part of the axillary artery and the smaller anterior circumflex artery surround the surgical neck. The posterior humeral circumflex vessel gives off branches to the shoulder joint and possibly to the humeral head through the rotator-cuff insertion. Both circumflex arteries anastomose at the lower border of the subscapularis. The anterior humeral circumflex gives off a twig(s) to the shoulder joint and a branch that ascends to the head of the humerus at the upper end of the bicipital groove, or branches may enter the lesser and greater tuberosities. This vessel has been described as the "arcuate artery."[30] Thus, any trauma that disrupts this arterial system and isolates the humeral head from its blood supply may lead to osteonecrosis of the humeral head segment.

Classification

Codman showed that fracture lines about the humeral head generally followed the old epiphyseal lines, delineating the tuberosities and anatomic head from the diaphysis.[31] He suggested that the proximal humerus be divided into four main segments or combinations of four parts including the humeral head, the lesser tuberosity, the greater tuberosity, and the shaft. Although other systems have been suggested,[32,33] Neer devised a classification of proximal humeral fractures that is now almost universally accepted.[34,35] The system is based on the displacement of one or more of the previously described four major segments. It differentiates the different kinds of fractures, predicts the status of the vascular supply, and provides useful information concerning the effects of the muscle attachments and continuity of the articular surface of the proximal humerus. There are six groups in Neer's classification.

Minimum Displacment. In this group, regardless of the level of the fracture or the number of fracture lines, no segment is displaced more than 1 cm or angulated more than 45°. These fractures account for a majority of fractures of the proximal humerus and are considered one-part fractures. Because the bone fragments usually are held together or impacted, early motion exercises can be started.

Articular Segment Displacement. This group represents fractures that occur entirely through the anatomic neck and are considered two-part fractures. Displacement of fractures at the anatomic neck without separation of the tuberosities is rare. Disability may result from malunion or osteonecrosis of the humeral head.

Shaft Displacement. In this group, fractures occur at the level of the surgical neck. The fragments are displaced more than 1 cm or are angulated more than 45°. The rotator-cuff attachment usually is intact, thereby allowing the humeral head to remain in a neutral position.

Greater Tuberosity Displacement. Any one of three facets or the entire tuberosity may be retracted more than 1 cm from the lesser tuberosity. This two-part fracture can be difficult to reduce by closed methods and may be associated with a longitudinal tear in the rotator cuff. In addition, in a fracture through the surgical neck of the humerus, a three-part injury results. With significant displacement to the surgical neck and retraction of the greater tuberosity, the articular segment is rotated internally by the action of the subscapularis. Because of the integrity of the anterior soft-tissue attachment, the blood supply to the humeral head is preserved.[34]

Lesser Tuberosity Displacement. An uncommon two-part lesion occurs with an isolated avulsion fracture of the lesser tuberosity. Three-part lesions occur when there is also a fracture of the surgical neck. Here, the articular segment may be rotated externally and abducted by the external rotators. The blood supply remains intact through the posterior soft-tissue attachments. In four-part fractures, both tuberosities may be retracted, and in this event, the blood supply to the humeral head usually is lost.

Fracture-Dislocation. This injury results in dislocation of the humeral head from its glenoid. The capsule and ligamentous structures are torn. The humeral head may be displaced anteriorly or posteriorly. The blood supply to the humeral head usually is adequate in two- and three-part fracture-dislocations because one of the tuberosities with its soft-tissue attachments remains intact with the articular segment. In an anterior fracture-dislocation, the lesser tuberosity remains attached to the humeral head (Fig. 25-1), whereas in posterior fracture-dislocations, the lesser tuberosity is displaced. In four-part anterior and posterior fracture-dislocations, the blood supply to the humeral head is destroyed since both tuberosities are detached. In this event, osteonecrosis of the humeral head is common. In unusual cases, the rotator cuff may be avulsed.[36]

The articular cartilage may be crushed against the glenoid, causing an extrusion of fragments from the glenoid. An impression defect (Hill-Sachs lesion) can occur in the posterolateral humeral head as a result of an anterior dislocation. An impression defect or reverse Hill-Sachs lesion sometimes occurs in the anteromedial humeral head as the result of a posterior dislocation.

Diagnosis

The majority of fractures of the upper humerus results from a force transmitted in the longitudinal axis of the arm.[37] The patient complains of pain in the shoulder. The surgeon should not depend on the physical examination alone to diag-

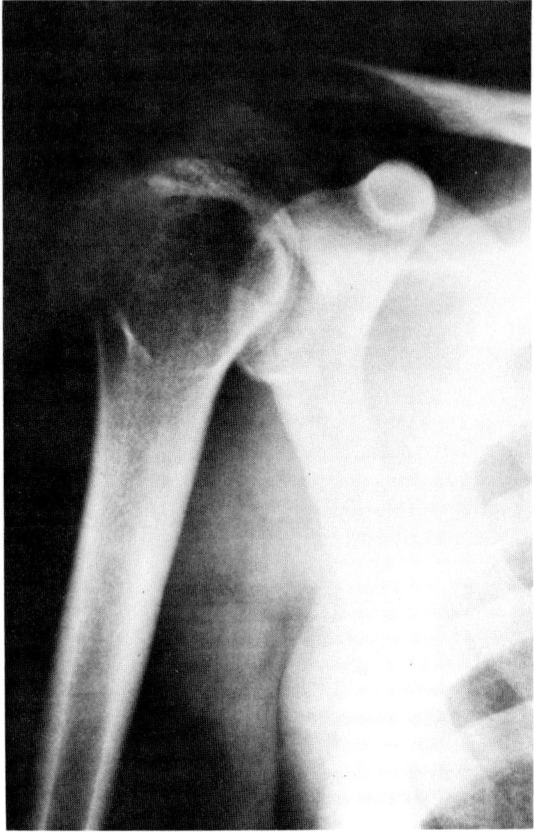

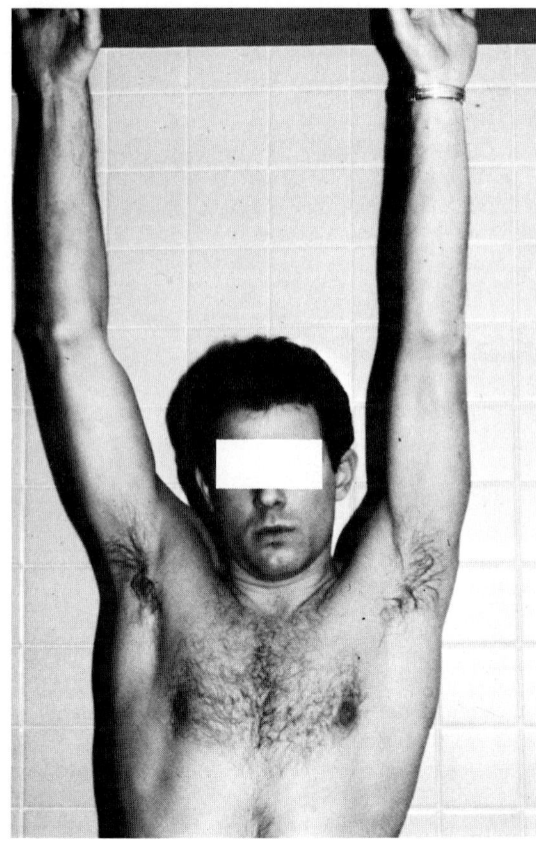

FIG. 25-1. *A*, A 20-year-old patient, injured in a motorcycle accident, sustained a complete brachial plexus palsy and abdominal injuries. *B*, Twenty days after closed reduction, the patient was placed in a plaster-of-Paris spica cast with dynamic splinting of the fingers for 5 weeks. Thereafter, gentle motion exercises were started. Note the active range of shoulder motion 8 months later. There was a 98% return of hand function.

nose the lesion, especially in well-developed individuals. Rather, the surgeon should rely on excellent-quality roentgenograms taken in multiple planes for a correct diagnosis. In addition, a thorough vascular and neurologic examination should be performed since neurovascular injury can be associated with proximal humeral fractures.

Treatment

Treatment should be individualized for each patient, selecting the method that is best for the patient. Most proximal humeral fractures, except for three- and four-part fractures, severe impression fractures of the humeral head, and some fracture-dislocations, can be treated by closed methods.

Closed. The use of a hanging cast is not recommended for most proximal humeral fractures because the cast may cause inferior subluxation and nonunion resulting from distraction of the fragments.[38] Excellent results can be achieved with manipulation, Velpeau's immobilization, shoulder spica casts, and, occasionally, traction methods when deemed necessary. Prolonged excessive traction may cause stiffness of the elbow and shoulder. Only enough traction weight to maintain reduction of the bone fragments should be added for a reasonable period of time.

When manipulation is employed to reduce displaced fractures, the surgeon should consider the deforming forces of muscles on the fracture segments. Bell described a closed method of reduction for posterior fracture-dislocation that has been used with excellent results, even when open reduction seemed likely (Fig. 25-2).[39]

Whatever method of management is selected, sufficient bone healing must occur before motion can be started. Failure to follow this principle

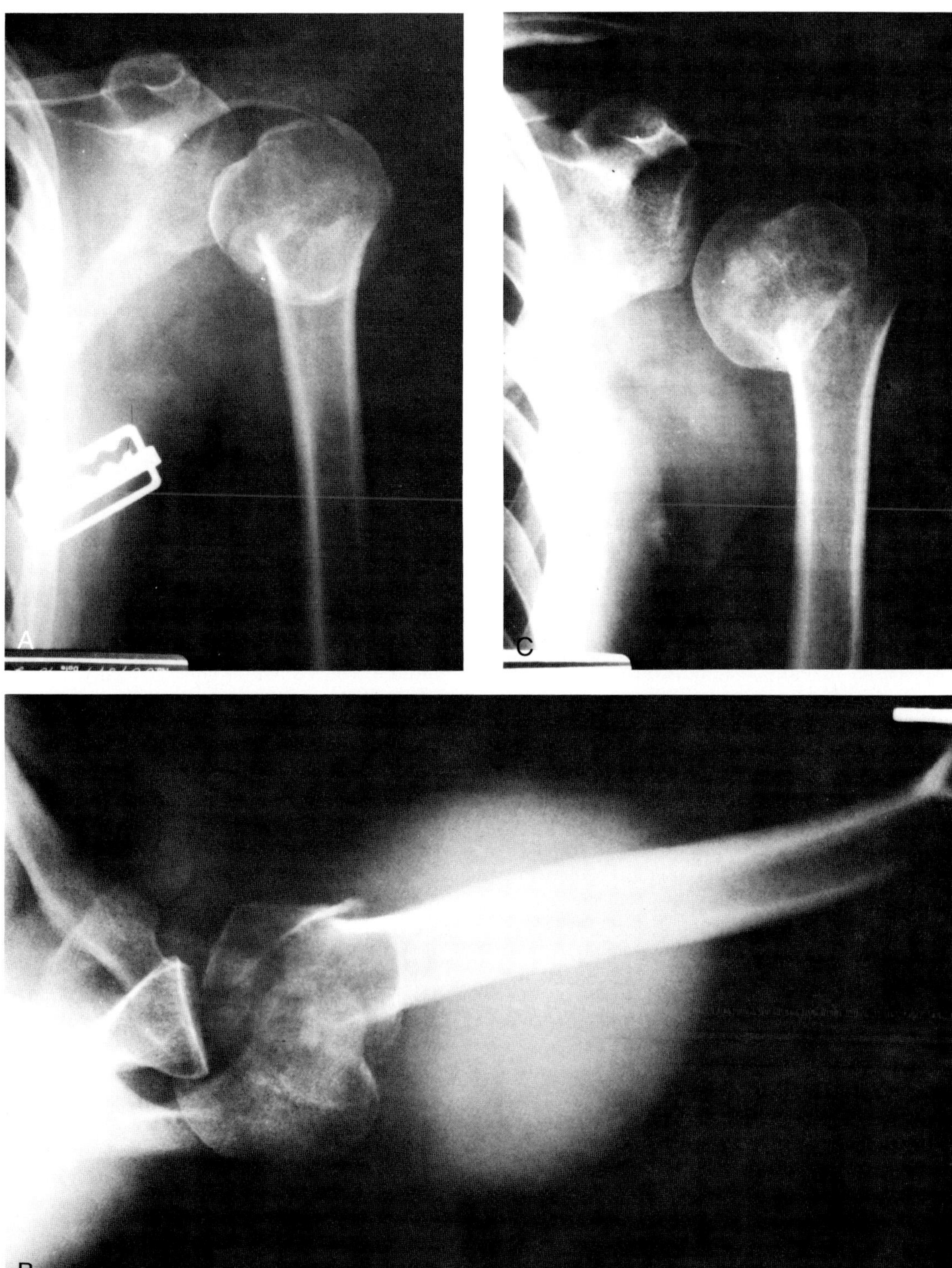

FIG. 25-2. *A* and *B*, Anteroposterior and axillary roentgenograms show a posterior fracture-dislocation in a 35-year-old woman. *C*, A closed reduction was achieved easily by using Bell's method. Note the healing fracture 6 weeks later. Transitory atony of the shoulder girdle muscles and inferior subluxation subsided during the rehabilitation period.

may cause angulation at the fracture site so that even a simple surgical neck fracture, for example, may become complicated.

Open. When an accurate reduction of the fracture fragments cannot be achieved by closed means, open methods may be considered. In an elderly, poor-risk patient, it is wise to accept a functional loss rather than subject such a patient to surgical treatment. Open treatment may become necessary when the long head of the biceps is interposed or when reduction of the fracture fragments is difficult to maintain by closed methods. Open methods of treatment include internal fixation methods, head resection and reattachment of the rotator cuff to the shaft,[40] and arthroplasty. Although use of prosthetic replacement has been reported as more successful in the acute than in the chronic phase,[41] the results of one method over the other have been inconsistent mainly because of scarring and contraction of the soft tissues.

The anterior surgical approach can be employed in open treatment for most proximal humeral fractures. This approach permits elevation of the deltoid from its clavicle if necessary. Internal fixation methods that provide good results include the use of a Rush nail driven through the proximal segment into the shaft to stabilize the humeral head in acute injuries or nonunion, the use of a lag screw to provide stability of the fracture fragments and thereby to permit early motion exercises, the use of multiple screws (Fig. 25-3), and the use of an AO shoulder plate. On occasion, a Nicola procedure is used in which the long head of the biceps tendon is transected in its groove and its proximal portion is threaded through a hole made in the humeral head, exiting near the proximal end of the bicipital groove.[42] Both cut ends of the tendon are secured to the shaft. The latter method should be avoided in patients with osteoporotic bone or when the humeral head has sustained a comminuted fracture. The first three methods usually require external support for varying periods to ensure sufficient healing to prevent displacement of the bone fragments (Fig. 25-3). Whatever method of internal fixation is used, the surgeon must be confident that the fracture fragments are stable at the close of the surgical procedure and will not displace postoperatively.

Head resection is performed infrequently because good, active, overhead motion ordinarily is lost, especially if the external rotator muscles are weak. Thus, the procedure frequently results in persistent pain and weakness about the shoulder. Prosthetic replacement may give good results when the humeral head is damaged irreparably. However, the functional results of hemiarthroplasty for these injuries are inconstant, especially in posterior fracture-dislocations.[43]

In the first 24 hours postoperatively, hemovac drainage is instituted to minimize the accumulation of hematomata. In most open procedures, preoperative, intraoperative, and postoperative intravenous administration of antibiotics is used for 3 days.

Specific Treatment

Minimally displaced fractures usually are stable and heal at 6 weeks. This fracture is treated in a sling for up to 3 weeks. As soon as the level of pain permits, gentle motion exercises are started and increased gradually. Overhead motion is best achieved if the patient is supine and reaches overhead while grasping a length of 1-inch diameter dowel with both hands.

In anatomic humeral neck fractures, the incidence of osteonecrosis of the articular segment is high. Nevertheless, severely displaced fractures should be reduced and internally fixed with two screws, if possible. Immediate prosthetic replacement is ill advised because a good result occasionally can be obtained when the humeral head is preserved. With minimal displacement, closed treatment and simple immobilization of the extremity for 4 or 5 weeks until adequate healing occurs are the sole treatment procedures necessary until gentle motion exercises can be initiated.

The majority of surgical neck fractures can be treated by closed methods. If the fracture is impacted and stable, the patient can be treated with Velpeau's immobilization and started on motion exercises at 3 weeks with the extremity in a sling. When the fracture is severely displaced or excessively angulated, or if there is an excessively angulated impacted fracture, manipulation under general anesthesia and traction are used to reduce the impaction and correct the angulation. Velpeau's immobilization for several weeks or longer may be needed before gentle motion exercises can be started. Mobilization started too early may cause a loss of the reduction. In any event, in an unstable or displaced two-part surgical neck fracture, inadequate immobilization may lead to a failure of treatment regardless of the initial reduction.

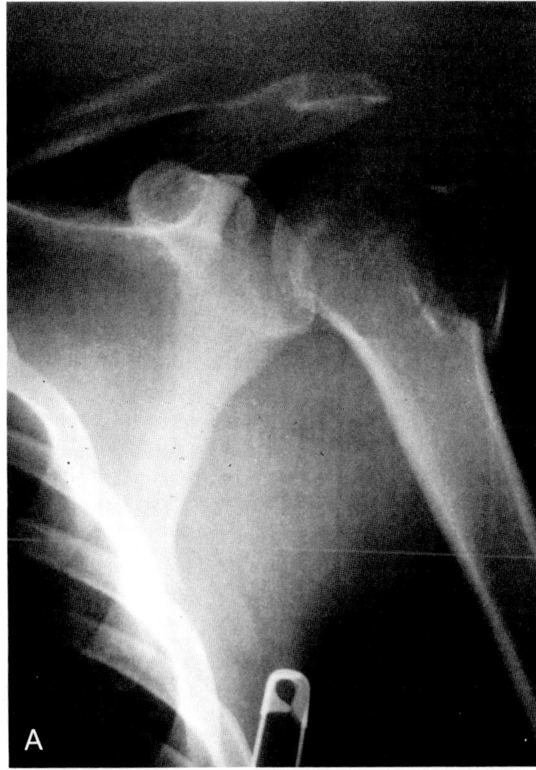

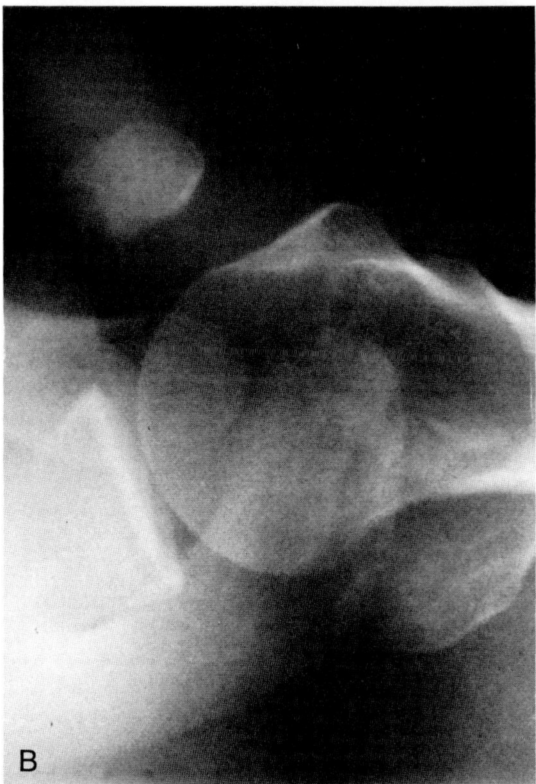

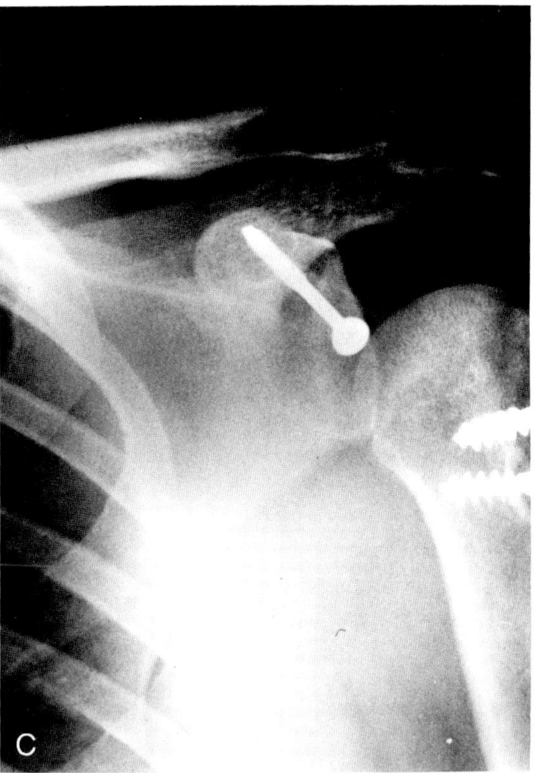

FIG. 25-3. *A* and *B*, A young adult sustained an anterior fracture-dislocation shown in the anteroposterior and axillary films taken after a closed reduction. Note the large greater tuberosity fragment. The fractured coracoid was discovered before manipulation on the modified axillary view. *C*, An open reduction and multiple screw fixation are shown at 3 weeks, during which time a Velpeau cast was used. Motion exercises were started thereafter. The result was excellent.

When treatment by traction is decided on, a threaded pin is placed through the olecranon and the arm is brought into 45 to 90° of abduction.[44] The traction is maintained for several weeks with just enough weight employed to maintain the reduction. Traction then is removed, and the extremity is treated in a sling or Velpeau's immobilization for up to several additional weeks until adequate bone healing has occurred to permit gentle pendulum and motion exercises. Premature use of vigorous exercise can lead to a loss of the initial anatomic reduction of the bone fragments.

Three-part surgical neck fractures often require open accurate reduction of the bone fragments and repair of the rotator cuff. Open reduction may be needed when the surgical neck is comminuted and reduction cannot be maintained by closed methods, or in the case of an interposed tendon of the long head of the biceps. The surgeon must be certain that the internal fixation device has truly stabilized the fracture fragments; otherwise, the reduction of the fracture fragments will be lost and a poor result obtained (Fig. 25-4). Postoperative immobilization and rehabilitation are the same as for other displaced two-part surgical neck fractures.

Most superiorly displaced fractures of the greater tuberosity require early open reduction and internal fixation. Occasionally, such a displaced segment can be maintained in a reduced position by closed methods.[45] However, when open reduction is needed, a greater tuberosity fragment may be replaced by using a suture or screw and the rotator-cuff defect repaired through an anterior or saber-cut surgical approach. With the saber-cut approach, only a small portion of the deltoid needs to be elevated from the anterior acromion and lateral clavicle. The upper inch of the deltoid muscle and its deep fascia are split to gain adequate exposure. Open reduction performed 2 to 3 weeks following the injury requires a more extensive surgical approach since scarring and contracture of the injured rotator cuff and capsular tissues make anatomic reduction more difficult. Nevertheless, restoration of function depends on the anatomic replacement of the fracture fragments with repair of the torn rotator cuff. In four-part fractures, good results have been reported when the cancellous bone has been scooped from the head and the remaining articular shell replaced on the reshaped proximal shaft.[46] However, initial prosthetic replacement is the preferred treatment method for such injuries.

When the lesser tuberosity is fractured, no additional treatment is ordinarily required. If the surgical neck also is fractured and displaced and the lesser tuberosity remains attached, the humeral head internally rotates. In this case, a closed reduction often is impossible to achieve. This type of fracture requires an open reduction through an anterior approach and replacement of both tuberosities with repair of the soft-tissue defect. After adequate healing has occurred, gentle motion exercises are initiated.

If the lesser tuberosity alone is avulsed and the fragment is small, the injury may be treated with a collar and cuff or sling. When the fragment is large and displaced, it is surgically reduced; when it is small and displaced and the surgeon believes that it will cause loss of function, it may be excised and the detached subscapularis tendon insertion repaired. The extremity is immobilized in Velpeau's position for 3 weeks before gentle motion exercises are started.

When a fracture-dislocation has occurred, it is best to reduce the dislocation as quickly as possible. The number of broken bone segments and the direction of the dislocation should be determined. If closed reduction is performed under general anesthesia, a gentle manipulation should be used to preserve any remaining blood supply to the humeral head. Force must be avoided when reducing any dislocation. If gentle closed reduction methods fail, open reduction and internal fixation should be performed. A neurovascular examination of the extremity should be carried out before and after the manipulation.

When an anterior fracture-dislocation is manipulated successfully, a displaced greater tuberosity fragment often reduces. If the fragment remains superiorly retracted, open reduction and internal fixation with repair of the rotator-cuff tear are necessary.[44,47] The extremity is placed in Velpeau's plaster-of-paris cast for 4 weeks. Thereafter, gentle motion exercises are started.

The uncommon posterior fracture-dislocation usually results from convulsive disorders, direct trauma, or other violence.[32,48] Posterior fracture-dislocation with avulsion of the lesser tuberosity may be treated by closed means if the patient is relaxed under general anesthesia while traction is placed on the extremity and the arm is flexed slowly, adducted, and, if needed, gently rotated internally.[39,49] Some pressure can be applied to the humeral head from behind. This technique of closed reduction unlocks the humeral head from behind the posterior glenoid rim. Following reduction, the arm is immobilized at the side in varying degrees of rotation, from slight external rotation to 50° of internal rotation, but is never fully internally rotated since this position may cause spontaneous posterior dislocation.

Three-part posterior fracture-dislocations are best treated by open reduction and suture of the reduced fragments with repair of the torn rotator cuff in most cases. However, in selected cases, closed reduction may be attempted first. Aftercare in a Velpeau's spica cast is the same as that with similiar three-part injuries without dislocations.

In four-part anterior fracture-dislocations, it is probably best to replace the head initially with a prothesis and to start early motion exercises.

Four-part posterior fracture-dislocations are

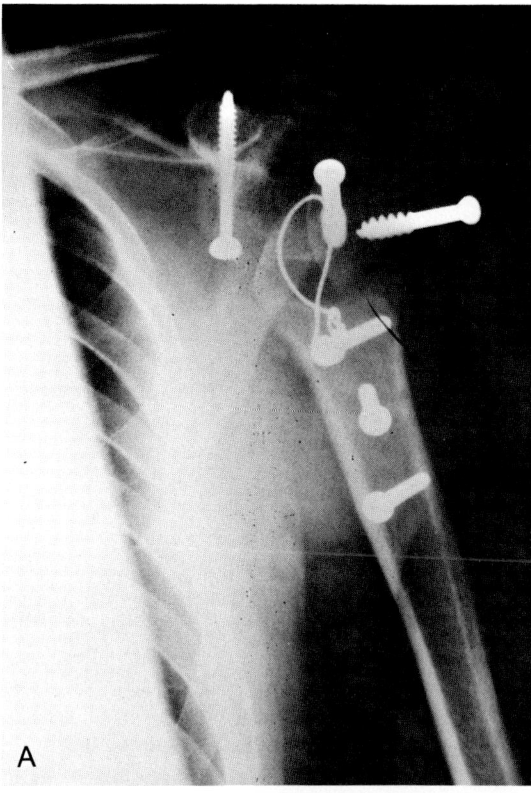

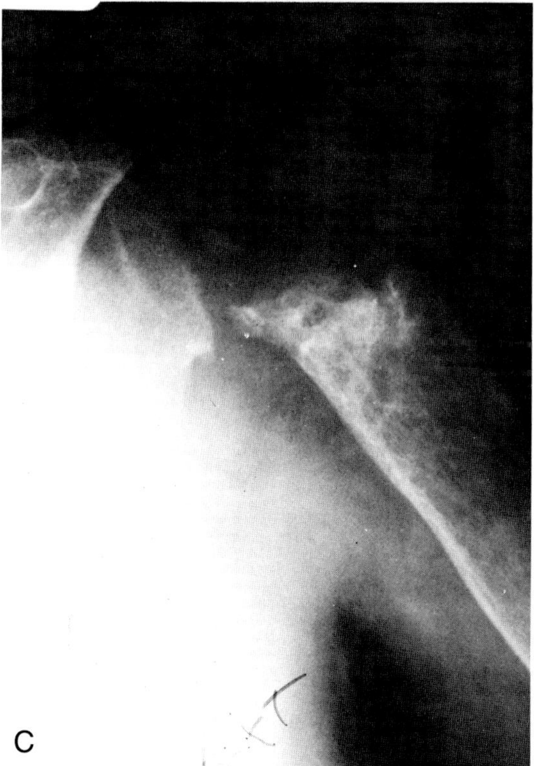

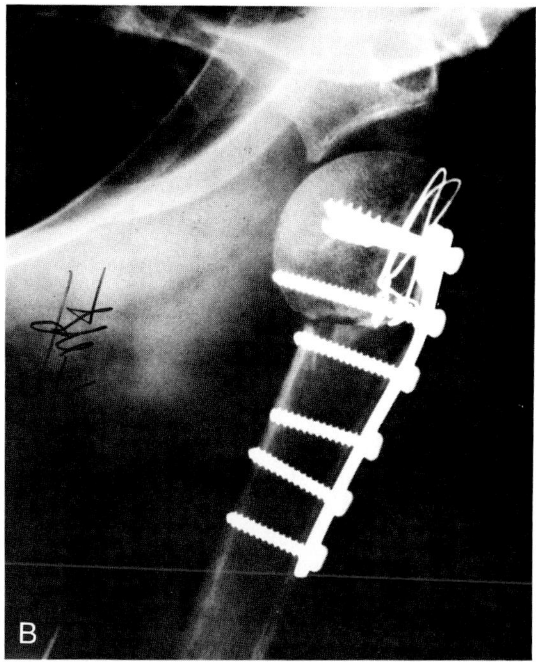

Fig. 25-4. *A*, An adult man sustained comminuted three-part surgical neck and coracoid fractures during a motorcycle accident. An excellent reduction, but inadequate stabilization, was attained in a first operation; a second operation was needed. Note the displacement of the fracture fragments following the second operation. *B*, A third operation using a "T" plate achieved stabilization of the bone fragments much later, but resulted in a deep joint infection. *C*, The proximal humeral fragments were resected, and the infection cleared. The shoulder was flail and painful.

rare and are best treated in the acute stage by prosthetic replacement of the humeral head because of a high incidence of osteonecrosis of the head. The elderly, poor-risk patient is best treated symptomatically with a sling.

Impression Defects

A posterolateral impression defect in the humeral head caused by an anterior dislocation usually does not cause the serious problem often noted with anteromedial defects in the head associated with posterior fracture-dislocations. In these injuries, defects of less than 20% of the articular surface may be reduced and immobilized as described previously for fracture-dislocations. Redislocations occur in most cases with a 20 to 40% impression defect unless the humeral head is stabilized by transplanting the subscapularis tendon into the anteromedial defect in the head, as suggested by McLaughlin.[50,51] When a defect of 50% or more of the head surface is present, the joint is unstable and dislocates regardless of any surgical reconstruction. In this event, prosthetic replacement of the humeral head may be performed early with acute posterior dislocation if the rotator-cuff structures are functioning. Recent experience has shown that good results are obtained in long-standing chronic dislocations by using a constrained total shoulder replacement. However, such a replacement should be avoided in patients who are subject to recurrent convulsive seizures.[52,53] The long-term results of such replacements (longer than 9 years) are unknown.

Complicated Fractures

In some severe three-part fractures, most four-part fractures, severe posterior fracture-dislocations not amenable to open reduction, large impression defects of the head, and cases of highly fragmented or split humeral heads, treatment often fails when inadequate closed or open methods of management are used. In these cases, special treatment is required. An early decision should be made regarding a definitive method of treatment to obviate the need for fruitless, subsequent multiple operations to rid the patient of pain and to restore function. These kinds of injuries are notorious for resulting in severe scarring of the damaged rotator cuff. Each added procedure greatly exacerbates this serious problem, usually increasing shoulder pain and reducing function. Missile wounds that destroy the humeral head carry an especially ominous prognosis (Fig. 25-5).

If the humeral head is greatly fragmented, it can be replaced with a prosthesis.[54] Results of such treatment vary with the status of the shoulder girdle muscles, particularly the deltoid and external rotators, at the time of implantation following trauma. When there is an associated brachial plexus injury, the results are especially poor in terms of restoration of function.

A split humeral head should be treated like a fragmented head—replaced with a prosthetic device and mobilized with early motion, particularly if the rotator-cuff tissues are healthy.[47]

Neurovascular Deficit

With displaced surgical neck fractures or fracture-dislocations, significant neurologic and vascular deficit may ensue. These injuries may damage a vessel and cause the development of an

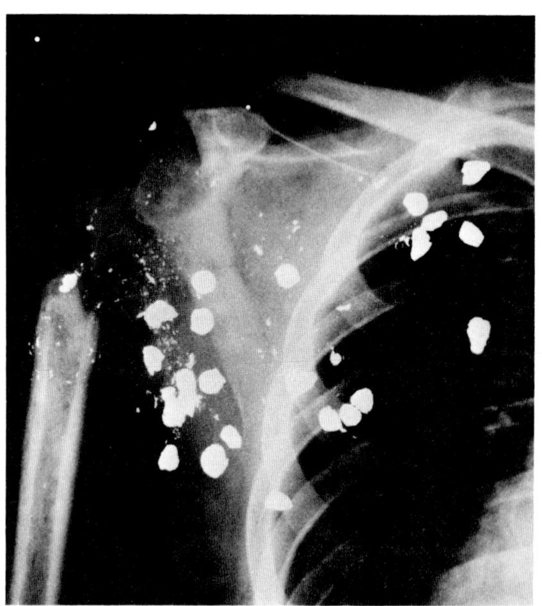

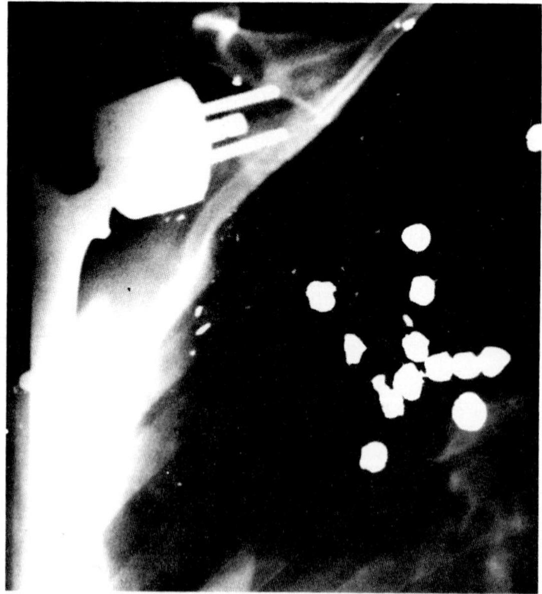

FIG. 25-5. *A*, A 38-year-old man sustained a severe gunshot wound and brachial plexus injury. After several operations, the proximal bone fragments were removed. *B*, A constrained total joint replacement stabilized the humerus. The result was satisfactory.

aneurysm or tear of a vessel. These injuries take precedence over the fracture itself and, in many instances, preclude early treatment of the bone injury (Fig. 25-6).

Dislocations of the Shoulder

The glenohumeral joint is an unstable joint that lends itself easily to traumatic dislocation. This injury is more frequent than fracture of the neck of the humerus in the 17-to-30-year-old age group. The great majority of dislocations occur in young men, although an increasing number of athletic injuries in women now are being observed. Nevertheless, shoulder dislocation in women is still not as common as that in males.

Rowe stated that recurring dislocations of the shoulder can be classified into a traumatic group accounting for 85% of the cases and an atraumatic group constituting 15% of the cases.[55,56] The atraumatic group includes the rare voluntary type of injury. Generally, results of treatment depend in large measure on the cause of the dislocation. Dislocations of the glenohumeral joint may be divided into four groups: anterior, posterior, inferior, and superior. The degree and mechanism of injury determine the degree of subluxation or complete joint dislocation.

Anterior Glenohumeral Dislocations

Anterior dislocation of the shoulder constitutes approximately 95% of all shoulder dislocations. The final resting position of the humeral head following dislocation depends primarily on the mechanism of injury and the delivered force. The most common type of anterior dislocation is subcoracoid anterior dislocation, in which the head of the humerus rests anteriorly to the coracoid process. Subglenoid anterior dislocation is the next most common type, although it occurs infrequently. In such injuries, the head of the humerus lies anteriorly beneath the inferior glenoid process. Other rare forms of anterior shoulder dislocation are the subclavicular and intrathoracic types. In the subclavicular type, the humeral head is medial to the coracoid and below the clavicle. In the exceptionally rare intrathoracic dislocation, a medially directed force drives the humeral head between the ribs into the thoracic cavity.

Mechanism of Injury

In most cases of anterior dislocation, a fall or blow upon the abducted arm has been sustained.[57] Thus, the humeral head is forced against a weakened anterior or anteroinferior aspect of the capsule when the force is transmitted on the outstretched hand with the elbow in an extended position. During the fall, the head of the humerus tilts downward and forward while the extremity is in abduction and in an externally rotated position. The greater the degree of hyperabduction, the more the head is forced downward on the inferior part of the capsule. As the fall is completed, the arm may be extended momentarily, and at this point, the posterolateral portion of the humeral head comes in contact with the glenoid rim. Less forceful similar trauma is required to cause a recurrence. Eventually, merely turning in bed or elevating and hyperabducting the arm can cause a dislocation.

The exact resting position of the head of the humerus is determined by the degree of force, its direction, and the movement of the arm during the dislocation. Moseley stated that there is a greater incidence of greater tuberosity fracture of the humerus and of rotator-cuff avulsion with subglenoid dislocation than with other types.[58] When a rotator-cuff avulsion is associated with a reduced fracture-dislocation, there is less likelihood of recurrent dislocation.

Pathology and Pathogenesis

There is no single cause for recurrent dislocation. According to Bankart, a tear in the fibrous capsule heals rapidly, whereas a detached capsule fails to unite spontaneously with the fibrocartilage, thus creating a permanent defect that permits the head to dislocate over the anterior glenoid even with minimal force. Others have stated that there is significant laxity of varying degrees in the musculotendinous cuff in all cases with erosion and eburnation of the anterior margin of the glenoid fossa in which labral detachment was found.[59-62] Reeves demonstrated that the capsule and subscapular tendon rupture occurred most frequently in the elderly person because these areas become the weakest with increasing age, whereas intracapsular dislocation resulted in younger patients because the weakest point in this age group is the glenoid labral attachment.[62] He concluded that the strength of the tissues rather than the mechanism of injury is an essential factor in anterior dislocation. Whatever

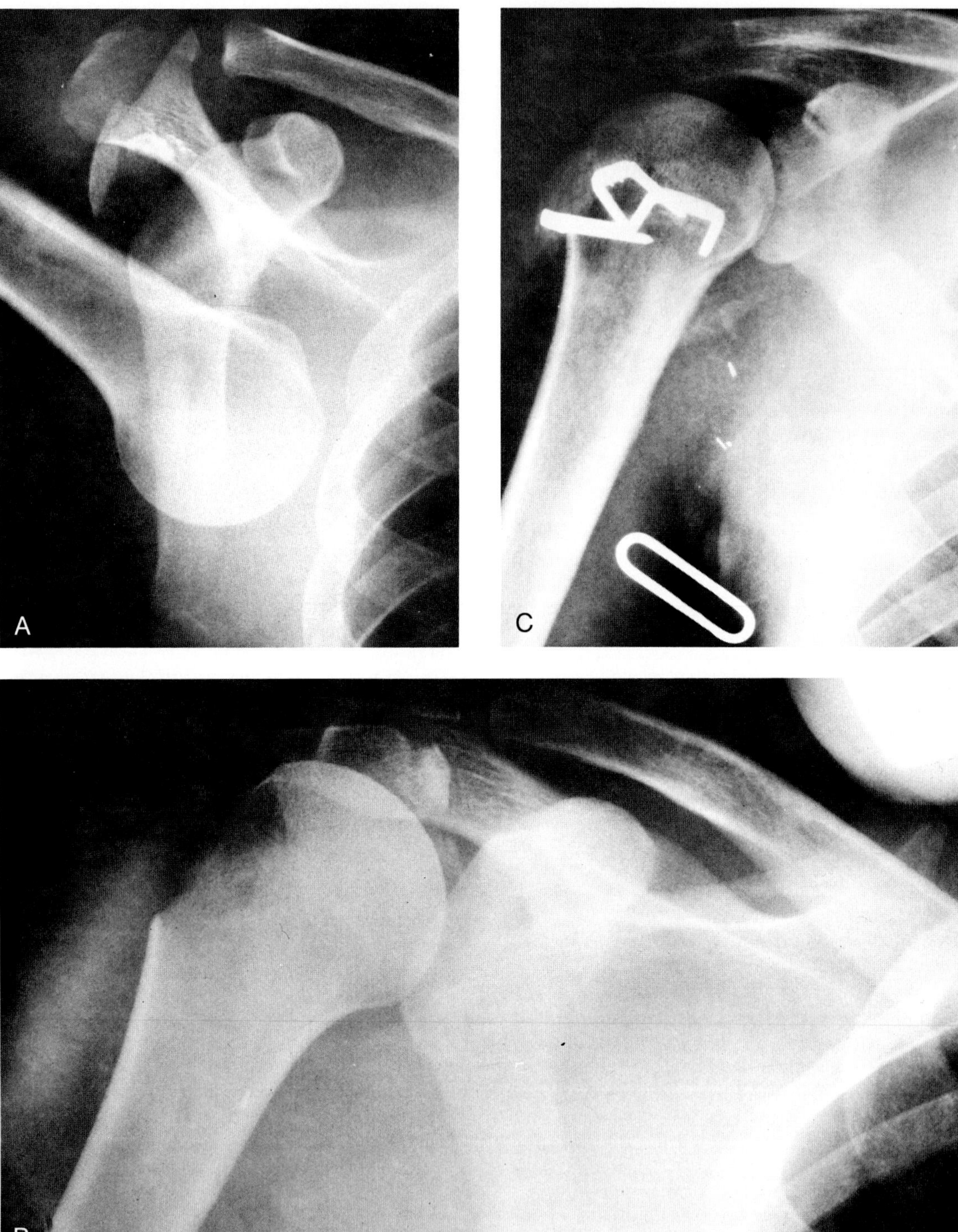

Fig. 25-6. *A*, A young adult sustained a two-part inferior fracture-dislocation and a tear of the axillary artery. *B*, Following a closed reduction, a Dacron tube graft was used to restore circulation to the extremity. The entire circumferential rim of greater tuberosity remained retracted for 6 weeks and resulted in a painful, stiff shoulder. *C*, An open reduction and staple fixation of the fragments with repair of the rotator cuff were accomplished. A plaster-of-Paris spica cast held the arm abducted 60° for 4 weeks, and the extremity was brought slowly to the side. The result was excellent.

the cause of the anterior dislocation, the stretching of the subscapularis that occurs during recurring dislocation decreases its power and results in lengthening and laxity, which predispose to dislocation.[58,63]

An abnormal force drives the head of the humerus from its shallow glenoid socket. The capsule may be stripped from the anterior scapular neck and may become detached. The posterolateral humeral head may be compressed by the anterior bony glenoid rim, thus causing an indentation or notch (the Hill-Sachs lesion).[64] Finally, the subscapularis tendon may be overstretched during dislocation and may remain lax. Laxity greatly diminishes the normal restraints that help to fix the humeral head in its socket. Thus, the musculotendinous structures of the shoulder joint and their dynamic relationship to one another are crucial in maintaining the integrity, stability, and normal function of the shoulder joint.

Diagnosis

A careful history should determine whether there have been previous dislocations or subluxations. Following the first acute dislocation, a patient may complain of subluxation or dislocation from simply abducting the arm. To minimize these occurrences, the patient may limit external rotation movement and splint the arm at the side.

During an anterior dislocation, the normal rounded contour of the shoulder disappears and is replaced by a flat, sharp outline over the lateral part of the shoulder joint. The acromion is prominent. Palpation reveals a depression or concavity beneath the acromion. In the acute state, the patient has considerable pain, but may experience little discomfort in a chronically dislocated shoulder. The extremity is abducted slightly. The patient may tilt slightly toward the affected side to keep the arm in a vertical position. Any attempt to bring the arm to the side causes pain and is resisted by the patient. A careful examination for any abnormal neurovascular findings should be made before and after manipulation.

Roentgenographic Interpretation

Roentgenograms should be obtained in at least two planes. In addition to the anteroposterior film, either an axillary, lateral transthoracic, or "Y" view should be obtained. Although the axillary view gives specific information, it may be more difficult to obtain because of pain, and therefore, the surgeon may need to rely on other views for diagnosis. In 80 to 90% of cases of anterior shoulder dislocation, a Hill-Sachs lesion may be seen when the arm is rotated internally between 50 to 80°; an anteroposterior film should be obtained in such instances. The surgeon should look for an erosion of the glenoid rim, other associated fractures, and loose bodies in the joint, which occur in about 8% of the patients.

Management

Mild sprains of the glenohumeral joint may be treated with simple sling support for as long as 7 days to permit the pain to subside. Gentle motion exercises can be started thereafter and gradually increased over the next several weeks. With a moderate sprain, a sling support or immobilizer should be worn for 3 weeks to allow adequate healing of the torn ligament fibers. If the pain is severe and the joint is stable, Velpeau's shoulder cast can be applied for 2 or 3 weeks, after which the patient is started on gentle motion exercises. With complete tearing of the anterior ligaments of the capsule, the shoulder injury should be treated like an anterior shoulder dislocation to avoid instability later.

Before treating an acute anterior dislocation, the surgeon should know the precise position of the humeral head, the condition of the humeral head and its glenoid fossa, whether there are any associated fractures, whether the dislocation is primary or recurrent, whether a congenital condition exists that might influence treatment, the length of time the shoulder has been dislocated, and whether there is a vessel or nerve injury.

Most acute shoulder dislocations can be reduced by closed methods if performed as soon as possible following the injury. In any event, force never should be used to accomplish a reduction since undue force may cause joint, vessel, or nerve injury or an iatrogenic fracture, which would complicate an otherwise simple injury. Following the reduction, the patient should be examined immediately, using whatever anesthesia is required to achieve relaxation, for any change in the neurovascular status. Roentgenograms should be obtained in two planes to prove that the reduction has been achieved. A variety of closed methods used to accomplish reduction have been described.

Whatever method is used to effect reduction of an acute dislocation, the extremity should be supported with a Velpeau's plaster cast or Velpeau's sling and swath. If the patient is younger than 50 years of age, the shoulder should be immobilized for up to 4 weeks to allow sufficient healing of the soft tissues; gentle motion exercises are started thereafter. In addition, rehabilitation should strive not only to increase motion but also to restore strength of the atrophied muscles about the shoulder girdle. A frozen shoulder may result following treatment, and therefore, a longer period of time than usual may be required to regain full motion.

Early violent extremes of motion and manipulation should be avoided. Rather, patience and frequent progressive exercises performed each day are the aims of treatment. After the age of 50 years, the incidence of recurrence is lessened, and the shoulder may be immobilized for 2 to 3 weeks in elderly patients. Pendulum exercises are started thereafter and motion gradually increased.

Irreducible Anterior Dislocation

Rarely, an acute anterior dislocation of the shoulder may not reduce by ordinary methods while the patient is under general anesthesia. In this most unusual event, an open reduction may be needed to unlock the humeral head by dividing the subscapularis that is stretched and taut over a locked humeral head within a notched defect over the anterior glenoid rim.

Unrecognized Anterior Dislocation

Unrecognized or chronic dislocation of the shoulder is common. Posterior dislocation is missed more easily than is anterior dislocation unless the diagnosis is suspected. There may be associated fractures and neurologic deficit. Closed manipulation may be attempted as long as 6 weeks after the time of injury. During this period, there is a chance that function can be restored. The earlier the reduction after injury, the better is the result. A rare satisfactory result with closed manipulation of an older chronic anterior dislocation can be obtained, but should not be expected. Force and repeated manipulation should be avoided.

If closed manipulation fails in these cases, open reduction in the young patient can be performed as long as 6 months after dislocation. An extensive dissection of the surrounding scarred tissues usually is required. The glenoid fossa must be cleared of all soft tissue before the humeral head can be replaced. In any event, a good result may not be obtained.

When open reduction fails and severe disability or pain results, other procedures now are being employed with greater frequency, including the newer techniques of total shoulder replacement. In the elderly patient, surgical treatment is best avoided unless there is intractable pain.

Associated Fractures

When an anterior shoulder dislocation is associated with an angulated or displaced fracture of the acromion, the dislocation must be reduced and any inferior angulation or displacement of the acromion corrected using internal fixation methods, such as intramedullary Steinmann's pins, to maintain the fracture fragments and thereby avoid inferior humeral head subluxation later. When an acromial fracture is left unreduced, glenohumeral reduction usually is blocked and overhead motion limited. Rarely, the humeral head may be displaced superiorly. In these cases, the rotator cuff may be sufficiently torn to require repair of the soft tissues and internal fixation of the acromial fracture.

Anterior dislocation and fracture of the greater tuberosity have been discussed previously. However, when an anterior dislocation of the shoulder is associated with a fracture of the greater tuberosity that is superiorly displaced, and the fragment does not reduce, open reduction and internal fixation should be performed.

When an anterior dislocation is associated with a fracture of the glenoid rim, the size of the rim fracture must be determined since small rim fragments should be treated closed, whereas larger rim fragments (more than 5 to 6 mm in thickness) should be treated surgically to avoid later recurrent dislocation.

Complications

Rotator-Cuff Injury

Rotator-cuff tear is common with anterior shoulder dislocation. When the humeral head is displaced severely, the rotator cuff is most certainly torn.[65] If pain persists following treatment and a massive rotator-cuff tear is suspected, early confirmation may be obtained by arthrograms. Pettersson showed that, in a series of patients with first-time traumatic dislocations who had undergone arthrography, 43.5% had no rotator-cuff rupture, whereas 31.3% exhibited rupture without bone injury.[56] The average age of the group with rupture was 63 years compared with an average age of 45 years in the group without rupture. He believed that the condition of the rotator cuff determines the type of joint injury that is associated with traumatic dislocation.

Vascular Injury[66–68]

Although injury to the axillary artery occurs most frequently in the elderly patient who shows arteriosclerosis, it also may occur in the young patient as a result of excessive manipulation and traction of the extremity. Increasing numbers of this serious complication in the young person have been observed recently as a result of motorcycle accidents (see Fig. 25-6). The most common sites of injury are the second and third parts of the axillary artery where the vessel is fixed by the pectoralis minor. An aneurysm may form and there may be an avulsion of the axillary artery, or complete rupture may result. The axillary vein may be affected also.

The diagnosis should be suspected when there is persistent pain and severe swelling in the shoulder. A bruit may be heard over the site of an aneurysm. The extremity may become hypesthetic and even paralyzed. The radial pulse disappears with complete rupture, diminished circulation to the hand may cause cyanosis, and the extremity becomes cold. An arteriogram should be obtained to confirm the diagnosis, locate the exact site of injury, and determine the degree of injury to the vessel. Whenever possible, every effort should be made to repair the torn vessel to restore circulation to the distal parts. Restoration of the circulation to achieve an adequate blood flow distally is especially important in the elderly patient.

Nerve Injury[69–72]

Nerve injury is common with an incidence reported as 10.5% for acute dislocation and 2% for recurrent dislocation. Rowe reported a spontaneous recovery in 23 of 27 patients with nerve injury.[57] Merely examining for sensory distribution of the axillary nerve when injury is suspected is unreliable. Thus, if every patient seen for shoulder dislocation were carefully examined for nerve injury, the incidence of such complications would rise.

With an isolated nerve injury, the nerve recovers within weeks to months since the damage usually is transitory. The axillary nerve is injured most often. Downward traction may injure the axillary, radial, and musculocutaneous nerves. Increased internal and external rotation may increase the pull on the nerves and exacerbate the damage. The axillary nerve is especially vulnerable when it is stretched over the humeral head while the arm is hyperabducted during dislocation. Other nerves may be injured, including the ulnar and median nerves, or combinations of these, and the whole of the brachial plexus, particularly when the dislocation force has been severe (see Fig. 25-1). Multiple nerve injuries tend to be more severe and permanent.

Postoperative Complications

In an uncooperative patient, the soft-tissue repair may be disrupted, or the coracoid and its conjoined tendon may be pulled from its transplanted site. If the shoulder is immobilized for an extended period, a good result may still be achieved.

Postoperative infection may cause much functional loss and may even require subsequent arthrodesis procedure to rid the patient of pain.

Other complications include osteonecrosis and cartilage necrosis of the humeral head and late severe arthritis of the shoulder joint. In patients who develop such late complications, reconstructive procedures, including total shoulder replacement may become necessary.

Inferior Dislocation of the Glenohumeral Joint

Inferior dislocation of the glenohumeral joint is rare, but is more common than intrathoracic or superior dislocation of the glenohumeral joint. The top of the humeral head is displaced inferiorly as a result of a severe hyperabduction force. This force results in displacement of the humeral head beneath the glenoid fossa, leaving the diaphysis in a displaced overhead position. Motorcycle accidents may cause this injury (see Fig. 25-6).

During examination, the arm is pointed overhead and locked. Any attempt to move the extremity causes severe pain. The elbow is held in a flexed position with the forearm usually overhead. Neurovascular deficit is commonly present.

Closed reduction is carried out by traction in the upward and slightly outward position; countertraction is applied across the top of the shoulder with a sheet. If the inferior capsule is ruptured and closed reduction fails, open reduction should be accomplished. Although this injury is severe, excellent results still can be achieved.

Posterior Dislocation

Posterior dislocation of the shoulder is frequently missed and may go unrecognized for months or years. A missed diagnosis can be most disabling and its complications difficult to treat.

Rowe reported a 2% incidence in 500 cases,[73] and McLaughlin reported a 3.8% incidence in his series of 581 shoulder dislocations.[74] A true incidence probably would be closer to 5% if all the missed unreported cases were included.

The degree of posterior shoulder instability resulting from trauma depends on the amount of ligamentous tearing and the extent of healing. With poor soft-tissue healing, the patient experiences recurrent posterior dislocation merely by adducting and internally rotating the extremity into certain positions. The head may be displaced in the subacromial, subglenoid, or subspinous positions in posterior dislocation. The subacromial type of injury accounts for the vast majority of posterior dislocations wherein the humeral head lies behind the glenoid and below the acromion (Fig. 25-7).

Mechanism of Injury

The patient usually relates a history of an indirect force applied as a result of a fall on the outstretched hand that causes sudden internal rotation, adduction, and flexion of the arm. A posterior dislocation may be associated with epilepsy and other convulsive disorders. Associated severe injuries take precedence over the joint injury. The posterior dislocation may not be recognized because of trauma sustained when a force is applied directly to the front of the shoulder, thereby displacing the humeral head posteriorly.

Pathology and Pathogenesis

As in anterior dislocations, there is no single cause of posterior dislocations. Pathologic changes may or may not be associated with congenital abnormalities. Pathologic lesions that may be associated with posterior dislocation include detachment and laxity of the posterior part of the capsule, detachment or erosion of the posterior labrum (a reverse Bankart lesion), an impression defect in the anteromedial part of the humeral head, fracture of the posterior glenoid fossa, congenital defects of the glenoid fossa (excessive retrotilt), and excessive retroversion of the head of the humerus.[75] The lesser tuberosity may be avulsed with traumatic posterior dislocation.

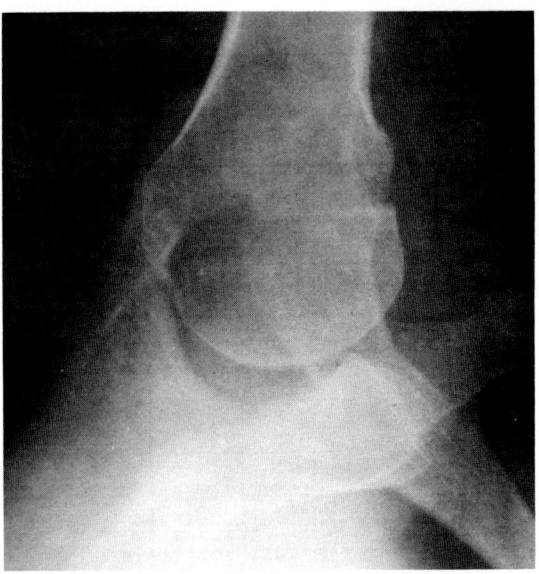

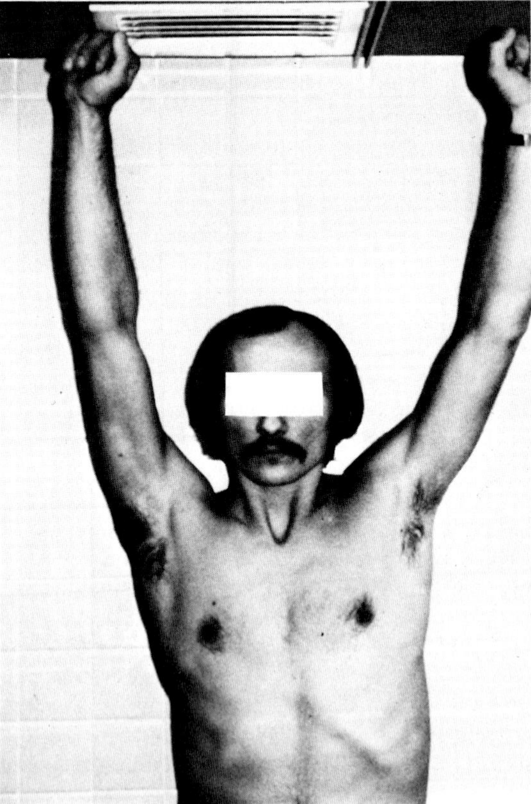

Fig. 25-7. *A*, A young adult sustained a chronic subglenoid posterior dislocation 21 months before this film was taken. Note the position of the humeral head behind the glenoid. *B*, Shoulder replacement or arthrodesis was not advised in view of the excellent motion and tolerable, mild-to-moderate pain with activity.

The subscapularis is stretched across the anterior glenoid rim during dislocation. The notched defect in the anteromedial humeral head results from impaction of the posterior glenoid rim against the spongy head of the humerus. Neurovascular deficit rarely results from posterior dislocation.

Diagnosis

To make a correct diagnosis, the physician must suspect the presence of a posterior dislocation of the shoulder. An inspection of both shoulders must be made because the shoulder contour in a posterior dislocation may appear normal if not compared to that of the opposite shoulder. In posterior dislocation, the anterior aspect of the shoulder is flattened, whereas the posterior portion may be prominent when viewed from behind. The coracoid may be more pronounced than usual and is palpated more easily, especially in the thin individual. The extremity is held in a fixed, neutral, internally rotated position with the arm adducted.[76] The arm cannot be abducted without increasing pain. In recurring posterior dislocation, however, there may be relatively little pain, especially in chronic dislocation.

Roentgenographic Interpretation[45,77]

Multiple roentgenograms, including an anteroposterior, lateral transthoracic, "Y", and modified axillary views, are all important in helping to evaluate posterior dislocation. The usual anteroposterior film does not reveal the maximum length of the anatomic neck. Since the extremity is held in the internally rotated position, little is revealed of the normal length of the anatomic neck. A significant finding is known as the "rim" sign. Here, the humeral head is rotated internally in posterior dislocation, and an increased space may be visible between the anterior glenoid rim and medial portion of the humeral head. A measurement of more than 6 mm between the medial aspect of the humeral head and the anterior glenoid rim is believed to occur only in posterior dislocation.[78] Fracture of the posterior glenoid, displacement of the posterior glenoid rim, and increased space may not be apparent during a cursory examination of the roentgenograms, even though a posterior dislocation exists. Another important finding of posterior dislocation in the anteroposterior film is the disappearance of a normal half-moon overlap. However, this finding is not pathognomonic since an angled projection of the normal shoulder may also show the disappearance of the overlap. The anteroposterior view may show the humeral head in the injured shoulder to be lower or higher than that of the normal shoulder. The true axillary view, "Y" view, and lateral transthoracic roentgenograms show the lesion and, when correctly interpreted, make the diagnosis of posterior dislocation quite clear.

Management

Mild and moderate sprains of the posterior shoulder joint can be treated like sprains of the anterior shoulder joint. Sling immobilization for 1 to 3 weeks is adequate treatment during the acute phase. In a severe sprain, such as an acute posterior shoulder dislocation, longer treatment is needed.

Acute Traumatic Posterior Dislocation

Successful reduction of an acute posterior dislocation requires relaxation of the surrounding shoulder muscles by general anesthesia or a slow intravenous injection of meperidine and hydroxyzine, as used for acute anterior dislocation. Excessive force must be avoided to obviate additional injury to the joint.

Gentle but firm traction is applied to the extremity while in the internally rotated, adducted position. The humeral head can be nudged and assisted over the posterior glenoid rim, if necessary. When the glenoid rim is locked into a notched defect on the anteromedial head of the humerus, gentle internal rotation of the arm with the elbow flexed can be added to the maneuver to unlock the head. Following reduction, the arm is rotated into approximately 50° of internal rotation to prevent backward slipping of the head. This position usually is the most stable and should be used. Thereafter, the patient should be placed in a plaster-of-paris shoulder cast to maintain position.

Chronic Unreduced Dislocation

When a posterior dislocation of the shoulder has been missed, the surgeon still may attempt closed reduction in a chronic unreduced shoulder dislocation as long as 2 to 4 weeks following injury. The longer the delay, the less likely that reduction can be achieved. Closed reduction fails after many months have passed. If open reduction is contemplated, one must be aware that the longer the delay in reduction, the more extensive must be the dissection of the surrounding scarred structures. If the patient does not have significant pain and is not significantly disabled, a long-standing posterior dislocation is best left alone, especially when an elderly, poor-risk patient experiences only minimal discomfort (Fig. 25-7). If the disability is great in a younger person, reconstruction, including a total shoulder replacement, may be performed.[53] Before arthrodesis is considered, the patient should be advised that limited mobility of the shoulder will result.

Acromioclavicular Joint

The acromioclavicular joint is commonly injured, and the main question is whether to treat the injury surgically or conservatively. If an operative method is decided upon, the procedure that is best for the patient is selected.

Allman classified sprains of the acromioclavicular joint into grades I, II, and III.[1] Grade I sprains result from a mild force with tearing only of a few fibers of the acromioclavicular ligament and capsule. There is no joint instability. Grade II sprains result from a moderate force that causes rupture of the capsule and acromioclavicular ligament and often causes a subluxation. The coracoclavicular ligament is not ruptured. Grade III sprains of the joint result from severe force that ruptures both the acromioclavicular and coracoclavicular ligaments. This injury produces a dislocation of the acromioclavicular joint.

Mechanism of Injury

Injury to the acromioclavicular joint usually results from a fall onto the point of the shoulder. The severity of the injury is determined by the amount of force that causes a sudden depression of the shoulder tip with the arm in slight internal rotation and abduction.[79,80] When the scapula is depressed suddenly and pulls the attached clavicle through the supensory coracoclavicular ligament, the medial part of the clavicle strikes the first rib, thereby causing an opposing resistance and concentration of force at the acromioclavicular and coracoclavicular ligament. The meniscus may be torn during dislocation.

Indirect force resulting in acromioclavicular injury may be caused by a transmitted force from a fall on the elbow or outstretched hand that forces the humeral head against the undersurface of the acromion.[81]

Rarely, a posterior displacement of the lateral clavicle may occur following a blow to the distal end of the clavicle or may result following closed treatment during which a superior dislocation is converted to a posterior displacement.

Diagnosis

The patient points to the area of pain at the acromioclavicular joint. The pain usually is local, and its severity relates to the degree of injury. The arm is commonly splinted at the side, and any movement increases the pain over the joint region.

Physical examination may show a swelling, abrasion, or deformity over the acromioclavicular joint. Local tenderness is present in grade I injuries, whereas exquisite tenderness is present in grade III injuries. Tenderness may also be present over the coracoid and in the lateral infraclavicular regions.

Anteroposterior roentgenograms should be taken, preferably with the patient in the standing or sitting position. This view may show widening of the joint space, subluxation, or complete dislocation.[79,82] There may be associated fractures of the acromion, coracoid, or lateral clavicle. If there is any question as to the grade of injury, a 5- to 10-pound weight should be suspended from the wrists and identical anteroposterior views taken of both acromioclavicular joints. If an operation is planned that requires an intact coracoid process for the placement of a loop or suture, polyester synthetic tape, or screw from the clavicle to the coracoid, the surgeon must first determine that there is no fracture of the coracoid and that the bone is not osteoporotic.

Management

Closed Methods of Grades I and II Sprains

Once the correct diagnosis is established, grade I sprains should be protected until most of the pain has subsided. Ice packs may be applied as tolerated to the injured joint for relief of pain in the first 24 hours, and warm packs may be applied thereafter. A sling support is used for 4 to 10 days, depending on the symptoms. Thereafter, a gradual increase in activities is allowed. Full activities are not permitted for several weeks, even if there is a full range of painless motion early.

Grade II sprains are immobilized for as many as 3 weeks. A variety of splints, harnesses, braces, and halters, as well as various adhesive taping methods have been recommended.[1,81,83–87] When conservative methods and an axillary pad are employed, the surgeon must be sure that a neurapraxia of the nerves in the high medial arm does not result. Adhesive taping treatment often causes irritation and excoriation of the skin, which may prevent completion of closed treatment methods. The Kenny Howard type of sling-halter works satisfactorily in a cooperative patient. After 3 weeks, immobilization is stopped, and gentle motion exercises are started, depending on the symptoms and the type of activity.

Grade III dislocations can be treated by closed methods if the patient can tolerate 6 to 8 weeks of conservative treatment.[88,89] The patient must be examined frequently and the reduction confirmed by roentgenograms taken periodically. For patients who cannot tolerate strap devices or in whom conservative treatment is not effective, open methods may be needed.

The main goal of any treatment is to achieve stability of a healed joint that is painless and has full motion. A number of procedures have been recommended and may be divided into coracoclavicular ligament repair, fixation or reconstruction,[78–80,90–93] acromioclavicular joint repair, internal fixation or reconstruction,[1,90,94–97] dynamic muscle transfers,[98–100] and excision of the lateral clavicle.[90,92,101–104]

An especially good method for holding the clavicle in a reduced position is that described by Harrison and Sisler in which the synthetic polyester tube or tape is placed through a hole in the clavicle and looped about the coracoid process.[105] Bosworth described his technique of holding a clavicle in a reduced position by placing a screw through the superior clavicle into the coracoid below.[82] Whatever method is employed, a torn meniscus should be removed from the acromioclavicular joint, and the torn deltoid trapezius aponeurosis should be repaired. The use of one or two smooth wires introduced across the joint in a retrograde manner may be dangerous (Fig. 25-8). The ends of the pins must be bent to avoid migration, and roentgenograms must be taken to confirm proper positioning of the pins. A number of open methods have been described in detail.

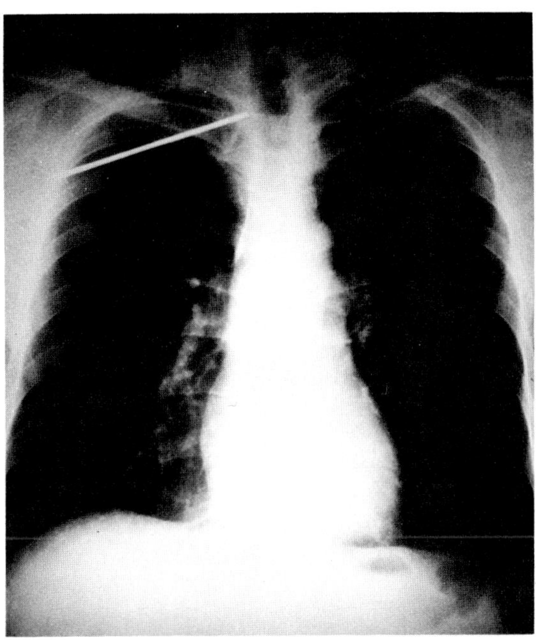

Fig. 25-8. Two threaded pins, which were not bent at the end, were used to stabilize a grade III left acromioclavicular dislocation. Two weeks later, the patient complained of fever and a cough. Note the migration of one pin into the right chest cavity. The problem was resolved with a thoracotomy. Meanwhile, the acromioclavicular dislocation healed in a dislocated position. There was no functional loss of motion and only slight discomfort.

Complications

Numerous complications after treatment of acromioclavicular joint injuries have been reported.[1,81,82,86,93,102,106] In closed methods, various complications, including deformity, degenerative arthritis, residual subluxation with or without symptoms, calcification of soft tissues, skin irritation and ulcers from joint stiffness and decreased function, may result. Complications seen with open methods include wound infection, traumatic arthritis, soft-tissue calcification, metal failure, migration of pins, loosening of the screw, inadequate reduction, iatrogenic fracture, residual deformity, pain, weakness, loss of motion, poor cosmetic scar, and anesthetic complications.

There is clearly no one best treatment. The injury of each patient must be assessed carefully and the appropriate method of treatment selected.

References

1. Allman, F. L.: Fractures and ligamentous injuries of the clavicle and its articulation. J. Bone Joint Surg., *49-A*:774, 1967.
2. Neer, C. S.: Fractures of the distal third of the clavicle. Clin. Orthop., *58*:43, 1968.

3. Weiner, D. S., and O'Dell, H. W.: Fractures of the first rib associated with injuries to the clavicle. J. Trauma, *9*:412, 1969.
4. Young, C. S.: The mechanisms of ambulatory treatment of fractures of the clavicle. J. Bone Joint Surg., *13*:299, 1931.
5. Howard, F. M., and Shafer, S. J.: Injuries to the clavicle with neurovascular complications. J. Bone Joint Surg., *47-A*:1335, 1965.
6. Jablon, M., Sutker, A., and Post, M.: Irreducible fracture of the middle third of the clavicle. J. Bone Joint Surg., *61-A*:296, 1979.
7. Miller, D. S., and Boswick, J. A.: Lesions of the brachial plexus associated with fractures of the clavicle. Clin. Orthop., *64*:144, 1969.
8. Neer, C. S.: Nonunion of the clavicle. J.A.M.A., *172*:1006, 1960.
9. Rowe, C. R.: An atlas of anatomy and treatment of midclavicular fractures. Clin. Orthop., *58*:29, 1968.
10. Sakellarides, H.: Pseudarthrosis of the clavicle. J. Bone Joint Surg., *43-A*:130, 1961.
11. Lee, H. G.: Treatment of fracture of the clavicle by internal nail fixation. N. Engl. J. Med., *234*:222, 1946.
12. Murray, G.: A method of fixation for fracture of the clavicle. J. Bone Joint Surg., *22*:616, 1940.
13. Penn, I.: The vascular complications of fractures of the clavicle. J. Trauma, *4*:819, 1964.
14. Lusskin, R., Weiss, C. A., and Winer, J.: The role of the subclavius muscle in the subclavian vein syndrome (costoclavicular syndrome) following fracture of the clavicle: A case report with a review of the pathophysiology of the costoclavicular space. Clin. Orthop., *54*:75, 1967.
15. Aston, J. W., and Gregory, C. F.: Dislocation of the shoulder with significant fracture of the glenoid. J. Bone Joint Surg., *55-A*:1531, 1973.
16. Bonnin, J. G.: A Complete Outline of Fractures. New York, Grune & Stratton, 1946.
17. Cooper, A.: Lectures on Principles and Practice of Surgery. 3rd Edition. Boston, Lilly & Walt, 1831.
18. Key, J. A., and Conwell, H. E.: Fracture, Dislocations and Sprains. 5th Edition. St. Louis, C.V. Mosby, 1951.
19. McLaughlin, H. L.: Trauma. Philadelphia, W. B. Saunders, 1959.
20. Imatani, R. J.: Fractures of the scapula: A review of 53 fractures. J. Trauma, *15*:473, 1975.
21. McGahan, J. P., Rab, G. T., and Dublin, A.: Fractures of the scapula. J. Trauma, *20*:880, 1980.
22. Nettrour, L. F., Krufky, E. L., Mueller, R. E., and Raycroft, J. F.: Locked scapula: Intrathoracic dislocation of the inferior angle. A case report. J. Bone Joint Surg., *54-A*:413, 1972.
23. Köhler, A., and Zimmer, E. A.: Borderlines of the Normal and Early Pathologic Skeletal Roentgenology. 3rd Edition. New York, Grune & Stratton, 1968.
24. Liberson, F.: Os acromiale-contested anomaly. J. Bone Joint Surg., *19*:683, 1937.
25. Kummel, B. M.: Fractures of the glenoid causing chronic dislocation of the shoulder. Clim. Orthop., *69*:189, 1970.
26. Benton, J., and Nelson, C.: Avulsion of the coracoid process in an athlete. J. Bone Joint Surg., *53-A*:356, 1971.
27. Landoff, B. A.: Hitherto undescribed injury of the coracoid process. Acta Clin. Scand., *89*:401, 1943.
28. Boyer, D. W.: Trapshooter's shoulder: Stress fracture of the coracoid process. J. Bone Joint Surg., *57-A*:862, 1975.
29. Protass, J. J., Stampfli, F. W., and Osmer, J. C.: Coracoid process fracture diagnosis in acromioclavicular separation. Radiology, *116*:61, 1975.
30. Laing, P. G.: The arterial supply of the adult humerus. J. Bone Joint Surg., *38-A*:1105, 1956.
31. Codman, E. A.: The Shoulder. Boston, Thomas Todd, 1934.
32. Roberts, S. M.: Fractures of the upper end of the humerus. An end result study which shows the advantage of early active motion. J.A.M.A., *98*:367, 1932.
33. Sever, J. W.: Fracture of the head of the humerus. Treatment and results. N. Engl. J. Med., *216*:1100, 1937.
34. Neer, C. S., II: Displaced proximal humeral fractures, Part I. Classification and evaluation. J. Bone Joint Surg., *52-A*:1077, 1970.
35. Neer, C. S. , II.: Displaced proximal humeral fractures, Part II. Treatment of the three-part and four-part displacement. J. Bone Joint Surg., *52-A*:1090, 1970.
36. Baker, D. M., and Leach, R. F.: Fracture-dislocation of the shoulder. Report of three unusual cases with rotator cuff avulsion. J. Trauma, *5*:659, 1965.
37. Hoyt, W. A.: Etiology of shoulder injuries in athletes. J. Bone Joint Surg., *49-A*:755, 1967.
38. DePalma, A. F., and Cantilli, R. A.: Fractures of the upper end of the humerus. Clin. Orthop., *20*:73, 1961.
39. Bell, H. M.: Posterior fracture-dislocation of the shoulder. A method of closed reduction. J. Bone Joint Surg., *47-A*:1521, 1965.
40. Michaelis, L. S.: Comminuted fracture-dislocation of the shoulder. J. Bone Joint Surg., *26*:363, 1944.
41. Knight, R. A., and Mayne, J. A.: Comminuted fractures and fracture-dislocation involving the articular surfaces of the humeral head. J. Bone Joint Surg., *39-A*:1343, 1957.
42. Baker, L. D.: The Nicola operation: A simplified technique. J. Bone Joint Surg., *22*:118, 1940.
43. Kraulis, J., and Hunter, G.: The results of prosthetic replacement in fracture-dislocation of the upper end of the humerus. Injury, *8*:129, 1976.
44. Post, M.: Fractures of the upper humerus. Orthop. Clin. North Am., *11*:239, 1980.
45. Post, M.: The Shoulder: Surgical and Nonsurgical Management. Philadelphia, Lea & Febiger, 1978.
46. Dewar, F. P., and Yabsley, R. H.: Fracture-dislocation of the shoulder. Report of a case. J. Bone Joint Surg., *49-B*:540, 1967.
47. Prillaman, H. A., and Thompson, R. C.: Bilateral posterior fracture-dislocation of the shoulder. J. Bone Joint Surg., *51-A*:1627, 1969.
48. Shaw, J. L.: Bilateral posterior fracture-dislocation of the shoulder and other trauma caused by convulsive seizures. J. Bone Joint Surg., *53-A*:1327, 1971.
49. Chattapadhyaya, T.: Posterior fracture-dislocation of the shoulder. J. Bone Joint Surg., *52-B*:521, 1970.
50. McLaughlin, H.: Trauma. Philadelphia, W. B. Saunders, 1959.
51. McLaughlin, H. L.: Posterior dislocation of the shoulder, J. Bone Joint Surg., *34-A*:584, 1952.
52. Post, M., Jablon, M., Miller, H., and Singh, M.: Constrained total shoulder joint replacement: A critical review. Clin. Orthop., *144*:135, 1979.

53. Post, M., Haskell, S. S., and Jablon, M.: Total shoulder replacement with a constrained prosthesis. J. Bone Joint Surg., *62-A*:327, 1980.
54. Aufranc, O. E., Jones, W. N., and Turner, R. H.: Bilateral shoulder fracture-dislocation, J.A.M.A., *195*:1140, 1966.
55. Perthes, G.: Über Operationen bei Habituell Schulterluxation. Deutsch. Ztschr. Chir., *85*:199, 1906.
56. Pettersson, G.: Rupture of the tendon aponeurosis of the shoulder joint in anterio-inferior dislocation. A study on the origin. Acta Chir. Scand., Vol. 10 (Suppl.), *77*:1, 1942.
57. Rowe, C. R.: Anterior dislocation of the shoulder. Surg. Clin. North Am., *43*:1609, 1963.
58. Moseley, H. F.: The basic lesions of recurrent anterior dislocation. Surg. Clin. North Am., *43*:1631, 1963.
59. DePalma, A. F.: Recurrent dislocation of the shoulder joint. Ann. Surg., *132*:1052, 1950.
60. DePalma, A. F.: Factors influencing the choice of a modified Magnuson procedure for recurrent anterior dislocation of the shoulder—with a note on technique. Surg. Clin. North Am., *43*:1647, 1963.
61. DePalma, A. F., Cooke, A. J., and Prabhakar, M.: The role of the subscapularis in recurrent anterior dislocation of the shoulder. Clin. Orthop. *54*:35, 1967.
62. Reeves, B.: Experiments on the tensile strength of the anterior capsular structures of the shoulder region. J. Bone Joint Surg., *50-B*:858, 1965.
63. Symeonides, P. O.: The significance of the subscapularis muscles in the pathogenesis of recurrent anterior dislocation of the shoulder. J. Bone Joint Surg., *54-A*:476, 1972.
64. Hill, H. A., and Sachs, M. D.: The grooved defect of the humeral head. A frequently unrecognized complication of dislocations of the shoulder joint. Radiology, *35*:690, 1940.
65. Reeves, B.: Arthrography of the shoulder. J. Bone Joint Surg., *48-B*:424, 1966.
66. Brown, F. W., and Navigato, W. J.: Rupture of the axillary artery and brachial plexus palsy associated with anterior dislocation of the shoulder. Clin. Orthop., *60*:195, 1968.
67. Curr, J. F.: Rupture of the axillary artery complicating dislocation of the shoulder. J. Bone Joint Surg., *52-B*:313, 1970.
68. Jardon, O. M., Hood, L. T., and Lynch, R. D.: Complete avulsion of the axillary artery as a complication of shoulder dislocation. J. Bone Joint Surg., *55*:189, 1973.
69. Barnes, R.: Traction injuries of the brachial plexus in adults. J. Bone Joint Surg., *31-B*:10, 1949.
70. Bonney, G.: Prognosis in traction injuries of the brachial plexus. J. Bone Joint Surg., *41-B*:4, 1959.
71. Gariepy, R., Derome, A., and Laurin, C. A.: Brachial plexus paralysis following shoulder dislocation. Can. J. Surg., *5*:418, 1962.
72. Milton, G. W.: The mechanism of circumflex and other nerve injuries in dislocation of the shoulder and the possible mechanism of nerve injuries during reduction of dislocation. Aust. N. Z. J. Surg., *23*:25, 1953.
73. Rowe, C. R.: Prognosis in dislocations of the shoulder. J. Bone Joint Surg., *38-A*:957, 1956.
74. McLaughlin, H. D.: Posterior dislocation of the shoulder. J. Bone Joint Surg., *34-A*:584, 1952.
75. Nobel, W.: Posterior traumatic dislocation of the shoulder. J. Bone Joint Surg., *44-A*:523, 1962.
76. McLaughlin, H. D.: Locked posterior subluxation of the shoulder—diagnosis and treatment. Surg. Clin. North Am., *43*:1621, 1963.
77. Arndt, J. H., and Sears, A. D.: Posterior dislocation of the shoulder. Am. J. Roentgenol., *94*:639, 1965.
78. Alldredge, R. H.: Surgical treatment of acromioclavicular dislocation. J. Bone Joint Surg., *47-A*:1278, 1965.
79. Bearden, J. M., Hughston, J. C., and Whatley, G. S.: Acromioclavicular dislocation: method of treatment. J. Sports Med., *1*:5, 1973.
80. Brosgol, M.: Traumatic acromioclavicular sprains and subluxation. Clin. Orthop., *20*:98, 1961.
81. Urist, M. R.: Complete dislocation of the acromioclavicular joint. The nature of the traumatic lesion and effective methods of treatment with an analysis of 41 cases. J. Bone Joint Surg., *28*:836, 1946.
82. Bosworth, B. M.: Acromioclavicular separation. New method of repair. Surg. Gynecol. Obstet., *73*:866, 1941.
83. Giannestras, N. J.: A method of immobilization of acute acromioclavicular separation. J. Bone Joint Surg., *26*:597, 1944.
84. Gibbens, M. E.: An appliance for conservative treatment of acromioclavicular dislocation. J. Bone Joint Surg., *28*:164, 1946.
85. Jordon, H. H.: An improved abduction splint for the upper extremity. J. Bone Joint Surg., *26*:600, 1944.
86. Kennedy, J. C., and Cameron, H.: Complete dislocation of the acromioclavicular joint. J. Bone Joint Surg., *36-B*:202, 1954.
87. Spigelman, L.: A harness for acromioclavicular separation. J. Bone Joint Surg., *51-A*:585, 1969.
88. Arner, O., Sandahl, U., and Ohrling, H.: Dislocation of the acromioclavicular joint—Review of the literature and report of 56 cases. Acta Chir. Scand., *113*:140, 1957.
89. Quigley, T. B.: Injuries to the acromioclavicular and sternoclavicular joints sustained in athletics. Surg. Clin. North Am., *43*:1151, 1963.
90. Bateman, J. E.: Athletic injuries about the shoulder in throwing and body-contact sports. Clin. Orthop., *23*:75, 1962.
91. Laing, P. G.: Transplantation of the long head of the biceps in complete acromioclavicular separations. J. Bone Joint Surg., *36-B*:202, 1954.
92. Mumford, E. B.: Acromioclavicular dislocation. J. Bone Joint Surg., *23*:799, 1951.
93. Wilson, F. C., Jr., and Prothero, S. R.: Results of operative treatment of acute dislocation of the acromioclavicular joint. J. Trauma, *7*:202, 1967.
94. Ahstrom, J. P., Jr.: Surgical repair of complete acromioclavicular separation. J.A.M.A., *217*:785, 1971.
95. Bundens, W. D., and Cook, J. I.: Repair of acromioclavicular separations by deltoid-trapezius imbrication. Clin. Orthop., *20*:109, 1961.
96. Moshein, J., and Elconin, K. B.: Repair of acute acromioclavicular dislocation, utilizing the coracoacromial ligament. J. Bone Joint Surg., *51-A*:812, 1969.
97. Neviaser, J. S.: Acromioclavicular dislocation treated by transference of the coracoacromial ligament. Clin. Orthop., *58*:57, 1968.
98. Bailey, R. W.: A dynamic repair for complete acromioclavicular joint dislocation. J. Bone Joint Surg., *47-A*:858, 1965.

99. Bailey, R. W., O'Connor, G. A., Tilus, P. D., and Baril, J. D.: A dynamic repair of acute and chronic injuries of the acromioclavicular area. J. Bone Joint Surg., *54-A*:1802, 1972.
100. Dewar, F. P., and Barrington, T. W.: The treatment of chronic acromioclavicular dislocation. J. Bone Joint Surg., *47-B*:32, 1965.
101. Gurd, F. B.: The treatment of complete dislocation of the outer end of the clavicle. An hitherto undescribed operation. Ann. Surg., *113*:1094, 1941.
102. Lazcano, M. A., Anzel, S. H., and Kelly, P. J.: Complete dislocation and subluxation of the acromioclavicular joint. End results in 73 cases. J. Bone Joint Surg., *43-A*:379, 1961.
103. Moseley, H. F., and Templeton, J.: Dislocation of acromioclavicular dislocation, utilizing the coracoacromial ligament. J. Bone Joint Surg., *51-B*:196, 1969.
104. Weitzman, G.: Treatment of acute acromioclavicular joint dislocation by a modified Bosworth method. J. Bone Joint Surg., *49-A*:1167, 1967.
105. Harrison, W. E., and Sisler, J.: Acromioclavicular separation treated by Dacron vascular graft loop beneath the coracoid and through the clavicle. Scientific Exhibit, American Academy of Orthopaedic Surgeons, Dallas, TX, Jan., 1974.
106. Norrell, H., and Llewellyn, R. C.: Migration of a threaded Steinmann's pin from an acromioclavicular joint into the spinal canal. A case report. J. Bone Joint Surg., *47-A*:1024, 1965.

Chapter 26 Complex Fractures of the Elbow

ROBY D. MIZE
BERND F. CLAUDI

The elbow joint is the most complicated major joint in the body, both anatomically and functionally. It is comprised of three major long bones, which function as two joints. The spool-shaped trochlea of the humerus articulates with the olecranon notch of the ulna providing flexion-extension movements, strength, and stability to the elbow. The spherical capitellum of the humerus articulates with the disc-shaped head of the radius to provide the unique pronation-supination motion so critical for the fine dexterous functions of the hand. The proximal ulna articulates with the proximal radius primarily to facilitate pronation and supination. These unique structural and functional aspects leave the elbow joint vulnerable to injury. There is almost always some permanent loss of motion following severe injuries. Fortunately, the elbow can function quite well with limitations in flexion and extension. The loss of pronation or supination can be compensated for by humeral abduction and adduction.

Although periarticular fractures of the elbow joint account for only about 6% of all fractures treated,[1,2] they nevertheless usually present serious problems in management. The prognosis is related to the mechanism of injury, general characteristics of the fracture, associated injuries, and age of the patient. Complex injuries of the elbow include intra-articular fractures with involvement of the distal humerus and/or the proximal forearm, severely comminuted fractures with defect of the supracondylar humeral area, fractures and/or fracture-dislocations of the proximal forearm, fractures, and/or dislocations associated with neurovascular damage, and open fractures with varying degrees of soft-tissue damage.

Because complex elbow injuries occur infrequently, few surgeons have sufficient individual experience to enable them to evaluate methods of treatment critically. The final decision regarding the form of treatment used depends on the results the surgeon believes he can reasonably achieve with his skills in his institution. Regardless of technique, the surgeon must be accurate and decisive in the initial evaluation and management of these difficult injuries. Failure to institute an appropriate treatment usually leaves the patient with some permanent functional impairment.

Methods of Treatment

As in other areas of orthopaedic traumatology, there is some controversy regarding optimum treatment of complex elbow injuries. There are basically two schools of thought concerning management: those who favor closed management and those who favor surgical treatment. The ultimate aim of both forms of treatment should be the restoration of the injured elbow to the best possible function without residual deformity.

Closed (Nonoperative)

For many years, Sir Reginald Watson-Jones was the primary influence on fracture management in the United States as well as in parts of

Europe.[3] He was vehemently opposed to any form of operative treatment for elbow injuries. He condemned operative treatment because "adhesions of the triceps, contracture of the capsule, avascular necrosis of loose fragments, and the irritative reaction of metallic foreign bodies contribute to dense adhesion formation and permanent stiffness."[3] Other authors argued against operative treatment because of additional soft-tissue damage superimposed on that already produced by the fracture.[4–6] The propagation of nonoperative treatment of elbow fractures was supported by numerous other well-respected surgeons of that time.[7–10]

The methods of nonoperative treatment include: (1) closed reduction and plaster immobilization, (2) traction, and (3) "bag-of-bones" or collar-and-cuff technique.

1. Closed manipulation and application of a plaster cast are limited as an appropriate method since the vast majority of complex fractures of the elbow have little intrinsic stability because the muscles produce persistent displacement of the fracture fragments. The closed method of treatment often requires extremes in positioning to achieve and maintain adequate reduction. In addition, elbow motion is difficult to regain following a long period of immobilization.

2. There are numerous advocates of skeletal traction with or without manipulative reduction.[5,6,8,11–13] The objective is to align the fracture fragments slowly over a period of a few days to several weeks. The traction device must be inspected and frequently readjusted by the attending physician. Furthermore, this method requires repeated x-ray controls during a lengthy hospitalization. The patient's mobility during this time is severely hampered while attempting to maintain the reduction. Paradoxically, patients who are poor candidates for surgery, e.g., the elderly patient, the uncooperative patient, patients with severe head injuries, or patients with multiple-system injuries, also are unable to tolerate the prolonged bed rest required with this method. Temporary skeletal traction may be indicated in the patient with contaminated or infected soft tissues or in the patient with massive swelling of the upper extremity. Skeletal traction is often abandoned because of inability to achieve or to maintain acceptable reduction at a time when open treatment is made more difficult technically because of soft-tissue contractures and partial healing of the fracture. If surgery is undertaken as a secondary measure several days or weeks after injury, the often irritated pin sites can also increase the risk of infection. Effectiveness of skin traction is limited, as only 5 to 7 pounds of traction can be tolerated over a short period of time.

3. In England during the 1930s, Eastwood popularized the "bag-of-bones" technique,[9] in which the arm is placed in a collar and cuff and the elbow hangs free in as much flexion as possible. The underlying principle makes use of the force of gravity in allowing the fracture fragments to settle into alignment. Perhaps the only indication for this type of technique is in the elderly patient with marked osteoporosis or massive comminution in whom internal fixation has a higher rate of failure because of soft bone quality. In these patients, however, early motion is nevertheless strongly desired. These patients cannot tolerate prolonged traction and bed rest. This technique allows for immediate hand and finger motion.

Open (Operative)

The treatment of fractures by open reduction and internal fixation in North America began in an attempt to treat disabling nonunions and malunions that occurred as a result of closed methods of treatment.[14] In recent years, the trend has moved toward a more aggressive surgical approach to complex fractures. Much of the widespread interest has resulted from the work of the Association for Study of Internal Fixation (ASIF) Group from Switzerland.[15–17] Their basic principles for successful results with open reduction and internal fixation include anatomic reduction of the fracture, atraumatic technique on soft tissue as well as bone, rigid internal fixation, and early active postoperative mobilization of the injured limb. Advocates of this method feel that stable internal fixation performed by an experienced surgeon offers the most successful results, shortens the treatment time, and decreases the incidence of significant permanent disability.

Our attention in this chapter will be focused primarily on open reduction and internal fixation as the preferred method of treatment for almost all the complex fractures of the elbow. Thus, more detail will be given to this mode of treatment in the interest of brevity rather than bias.

Fractures of the Distal Humerus

Distal humeral fractures are seen more commonly in children than in adults. These injuries almost always present serious problems in management. According to Miller,[18] the severity of this type of fracture makes the incidence of these cases seem greater than it is in actuality. He found fewer than ten of these fractures per year at his hospital. Other authors with active trauma services report an average incidence of only four or five cases of distal humeral fractures per year.[1,19] This type of fracture in the adult was seen most often in the middle-age and elderly patient.[18] In these age groups, precipitating trauma usually is not severe. The patient may simply fall directly on the elbow, forearm, or the outstretched hand. The extent of damage is often disproportionate to the degree of trauma. Our experience shows that these fractures occur more often in patients of the younger generation, who are more prone to serious injuries, such as motor-vehicle accidents or falls from a height. The mechanism of injury involves complex forces; usually the wedge-shaped crest of the proximal arm strikes the waist of the spool-shaped trochlea, thereby splitting and separating the condyles.

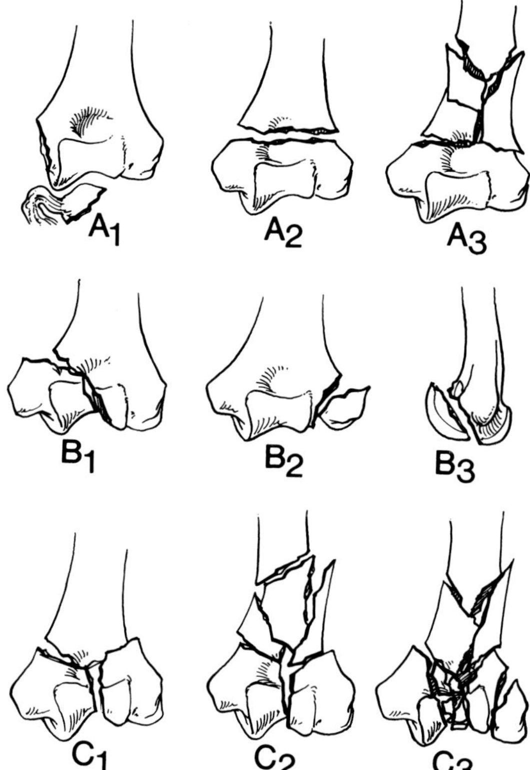

Fig. 26-1. Classification of distal humeral fractures according to M. E. Mueller. The fractures are split into three groups, each of which is subdivided from 1 through 3 according to the severity of the fracture pattern. Group A presents extra-articular fractures. In group B, unicondylar intra-articular fractures are gathered. Group C contains bicondylar intra-articular fractures with all different types of bone damage.

Classification

As with most types of complex fractures, it is difficult to apply a simple anatomic classification to distal humeral fractures. The classification by Mueller and associates seems to be the most comprehensive (Fig. 26-1).[16] When formulating a plan of treatment for these elbow injuries, all the following characteristics must be considered: bone quality (osteoporosis), associated neurovascular damage, extent and degree of soft-tissue damage, and presence of concomitant ipsilateral fractures.

Treatment Options

Treatment of distal humeral fractures should be individualized. One treatment that may work well in an adult may be highly inappropriate for a child or an elderly patient. There are advantages and disadvantages to each of the treatment modalities previously described and strong advocates of each.

Closed reduction and plaster immobilization are not recommended, as the vast majority of the distal humeral fractures have little intrinsic stability. Maintaining the reduction requires almost full extension in plaster. Elbow motion following immobilization and extension is difficult to regain. Evans recommended restoration of the articular surface by fixing the split condyles with a screw through a medial or lateral incision and then treating the supracondylar component in traction or closed manipulation and external immobilization.[10] Although this technique is still used by many surgeons, it should not be recommended any more. It combines the major disadvantages of both open and closed treatment by exposing the patient to infection and additional tissue trauma while preventing early motion of the joint, thereby increasing the risk of stiffness, muscle atrophy, and disuse osteoporosis (fracture disease). Evans reported good results in 5 of 6 patients, but 3 of the 5 good results were in patients less than 15 years of age.

Numerous authors support internal fixation for fractures of the distal humerus.[16,20–28] The recent study by Horne,[28a] however, reported better results with closed rather than open management. Although ASIF instruments were used in his series, the basic objectives of anatomic reduction and stable fixation were not achieved, thereby necessitating prolonged postoperative immobilization. Horne's work clearly demonstrates that the availability and use of excellent equipment do not ensure good results. It rather emphasizes the difficulty in application of the principles of internal fixation to these fractures.

Definitive Indications for Open Reduction and Internal Fixation

Providing the surgeon has the necessary facilities and the supporting staff, experience, and surgical skills, and there are no general medical contraindications for surgery, the following are definitive indications for internal fixation of fractures of the distal humerus:

1. Displaced intra-articular fractures.
2. Fractures with associated neurovascular injuries.
3. Open periarticular fractures.
4. Fracture-dislocations of the elbow.
5. Defect fractures of the supracondylar humerus.
6. Fractures associated with other ipsilateral fractures.
7. Periarticular elbow fractures in multiply injured patients.

Relative Indications for Open Reduction and Internal Fixation

Relative indications for internal fixation in distal humeral fractures may be given in elderly patients or seriously contaminated open fractures. Advanced age in itself should not be regarded as a contraindication to surgery. On the contrary, elderly patients need reliable fracture fixation allowing for postoperative mobilization as early as possible. Therefore, open reduction and internal fixation should be performed within hours after injury whenever possible. The necessary evaluation of each individual patient, however, must consider such characteristics as quality of bone, degree of comminution, and general status of the patient. If the surgery is not feasible, the treatment of choice should be to apply a collar and cuff in an attempt at early motion.

Seriously contaminated open fractures, particularly those referred for a delayed operative procedure, usually present their own problems. If thorough debridement and cleansing of the infection can be obtained, internal fixation with minimal application of hardware might be regarded as the appropriate treatment, e.g., an open contaminated intra-articular fracture that needs an early restoration of the articular surface by means of lag-screw fixation or by means of Kirschner wire pinning. In such situations, an additional temporary fixation device is needed to improve the healing conditions of both the soft tissues and the bone. To serve that function best, we strongly recommend the use of an external fixation device in combination with minimal internal fixation.

The application of an external fixation device in general presents a demanding operative technique. Its use must be handled in a most flexible manner, since its mechanics have to be adapted permanently to the actual needs of the course of soft-tissue and bone healing. According to Schatzker[29] and others, external fixation devices serve best when applied only as temporary devices. As soon as soft tissues and bone allow for further procedures, such as additional internal or external supporting fixation (e.g., a customized orthotic device), the external fixation device should be removed. Chapman and Mahoney argue against the use of external fixation devices in the upper extremity because the pins tend to tie down the forearm musculature, thus hampering the rehabilitation of the hand.[30] We believe an external fixation device is an excellent *temporary* device for patients with a severe open fracture associated with marked soft-tissue loss or contamination, periarticular fractures, fractures with severe neurovascular damage, burns, or shotgun fractures.

Although treatment of open fractures by open reduction and internal fixation remains controversial, we are convinced that this technique is the best prophylaxis against infection. The technique, however, requires critical surgical judgment and compulsive postoperative care. Rittmann and co-workers[17] achieved excellent functional results using internal fixation or a combination of external fixation and minimal internal fixation in patients with open fractures. Chapman[30,31] and others[15,32,33] also have emphasized the importance of immediate internal fixation in open fractures, in most intra-articular fractures, in patients with massive trauma or multiple-system injury, and in the elderly patient. For an open injury that can be debrided adequately, we prefer to perform internal fixation as an emergency procedure. Regardless of the method of fixation, meticulous wound debridement remains the cornerstone of successful open-fracture treatment. In severe open fractures with extensive loss of soft tissues, soft-tissue contamination, or associated serious neurovascular damage, burns, or gunshot injuries, we believe in temporary application of external fixation devices. When deciding whether to perform a primary elbow fusion, one should always consider the advantages of applying an external fixation device as a temporary device first, thus allowing for the overall rehabilitation instead of rushing into a surgical procedure that cannot be undone. In general, a fusion should not be regarded as the optimal primary treatment.

Contraindications for Open Reduction and Internal Fixation

In general, surgery is difficult to perform in the elderly, fragile patient with severe osteoporosis and massive comminution. These fractures often are impossible to fix regardless of the surgeon's skill; when these fractures are treated late, it is almost always impossible to get enough purchase in the brittle bone. Internal fixation is not advised when the soft tissues are seriously contaminated as, for example, in the shotgun wound or the burn patient. Although skeletal traction may be used in these patients, we prefer to use an external fixation device to immobilize the fracture site, thus facilitating general care of the soft tissues.

Our Preferred Method

As already outlined, we prefer internal stabilization of complex fractures of the distal humerus unless there is some contraindication to surgery. Following the basic principles of ASIF technique, we aim for early postoperative active mobilization of the elbow joint. We believe such mobilization can be obtained in the majority of these difficult injuries. The patient should be appraised of the potential hazards and complications of both open and closed methods of treatment and should participate in the decision for treatment whenever possible.

Preoperative Planning

Thorough preoperative planning is essential for a successful result in the complex elbow fracture. Complete sets of small- and large-fragment instruments and implants should be available prior to surgery.[16,34] We have found the small-fragment set to be ideal for fixing the uniquely shaped distal humerus. The preoperative radiographs should include good-quality anteroposterior and lateral views centered on the joint. Comparison radiographs of the normal elbow are helpful also. Careful scrutiny of the radiographs may reveal defects or gaps in both the supracondylar area and the articular joint surface. If any doubt exists, prepare the patient for a possible bone-graft procedure. A review of the anatomy of the distal humerus on a skeleton is helpful in determining the proper selection and placement of the fixation device. When the appropriate instruments and implants are anticipated, the procedure proceeds smoothly and the operative time is decreased significantly. The procedure should be undertaken only after a thorough review of the radiographs, operative approach, soft-tissue anatomy, and proposed fixation devices. We prefer to fix distal humeral fractures as soon as reasonably possible. In the absence of adequate preliminary preparation, however, the procedure should be delayed.

Operative Technique

With the patient in the prone position (Fig. 26-2), the arm is flexed over a well-padded arm holder, allowing almost full flexion of the elbow after draping is completed. We believe the prone position offers the following advantages: the surgeon may sit, less effort is required by the assistant, and the reduction is easier. A pneumatic tourniquet should be applied whenever feasible to provide a dry field.

Surgical Approach

The surgical approach deserves special mention. Fractures of the distal humerus require excellent visualization to accomplish internal fixation. We believe that many of the disastrous results described in the literature are the results of attempts to fix these difficult fractures through a limited medial and/or lateral incision. These limited approaches are useful only in the unicondylar fracture, which is not categorized as a complex injury. We routinely utilize a posterior approach for these fractures except in rare cases of fractures with associated vascular injury. There are basically two posterior approaches: Campbell's approach through the triceps for the more proximal supracondylar fracture without intra-articular extension[35] and Cassebaum's transolecranon approach for intra-articular fractures.[36] Although both approaches are useful and have specific indications and advantages, we have more experience with the transolecranon approach.

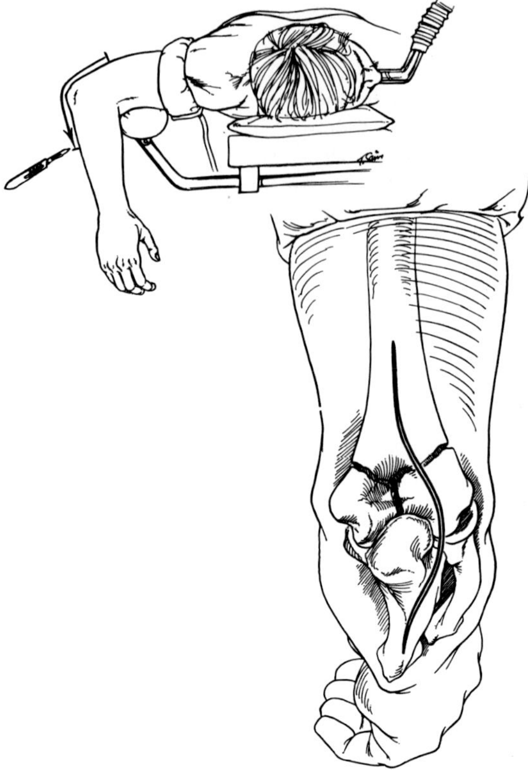

Fig. 26-2. Preferable position for operative treatment of distal humeral fractures. The patient is in a prone position, and the arm is placed on an arm holder. This position should allow for full extension as well as 20 to 30° of additional flexion in the elbow joint intraoperatively. The skin incision may be either straight or slightly curved around the lateral aspect of the olecranon.

Campbell's Approach for Extra-articular Fractures

Campbell, in 1939,[35] and Van Gorder, in 1940,[37] described an approach in which a posterior midline incision is made through the skin (Fig. 26-3), starting approximately 10 cm proximal to the olecranon and extending distally about 3 cm to its tip. The skin and subcutaneous layers should be dissected only as far as to provide identification of the ulnar nerve, which is retracted with a soft rubber band. Furthermore, dissection of the superficial layers should allow for incision of the superficial fascia covering of the triceps muscle. (For more details, see legend to Fig. 26-3.) Campbell's approach guarantees an appropriate visualization of the entire posterior surface of the distal humerus, including its medial and lateral borders, the olecranon fossa, and a portion of the articular surface. We have reserved this approach for the supracondylar fracture without intra-articular extension.

Technique of Fixation in Supracondylar (Extra-articular) Humeral Fractures

The fracture pattern and degree of comminution dictate the type of fixation device to be used. We prefer the small-fragment instruments and implants for fixation of these fractures.[16,34,38] The one-third tubular and the 3.5-mm dynamic compression plate (DCP) have been the most useful implants for this type of fracture (Fig. 26-4). Our experience with a Y-shaped plate, offered particularly as an advantageous implant for these fractures, is rather limited. Placed on the dorsal aspect, the Y-shaped plate must withstand most of the cyclic loadings produced by flexion-extension movements in the elbow joint. Thus, any implant placed posteriorly is prone to early fatigue and, consequently, failure. For supracondy-

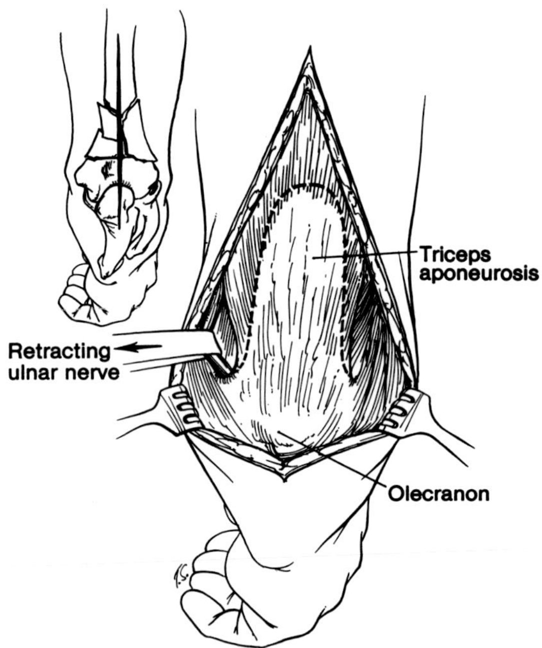

Fig. 26-3. Campbell's approach for extra-articular distal humeral fractures. A straight posterior midline incision over the distal third of the humerus is made down to the superficial fascia. The ulnar nerve must be identified and retracted by a soft rubber band. The dissection of the subcutaneous tissue is limited to the extent necessary to separate the tendinous from the muscular part of the distal triceps. This separation, representing a tongue-fashioned flap, should be performed strictly within the confines of the fascia itself. The flap is retracted distally, thus guaranteeing a sufficiently wide exposure to the distal extra-articular humerus (see Fig. 26-4).

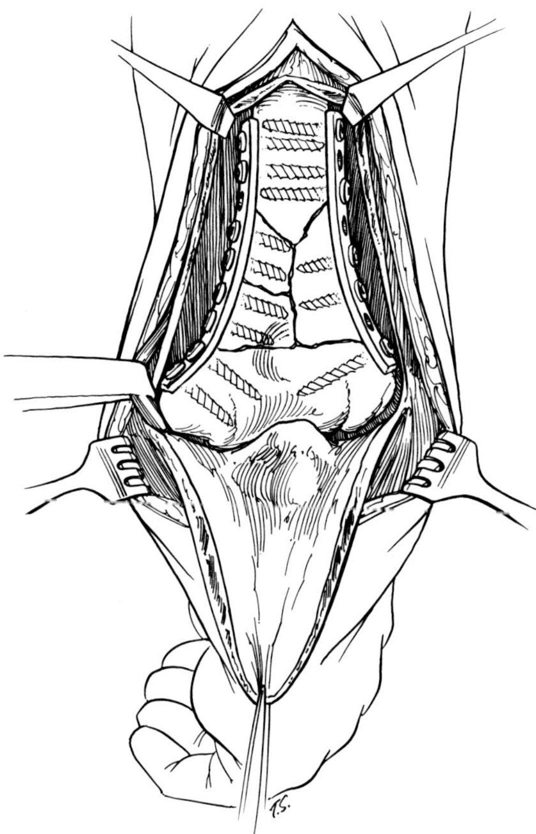

Fig. 26-4. Supracondylar extra-articular humeral fracture exposed through Campbell's approach. The multifragmented fracture is reduced anatomically, and the reduction is secured by a medially and a laterally placed 3.5-mm DCP. Note that there is no protrusion of any screwtip into the olecranon fossa. The medial and lateral placement of the implants makes them more resistant to cyclic loadings when early active mobilization is initiated.

lar humeral fractures, in particular those with marked comminution, we prefer the 3.5-mm DCP over the one-third tubular plate because the DCP is stronger and provides more stability. Most of the fractures at this level, however, can be managed best by using the one-third tubular plates applied unilaterally or bilaterally. The plates must be contoured exactly to fit the medial and lateral borders of the distal humerus. More technical details may be taken from the descriptions in the ASIF textbooks on internal fixation.[16,34] We recommend using plates on both the medial and lateral borders when necessary as this method greatly enhances the stability of fixation. The common error is to place a screw that crosses or protrudes into the olecranon fossa. This mistake must be avoided since it interferes with normal range of motion of the elbow joint. Remaining significant defects must be filled with cancellous bone graft, particularly in bone defects opposite an implant. When closing the incision, the fascial tongue is approximated to the retained fascial edge of the triceps with strong suture material. The wound then is closed carefully over a suction drain.

Cassebaum's Transolecranon Approach for Intra-articular Humeral Fractures

Most fractures of the distal humerus in adults extend into the joint space. To fix these fractures, we prefer a modification of the transolecranon approach described by Cassebaum in 1952 (Fig. 26-5).[36] With the patient in the prone position, a long posterior skin incision is made 8 to 10 cm proximal to the olecranon, skirting the radial side of the olecranon and extending distally 4 to 6 cm to its tip. The skin and subcutaneous layers are dissected on both sides to expose the distal triceps muscle and its insertion, the olecranon, and the fascia covering of the proximal ulna. The ulnar nerve is identified and retracted with a soft rubber drain.

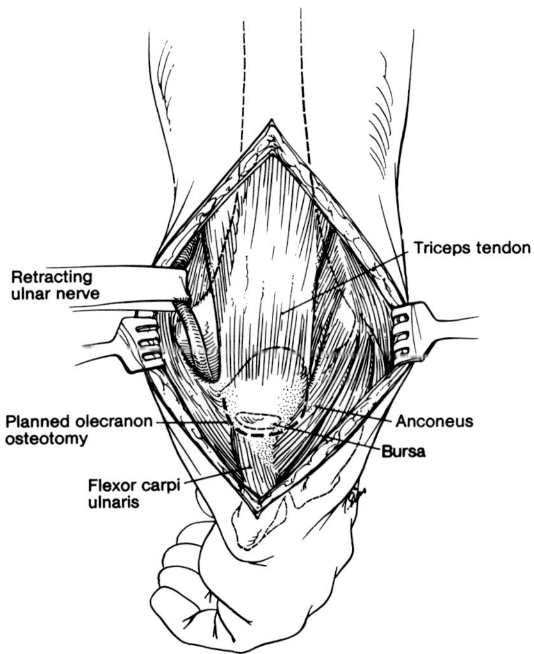

Fig. 26-5. Cassebaum's transolecranon approach in distal intra-articular humeral fractures. With the patient in a prone position and the injured arm supported by an arm holder, the straight posterior incision skirts the radial side of the olecranon and extends to the proximal forearm. Identification and protection of the ulnar nerve are obligatory.

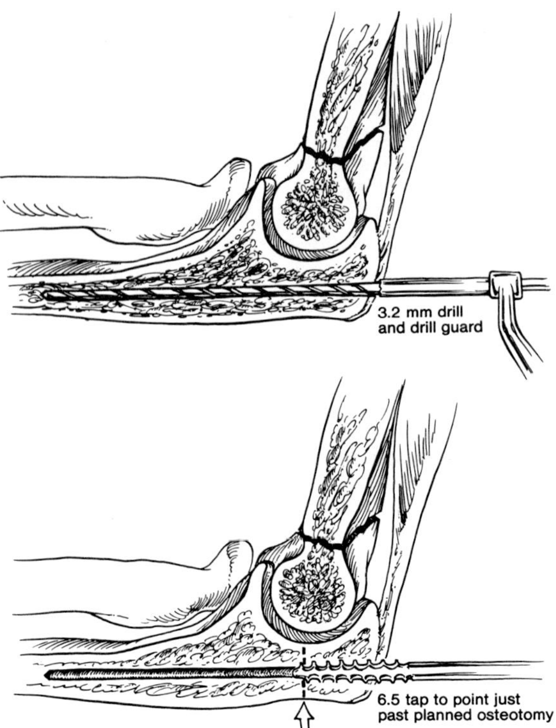

Fig. 26-6. Cassebaum's transolecranon approach: preparation of the olecranon osteotomy. Dissection of the subcutaneous tissues from the superficial arm fascia should be done only as far as is necessary to facilitate the approach to the osteotomy site and the later dissection of the triceps tendon. The screw placement is prepared by predrilling and partly pretapping prior to the osteotomy.

The olecranon osteotomy may be placed in a variety of locations. We prefer to place the osteotomy about 2 cm distally from the tip of the olecranon. A hole is first drilled with a 3.2-mm drill through the olecranon and down the medullary canal (Fig. 26-6). This hole is tapped with a large 6.5-mm tap to a point just distal to the proposed osteotomy site. The tips of two hemostats are placed in the trochlea notches of the olecranon (Fig. 26-7) on both the radial and ulnar sides to lift up and widen the joint space and serve as heels to prevent damage to the articular surface of the trochlea. A reciprocating power saw is used to make a transverse cut in the olecranon to the level of the subchondral bone. A straight osteotome is then used to carefully complete the division of the olecranon by wedging (Fig. 26-8). The medial and lateral distal expansions of the triceps insertion are divided before reflecting the olecranon-triceps mechanism. The olecranon with the attached triceps mechanism is reflected proximally to give complete exposure to the articular surface of the distal humerus.

Fixation of complex fractures of the distal humerus with split condyles should follow the same sequence each time. First, the articular surface, most particularly the trochlea, must be restored anatomically. The reconstructed articular component then is stabilized firmly to the metaphysis and the shaft. We believe the 4-mm cancellous screw is ideal for fixation of the condyles. We prefer this screw to the more commonly recommended malleolar screw. The large 6.5-mm cancellous screw should be used in this area only in special circumstances. Ideally, two of the 4-mm cancellous screws should be used. Correct placement of these screws is critical. A drill hole is placed from the lateral to the medial side using the 2-mm drill bit (Fig. 26-9). The near cortex

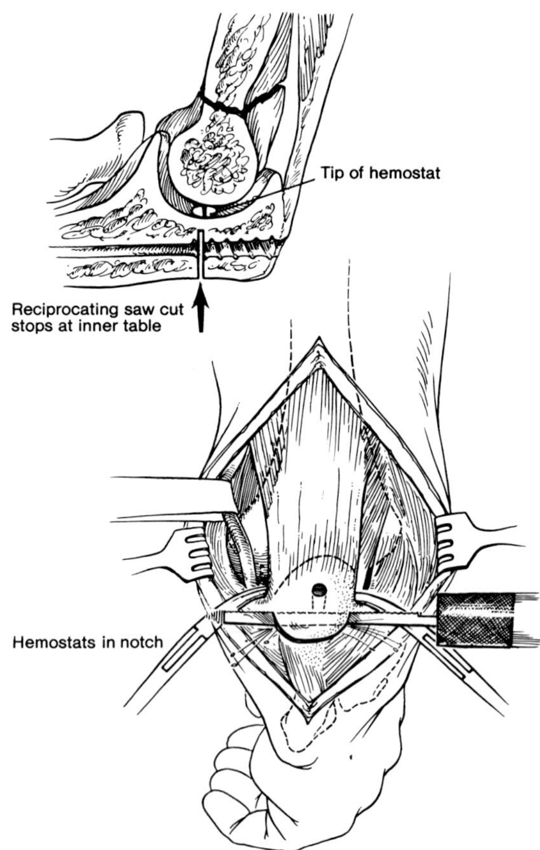

Fig. 26-7. Cassebaum's transolecranon approach: olecranon osteotomy. Two hemostats are placed into the joint space, which consequently is widened to avoid cartilagenous damage of the trochlea when the osteotomy is performed. Note that the osteotomy cut is extended only into the subchondral bone.

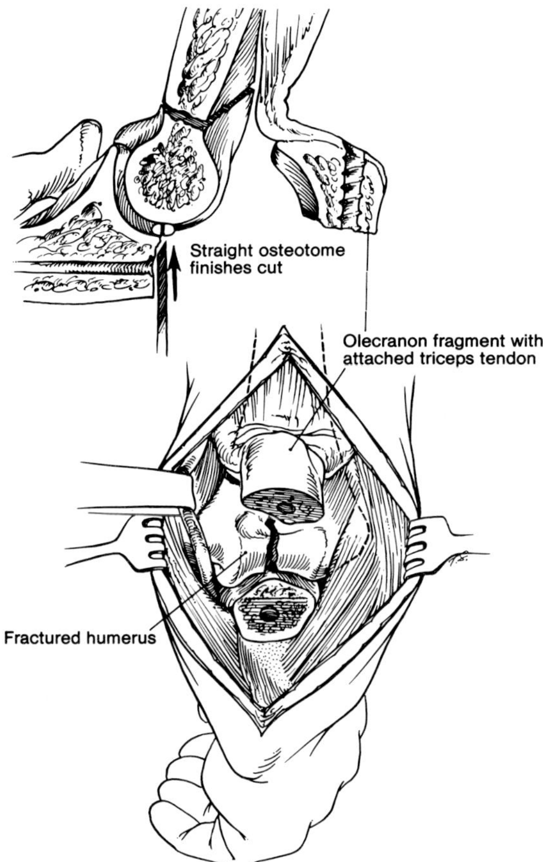

Fig. 26-8. Cassebaum's transolecranon approach: completion of the olecranon osteotomy. An oscillating power saw is used to extend the osteotomy into the subchondral bone. It is completed by carefully wedging the olecranon, using a straight osteotome. Dissection of the triceps follows bilaterally so that the olecranon-triceps mechanism can be reflected completely.

and the lateral fracture fragment are tapped with a 3.5-mm tap to a point just past the fracture line. Two 4-mm cancellous screws of appropriate length are placed with the screw threads located entirely in the far or medial fragment to give a lag effect (Fig. 26-10). The tip of the screws should barely penetrate the far cortex, if at all. Should the tip protrude into an area near the normal location of the ulnar nerve, transpose the nerve anteriorly before completing the procedure. The screw heads always should be located laterally to simplify removal at a later date through a small stab wound. Before compressing the condyles together, one must be sure there is no defect or gap in the articular surface of the trochlea. Closure of this gap with a lag screw is disastrous because it narrows the spool of the trochlea and creates incongruity in the articulation with the olecranon. The method to avoid this calamity is discussed in a later section of this chapter.

Occasionally, the articular surface is split into three major fragments, thus making anatomic reduction difficult. Before reducing the fragments, start a smooth Kirschner wire through the exact center of the capitellar fragment, beginning from the fracture surface and proceeding to the lateral cortical surface (Fig. 26-11). Change the power drill to the opposite end of the K-wire, cut a sharp point on the other end of the wire, and back the wire out laterally until only the sharp point is protruding. Reduce the medial fragment anatomically by running the K-wire through it until the sharp point is protruding. Then, reduce the medial (trochlea) fragment anatomically, continuing to drive the K-wire until the medial cortex is penetrated. The 2-mm triple drill guide is placed over the K-wire to direct a drill hole with a 2-mm drill bit (Fig. 26-12). This hole is tapped with a 3.5-mm tap just past the second fracture line. The correct length 4-mm cancellous screw is used to lag all three fragments together. A second 4-mm cancellous screw is added for more rigid fixation and to provide rotational stability.

The next step is to fix the conjoined stabilized articular component firmly to the metaphysis. Anatomic reduction is achieved and temporarily held with multiple crossed K-wires (see Fig. 26-10). Final fixation is accomplished in the manner previously described for the pure supracondylar fracture (see Fig. 26-4). The one-third tubular plate or 3.5-mm DCP is contoured to fit the medial and lateral surface of the distal humerus. The one-third tubular plate is somewhat easier to contour to the medial and lateral borders, which are the most favorable sites from a mechanical standpoint. When placed on the medial or lateral borders of the distal humerus, the plates withstand cyclic loadings best (compare with earlier comments on the Y-shaped plate in this chapter). Sometimes at least one of the cancellous screws used for the fixation of the condyles must be applied through the most distal plate hole. We prefer two plates and attempt to lag as many cortical screws through the plate as possible. Again, obstruction of the olecranon fossa must be avoided. Defects or gaps should be filled in with cancellous bone graft. The joint is inspected and irrigated to remove any loose bone fragments before it is closed.

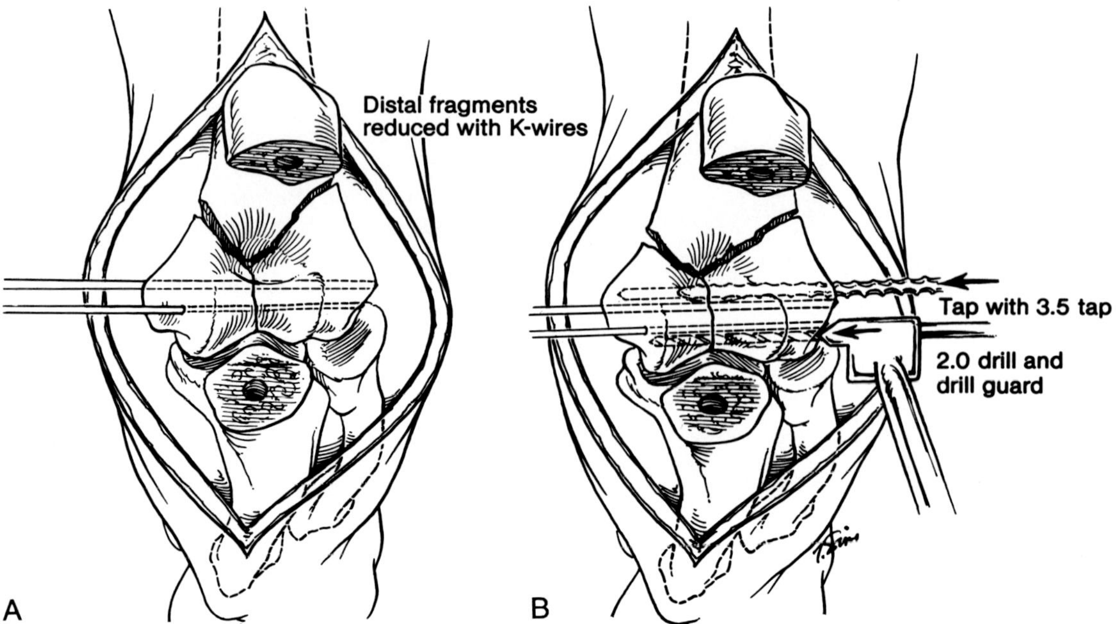

Fig. 26-9. Open reduction and internal fixation in distal intra-articular humeral fractures: restoration of the trochlea. The fracture site now is widely exposed. Reduction begins with the restoration of the articular surface. Appropriate reduction forceps or towel clamps should be used to reduce the joint fragments, which then are held temporarily with K-wires (*A*). Predrilling and pretapping with corresponding drill bits and taps in the technique outlined for the use of the small fragment set[16,35] always are performed in the same sequence (*B*).

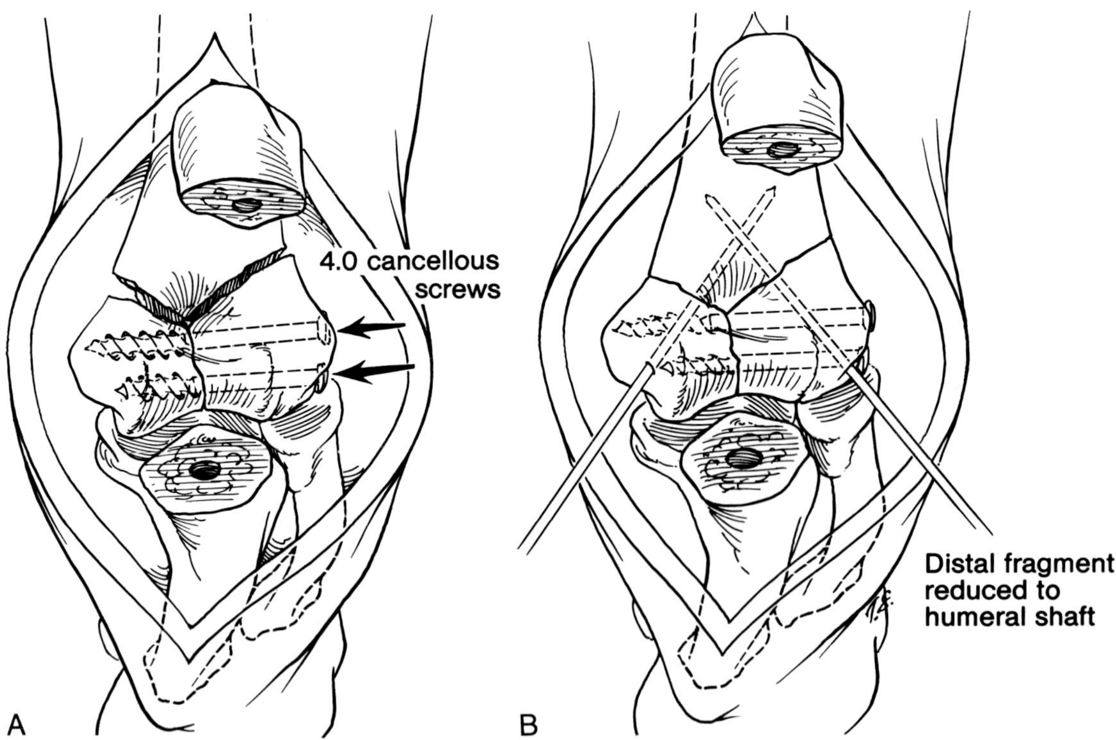

Fig. 26-10. Open reduction and internal fixation in distal intra-articular humeral fractures. *A*, The K-wire fixation subsequently is replaced by insertion of two 4.0-mm cancellous screws. *B*, Reduction of the distal fragment is followed by temporarily connecting the distal fragment with K-wires to the proximal humeral fragment. Fixation is completed according to Figs. 26-4 and 26-16.

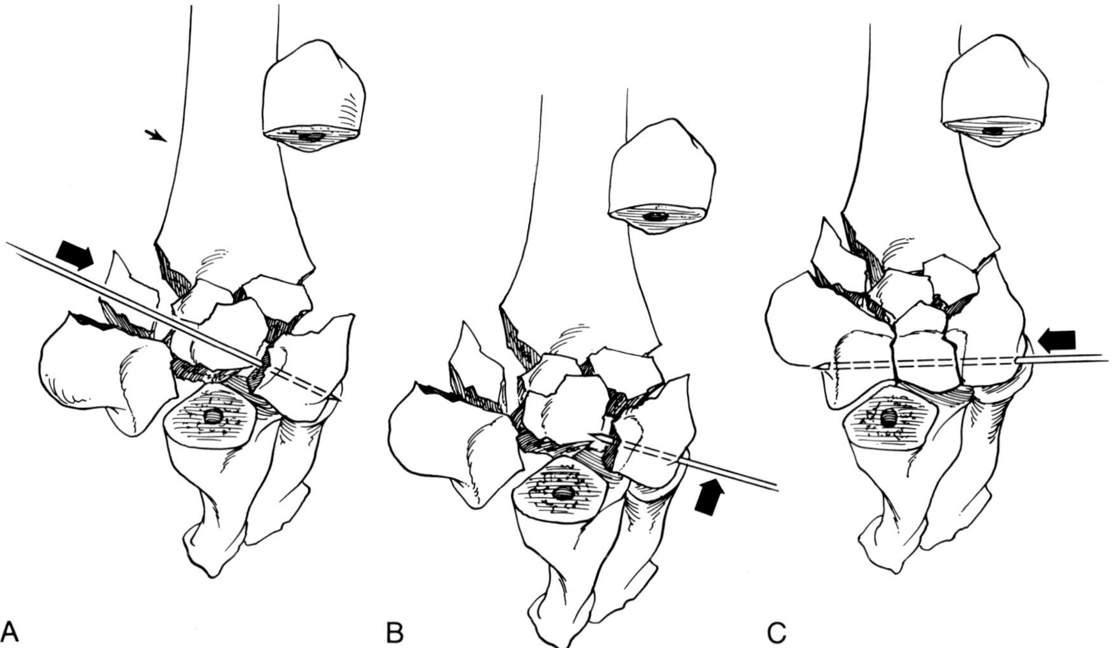

FIG. 26-11. Open reduction and internal fixation in distal intra-articular humeral fractures: restoration of a multifragmented trochlea. During an "inside-out" technique, the radial fragment is centrally pierced with a smooth K-wire (*A*), which then is driven back as soon as the rest of the fragments are lined up anatomically (*B* and *C*). The articular surface then can be restored.

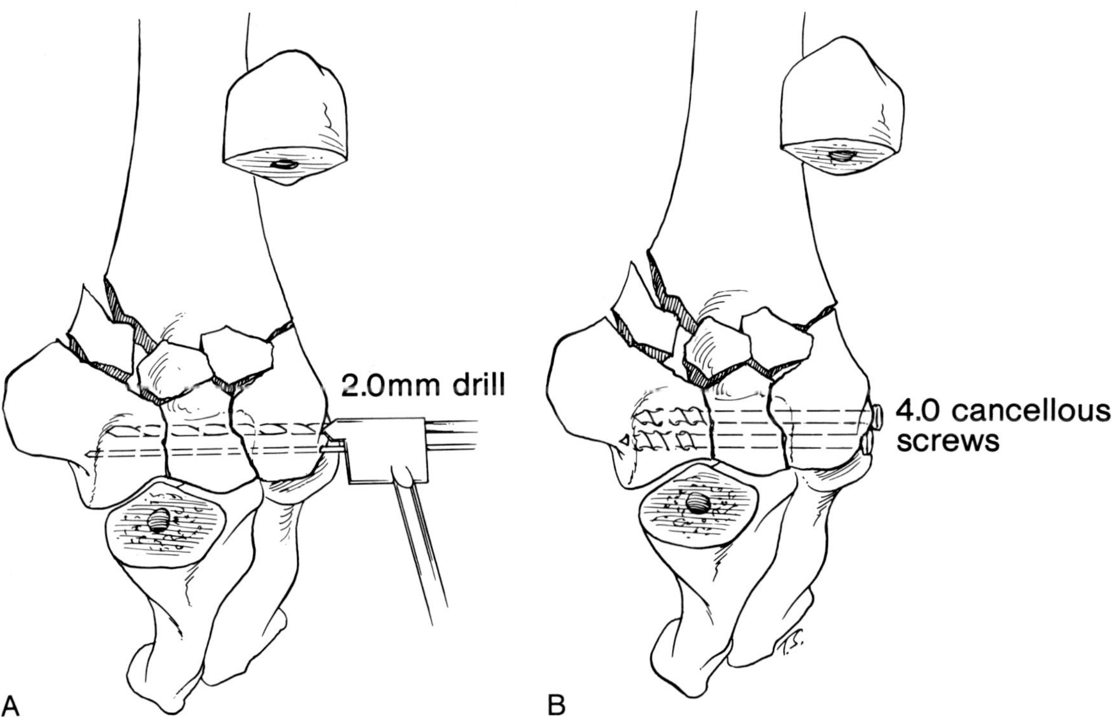

FIG. 26-12. Open reduction and internal fixation in distal intra-articular humeral fractures with a multifragmented trochlea. *A*, The triple guide is placed laterally over the K-wire which is used as a guideline. The screw site is prepared in the manner outlined in Figure 26-9. When one screw has been inserted, the K-wire is replaced by a second 4.0-mm cancellous screw (*B*). Note that the threads do not cross the fracture lines (lag-screw principle). The open reduction and internal fixation must be accomplished as demonstrated in Figures 26-4 and 26-16.

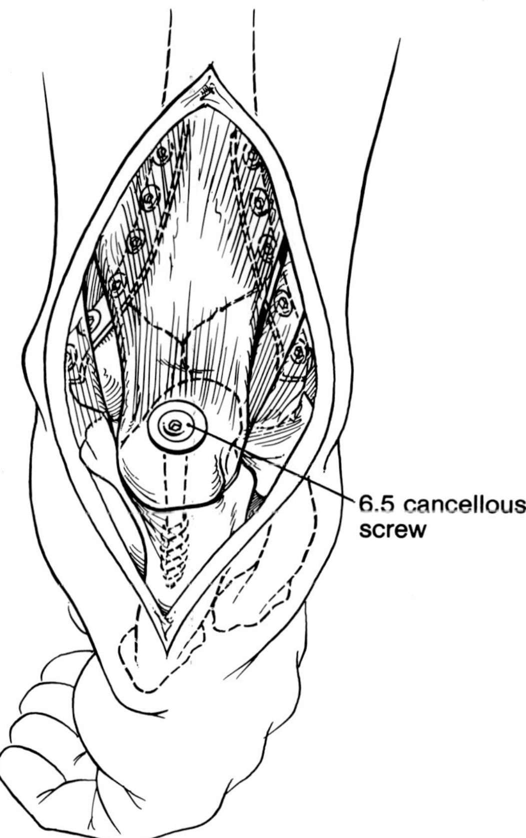

Fig. 26-13. Open reduction and internal fixation in distal intra-articular humeral fractures: fixation of the olecranon osteotomy. The reduced olecranon is held by means of a 6.5-mm cancellous screw applied with a washer. The dissected parts of the triceps tendon are sewn back.

The olecranon is reduced anatomically and fixed with a large 6.5-mm cancellous screw with a washer through the previously prepared hole (Fig. 26-13). The screw should measure 80 to 90 mm in length and should be the long thread-length type of screw (32-mm-length threads). The threaded part should never cross the osteotomy side, otherwise the lag-screw effect will not be accomplished. The screw fixation must be secured by means of an additional tension-band wire. Therefore, a 2-mm hole is drilled transversely across the ulna about 3 to 4 cm distal to the osteotomy site (Fig. 26-14). A 1.5-mm wire is passed through this hole, around and over the triceps tendon insertion, and is tightened in a figure-of-eight fashion to further amend fixation of the olecranon. Suction drainage is placed, and the skin is finally closed.

Special Operative Techniques in Defect Fractures of the Distal Humerus

Special problems involving osseous defects or gaps may occur in the distal humerus and deserve special comments. The first problem involves defects in the articular surface (Fig. 26-15). In stabilization of split condyles, one will occasionally note the existence of a gap, usually on the trochlea site. All the other fracture lines appear well reduced except for the persistent gap. Most orthopaedic surgeons naturally are tempted to compress or close the gap with lag screws. However, such treatment results in narrowing of the trochlea spool and creates an incongruity in articulation with the olecranon. To avoid this potential disaster, the surgeon must reduce the fragments anatomically and must temporarily maintain the reduction of the gap with multiple crossed K-wires. Place a 3.2-mm drill hole from the lateral to the medial side through both cortices (Fig. 26-16). Determine the proper length of screw and tap the drill hole with a 4.5-mm tap completely through both cortices without changing the gap. The 4.5-mm cortical screw—serving in this situation as a positioning

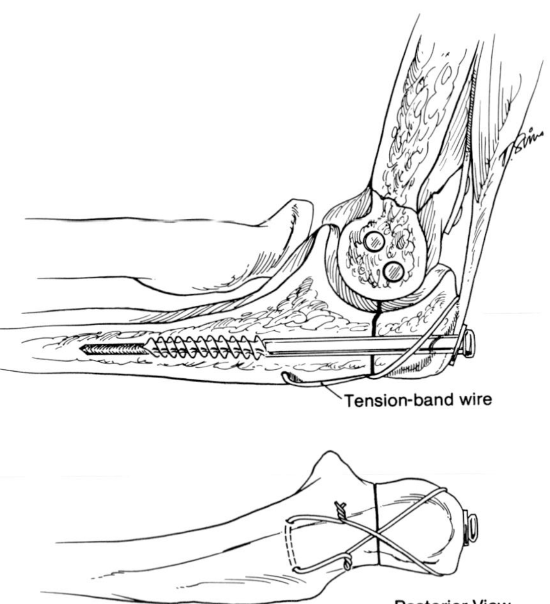

Fig. 26-14. Open reduction and internal fixation in distal intra-articular humeral fractures: fixation of the olecranon osteotomy. The screw fixation of the osteotomy finally is secured by a tension-band wire applied in a figure-of-eight fashion. For better distribution of the forces across the osteotomy site, it is preferable to rely on two inbuilt loops with which the tension-band wire is tightened.

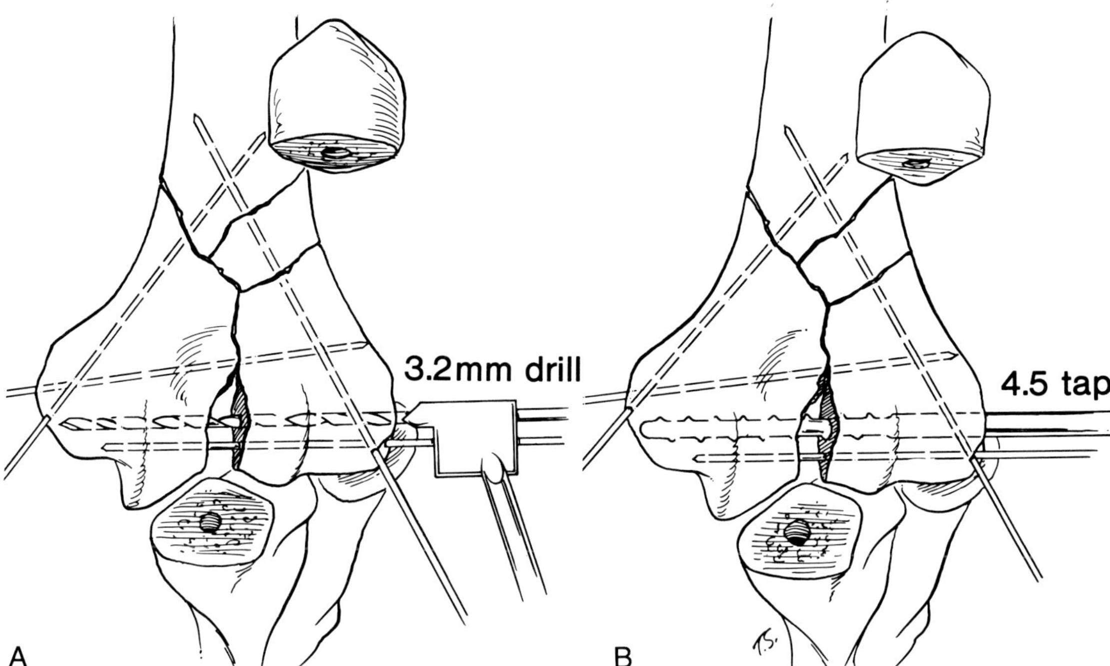

Fig. 26-15. Open reduction and internal fixation in distal intra-articular humeral fractures: bony defect in the trochlea. Anatomic reduction of the fracture site and preliminary K-wire fixation of the fragments are performed. *A*, Predrilling of the intratrochlear screw site, which is tapped with a corresponding tap throughout the length of both fragments (*B*). Note the bone loss causing the trochlear gap.

screw—is inserted in the two condyles, thus maintaining their proper position. The gap then is filled with a cancellous bone graft.

The second problem involves relatively large segmental defects in the supracondylar area of the distal humerus and can be handled only with careful planning. The olecranon should be osteotomized to obtain sufficient exposure. Cortical cancellous bone graft, about 3 to 4-mm thick and usually taken from the inner table of the iliac crest, is required to fill the gap (Fig. 26-17). Special preparation, which is provided with multiple 2-mm drill holes, is given to the graft before it is trimmed to bridge the gap (Fig. 26-18). Small notches made at each corner of the graft ensure a tight fit. The graft should be placed in the gap with the cancellous surface facing posteriorly, thus guaranteeing exposure to well-vascularized muscle tissue of the triceps. The multiple drill holes serve to ease the ingrowth of new vessels into the total graft. The remaining anterior portion of the defect is filled with cancellous bone as an onlay graft, which is widely exposed to the muscle tissue of the elbow flexors. The basic technique of internal fixation of these defect fractures by and large is the same as already outlined for the other complex fractures of the elbow.

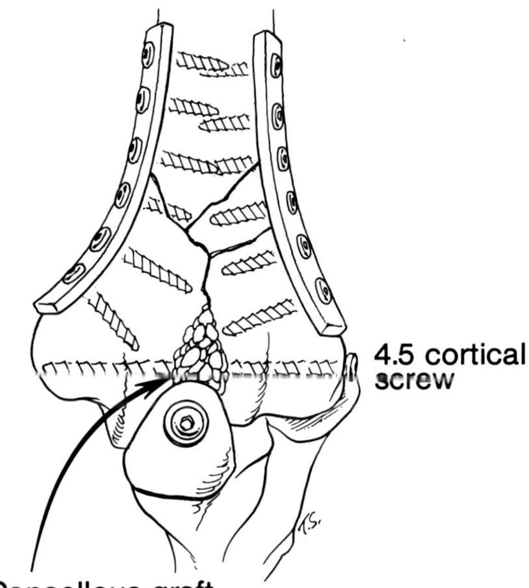

Fig. 26-16 Open reduction and internal fixation in distal intra-articular humeral fractures: bony defect in the trochlea. Accurate anatomic position of the main fragments is guaranteed by the insertion of a 4.5-mm cortical screw, which serves as a positioning screw. The gap is packed with pure cancellous bone, which must be contoured according to the shape of the trochlea. The internal fixation is accomplished in the usual manner (see Fig. 26-4).

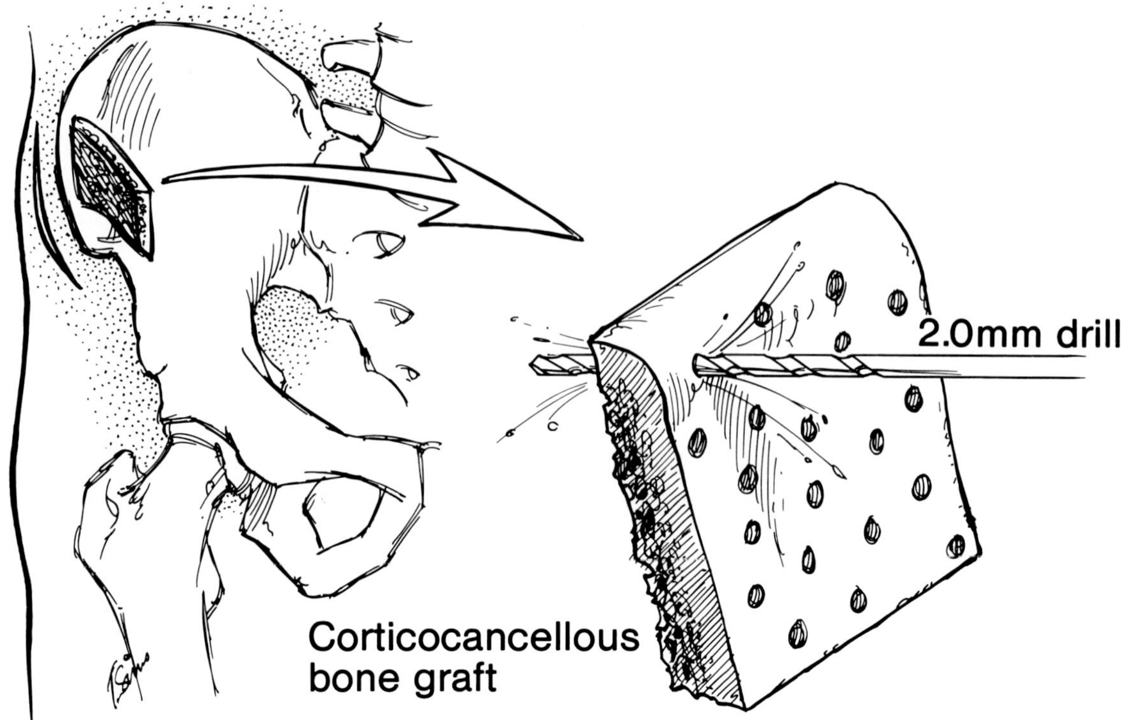

Fig. 26-17. Harvesting of a corticocancellous bone graft from the inner iliac table. The graft is trimmed to the size needed to fill a defect in the supracondylar humerus area. The graft should be 4 to 5 mm thick. Further preparation of the graft consists of the placement of as many drillholes as possible in the graft, aiming for an easier ingrowth of new vessels when the graft is implanted.

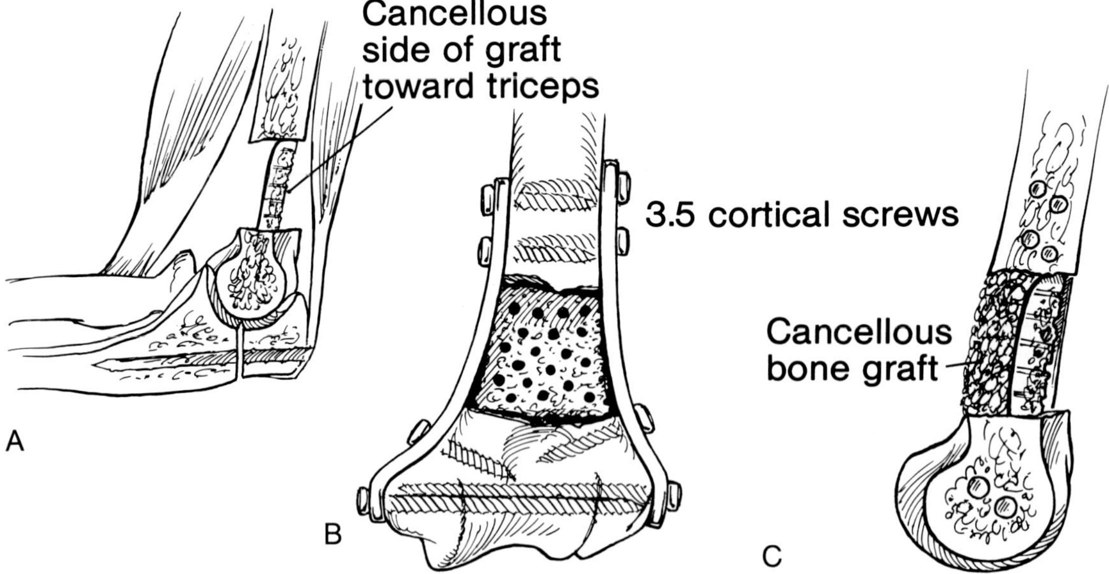

Fig. 26-18. Bone grafting and open reduction and internal fixation in supracondylar humeral fractures with bone loss. *A*, The corticocancellous graft, trimmed to the size and shape of the defect, is squeezed between the main fragments. The cancellous surface faces the well-vascularized triceps muscle. The remaining anterior defect consequently is filled with pure cancellous bone (*C*), which is exposed to the flexor muscles. The graft finally is secured by bilateral plating, as shown earlier (*B*).

Postoperative Management

The arm usually is placed in a well-padded posterior plaster splint with the elbow at an approximate 90° angle. Continued elevation of the arm is essential for the first 4 or 5 postoperative days. Although a variety of overhead slings is available, such slings are uncomfortable. We have found two or three pillows to be sufficient to maintain elevation. The patient may be allowed out of bed as long as elevation is not sacrificed. We apply suction drainage to prevent hematoma formation. These drains are removed within 24 to 48 hours after the operation. The neurovascular status of the extremity must be monitored closely. Gentle active motion of the shoulder and fingers is started as soon as possible to reduce swelling and prevent stiffness. On the third or fourth postoperative day, all splints and dressings are removed, and a right-angle plastic or plaster slab is applied. This slab is removed four to five times a day for gentle active assisted motion under the direction of a physical therapist. The need for external support and protection is critical during the initial rehabilitation phase. Sequential radiographs usually are obtained at 4, 8, and 12 weeks postoperatively. Depending on the stability of fixation, the splint is continued for 2 to 4 additional weeks postoperatively with continued emphasis placed on daily supervised physical therapy. For unreliable patients or those with tenuous fixation or marked comminution, the use of a functional hinged plastic orthotic device may be necessary. The patient and his family must be well informed regarding daily range-of-motion exercises, as the advantages of stable fixation and early joint mobilization are lost without maximum attention to aggressive postoperative therapy. In general, full weight-bearing of the elbow joint should not be allowed before 3 to 4 months after internal fixation.

Removal of the implant is not necessary unless complaints are specifically related to the device. The implants should be left in place for about 1 year to ensure solid union and to prevent refracture.

Fracture-Dislocations of the Elbow

Fracture-dislocations of the elbow are common injuries. They vary considerably in clinical presentation depending on the type and severity of the fracture. According to O'Hara and associates,[38] the most common fractures associated with elbow dislocations are, in order of decreasing frequency, fractures of the medial epicondyle, head and neck of the radius, the coracoid process, the lateral condyle of the humerus, and the capitellum. The dislocation should be treated as a true emergency and reduced as soon as possible. To minimize the chances of new bone formation in the periarticular tissue, we highly recommend fracture fixation at the earliest time after the reduction of the dislocated joint. The later the surgery, the higher the incidence of periarticular calcification.

Monteggia's Fracture-Dislocation

Monteggia's fracture-dislocation deserves special emphasis because of the difficulty in management and reputation for poor results.[28] Watson-Jones stated, "No fracture presents so many problems; no injury is beset with greater difficulty; no treatment is characterized by more general failure."[3] He reported that 95% of patients with Monteggia's fractures had permanent disability. Giovanni Monteggia first described this injury in 1814 as an anterior dislocation of the radial head associated with a fracture of the proximal ulna. This type of fracture has been noted in all age groups; however, the fracture is rare, occurring in about 0.7% of elbow fractures and dislocations and in 7% of fractures of the radius and ulna.[39] Actually, the dislocation of the radial head may occur in any direction, depending on the mechanism of injury.[40] This injury initially was thought to result from direct trauma to the proximal forearm, causing a fracture of the ulna and driving the radial head anteriorly out of its articulation. Fracture-dislocations, however, may have different mechanisms of injury, such as a fall on the outstretched hand while simultaneously twisting the trunk, resulting in a violent forced pronation of the forearm.

Classification

In 1967, Bado classified this fracture-dislocation into four types, mainly associating the types with the direction of the dislocation of the radial head.[40] Regardless of the type of injury, these fracture-dislocations should be treated operatively.

Pitfalls in Diagnosis

Failure to recognize the radial-head dislocation is the major problem in the diagnosis of Monteggia's fracture-dislocation. One always should be suspicious of a radial-head dislocation in all ulnar shaft fractures regardless of how benign the ulnar fracture appears. A good-quality true lateral radiograph of the elbow is necessary to confirm the diagnosis. The radial head is displaced and reduction is necessary when a line that bisects the center of the radial head does not go through the center of the capitellum.

Careful evaluation of the neurovascular status of the limb should be performed, as a high incidence of neurologic damage has been reported in Monteggia's lesion. A review of several series revealed associated nerve damage occurring in between 13 and 43% of patients.[39–42] The radial nerve is the nerve most frequently injured. Fortunately, most nerve palsies are transient in nature.

Our Preferred Method of Treatment

We believe that Monteggia's fracture-dislocation in the adult should be treated surgically. It is wise to gently attempt closed reduction of the radial head initially. This reduction frequently fails because of interposition of the ruptured annular ligament and capsule.

Operative Technique

The patient is placed in the supine position with the arm resting on a hand board. We prefer the surgical approach described by Boyd,[43] which exposes both the radial head and the fractured ulna through a single incision. The ulna is stabilized with a 6- to 7-hole 3.5-mm DCP. We do not recommend the use of shorter or thinner implants. Fixation of the ulna frequently results in a spontaneous reduction of the radial head. If dislocation of the radial head is persistent, one should extract the interposed annular ligament capsule, reducing it by means of direct visualization. An early attempt to repair the ligament by direct suture should be undertaken. Late reconstruction of the annular ligament with a strip of fascia often is associated with a tendency for calcification to develop in the repair, thereby resulting in restriction of pronation-supination motion.

Fractures of the Proximal Forearm

Fractures of the radial head or the olecranon rarely occur in combination with complex distal humeral fractures. Usually, they present isolated fractures as the result of an injury to the elbow area. These fractures require special attention since most of them demonstrate involvement of the elbow joint. Thus, following the basic principles applied in internal fixation of joint fractures, these fractures should be repaired surgically. Again, when properly done, internal fixation allows for earlier active rehabilitation of the involved elbow joint. The surgical approaches for isolated radial head or comminuted olecranon fractures differ only insignificantly from the incisions already outlined earlier for periarticular elbow fractures.

Fractures of the Radial Head

Dislocated fractures of the radial head are best treated by surgical procedures. The treatment option depends on the fracture pattern. Severe comminution of the radial head is best handled by an early excision of the fractured parts. We usually take off the proximal 10 to 15 mm of the radius. Reconstructive procedures for this fracture often fail, leaving behind an incongruent part of the elbow joint. Thus, the risk of early onset of posttraumatic arthritic changes increases. However, the resection of the severely comminuted radial head is not regarded as an ideal solution since late follow-up, particularly in young patients, frequently is accompanied by pain and functional disorders in the distal radioulnar joint caused by increasing incongruity at this level.[44,45] On the other hand, prosthetic replacements have not proved to have an outstandingly good long-time prognosis.[46,47] Pure wedge fractures of the head are treated by lag-screw fixation, either using a 4-mm cancellous screw or a 2.7-mm small-fragment screw. In the case of a depressed fracture, an attempt to elevate the depressed part should be undertaken. A local bone-graft transfer usually helps to keep the elevated part in the reduced position. Additional screw fixation rarely is indicated. When performing reconstructive procedures in radial head fractures, attention should be given to an associated avulsion fracture of the coronoid process of the ulna. The fracture should be fixed if possible. Small fragments must be removed to avoid later joint disorders, such as interpositioning of the fragment or chronic anterior joint instability. The surgical repair of a torn annular ligament remains controversial. Even when the ligament is sutured at the first attempt, long-term results do not seem to differ from those in whom the torn ligament is left behind without any suture repair.[48]

Fractures of the Olecranon

The majority of olecranon fractures may be fixed by tension-band wiring. With this technique, the two Kirschner wires provide the fracture site with enough rotational stability, whereas the tension-band wire withstands the tensile forces acting on the outer ulnar cortex as long as the elbow joint is brought into a flexed position.

In the more comminuted olecranon fracture or the comminution of the proximal forearm, tension-band wiring alone often fails to achieve reduction and to maintain appropriate fixation of the fracture site. In such instances, the combined technique using K-wires, lag screws, small-fragment implants, such as a one-third tubular plate or a laterally placed 3.5-mm DCP, or, if indicated by the size of the bone, a semitubular plate, dorsally applied with the instruments of the large-fragment set, should be recommended. Sufficiently wide exposure, appropriate instrumentation, excellent technical skills, and an experienced surgeon in charge are required to master this demanding problem.

Postoperative Management for Radial Head and Olecranon Fractures

The arm is placed in a well-padded posterior plaster splint with the elbow in neutral supination and 90° of flexion. The postoperative regimen as previously described for the distal humeral fractures is followed. Repeated radiographs are necessary to ensure the maintenance of the reduction of the radial head. The splint is removed when the positioning of the radial head and its fixation mode is sufficiently secure to maintain the result of the reduction.

Conclusion

Certain common as well as individual prerequisites must be fulfilled before the problem of a complex fracture of the elbow region should be tackled. Despite some surprising reports about excellent results in complex elbow fractures by means of initial traction followed by early mobilization, we must emphasize that a skilled technical repair applying stable internal fixation and early functional aftercare of the elbow joint give the best result.

References

1. Conn, J., Jr., and Wade, P. A.: Injuries of the elbow. A ten-year review. J. Trauma, *1*:248, 1961.
2. Wilson, P. D., and Cochrane, W. A.: Fractures and Dislocations. Philadelphia, J. B. Lippincott, 1938.
3. Watson-Jones, R.: Fractures and Joint Injuries. Baltimore, Williams and Wilkins, 1955.
4. Boehler, L.: Textbook on the Treatment of Fractures. 4th Edition. Baltimore, William Wood and Co., 1935.
5. Charnley, J.: The closed treatment of common fractures. Edinburgh, Livingstone, 1957.
6. McLaughlin, H. L.: Trauma. Philadelphia, W. B. Saunders, 1959.
7. Cave, E. F.: Fractures and Other Injuries. Chicago, Yearbook Medical Publishers, 1958.
8. Compere, E. L., Banks, S. W., and Compere, C. L.: Pictorial handbook of fracture treatment. Chicago, Yearbook Medical Publishers, 1958.
9. Eastwood, W. J.: The T-shaped fracture of the lower end of the humerus. J. Bone Joint Surg., *19*:364, 1937.
10. Evans, E. M.: Supracondylar Y fractures of the humerus. J. Bone Joint Surg., *35-B*:381, 1953.
11. Keon-Cohen, B. T.: Fractures at the elbow. J. Bone Joint Surg., *48-A*:1623, 1966.
12. Patterson, R. F.: A method of applying traction in T and Y fractures of the humerus. J. Bone Joint Surg., *17*:476, 1935.
13. Riseborough, E. J., and Radin, E. L.: Intercondylar T fractures of the humerus in the adult. A comparison of operative and nonoperative treatment in twenty-nine cases. J. Bone Joint Surg., *51-A*:130, 1969.
14. Robinson, R. A.: The historical background of internal fixation of fractures in North America. Bull. Hist. Med., *52*:354, 1978.
15. Matter, P., and Rittmann, W. W.: The Open Fracture. Bern, Hans Huber, 1978.
16. Mueller, M. E., Allgoewer, M., Schneider, R., and Willenegger, H.: Manual of Internal Fixation. Berlin, Springer-Verlag, 1979.
17. Rittmann, W. W., Schibli, M., Matter, P., and Allgoewer, M.: Open fractures—long-term results in two-hundred consecutive cases. Clin. Orthop., *138*:132, 1979.
18. Miller, W. E.: Comminuted fractures of the distal end of the humerus in the adult. J. Bone Joint Surg., *46-A*:644, 1964.
19. Wilson, P. D.: Fractures and dislocations in the region of the elbow. Surg. Gynecol. Obstet., *56*:335, 1933.
20. Bandi, W.: Die gelenknahen Frakturen des Oberarmes. Chirurg, *40*:193, 1969.
21. Burri, C., et al.: Behandlungsergebnisse nach operativer Versorgung distaler intraarticulaerer Humerusfrakturen. Chirurg, *44*:78, 1973.
22. Burri, C., and Rueter, A.: Distale Humerusfrakturen. Aktuel. Traumatol. *8*:79, 1978.
23. Bush, L. F., and McClain, E. J., Jr.: Operative treatment of fractures of the elbow in adults. *In* Instructional Course Lectures. Vol. 16. The American Academy of Orthopaedic Surgeons, 1969.
24. Cassebaum, W. H.: Open reduction of T and Y fractures of the lower end of the humerus. J. Trauma, *9*:915, 1969.
25. Knight, R. A.: The management of fractures about the elbow in adults. *In* Instructional Course Lectures. Vol. 14. The American Academy of Orthopaedic Surgeons, 1957.

26. Merle d'Aubigne, R.: Fractures suset intracondyliennes récentes de l'adult. Rev. Chir. Orthop., *50*:279, 1964.
27. Schmelzeisen, H., and Weller, S.: Operationstechnik und Taktik bei Frakturen der Trochlea humeri. Aktuel. Traumatol., *7*:177, 1977.
28. Speed, J. S., and Boyd, H. B.: Treatment of fractures of the ulna with dislocation of the head of the radius (Monteggia fractures). J.A.M.A., *115*:1699, 1940.
28a. Horne, G.: Supracondylar fractures of the humerus in adults. J. Trauma, *20*:71, 1980.
29. Schatzker, J.: Principles of stable internal fixation. Can. J. Surg., *23*:232, 1980.
30. Chapman, M. W., and Mahoney, M.: The role of internal fixation in the management of open fractures. Clin. Orthop., *138*:120, 1979.
31. Chapman, M. W.: The use of immediate internal fixation in open fractures. Orthop. Clin. North Am., *2*:579, 1980.
32. Anderson, J. T., and Gustilo, R. B.: Immediate internal fixation in open fractures. Orthop. Clin. North Am., *11*:569, 1980.
33. LaDuca, J. N., Bone, L. L., Seibel, R. W., and Border, J. R.: Primary open reduction and internal fixation of open fractures. J. Trauma, *20*:580, 1980.
34. Heim, U., and Pfeiffer, K.: Small Fragment Set Manual. Berlin, Springer-Verlag, 1974.
35. Campbell, W. C.: Operative Orthopaedics. St. Louis, C. V. Mosby, 1939.
36. Cassebaum, W. H.: Operative treatment of T and Y fractures of the lower end of the humerus. Am. J. Surg., *83*:265, 1952.
37. Van Gorder, G. W.: Surgical approach in supracondylar T fractures of the humerus requiring open reduction. J. Bone Joint Surg., *22*:278, 1940.
38. O'Hara, J. P., Morrey, B. F., Johnson, E. W., Jr., and Johnson, K. A.: Fracture conference: dislocations and fracture dislocations of the elbow. Minn. Med., *58*:697, 1975.
39. Bruce, H. E., Harvey, J. P., Jr., and Wilson, J. C., Jr.: Monteggia fractures. J. Bone Joint Surg., *57-A*:1563, 1974.
40. Bado, J. L.: The Monteggia lesion. Clin. Orthop., *50*:71, 1967.
41. Galbraith, K. A., and McCullogh, C. J.: Acute nerve injury as a complication of closed fractures or dislocations of the elbow. Injury, *11*:159, 1979.
42. Jessing, P.: Monteggia lesions and their complicating nerve damage. Acta Orthop. Scand., *46*:603, 1977.
43. Boyd, H. B.: Surgical exposure of the ulna and proximal third of the radius through one incision. Surg. Gynecol. Obstet., *71*:86, 1940.
44. Kirschner, P., Gamstaetter, G., and Schweikert, C. H.: Veraenderungen am Ellbogen- und Handgelenk nach Radiuskoepfchenresektion. Aktuel. Traumatol., *8*:123, 1978.
45. Radin, E. L., and Riseborough, E. J.: Fractures of the radial head. J. Bone Joint Surg., *48-A*:1055, 1966.
46. Beck, E.: Silastikprothese zum Ersatz des resezierten Speichenkoepfchens bei Truemmerbruechen. Arch. Orthop. Unfallchir., *80*:143, 1974.
47. Tietze, A.: Speichenkoepfchenbrueche—Ersatz durch Vitalliumprothese. Hefte Unfallheilkd., *114*:73, 1973.
48. Vollmar, D., Hecht, L., Groitl, H., and Glueckert, K.: Monteggiafrakturen, Behandlung und Spaetergebnisse. Aktuel. Traumatol., *8*:115, 1978.

Chapter 27 Complex Injuries of the Wrist and Hand

SIGURD C. SANDZÉN, JR.

The upper extremity is basically a series of graduated lever arms specifically designed to place the hand in the best functioning positions.

The hand itself represents the most complex integration of strength, stability, mobility, dexterity, and acute sensibility in the human body. The goal in treating a complex skeletal injury of the wrist and/or hand is to restore physiologic structures to as near normal as possible. The general basic functions of the wrist and hand include thumb opposition, synchronous digital flexion (index through little finger) with synergistic wrist extension, and digital extension with wrist flexion.

The general principles of management become increasingly important with the severity of the injury. These principles include:

1. primary wound care.
2. salvage and protection of viable tissue and amputated parts.
3. restoration of skeletal anatomy.
4. conversion of an open, contaminated wound to a closed, clean area as soon as possible.
5. primary, delayed primary, or secondary reconstruction.
6. physiologic immobilization and mobilization.
7. awareness of possible concomitant injuries in the ipsilateral and contralateral upper extremity and the entire musculoskeletal system.

Primary wound care is a salvage procedure, and its most important aspect is meticulous wound toilet—cleansing, irrigation, and debridement.

All viable tissue should be protected and handled gently for use at initial treatment or during secondary reconstruction of other areas in the severely injured hand (e.g., portions of a severely damaged digit, including pedicled skin, tendon, nerve, and bone).

The decision for deletion usually is deferred until after initial healing to permit profitable use of the selected elements previously illustrated. Generally, if three or more systems (integument, skeleton, musculotendinous system, vascular and nerve supply) are irreparably traumatized, digital deletion may be preferred to a prolonged, multiply staged reconstruction that would result in a marginally functional digit (see Figs. 27-18 and 27-19).

Replantation of completely amputated parts demands a serious consideration of logical indications and contraindications. Priorities for replantation include the thumb, as many digits as possible in multiple amputations, usually any digit in a child, and, in selected instances, a single digit in the adult.

Contraindications include amputation at the distal interphalangeal (DIP) joint level or distally in index through little fingers, at the interphalangeal (IP) joint or distally in the thumb, a single digit in the adult, amputations sustained in severe crush or avulsive types of injuries in which massive soft-tissue trauma occurred, and if longer than 8 hours have passed since injury with no cooling of the amputated segment. Though these are the general rules, each patient should be considered individually with regard to patient preference and medical and surgical considerations.

The amputated segment should be wrapped in sterile gauze saturated in normal saline or other physiologic solution and placed in a plastic bag. The plastic bag is placed on ice in an ice chest and taken with the patient to a center specifically prepared for replantation. The amputated segment should not be placed on dry ice, should not be frozen, and should not be allowed to remain at room temperature.

In all severe injuries, skeletal stability should be achieved at primary treatment, if possible. Thereby, a stable foundation and framework are provided for more extensive delayed primary or secondary reconstruction.

The open wound should be converted to a closed, clean area as soon as possible; however, primary closure need not always be attempted. Certain wounds and mechanisms of injury require initial open treatment, followed by delayed primary closure or resurfacing or secondary closure. Such situations will be discussed later.

Complicated reconstructive procedures generally are contraindicated initially because of the possibility of persistent wound contamination, marginal viability of severely damaged tissue, and greater jeopardy of tissue viability by additional surgical exposure and prolonged operative time. Generally, therefore, reconstruction of any complexity is better performed as a delayed primary or secondary procedure(s) at appropriately staged intervals.

Physiologic immobilization in the functional position of wrist extension, metacarpophalangeal joint flexion, interphalangeal joint extension, and wide thumb abduction and opposition, supplemented by elevation, is vitally important. Mobilization should be commenced when there is no danger of fracture redisplacement or joint redislocation.

If priority of treatment is centered on the obvious acute injury, diagnosis of other injuries, sometimes occult, can be made only by careful examination of the entire ipsilateral extremity. Systematic initial examination and periodic reexamination of the entire skeletal system frequently yield additional diagnoses initially unsuspected (Fig. 27-1).

Initial Patient Management

The sequence of priorities of general management of the patient with a severe upper extremity injury include:

1. resuscitation.
2. simultaneous hemostasis.
3. re-establishment of circulation.
4. diagnosis of a closed space or closed compartment compression syndrome.
5. immobilization.
6. general history and physical examination of the patient.
7. appropriate laboratory determinations.
8. tetanus prophylaxis and antibiotics.

Resuscitation of the patient is obvious, and details are not discussed here.

Generally, hemostasis can be achieved by proper application of a massive sterile, or at least clean, compressive dressing, augmented by external immobilization and vertical elevation. If a pneumatic tourniquet or blood-pressure cuff is necessary, the time of application must be noted on a strip of adhesive tape applied directly to the tourniquet.

"Clamping a bleeder" is contraindicated unless the vessel ends are visibly protruding from the wound; otherwise, additional contamination and often crushing of an adjacent nerve result (e.g., median nerve in the antecubital area and either median or ulnar nerve at the wrist).

Impaired circulation distal to the injury requires immediate fracture or joint reduction in both the open and closed wound. Continued impaired circulation requires vascular surgical consultation.

Immediate and accurate diagnosis of an impending closed space or compartment compression syndrome is important. Progressive sustained ischemia distal to the site of trauma, not relieved by conservative treatment, mandates adequate decompressive fasciotomy(ies). Areas commonly involved include the volar aspect of the forearm (Volkmann's ischemia), the dorsal forearm, the metacarpus, and the pulp of the distal phalangeal segments. Mechanisms of injury that cause this complication include skeletal trauma (dislocation or displaced fracture in the area of the elbow or proximal or middle forearm), crushing trauma, circumferential full-thickness burn, high-voltage electrical burn, high-pressure injection injury, high-velocity projectile injury, vascular accident, and, occasionally, infection and venomous reptile or insect bite.

The two most important diagnostic criteria include progressively increasing pain on attempted passive digital motion (passive digital extension

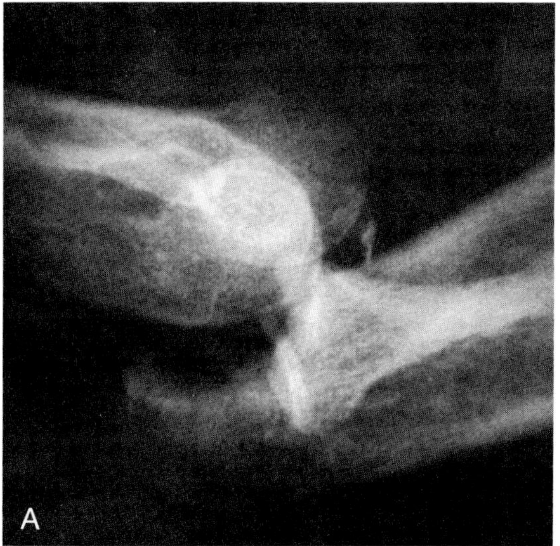

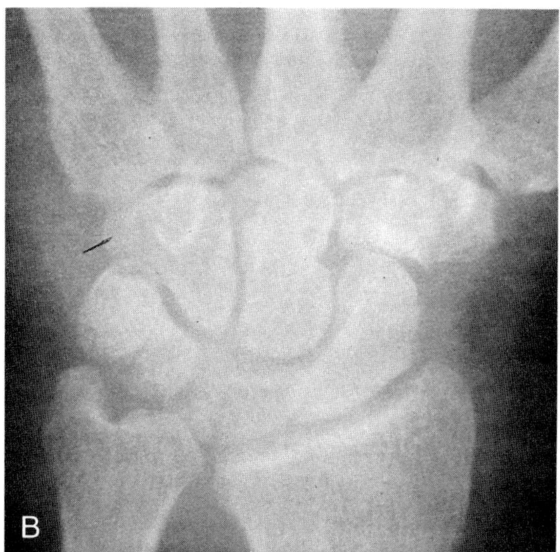

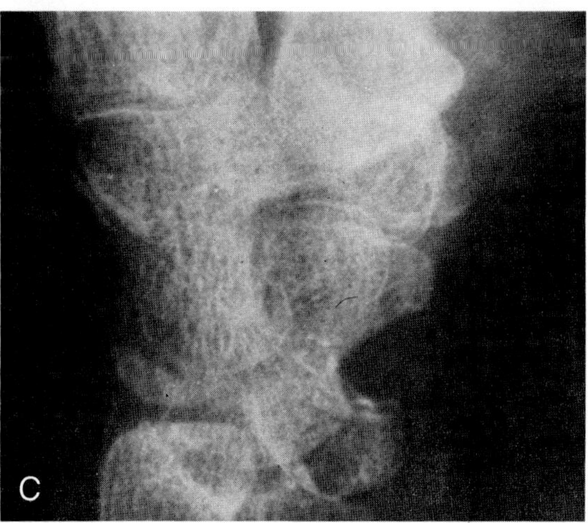

with volar forearm involvement and passive digital flexion with dorsal forearm involvement, and passive digital extension, particularly the MP joint, and abduction and adduction of digits provoking pain in the interosseous area of the metacarpus), and decreasing or absent superficial palmar arch pulse (usually determined by the Doppler ultrasonic flow meter). An indepth discussion of these criteria may be found in Chapter 8.

Physiologic immobilization includes the functional position of the wrist and hand, previously noted, combined usually with elbow flexion and elevation—the fingertips should point up and the hand should be palm up.

The general patient history includes pertinent information on possible drug sensitivities, particularly to local anesthetic agents, antibiotics, analgesics, and so forth, and on current medications (anticoagulants, mood elevators or depressants, antihypertensive drugs, insulin, steroids—particularly those taken for any prolonged period of time within 1 year prior to injury—and medications for chronic illnesses, including cardiovascular disease, chronic lung disease, and chronic renal disease). Any significant past or current medical disorder, familial or drug-related bleeding tendency, anticoagulation regimen, or current infection also must be noted.

A general history of previous trauma to the musculoskeletal and nervous systems is necessary with particular attention paid to involvement of the injured extremity.

General physical examination is especially important in patients who have sustained multiple injuries in a motor-vehicle accident, fall from a high place, or similar type of injury. Again, initial examination, followed by re-examination at

Fig. 27-1. *A*, Lateral roentgenograph shows a posterior fracture-dislocation of the right elbow. *B*, Seven weeks after injury, this posteroanterior view of the ipsilateral right wrist shows rarefaction of the lunate and indistinct articulations of the lunate with adjacent carpals and the distal radius. The distal ulna is abnormally longer than the distal radius, and the distal radioulnar articulation is incongruous. *C*, Lateral view of the right wrist shows complete anterior dislocation of the lunate with a volar tilt of approximately 65°. The concomitant anterior dislocation of the lunate was not recognized until 7 weeks after the injury occurred. This case illustrates the importance of careful initial examination of the entire injured extremity and examination at periodic intervals thereafter to avoid unnecessary and tragic complications. (From Sandzén, S. C., Jr.: Atlas of Wrist and Hand Fractures. Littleton, MA, PSG Publishing, 1979.)

periodic intervals, often is rewarding in diagnosing less severe, often occult trauma, particularly as the patient becomes more responsive and alert after stabilization of a potential or actual life-threatening situation.

Appropriate laboratory determinations include those necessary preoperatively for general anesthesia and evaluation of vital body functions (e.g., PA of the chest, complete blood count, urinalysis, EKG, and potassium determinations).

Tetanus prophylaxis is administered as recommended by the Committee on Trauma of the American College of Surgeons.[1] Generally, if the patient has received adequate initial prophylaxis and has had a toxoid booster within 5 years prior to injury, no treatment is necessary. If more than 5 years have passed since the last tetanus toxoid booster, 0.5 ml of tetanus toxoid are required. Patients suspected of having incomplete or no initial prophylaxis (elderly females, males who have not served in the military service, and foreigners—particularly those not speaking English) require administration of tetanus toxoid booster and 250 units of tetanus immune globulin, followed by completion of the recommended tetanus prophylactic regimen by their family physician.

Antibiotics are indicated in any severe open injury of the upper extremity involving the skeletal system, particularly if the injury was incurred in a contaminated environment or if large amounts of soft tissue remain with precarious viability.

Specific Wound Treatment

The sequential stages of primary wound care are:

1. accurate history of injury.
2. initial wound evaluation.
3. appropriate roentgenographs.
4. anesthesia.
5. wound culture and gram stains.
6. meticulous wound toilet.
7. decision of initial wound care: open treatment, primary closure or resurfacing, or delayed primary closure or resurfacing.
8. accurate indepth wound examination.
9. management of deeper structures: vascular system, tendons and nerves, and skeletal system.
10. immobilization.
11. mobilization and rehabilitation.

History

Initial history and evaluation of structures distal to the injury are often incomplete or inaccurate because of the patient's anxiety, pain, lack of cooperation, or obtunded mental status (alcohol or drug related or from head trauma). Nevertheless, all findings must be documented in writing. Only by doing so can the physician evaluate later whether nerve or vascular damage existed prior to initial treatment. Specific information includes the mechanism of injury and environment in which the injury was sustained to ascertain type and extent of trauma and the degree of contamination. Wounds generally considered contaminated involve human and most animal bites, those sustained in a particularly contaminated environment (e.g., farmyard, garbage truck, or garbage compactor), and those that have remained open for 10 hours or longer. Any first-aid treatment, particularly medications, attempted manipulations, and the last time and contents of oral intake are noted.

Initial Examination

Often it is unnecessary to disturb dressings and immobilization at the time of initial wound examination, particularly in massive injuries. At this time, a pneumatic tourniquet should be in place on the upper arm and ready to inflate in case of unexpected hemorrhage.

Early accurate diagnosis of progressive ischemia resulting from a closed space (compartment) compression syndrome again is stressed with particular attention paid to the superficial palmar arch pulse.

The "soaking" of an open wound in soapy water or similar solution is not indicated. A hypotonic "soaking solution" causes tissue edema, which is particularly troublesome in massive injuries and, perhaps more importantly, may lead the attending physician into a dangerous false sense of security that the wound, particularly the small wound, has been cleansed when, indeed, this assumption is completely false.

If the open wound is examined, "blind probing" with a hemostat definitely is contraindicated because of the risk of additional contamination, injury to marginally viable structures, nerve and tendon damage, and unnecessary pain incurred.

Vascular supply, nerve innervation (sensory and motor), and tendon function distal to the wound are examined accurately.

Each specific musculotendinous unit of each separate digit is evaluated in detail. Sensory and motor modalities of median, ulnar, radial, anterior, and posterior interosseous nerves are examined, and if crossed innervation of any major nerve is suspected, a selected nerve block may be valuable.

Skeletal involvement usually is obvious in the more severe injuries, sometimes with characteristic deformities. However, these characteristic lesions become obscured by diffuse swelling of the area a few hours after injury. Point tenderness and stress testing of ligaments prior to anesthesia may afford helpful diagnostic clues.

Roentgenographs

Roentgenographic evaluation includes, minimally, a posteroanterior, lateral, and two oblique views, centered specifically at the site of injury determined at initial evaluation. In the skeletally immature patient and in patients with wrist injuries, roentgenographs taken of the contralateral normal extremity may be helpful for comparison. If possible, intact dressings and immobilizations are not disturbed during roentgenographic examination.

Any severe injury of the wrist and/or hand must be treated in an adequately equipped and staffed surgical suite. Any additional roentgenographic views or supplementary studies can be obtained in the suite.

Anesthesia

Adequate anesthesia must precede initial primary wound care. Brachial plexus anesthesia, either from the axillary or supraclavicular approach, is excellent if trauma is restricted to a single upper extremity. However, the possibility of producing a pneumothorax accompanies the use of the supraclavicular approach.

Bier's block intravenous regional anesthesia usually is not feasible on extensive upper extremity injuries and is not applicable for open wounds of any extent since the tourniquet should be released following wound toilet to reevaluate circulation and tissue viability.

Three important principles in upper extremity nerve block anesthesia are:

1. Epinephrine must be excluded from all anesthetic agents administered distal to the wrist because of the possibility of vascular constriction causing irreversible ischemic changes in already severely traumatized digits.

2. If there is any suspicion of a progressive closed space (compartment) compression type of syndrome, the use of long-acting anesthetic agents (Marcaine) is contraindicated. The paramount signs and symptoms of progressive ischemia are obscured, and because of delayed diagnosis, irreversible ischemic changes may occur,

3. General anesthesia often is preferable in the young child, the extremely agitated patient, the elderly person, the uncooperative patient, the mentally retarded person, those unfamiliar with the English language for whom no interpreter is available, and in persons with concurrent infections of the hand or digits.

Wound Culture and Gram Stains

Prior to wound toilet, specimens are taken for appropriate bacterial determinations and gram stain. A pneumatic tourniquet, if not in place already, is applied to the upper arm to be inflated when necessary.

Wound Toilet

Meticulous wound toilet is by far the most important aspect of primary care in the open, acute, upper extremity injury. Wound toilet includes meticulous, gentle cleansing, copious irrigation with sterile isotonic solution, and meticulous debridement of foreign bodies and nonviable tissue while protecting all viable elements.

Cleansing is effected by gentle mechanical washing of all surrounding normal skin areas that will be within the surgical field prior to directing attention to cleansing the open wound. Wound cleansing should continue for a minimum of 10 to 20 minutes in the average wound, and the use of sterile gloves and 4-by-4-inch gauze sponges or their equivalent is necessary. In particularly extensive or contaminated injuries, two separate scrubs, each a minimum of 15 minutes with completely separate scrub solutions and sterile glove changes, are recommended.

Irrigation must extend to the depths of the wound with a minimum of 2 to 3L of sterile isotonic solution (e.g., sterile isotonic saline). The use of sterile water or ordinary tap water is contraindicated in larger wounds because the hypotonicity causes excessive soft-tissue edema. The use of a water pik or a genitourinary sterile irrigation system (3L sterile saline irrigating unit) may be preferred.

Precise debridement of all foreign matter and nonviable tissue includes loose segments of epithelium, crushed nonviable skin, segments of completely avulsed tendon or ligament, elevated portions of nailplate or completely elevated nailplate, and small free bone fragments unattached to soft tissue. Any contaminated exposed bone is cleaned meticulously down to normal-appearing clean bleeding bone, and any viable bone segment of significant size attached to soft tissue, particularly a collateral ligament or volar plate, is meticulously cleaned and retained.

If prior immediate reduction of an open dislocation or displaced fracture was necessary to restore circulation distally, redislocation or redisplacement at this time permits effective adequate wound toilet and prevents sequestration of contaminated material prior to definitive reduction.

Vessels previously clamped and ligated are reclamped and religated with excision of the segment distally.

Salvage and protection of all viable tissue, continued irrigation, and redirection of the overhead spotlight away from the open wound to prevent unnecessary desiccation are performed simultaneously with debridement.

There is no shortcut to meticulous wound toilet. Unnecessary delay or inadequate technique is responsible minimally for prolonged morbidity (Fig. 27-2).

Evaluation of Wound and Integument

Closed Space (Compartment) Compression Syndrome

The early diagnosis of a progressive closed space (compartment) compression syndrome necessitating surgical intervention with appropriate fascial lyses cannot be overemphasized. Fasciotomies must be extensive enough to relieve internal pressure completely and should extend into normal tissues proximally and distally. In high-voltage electrical injuries, escharotomy alone usually is insufficient to release pressure; consequently, fasciotomy is indicated. Physiologic skin incisions, performed with care to avoid damage to deeper structures (ulnar nerve at the elbow and median and ulnar nerves at the wrist), prevent unnecessary secondary scar contractures. Compartmental fascial lysis occasionally must be augmented by lysis of the fascial covering of individual muscles (epimysium). Decompression of the interossei is effected by dorsal longitudinal incisions between each pair of metacarpals. Release of the distal phalangeal pulp space is brought about by an incision similar to that used to decompress and evacuate an extensive pulp-space abscess.

Open Wounds

In the open wound, the condition of the skin in and about the injury, as well as the mechanism and environment of injury, determines whether primary closure or coverage, or initial open treatment with delayed primary or secondary closure or coverage, is preferred.

Open Treatment

Initial open treatment is mandatory in all human and most animal bites. Other indications for initial open treatment are a wound that is judged either by history, physical examination, or both to be severely contaminated; a wound that has much marginally viable tissue retained after initial wound toilet; following fascial lysis of a closed compartment type of syndrome; a massively edematous wound; and any wound in which additional hemorrhagic oozing or edema probably will continue.

Primary Wound Closure

Primary wound closure is obviously the preferred treatment, but often the skin in a complex injury is insufficient to permit closure under no tension. If skin of precarious viability is primarily closed under tension, additional vascular compromise is caused both by impeded venous drainage and arterial supply, compounded by progressive edema, and results in necrosis of the wound edges, usually with diastasis and often with subsequent infection.

However, if all viable irregular skin tags have been preserved and protected, they often can be interdigitated to afford satisfactory primary closure.

Primary Resurfacing

Particularly in blast injuries and injuries in which skin and subcutaneous tissue have been avulsed completely or must be debrided because of nonviability, a gaping wound persists that may be suitable for primary resurfacing by a split-thickness skin graft. The split-thickness graft may be applied directly to viable bone, tendon sheath, muscle, or fascia but cannot be expected to "take" on articular cartilage, nonviable bone, or abraded rough tendon or nerve. The graft

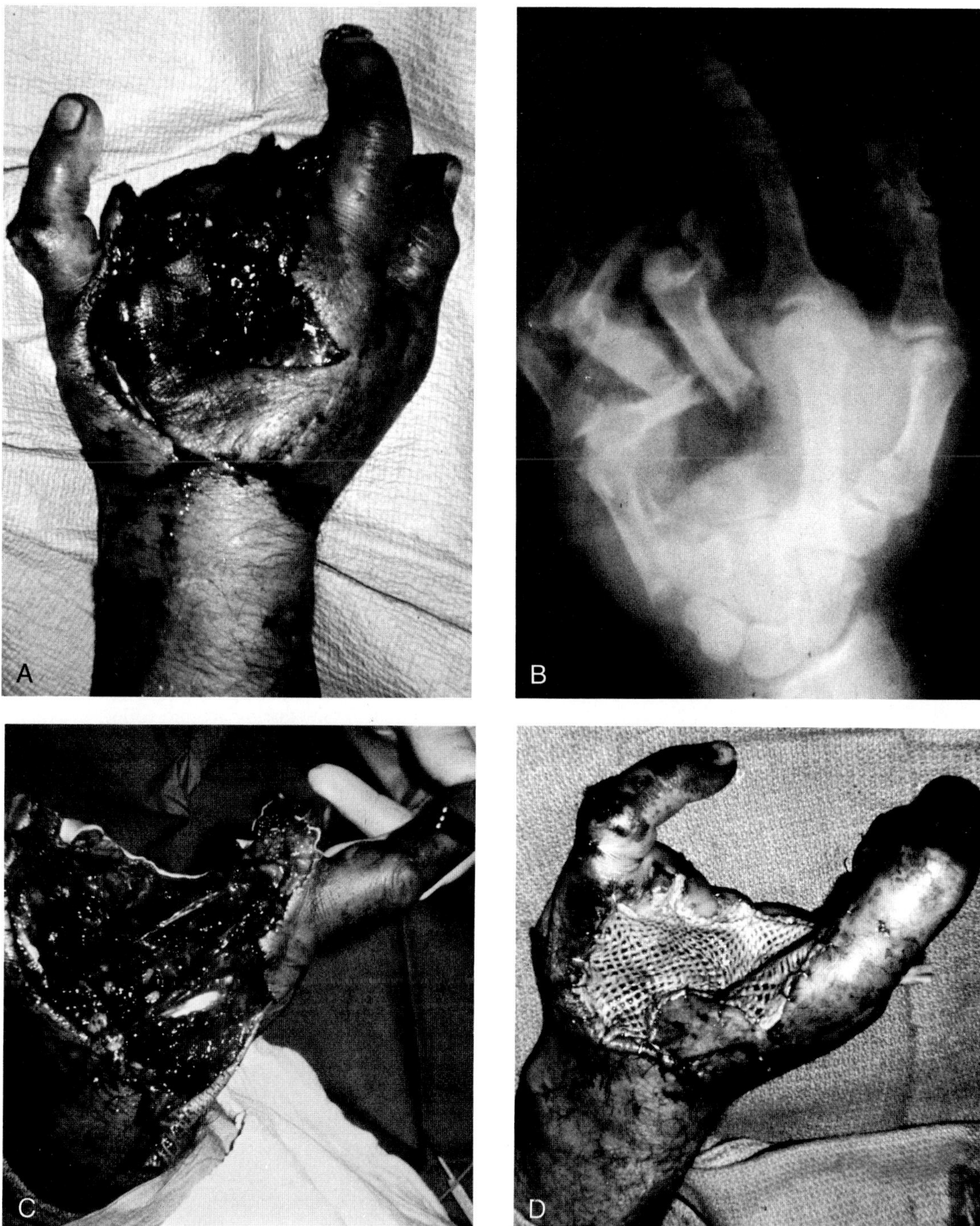

Fig. 27-2. *A*, This patient sustained severe blast injury to his left hand; wound toilet was not effected until 72 hours post-trauma (the time of this photograph). *B*, The roentgenograph shows marked destruction of the central portion of the hand with displaced fractures of the metacarpal bases of the index and little finger. *C*, After debridement of the foul-smelling necrotic central portion of the hand, remaining viable elements included skin tags, little finger, thumb, and index ray. *D*, After four staged debridements, the wound was clean enough to receive a meshed, split-thickness skin-graft resurfacing, applied 20 days after injury. This case illustrates the necessity of proper effective primary care with meticulous wound toilet. The delay of 72 hours caused more than 2 weeks of additional morbidity before the split-thickness graft could be applied.

should be .016 to .018 of an inch in thickness and may be fenestrated or "meshed" if one is concerned about future transudate, exudate, or oozing hemorrhage. The meshed graft, applied in a ratio of 1.0 to 1.5 length to 1.0 width, also assures accurate application to irregular surfaces. The eventual durability of the initial resurfacing of the split-thickness graft usually obviates the need for reconstructive grafting except when extensive deeper reconstructive procedures are necessary.

Occasionally, a local rotational pedicle graft may be indicated primarily, but a distant pedicle graft rarely is recommended. By far, it is better to provide initial resurfacing by split-thickness skin graft, applying distant pedicle graft coverage later, only if necessary. Either initial application of a split graft or initial open treatment is strongly recommended for surgeons not thoroughly acquainted with indications for and principles and techniques of proper distant pedicle utilization.

Delayed Primary Closure and Resurfacing

Delayed primary closure or resurfacing is the method of choice for all wounds treated initially by open treatment. Often, delayed primary closure may be accomplished 24 to 48 hours after injury if no additional tissue necrosis or contamination is found at the first dressing change. If necessary, the wound is redebrided and treated open for an additional 24 to 48 hours prior to the second dressing change and re-evaluation. Closure should be contemplated only when one is as sure as possible that the wound is clean with no evidence of infection and no further tissue necrosis. Delayed primary resurfacing is indicated when hemorrhagic oozing or redebridements prevent initial use of a split-thickness skin graft (see Fig. 27-2).

Occasionally, a homograft (cadaver skin) or xenograft-heterograft (porcine skin) may be valuable for either primary or delayed primary resurfacing when deeper structures must be protected or when infection or further tissue necrosis is suspected. These grafts act as a physiologic dressing until the wound is entirely acceptable for a graft.

Secondary Closure and Resurfacing

Secondary closure indicates a longer time interval between injury and wound closure. The margins of the skin edges in a clean wound are debrided to healthy viable tissue, and skin closure is accomplished with elimination of any dead space and under no tension.

Secondary resurfacing usually employs a pedicle type of procedure (local pedicle, rotational pedicle, distant pedicle, or free pedicle graft) to provide sufficient subcutaneous tissue enabling extensive deeper reconstruction (e.g., bone graft, tendon transfer). The best sources for distant pedicle resurfacing, and the most predictable, are random pedicles from the contralateral lower abdominal quadrant or supraclavicular or deltoid areas. If an extensive distant pedicle graft is required, it should be based on a known vascular supply.

The specific problems of a distally based, partial skin crush avulsion and interdigital web injuries will be discussed in the sections entitled Crush Injuries and Blast Injuries.

Indepth Wound Evaluation

It is important to stress again that only after meticulous wound toilet should an indepth examination of the wound be carried out with accurate assessment of injuries to deeper structures for precise diagnoses.

Though inflation of the tourniquet may have been unnecessary during wound toilet, it usually is utilized for accurate indepth wound evaluation.

Generally, the repair of deeper structures (skeleton, nerves, tendons, and vessels) should be accomplished only if the wound is clean and if primary closure is feasible.

Management of Deeper Structures

Vascular System

Following fracture or joint reduction, if ischemia of structures distal to the injury persists, direct examination of the vascular supply becomes necessary, usually following appropriate arteriographic studies. Arterial and/or vein repair or graft often restores satisfactory circulation. The general concept of vascular repair in replantation of parts is currently one vein for each artery.

If either the radial or ulnar artery is in continuity, satisfactory circulation usually persists; however, each damaged artery must be evaluated individually. If both radial and ulnar arteries are damaged, both should be repaired.

Generally, if one volar proper vascular bundle remains intact, digital viability is assured and primary vascular repair is not necessary.

Tendon and Nerve Injuries

If a tendon or nerve injury is suspected, either at initial physical examination or because of the specific anatomic area of the injury, meticulous wound examination is necessary for accurate diagnosis, particularly to properly diagnose a partial major nerve laceration.

Primary repairs are contraindicated in massively contaminated wounds or when skin coverage is unsuitable.

The more severe the injury, the more indication there is for delayed primary or secondary tendon and nerve repair. Primary repairs often necessitate somewhat extensive surgical exposure, which may further jeopardize soft tissue of already precarious viability.

During open reduction and internal fixation of fractures and dislocations, any sharp bone spicules adjacent to tendons or nerves must be removed and anatomic fracture or joint reduction achieved to prevent abrasion or actual severance of these structures later. Repair of a partially lacerated major nerve or tendon is important, either primarily or as a delayed primary procedure. Repair of the partially lacerated major nerve is much more important since later reconstruction is technically difficult and requires protection of the intact nerve fibers, excision of the neuroma in continuity, and either secondary repair or interposition of a nerve graft with often less than desired functional result.

Partially lacerated tendons may rupture at a later time or resultant scar formation may restrict tendon gliding, particularly of the long flexor tendons (profundus and superficialis) within the flexor sheaths. Severe direct trauma to a tendon may cause local avascularity significant enough to result in secondary rupture; severe direct trauma to a nerve may cause varying degrees of neurapraxia requiring later neurolysis.

In massive trauma, primary repair of the flexor tendons within the flexor sheaths rarely is advisable.

If median or ulnar nerve repair and/or flexor tendon repairs in the area of the carpal tunnel are effected, lysis of the transverse carpal ligament is recommended.

Crush injuries sustained to the proximal phalanges invariably bind down the superficial flexors (which are deep to the profundi at this point) in callous and cicatrix to the palmar aspect of the proximal phalanges. Usually, profundus tendolysis, and often resection of the superficialis tendon, is necessary later to provide effective profundus action.

The extensor tendons are particularly vulnerable to injury at the proximal interphalangeal (PIP), DIP, and wrist joint levels.

Recognition and repair of a laceration or of an open avulsion fracture of the central slip of the extensor tendon insertion dorsal to the PIP joint is important to prevent a boutonnière lesion from developing. The PIP joint should be maintained in extension by temporary oblique or longitudinal Kirschner wire fixation for approximately 4 to 5 weeks.

Avulsion of long flexor tendon insertions (flexor digitorum profundus and flexor pollicis longus tendons) requires surgical treatment of reinsertion or tendon advancement; however, conservative treatment by 6 to 8 weeks of immobilization of the DIP joint in extension is indicated for long extensor tendon insertion avulsions (drop or mallet finger).

Significant fracture avulsions, generally over 25% of the articular surface, of both long flexor and extensor tendon insertions require open reduction and anatomic fixation (Blalock's technique is most effective to anatomically reduce and securely fix the articular fracture fragment avulsion, which usually is "flipped over" 60 to 90° (Fig. 27-3)).

Small fragments may be debrided from the long flexor tendon insertions and that tendon insertion advanced, but a comparable lesion of a long extensor tendon insertion should be treated conservatively, as previously noted.

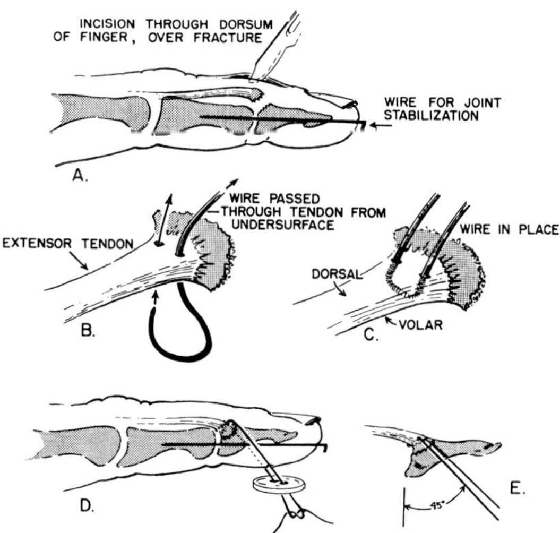

FIG. 27-3. *A* through *E*, The Blalock technique effectively reduces and securely fixes virtually any tendon or ligament fracture avulsion. (From Blalock, S. H.: Technique for reattachment of extensor fracture avulsion.)

In multiple-system trauma, open or closed reduction of joints and displaced fractures, usually with internal fixation or percutaneous Kirschner wire fixation, should precede any attempt at either primary or delayed primary tendon or nerve repairs.

Reconstruction of tendons and nerves requires satisfactory skin and subcutaneous tissue overlying the wound. Therefore, appropriate resurfacing must be provided as soon as possible to enable early repair of deeper structures.

Skeletal System

The gross configuration often is suggestive of a specific skeletal injury. Accurate diagnosis is assured by routine roentgenographs and supplemented by distraction views, tomographs, and carpal tunnel view. Stability is evaluated by gross stress-test examination of specific ligaments and direct examination in the open injury.

The image intensifier is useful to monitor manipulations in fracture and joint reduction but cannot be relied on for detailed information (articular fractures). Posteroanterior and lateral views taken after distractive forces have been applied can be helpful to separate the various components in a complex skeletal trauma (see Fig. 27-7, *B*).

Closed manipulation and reduction is the preferred treatment; however, this treatment is often insufficient with marked skeletal distortion, and open reduction and internal fixation are necessary.

If anatomic reduction can be achieved but not maintained, closed reduction and multiple percutaneous Kirschner wire fixations may be the solution.

Failed closed reduction necessitates open reduction and fixation, achieved by the most applicable technique or techniques: percutaneous Kirschner wire fixation and/or internal fixation with Kirschner wires, screws, plates, or wires.

Extensive segmental bone loss usually is not treated definitively initially unless a segment of bone from a nonviable area, which would otherwise be discarded, can be inserted as a primary autogenous bone graft (see Fig. 27-14).

Segmental bone loss usually is managed by one of the following methods, only if vascularity is not impaired: dynamic skeletal traction through a transverse Kirschner wire placed through the phalanx distal to the injury; "pins-and-plaster" fixation; Stader splint, Hoffman, or Roger Anderson external immobilization or modification thereof; and occasionally by an interpositional Kirschner wire spreader placed in the bone defect to exert pressure proximally and distally.

Reinsertion of a complete ligament avulsion or anatomic replacement of an articular fracture avulsion by the Blalock technique is indicated in the following important areas: the radial and ulnar collateral ligaments of the thumb metacarpophalangeal (MP) joint, the radial collateral ligament of the index finger MP joint, the radial collateral ligament of the index finger PIP joint, and both the radial and ulnar collateral ligaments of the little finger PIP joint.

Particularly important is restoration of proper rotational alignment in displaced metacarpal and phalangeal fractures and correction of angulation deformities and shortening of proximal and middle phalangeal fractures.

Articular Fractures. Only by precise roentgenographic evaluation can one accurately evaluate a joint injury. The image intensifier is not useful in recognizing anatomic incongruity of an articular fracture because the detail is unsatisfactory.

Articular fractures must be differentiated accurately from periarticular fractures since articular fractures, if displaced, often require surgical intervention for anatomic reduction, but periarticular fracture injuries often may be reduced closed and treated conservatively.

Displaced, irreducible, or unstable fractures involving generally 25% or more of the articular surface require open reduction and internal fixation.

As noted, a displaced articular fragment attached to a collateral ligament should be anatomically reduced and fixed, if possible, but if this fragment is too small, it should be debrided and the collateral ligament reattached to its normal anatomic location.

When multiple severe injuries involve many areas in the wrist and hand, gross realignment of the digits by longitudinal Kirschner wire fixation, or occasionally by using dynamic skeletal traction to align joints, often is all that can be realistically achieved. Primary arthrodesis rarely is indicated, even for severe comminuted articular injuries. Surprisingly, acceptable function often can be salvaged in such cases by commencing early active and passive range of motion exercises.

If stable reductions are achieved and maintained, particularly by skeletal fixation, gentle range of motion exercises should be commenced as soon as possible (e.g., following subsidence of edema and hemorrhage of trauma and surgery—approximately 5 to 7 days postinjury). Once again, the functional position of immobilization is stressed.

Injuries to the Skeletally Immature Extremity. Injuries to the epiphyseal growth plates, or physes, often occur more frequently than fractures and dislocations in the skeletally immature patient (see Fig. 27-16, *B*). The Salter-Harris classification is acceptable (Fig. 27-4) and signifies that anatomic reduction is essential in types III and IV injuries to restore acceptable articular surfaces. With the frequency of epiphyseal growth-plate injuries, more growth disturbances surprisingly do not result unless extensive crushing trauma to the physis occurs (Salter V injury).

The same general principles are recommended in treating fractures and dislocations in children as those for comparable injuries in adults. Fortunately, nature is forgiving in fracture healing in the young. Adaptive remodeling of the healing fracture site responds to functional stresses and demands (Wolff's law); however, rotational deformities are permanent, and any malrotation not corrected initially persists.

Angulation deformities spontaneously correct with the following considerations:

1. The younger the child, the more rapid and better the correction.
2. The angulation must be in line with motion of an adjacent hinge joint.
3. The closer the angulation is to the metaphysis and adjacent joint, the more rapid and better the correction.
4. The least severe angulations correct most rapidly and most completely.

Open reduction (often with internal fixation), though less frequently utilized, is necessary to treat irreducible fractures or dislocations and to fix unstable situations. Care must be taken, however, to avoid damage to epiphyseal growth plates and to provide effective external immobilization, usually with a long-arm cast with soft Velpeau's cast and sling (mandatory in the hyperactive child).

Immobilization

Physiologic immobilization in the functional position is strongly recommended in virtually all instances and is important following extensive trauma. This position includes wrist extension, wide thumb abduction and opposition, metacarpophalangeal joint flexion, and proximal and distal interphalangeal joint extension. Any portion of the hand and digits not necessary for immobilization should be moved immediately. Mobilization of the injured areas commences as soon as there is no danger of fracture redisplacement, joint redislocation, or avulsion at the site of vascular anastomosis, tenorrhaphy, neurorrhaphy, or ligament repair.

Mobilization and Rehabilitation

The entire upper extremity must be considered. Mobilization includes shoulder circumduction exercises to prevent needless adduction contracture following injudicious prolonged immobilization. The elbow must be exercised actively to regain extension and flexion, pronation and supination; passive stretching exercises, however, are contraindicated. Active and gentle passive exercises must involve every joint of every digit and the wrist. All active exercises should be carried out aggressively "to the full count of 10 or 15." If dependent edema can be avoided, whirlpool therapy may be helpful.

Most importantly, the patient must realize that his rehabilitation, and ultimate functional result, depends on utmost cooperation in carrying out the specific rehabilitative exercises prescribed by the physician and therapist at specifically designated times during all waking hours.

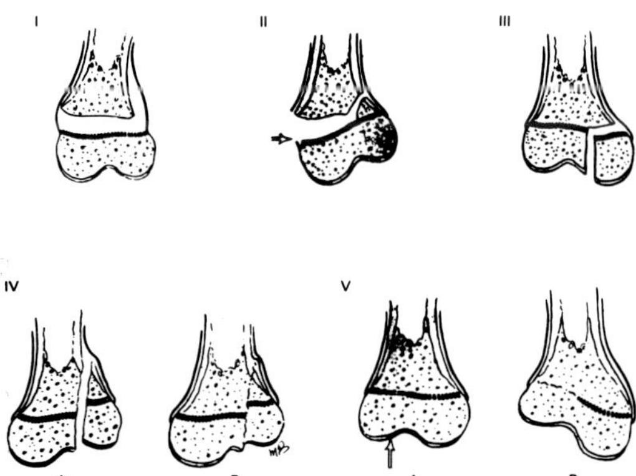

FIG. 27-4. The Salter-Harris classification of epiphyseal growth-plate injuries illustrates possible complications of types III, IV, and V. (From Salter, R. B., and Harris, W. R.: Injuries involving the epiphyseal plate. J. Bone Joint Surg., *54-A*:587, 1963.)

Specific Areas of Trauma

Distal Forearm

Fractures of the distal radius are divided into two distinct categories: (1) distal metaphyseal and (2) articular.

Distal metaphyseal fractures include: Colles', Smith's or reversed Colles', Colles' or Smith's fracture complicated by marked comminution of the metaphysis involving the distal articular surface, and any of the aforementioned fractures complicated by disruption of the distal radioulnar joint (Fig. 27-5). In the skeletally immature person, a slipped epiphysis is the equivalent injury.

Articular fractures of the distal radius include: dorsal Barton's, volar Barton's, and Chauffeur's fractures (Fig. 27-6). Differentiation between the distal metaphyseal, or nonarticular fractures, and the intra-articular fractures is important because of treatment.

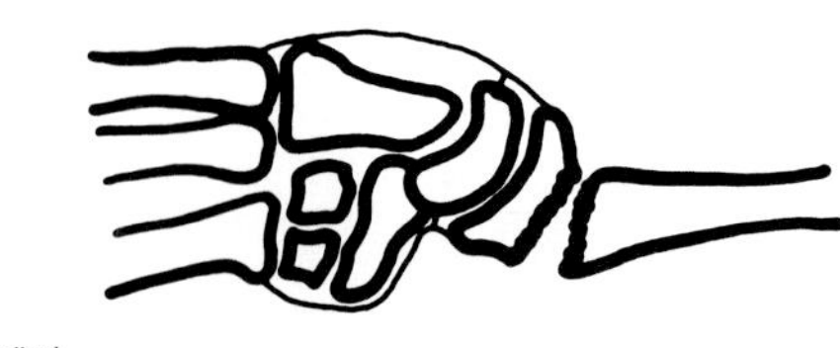

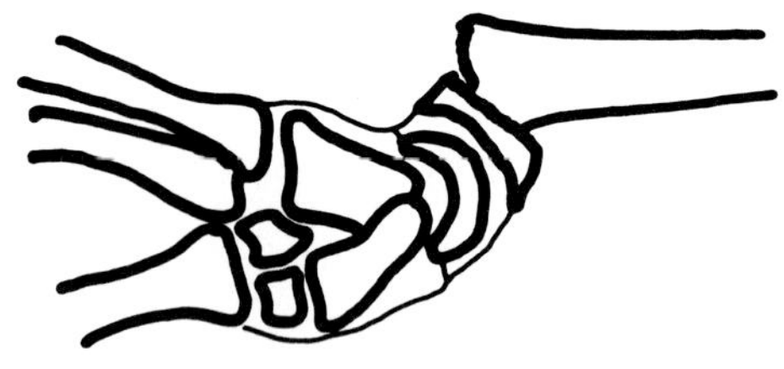

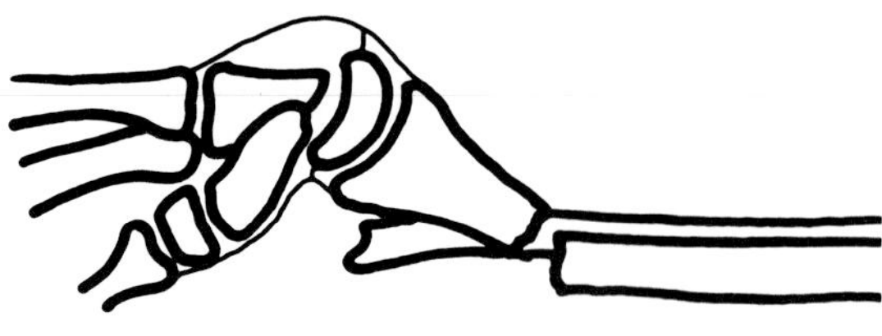

Fig. 27-5. The Cautilli classification of metaphyseal fractures of the distal radius includes Colles', Smith's, and Galeazzi. (From Cautilli, R. A., Joyce, M. F., Gordon, E., and Juarez, R.: Classification of fractures of the distal radius. Jefferson Orthop. J., *111*:46, 1974.)

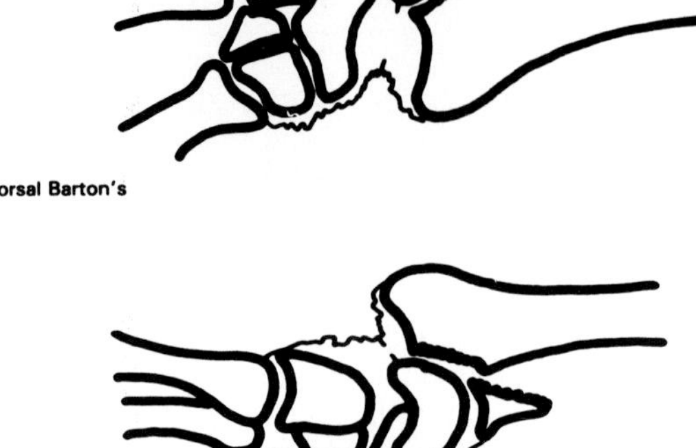

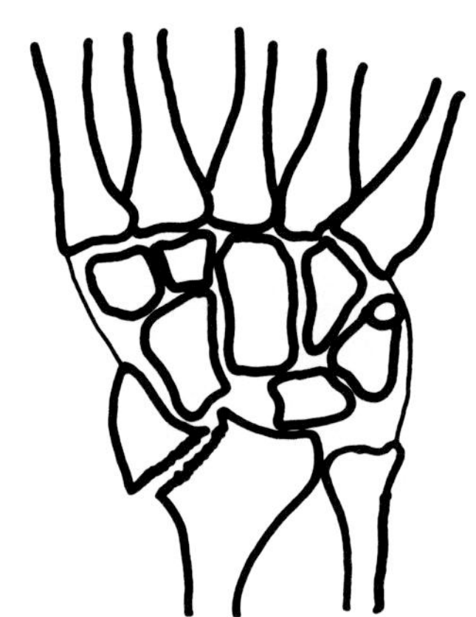

Fig. 27-6. The Cautilli classification of articular fractures of the distal radius includes dorsal Barton's, volar Barton's, and Chauffeur's fractures. (From Cautilli, R. A., Joyce, M. F., Gordon, E., and Juarez, R.: Classification of fractures of the distal radius. Jefferson Orthop. J., *111*:46, 1974.)

Closed manipulation and reduction of the stable distal radial metaphyseal fracture usually suffice. If unstable, particularly in physiologically young people, closed manipulation and reduction combined with "pins-and-plaster" immobilization achieve and maintain satisfactory position and length. Both Colles' and dorsal Barton's fractures are reduced in essentially the same manner, but immobilization is opposite. Colles' fracture is immobilized in some flexion and ulnar deviation, but dorsal Barton's fracture must be immobilized in some wrist extension to maintain fracture reduction. Opposite and comparable treatment principles are true for Smith's and volar Barton's fractures, which are mirror-image lesions of their dorsal counterparts.

Large segmental displaced articular fractures of the distal radius should be reduced anatomically. The method of closed reduction alone may suffice, but often anatomic reduction is impossible, requiring open reduction combined with either percutaneous Kirschner wire fixation or internal fixation of some sort to provide necessary stability.

In any complex skeletal injury of the distal upper extremity with multiple fractures, it is necessary first to reduce and stabilize the distal forearm fractures prior to treating injuries of the carpus and/or hand.

Chauffeur's fracture is often associated with a fracture of the scaphoid or scapholunate dissociation because the cleavage line of force passes through either the scaphoid itself or the scapholunate joint (Fig. 27-7).

Solitary fracture of the distal third of the radius (Piedmont fracture) often must be treated by open reduction and internal plate fixation because of the distorting forces of the brachioradialis augmented by the pronator quadratus. Solitary fracture of the distal ulnar shaft, however, usually is stable and does not require surgery. However, in complex injuries involving the carpus and/or hand, and certainly in both bone fractures of the distal forearm, internal fixation generally is necessary.

Galeazzi's fracture generally is treated by open reduction and internal plate fixation of the fracture of the distal radius and re-establishment of the distal radioulnar articulation.

Wrist

The wrist is suspended from the radius primarily by two important ligaments: radially, the volar radiocarpal ligament, originating radially and volarly from the distal radius, and, ulnarly, the ulnocarpal ligament complex (including the ulnocarpal meniscus, the triangular fibrocartilage, and the ulnolunate ligament), originating ulnarly and dorsally from the distal radius. These two ligaments converge distally to attach primarily to the capitate, lunate, triquetrum and scaphoid.[2]

The wrist joint articulates the distal radial articular surface proximally, which angulates volarly 10 to 12° and ulnarly 12 to 14° with the scaphoid and the lunate distally. The ulna is secured distally to the radius primarily by the triangular fibrocartilage but does not enter into the wrist joint itself; two separate, contiguous, and continuous structures, the triangular fibrocartilage and the ulnocarpal meniscus, separate the distal ulna from the triquetrum.

The eight carpal bones are arranged roughly into a proximal and distal row with the scaphoid as the integral coordinating, connecting osseous link. To understand wrist disorders, one must appreciate that the distal carpal row (trapezium, trapezoid, capitate, and hamate), combined with the second and third metacarpals, is functionally a single osseoligamentous unit comprising the stable portion of the hand. The midcarpal joint between the proximal and distal carpal rows is essentially an extended ball-and-socket joint. The head of the capitate and proximal pole and ulnar border of the hamate are the "ball" and the contiguous articular surfaces of the scaphoid, lunate, and triquetrum form the "socket." The midcarpal joint extends radially between the scaphoid and the trapezium and trapezoid.

The proximal carpal row is more complex and represents an intercalated segment between the distal radius and the distal carpal row. Most importantly, the lunate is the central point of the carpus and forms both a significant portion of the "socket" of the midcarpal joint distally and a significant portion of the wrist joint proximally.

The 45° volar angulation of the scaphoid from proximal to distal pole is responsible for the basic configuration of the transverse arch of the hand that is fundamental to thumb abduction and opposition.

Diagnosis

Diagnosis of any wrist injury is based on the gross appearance of the acute injury, point tenderness, and most importantly, on accurate roentgenographic evaluation. When seen shortly after trauma, significant carpal injury is suspected with either dorsal displacement of the carpus or volar protusion of the lunate, combined with median neurapraxia, impaired ability to flex actively or to extend the digits, and pain on passively attempting to extend the digits. If the injury is not seen until some hours after trauma, identifying characteristics are obscured by moderate to massive edema. Posteroanterior, lateral,

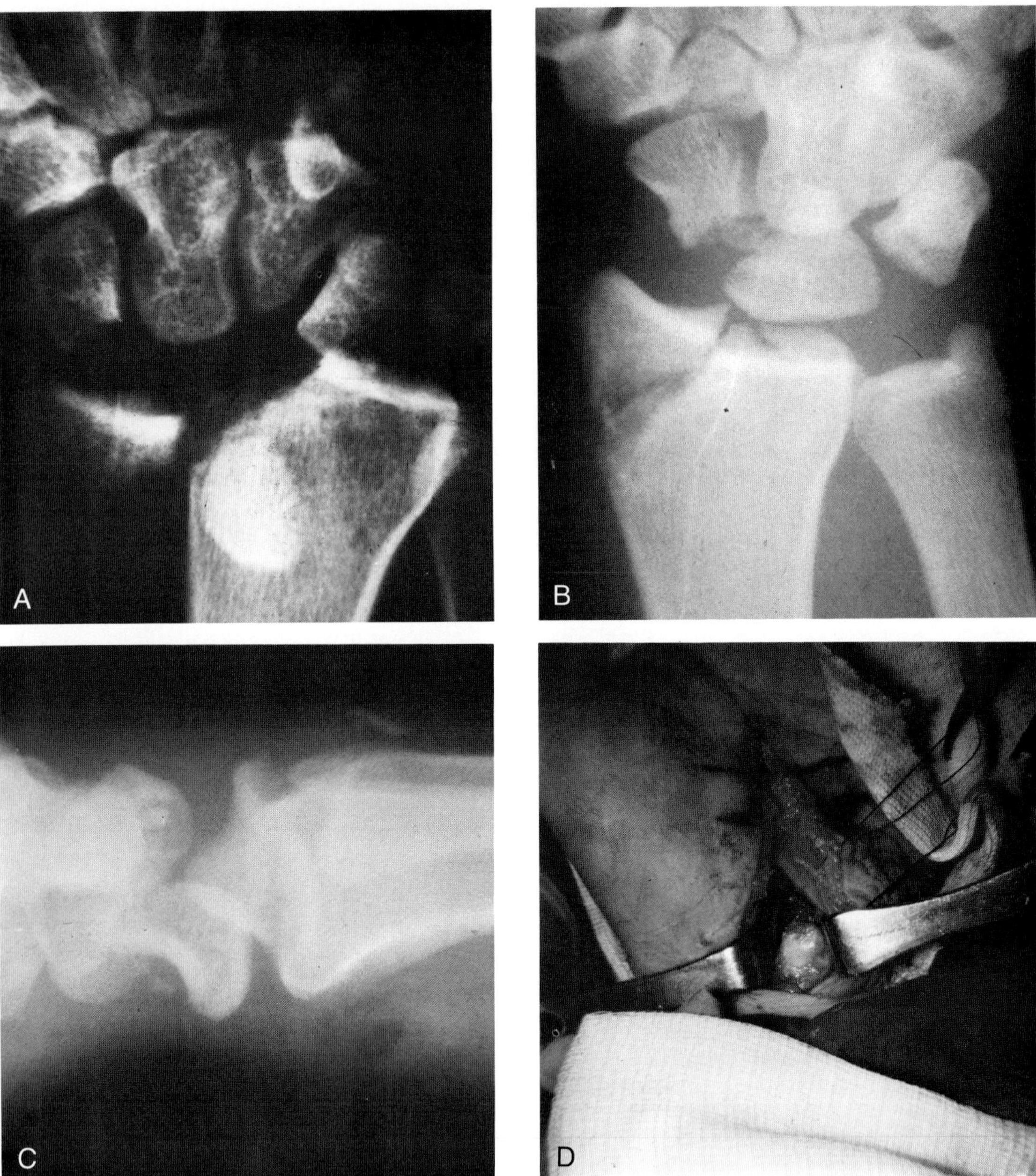

Fig. 27-7. *A*, This posteroanterior roentgenograph shows damage sustained to both the distal radius and carpus in a fall on the outstretched right hand. Injuries of this severe, open, fracture-dislocation of the wrist include completely displaced Chauffeur's fracture of the distal radius, dorsal subluxation of the distal ulna, complete volar proximal dislocation of the lunate, and fracture at the junction of the proximal and middle thirds of the scaphoid with marked displacement of the proximal fragment. *B*, The various components of this complex injury are visualized better in this distraction view taken at the time of initial treatment. The proximal third of the scaphoid has been debrided, the lunate has a "pie-shaped" configuration, the Chauffeur's fracture is in much better position, and the dorsal subluxation of the distal ulna is reduced. *C*, Simultaneous lateral roentgenograph shows persistent volar dislocation of the lunate. Initial treatment included meticulous wound toilet and "pins-and-plaster" immobilization for the reduced Chauffeur's fracture and dorsal subluxation of the distal ulna. *D*, Volar lunate dislocation was not reduced at initial treatment, but was carried out as a reconstructive procedure approximately 3 weeks later, after successful wound healing and patient referral for consultation. The volar approach allowed exploration of the ulnar nerve with neurolysis for persistent ulnar neurapraxia and exposure of the volar dislocation of the lunate as seen in this photograph.

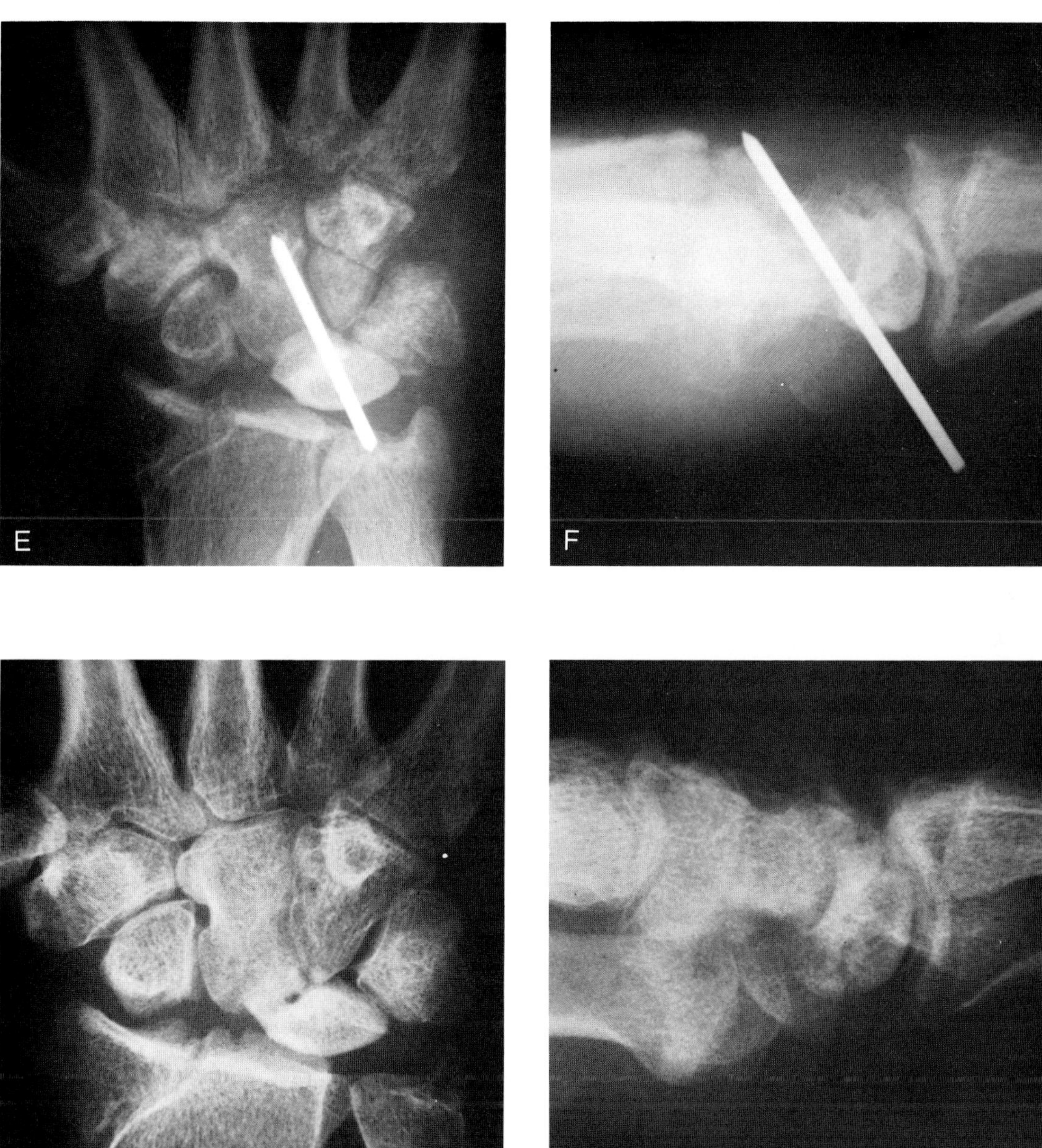

Fig. 27-7 (*continued*). *E*, Posteroanterior roentgenograph following open reduction and Kirschner-wire fixation of the lunate 2 months postoperatively. One or more Kirschner wires may be necessary to achieve stability and, preferably, should not cross the wrist joint. Moderate aseptic necrosis of the lunate is evident. *F*, Corresponding lateral view shows generally acceptable carpal structure, including position of the lunate. *G*, Posteroanterior roentgenograph taken 8 months after injury illustrates healed Chauffeur's fracture in good position and acceptable anatomy of the distal radioulnar joint and carpus. (Structural changes include absence of the proximal half of the scaphoid, a somewhat flattened and sclerotic lunate ulnarly displaced and autofused to the head of the capitate, and irregularities of the distal radial articular surface). *H*, Corresponding lateral view shows similar findings with some dorsal rotation of the lunate. This case illustrates the importance of anatomic restoration of the distal radius and ulna before that of the carpus (despite the 4-week delay before reduction of the lunate). (From Sandzén, S. C., Jr.: Atlas of Wrist and Hand Fractures. Littleton, MA, PSG Publishing, 1979.)

and two oblique roentgenographs, centered accurately on the point of tenderness and/or disfiguration, are essential for accurate diagnosis of carpal injuries. The key view is the lateral, and the lunate is the focal point. A posteroanterior view with traction applied to the digits often separates and clarifies superimposed components of distorted carpal anatomy (Fig. 27-7, *A* and *B*). Tomographs occasionally may help.

Wrist Joint

Dislocation of the wrist is rare since the entire ligamentous suspension, including the strong volar radiocarpal ligament and the ulnocarpal ligament complex, must be avulsed completely. However, fracture-dislocations of the wrist, including dorsal and volar Barton's fractures and Chauffeur's fractures, are common. Again, reduction and effective immobilization of the distal radial segment should precede treatment of the carpal disorder.

Carpal Injuries

Severe trauma usually divides the carpus into two segments: (1) the lunate with the proximal portion of the scaphoid (e.g., transscaphoid perilunate fracture-dislocation) or the lunate without the proximal scaphoid segment (e.g., perilunate dislocation or lunate dislocation) and (2) the remainder of the carpus. This pattern of carpal disruption is primarily due to the anatomic attachments and great strength of the volar radiocarpal ligament and the ulnocarpal ligament complex. The most common significant wrist disorder is dorsal transscaphoid perilunate fracture-dislocation.

The lunate is the focal point in diagnosis and treatment of all carpal trauma (Figs. 27-7 and 27-10, *B* through *E*). Diagnosis is facilitated by considering separately each of the four borders of the lunate. Disorders on the radial aspect include scaphoid fracture, scapholunate dissociation, usually accompanied by scaphoid rotational deformity, or a combination of both. Distortion of the distal border indicates fracture of the capitate neck with or without scaphoid fracture (naviculocapitate syndrome). Disorders on the ulnar aspect of the lunate include lunate-triquetrial joint instability and/or fracture of the triquetrum, and on the proximal border, wrist dislocation.

Simultaneous distortion of three borders of the lunate indicates either dorsal transscaphoid perilunate fracture-dislocation or dorsal perilunate dislocation. Involvement of all four lunate borders indicates dislocation of the lunate.

Any combination of carpal fractures, subluxations, dislocations, and ligamentous injuries may occur, depending on the mechanism and severity of injury, age of the patient, and local and systemic disorders (e.g., enchondroma or osteoporosis).

Scaphoid fracture is common because of the vulnerable position of the scaphoid as the connecting osseous link between the proximal and distal carpal rows associated with its palmar angulation of 45°. Fracture, however, may be either isolated or part of a complex that may include dorsal transscaphoid perilunate dislocation, naviculocapitate syndrome, or association with Chauffeur's fracture.

The functional distortion following scaphoid fracture is that the distal scaphoid segment becomes a part of and moves with the distal carpal row and the proximal scaphoid segment remains with the proximal carpal row. Therefore, an unstable or displaced scaphoid fracture causes carpal instability, and conversely, carpal instability is often responsible for scaphoid fracture nonunion.

Generally, displacement or rotation of a scaphoid fracture indicates more complex trauma to the wrist than does merely an isolated scaphoid fracture.

The most frequent causes for delayed union or nonunion of a scaphoid fracture are:

1. Inaccurate or incomplete reduction.
2. Instability.
3. Improper or inadequate immobilization.
4. Undetected and concurrent subluxation, dislocation, or fracture-dislocation of other carpal elements.

An isolated scaphoid dislocation is rare and is caused by severe localized trauma. Scaphoid dislocation usually is associated with other severe carpal trauma.

Lunate fracture of any significance usually forbodes the complication of avascular necrosis (Kienböck disease) with progressive distortion of carpal architecture, compression of the proximal scaphoid, and proximal migration of the entire distal carpal row, ultimately resulting sometimes in articulation of the capitate head with the distal radius.

Fracture of the neck of the capitate with or without displacement follows significant trauma to the midcarpal area. The longitudinal orientation of the capitate head becomes reversed 180°, resulting in the articular surface facing distally and the fractured surface facing proximally. When this combination occurs with scaphoid fracture, the entity is referred to as the naviculocapitate syndrome.

Severe trauma noted in either the hamate or triquetrum should lead one to suspect associated injuries to other areas of the carpus, distal forearm, and/or hand.

Treatment. The best functional result following severe wrist trauma is achieved by anatomic reduction of fractures and dislocations. The image intensifier greatly aids reaching precise diagnoses, manipulating, and achieving accurate reduction.

Unsuccessful closed reduction and open reduction require either percutaneous or internal Kirschner wire fixations. The volar approach is recommended in the majority of instances, particularly volar dislocation of the lunate, but may be supplemented by dorsal exposure when necessary. As many Kirschner wires as necessary should be employed to achieve accurate and stable fixation, placing them either at the surgically exposed fracture or dislocation site, employing them percutaneously, or using both methods. The surgeon should attempt to avoid crossing the wrist joint with Kirschner wire fixation unless, of course, that fixation is necessary to maintain wrist joint stability itself (Figs. 27-7, *E* and *F*; Fig. 27-10, *E*).

Following reduction and fixation, external long-arm cast immobilization for a period of 6 to 8 weeks usually suffices, but, particularly in the case of scaphoid fracture, may be much longer. The most secure and reliable cast is the long-arm cast incorporating a thumb spica and immobilizing the index and long fingers with the MP joints flexed and PIP joints extended. Adequate thumb-index web space must be maintained by physiologic thumb abduction and opposition. After a period of 4 to 6 weeks, if healing is progressing, the cast may be altered to a short-arm thumb spica cast. If delayed union persists, particularly with scaphoid fracture, the long-arm thumb spica modified cast, noted previously, should be retained until either union is achieved or bone graft becomes necessary.

Occasionally, despite distorted carpal anatomy, acceptable function with minimal pain may result (Fig. 27-7). If, however, posttraumatic arthritis of the wrist becomes incapacitating, the alternatives of arthroplasty (proximal row carpectomy with or without silastic hinged implant interposition) or arthrodesis may be indicated.

Ligamentous Injuries

Carpal instability from complete ligamentous avulsions and fracture avulsions may occur as an isolated injury, but often follows reduction of either a dorsal perilunate dislocation or a volar lunate dislocation.

Findings may include volar rotational instability of the scaphoid, dorsal rotational instability of the lunate, or occasionally volar rotational instability of the lunate, all often associated with scapholunate dissociation. For a thorough discussion of these entities the reader is referred to the writings of Dobyns and associates[3] and Linscheid and associates.[4]

Technically, the diagnosis of scapholunate dissociation is made by discrete tenderness localized over that joint dorsally and a greater than 3-mm space between the scaphoid and lunate on the anteroposterior roentgenograph. The anteroposterior roentgenograph is the diagnostic view taken with the hand supinated and the wrist in marked ulnar deviation.

Rotational instabilities are diagnosed by tenderness in the anatomic areas of the scaphoid and the lunate and principally by the lateral roentgenograph showing abnormal increase in the volar tilt of the scaphoid and either dorsal or volar tilt of the lunate. In volar rotational instability of the scaphoid, the posteroanterior roentgenograph shows an abnormally short scaphoid caused by the increase of its volar inclination.

These ligamentous problems must be diagnosed following successful reduction of a dorsal perilunate dislocation or a volar lunate dislocation. Roentgenographs should be made prior to cast application and at weekly intervals thereafter for approximately 4 to 5 weeks after anatomic reduction and during cast immobilization. If rotational instability is diagnosed at any time, it should be treated in one of two ways: (1) percutaneous Kirschner wire fixation of the lunate, scaphoid, and capitate not crossing the wrist joint, following successful closed reduction, or (2) open reduction, ligamentous repair, and percutaneous Kirschner wire fixation in the same manner if closed reduction does not achieve normal anatomy.

The volar approach is recommended to repair the all-important volar radiocarpal ligament and is often augmented by the dorsal approach to repair the dorsal radiocarpal ligament and the dorsal capsule, if necessary.

Cast immobilization, as previously noted, should persist for a minimum of 6 weeks postoperatively after either closed reduction or open reduction and pin fixation.

Hand

The hand has two basic functional arches, the transverse and the longitudinal, both palmarly concave. These arches are responsible for coordinated synergistic index-through-little-finger digital flexion and extension and thumb-little finger opposition. The transverse arch, originating from the central carpus (specifically the capitate head), flares out from proximal to distal in an open, cone-shaped configuration terminating at a second transverse arch located at the metacarpophalangeal joints and centered at the index and long metacarpal heads.

The longitudinal arch or arches (since each digit forms its own separate arch) is centered at the metacarpophalangeal joints of the index through little fingers. The long finger ray and the capitate comprise the central focal point.[5]

The stable portion of the hand was noted previously to consist of the distal carpal row and index and long metacarpals. The most mobile portions of the hand involve its radial and ulnar borders, both of which are capable of opposition. The most mobile is the thumb ray (metacarpal, proximal, and distal phalanges) at its carpometacarpal articulation. The second-most mobile portion is the little finger and the third (the ring) finger, each digit's motion centered at its specific carpometacarpal articulation.

There are two centers of power grip: one includes the ulnar aspect of the hand, comprising the hypothenar muscles and the ring and little fingers, motored by ulnar nerve innervation; the other centers on the radial aspect of the hand, including the thumb, thenar eminence, index finger, and intervening intrinsic muscles, motored by median and ulnar nerve innervation.

Intricate motions of the hand usually are centered on the radial aspect—thumb, index, and long fingers.

Gross distortion of any portion of this precise integrated skeletal anatomy of the hand incapacitates general physiologic function.

Long Bones of the Hand

The long bones of the hand include metacarpals and phalanges.

Metacarpals. Markedly displaced unstable metacarpal base fractures or dislocations are treated by closed reduction and similar types of irreducible lesions by open reduction combined with multiple percutaneous Kirschner wire fixations into adjacent stable metacarpals or into the carpus (Fig. 27-8).

An obvious fracture, fracture-dislocation, or dislocation of one metacarpal base should alert the physician to possible disorders of an adjacent metacarpal base or bases, particularly on the ulnar aspect of the hand since multiple injuries of this type are common in this area.

Grossly displaced or severely angulated irreducible or unstable metacarpal shaft fractures ("pick-up sticks") require anatomic reduction (Fig. 27-9).

Closed reduction, if possible, or open reduction from the dorsal aspect accompanied by multiple Kirschner wire fixations to adjacent metacarpals if some stability persists, or obliquely across the fracture sites, may be sufficient. However, the most effective immobilization is accomplished by surgical exposure of the metacarpal shaft fracture, retrograde passage of a double-ended Kirschner wire proximally intramedullary, reduction of the fracture, and, finally, drilling of the Kirschner wire across the reduced fracture into the distal metacarpal metaphysis without impinging upon the MP joint.

Plate fixation of an unstable transverse metacarpal shaft fracture may be preferred.

An oblique metacarpal shaft fracture that impinges on the MP joint must be reduced, and fixation is provided either by Kirschner wires or screws.

Segmental bone loss is treated by insertion of an internal spacer, skeletal traction, or transverse Kirschner wire fixation to intact metacarpals, only if circulation is not impaired.

Internal fixation for distal metaphyseal fractures (boxer's fractures) usually is reserved for displaced irreducible or grossly unstable fractures.

The important point is to restore metacarpal anatomy as accurately as possible, correcting malrotation and accomplishing stability often by mixture of varied techniques, to permit early digital motion (Fig. 27-8).

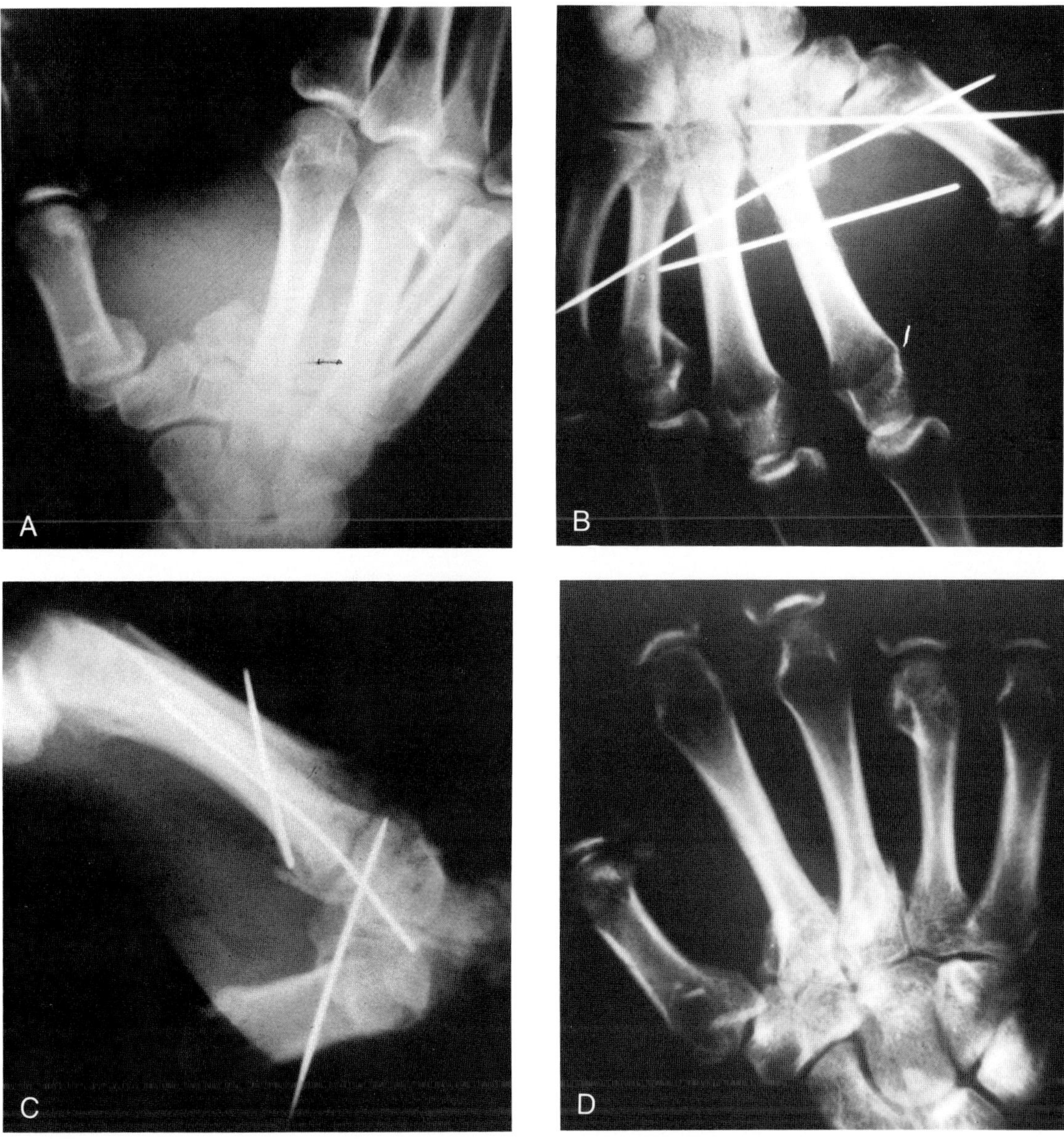

FIG. 27-8. *A*, This oblique roentgenograph shows dorsally displaced fractures of the thumb, index, and long-finger metacarpal proximal metaphyses and volarly angulated, displaced fracture of the ring finger metacarpal distal metaphysis or neck (angulated displaced boxers' fracture). *B*, Acceptable positions noted after closed manipulation and reduction of the ring-finger distal metaphyseal fracture, open reduction and transverse percutaneous Kirschner-wire fixations of the index and long metacarpal fractures, and closed manipulation and reduction with percutaneous Kirschner-wire immobilization of the thumb proximal metacarpal fracture to the carpus. *C*, Corresponding lateral roentgenograph shows good anatomic alignment of all metacarpal shafts and acceptable reduction of all fractures. *D*, Posteroanterior view shows good healing 3 months after injury with some shortening of the ring-finger metacarpal caused by the extensive comminution of the original distal metaphyseal fracture. This case illustrates different techniques utilized simultaneously to achieve acceptable reduction and fixation of multiple displaced metacarpal fractures. (From Sandzén, S. C., Jr.: Atlas of Wrist and Hand Fractures. Littleton, MA, PSG Publishing, 1979.)

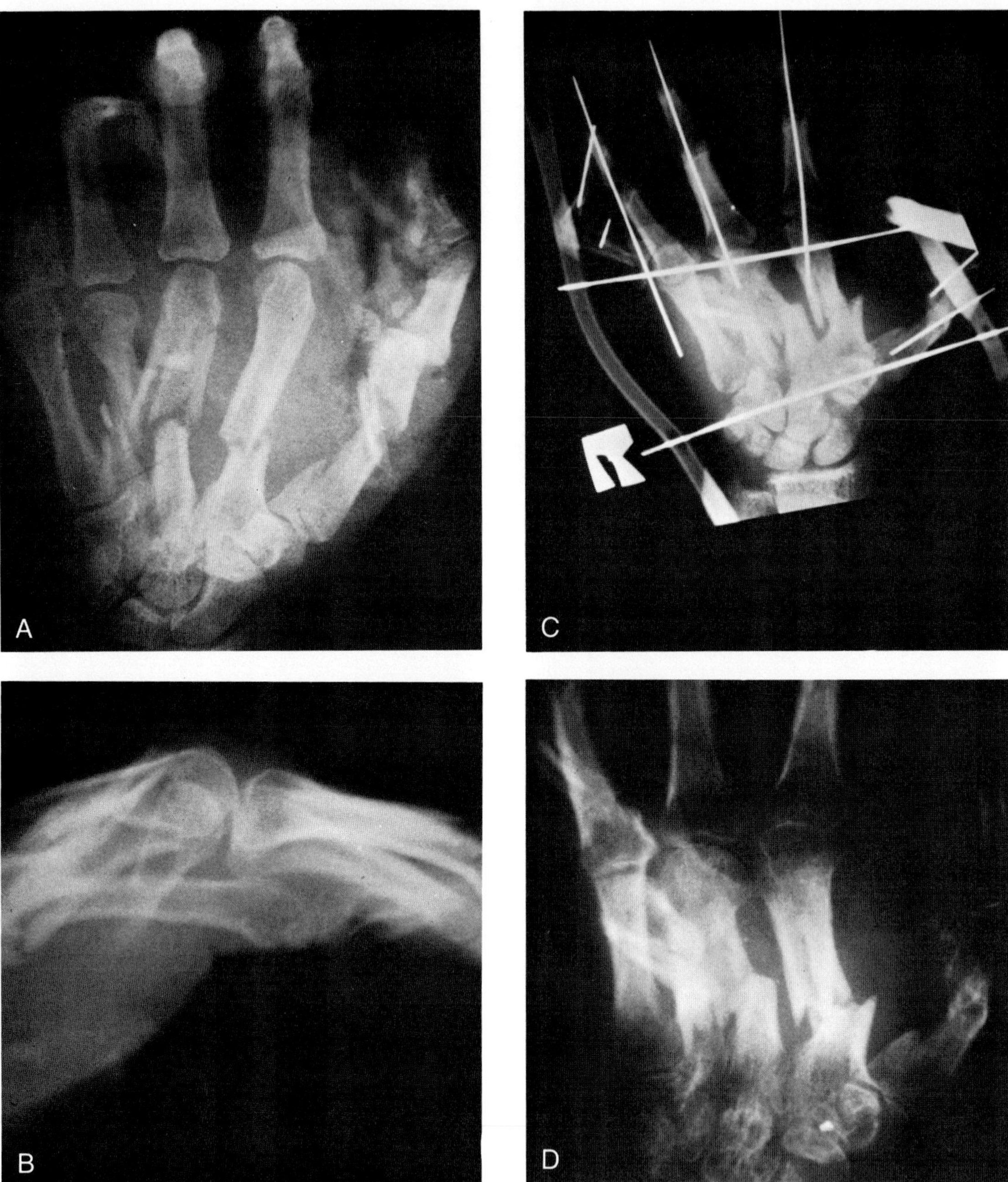

Fig. 27-9. *A*, Multiple comminuted fractures of the thumb, index-finger, long-finger, and ring-finger metacarpal shafts are seen in this posteroanterior roentgenograph. Associated fractures of the thumb metacarpal proximal metaphysis and distal phalanx, fracture-dislocation of the thumb IP joint, and comminuted fracture of the little-finger proximal phalanx are all open and severely crushed. *B*, This simultaneous lateral roentgenograph shows complex distortion of metacarpal anatomy with a markedly displaced and angulated ring-finger metacarpal shaft fracture. *C*, This posteroanterior roentgenograph shows attempted reduction and fixation of these multiple fractures with the use of transverse Kirschner wires attached to external fixers and augmented by longitudinal Kirschner wires. *D*, This posteroanterior roentgenograph taken 5 months after injury illustrates gross malunion at virtually all fracture sites primarily caused by improper and inadequate initial attempts at reduction and fixation in this extensive injury.

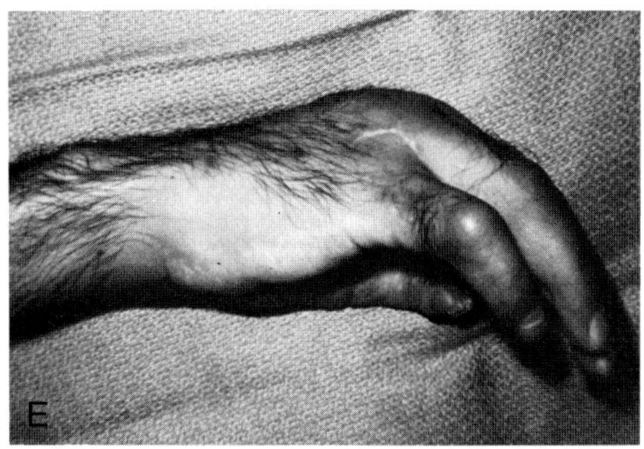

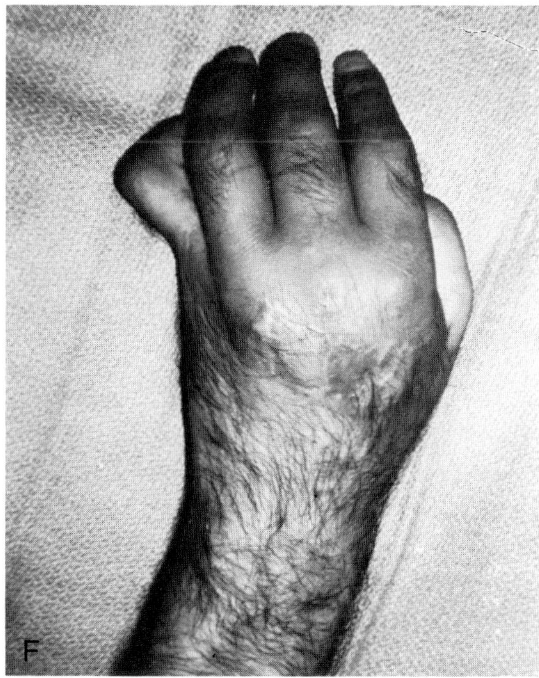

FIG. 27-9 (*continued*). *E*, This lateral photograph of the patient's hand, taken the same time as was the roentgenograph in Figure 28-9, *D*, shows flexed attitude of the wrist and abnormal digital configuration, particularly that of the little finger, with approximately 5 to 10° of active and passive motion at each joint. *F*, Corresponding dorsal view shows marked distortion of the little-finger ray, but does not show adequately the severe adduction contracture of the thumb-index web. This case illustrates the importance of appropriate primary care that emphasizes anatomic fracture reduction and effective fixation. (However, fracture reductions were not achieved in this instance, and the subsequently attempted, inappropriate skeletal fixation was unacceptable. The results were inability to commence early rehabilitation therapy and, consequently, an essentially nonfunctioning hand. Reconstruction would include realignment of metacarpal-shaft malunions, release of the thumb-index web adduction contracture with distant pedicle resurfacing, and intensive therapy to regain all motion possible in each individual joint.)

External immobilization must achieve metacarpophalangeal joint flexion and interphalangeal joint extension.

Closed space compression problems in the metacarpal area were discussed previously.

Phalanges. Treatment of proximal and middle phalangeal fractures can be most perplexing since normal anatomic restoration is necessary to restore the proper synergistic balance between the long flexors and long extensors coordinated by the intrinsic muscles. Proper rotational alignment is paramount, but restoration of length and correction of significant angulation are also important.

Any impingement on either PIP or DIP joint by a spicule of a proximally displaced oblique shaft fracture must be corrected, usually by open anatomic fracture reduction and percutaneous or internal fixation.

Torsional forces, though often responsible for metacarpal and proximal phalangeal fractures (often oblique), rarely injure middle and distal phalanges. The latter bones are injured most frequently by crush, blast, and avulsive crush lacerations (e.g., lawn mower and power saw). Therefore, treatment of the soft-tissue injuries often takes precedence over fracture treatment.

Closed space compression syndrome of the pulp of the distal phalanx was also discussed previously.

When devastating injury occurs to a finger, temporary longitudinal internal Kirschner wire stabilization may be the best initial solution. If the digit remains viable, the appropriate reconstructive procedures can be effected later.

Fracture-Dislocations and Ligamentous Injuries

Carpometacarpal joint disorders have been discussed.

Displaced articular fracture of the little finger metacarpal base will be covered later in the discussion of Bennett's fracture of the thumb since it is the mirror image of that lesion.

Because of the massive trauma necessary to cause multiple metacarpophalangeal joint dislocations, these injuries often are reducible by closed manipulation (Fig. 27-10). If irreducible, unstable, or open, open reduction from the palmar approach is recommended to achieve reduction and/or repair volar plate insertions; however, great care must be taken to avoid injury to the

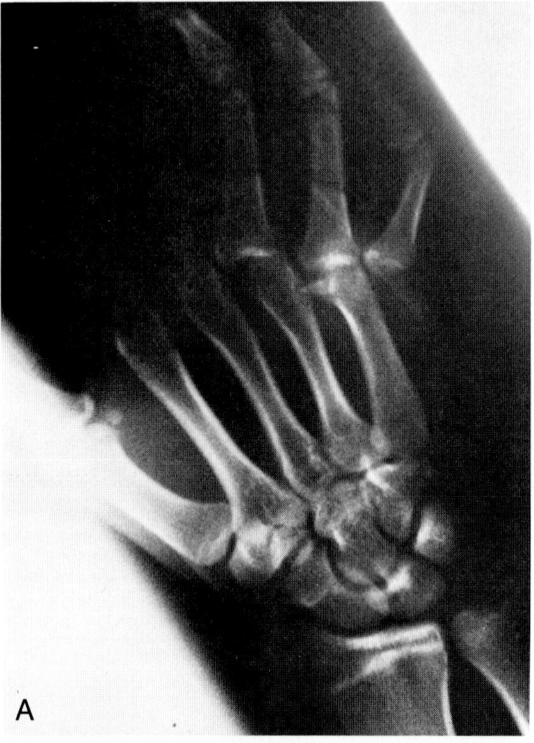

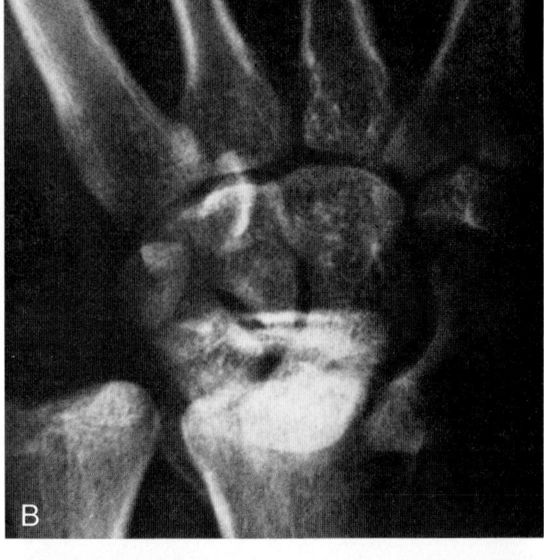

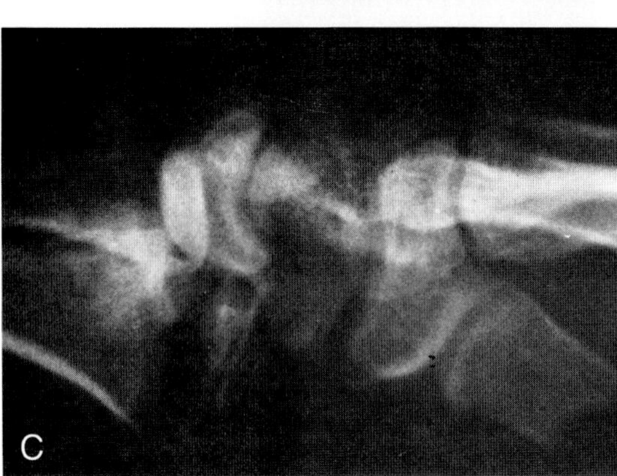

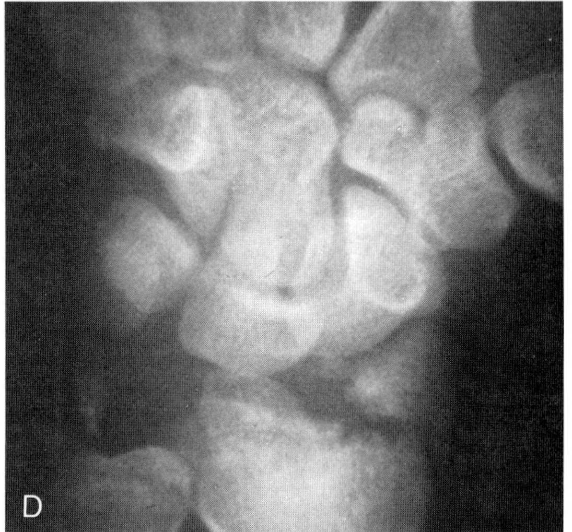

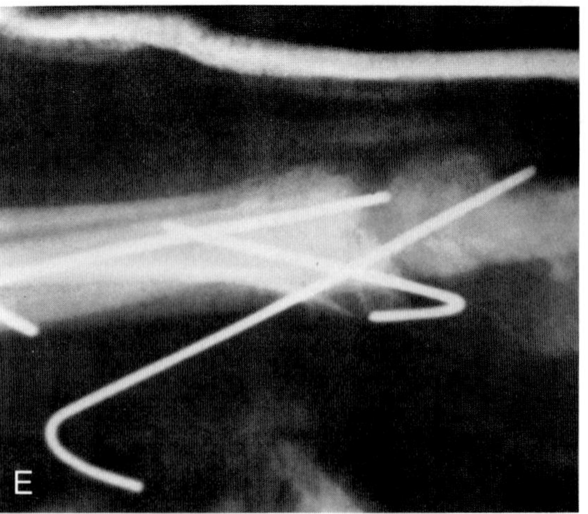

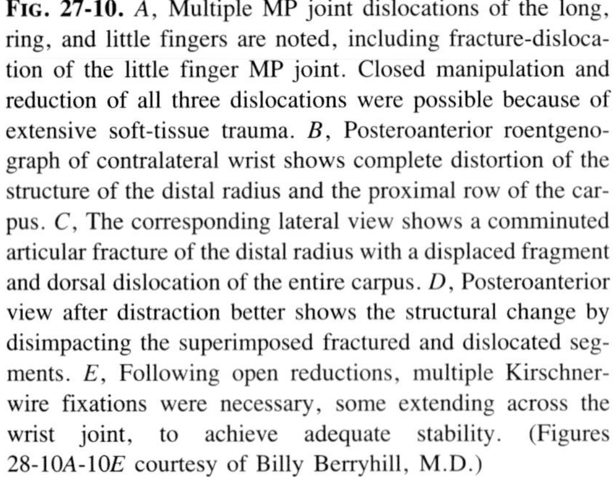

FIG. 27-10. *A*, Multiple MP joint dislocations of the long, ring, and little fingers are noted, including fracture-dislocation of the little finger MP joint. Closed manipulation and reduction of all three dislocations were possible because of extensive soft-tissue trauma. *B*, Posteroanterior roentgenograph of contralateral wrist shows complete distortion of the structure of the distal radius and the proximal row of the carpus. *C*, The corresponding lateral view shows a comminuted articular fracture of the distal radius with a displaced fragment and dorsal dislocation of the entire carpus. *D*, Posteroanterior view after distraction better shows the structural change by disimpacting the superimposed fractured and dislocated segments. *E*, Following open reductions, multiple Kirschner-wire fixations were necessary, some extending across the wrist joint, to achieve adequate stability. (Figures 28-10*A*-10*E* courtesy of Billy Berryhill, M.D.)

volar proper digital nerves and vessels and the flexor tendons (Fig. 27-11). Generally, if these injuries are irreducible, the volar plate is the culprit and is found impinged in the subluxed or dislocated MP joint. After excision of a segment of the flexor sheath palmar to the MP joint area, the volar plate may be released, and joint debridement precedes satisfactory reduction.

Any significant displaced segment of a metacarpal head articular surface or base of a proximal phalanx (usually attached to an insertion of the MP joint collateral ligament) should be reduced anatomically (usually surgically) and fixed by Kirschner wires.

Proximal interphalangeal joint dislocations usually are easily reduced closed, but fracture subluxations or dislocations, which are more common dorsally, often require surgical intervention (Fig. 27-12). Either fracture reduction of the volar aspect of the middle phalangeal base or volar plate advancement according to the technique of Eaton is often necessary to prevent persistent dorsal PIP joint subluxation. For a volar fracture subluxation of the PIP joint, the central slip of the extensor tendon or the articular segment to which it is attached must be replaced anatomically into the dorsal aspect of the middle phalanx base to prevent a chronic boutonnière type of deformity.

Thumb

Ideally, initial treatment of severe trauma to the thumb skeleton (trapezium, metacarpal, proximal and distal phalanges) should restore physiologic thumb abduction and opposition by providing acceptable stability, mobility, sensibility, and motor power. At the worst, the attempt must be made to retain as functional a thumb unit as possible based on remaining viable tissues. Often, later reconstructions can restore surprisingly good function (see Figs. 27-14; 27-16).

Though carpometacarpal dislocation of the thumb usually reduces easily, instability often persists, thereby necessitating closed rereduction, percutaneous Kirschner wire fixation from metacarpal to carpus augmented by external splint, or cast immobilization for approximately 4 weeks.

Fractures of the base of the thumb metacarpal are divided into (1) metaphyseal or nonarticular and (2) articular fractures (Fig. 27-13). The metaphyseal fractures (transverse, oblique, and epiphyseal separation) generally can be treated by closed methods although percutaneous Kirschner wire fixation may be necessary. Articular fractures include Bennett's fracture, fracture of Rolando, and extremely comminuted articular fractures of the carpometacarpal joint. In Bennett's fracture, the small articular fragment (volar beak) remains in its normal anatomic position and the remainder of the thumb ray is displaced proximally by the pull of the abductor pollicis longus augmented by adductor pollicis. A similar situation exists with the Bennett's type of fracture of the little finger metacarpal base; the distracting force is the extensor carpi ulnaris augmented by the flexor carpi ulnaris. Following reduction of the entire metacarpal shaft to the small undisplaced fragment, fixation of some type is necessary and may include percutaneous transverse Kirschner wire fixation, open reduction with internal fixation, or, occasionally, dynamic physiologic skeletal traction for a severe fracture of Rolando or comminuted articular fracture.

In shaft fractures of the thumb metacarpal, the adduction flexion deformity of the transverse fracture and the loss of length of the oblique fracture should be reduced and treated by skeletal fixation if necessary, particularly if the MP joint or carpometacarpal joint is impinged on.

If a thumb MP joint dislocation, which is the most common dislocation in the hand, cannot be reduced by closed methods, open reduction from the volar approach is indicated with care to protect the flexor pollicis longus tendon and the two proper neurovascular bundles during exposure.

Complete avulsion of either the ulnar collateral ligament (gamekeeper's thumb) or the radial collateral ligament (reverse gamekeeper's thumb) or complete avulsion of the volar plate with hyperextension instability of the MP joint should be repaired, along with their displaced articular fracture counterparts, in anatomic reduction for the most predictable result.

Fractures of the proximal and distal phalanges of the thumb are compared to injuries of the proximal and distal phalanges of the other digits, and the thumb IP joint is compared to the DIP joint of other digits with comparable treatment, as indicated.

Massive Injuries

The primary treatment of massive injuries to the distal forearm, wrist, and hand is a salvage procedure of all remaining viable elements. Important aspects of care are stressed again:

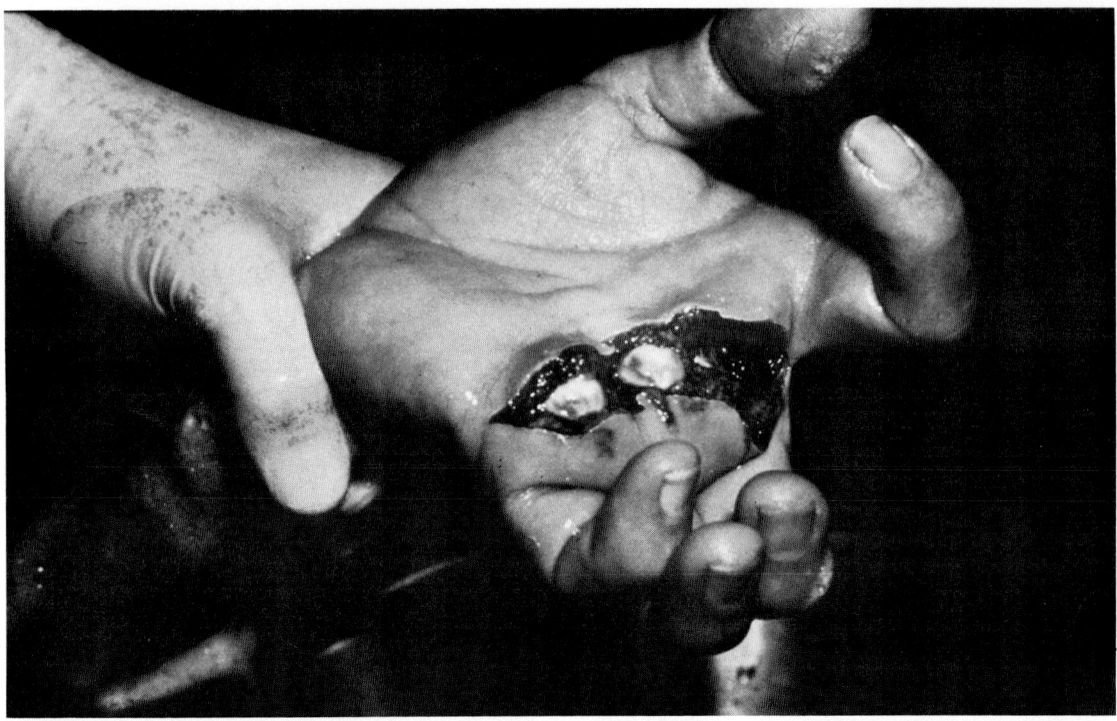

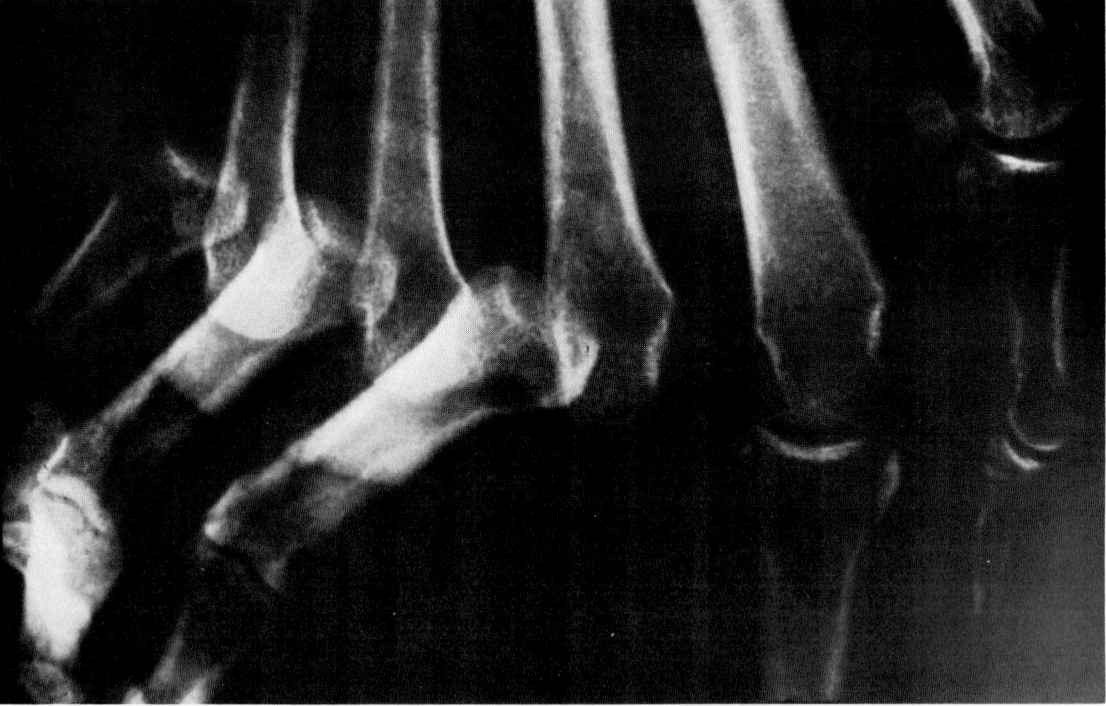

FIG. 27-11. *A*, Multiple open MP joint dislocations of the long, ring, and little finger with jagged volar avulsion laceration treated by meticulous wound toilet, open reduction of the dislocations, and repair of the volar plates. The ring- and little-finger metacarpal heads can be seen protruding from the wound, and the hyperextension deformities of the involved MP joints can be appreciated. *B*, Corresponding roentgenograph shows dorsoulnar long-, ring-, and little-finger MP joint dislocations with the characteristic hyperextension deformities. (Figures 28-11*A* and 11*B* courtesy of John Weber, M.D.)

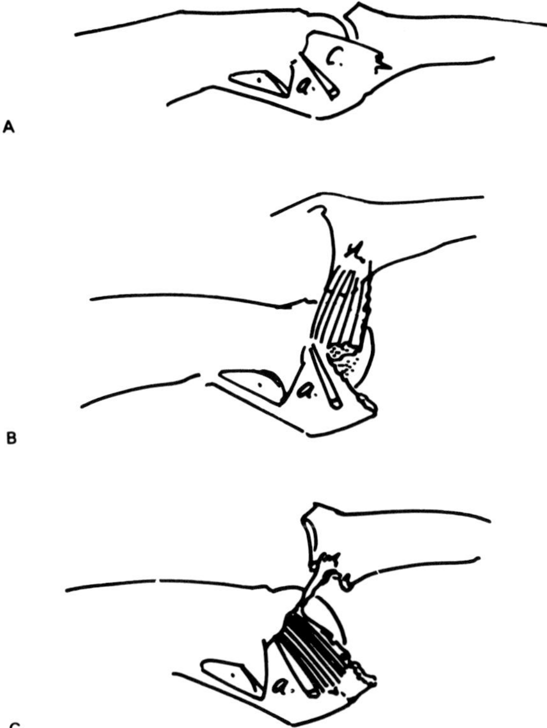

Fig. 27-12. Normal structure (*A*), dorsal dislocation (*B*), and dorsal fracture-dislocation (*C*) of the proximal interphalangeal joint. (From Eaton, R. G., and Littler, J. W.: Joint Injuries of the Hand. Springfield, IL, Charles C Thomas, 1971.)

1. Meticulous wound toilet, debridement of all foreign bodies and nonviable tissue, and preservation and protection of all viable tissue.
2. Re-establishment of circulation, if necessary.
3. Restoration of basic skeletal anatomy to as near normal as possible.
4. Initial open treatment in the majority of instances.

Crush Injuries

The immense pressure sustained in a severe crush injury (e.g., by punch press or rollers) often bursts the skin of the interdigital webs, thereby extruding the interosseous muscles in a manner similar to squeezing a grape between one's fingers or crushing a tomato. Particularly impressive is extrusion of the first dorsal interosseous, adductor pollicis, and deep head of the flexor pollicis brevis muscles from the thumb-index web area. Despite the enormous pressure sustained, much soft tissue often remains viable (Fig. 27-14).

Primary closure usually is impossible, and delayed primary or secondary closure is indicated to allow positive demarcation between viable and nonviable tissue, which may not be evident until sometime after injury. Initial debridement, therefore, is restricted to removal of foreign matter and only definitely nonviable tissue; all marginally viable tissue must be protected by delicate handling and repeated application of physiologic moistening (e.g., physiologic saline). Distally based partial pedicled skin avulsion often occurs on the dorsum of the hand and requires conservative treatment. Generally, a portion of the periphery of the pedicled skin does not survive, primarily because of impaired venous and lymphatic drainage but also, to a more limited degree, because of decreased arterial supply.

Therefore, repeated dressing changes and debridements at approximately 2-day intervals precede any attempt at delayed primary or secondary closure or resurfacing.

Bursting lacerations occur transversely in the webs. Adduction contractures can be expected, but no attempt should be made to prevent such contractures by primary Z-plasty skin revisions.

Massive edema of both subcutaneous and interstitial areas involves the entire hand and wrist, combined with diffuse oozing of blood in soft

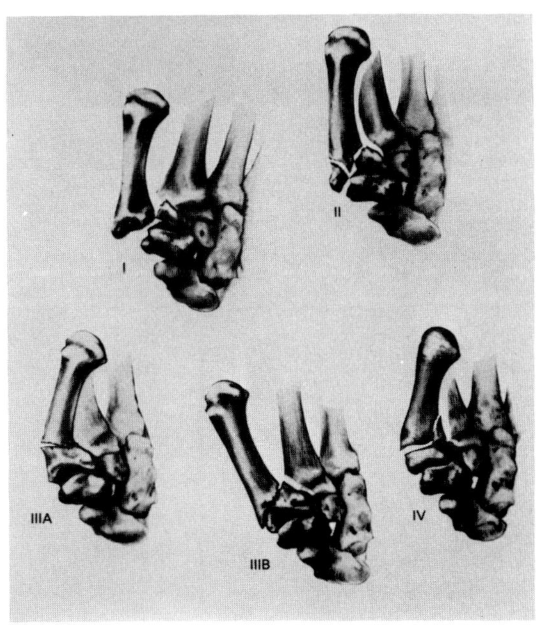

Fig. 27-13. Classification of thumb proximal metacarpal fractures differentiates proximal metaphyseal from articular. (From Green, D. P., and O'Brien, E. T.: Fractures of the thumb metacarpal. South. Med. J., *65*:807, 1972.)

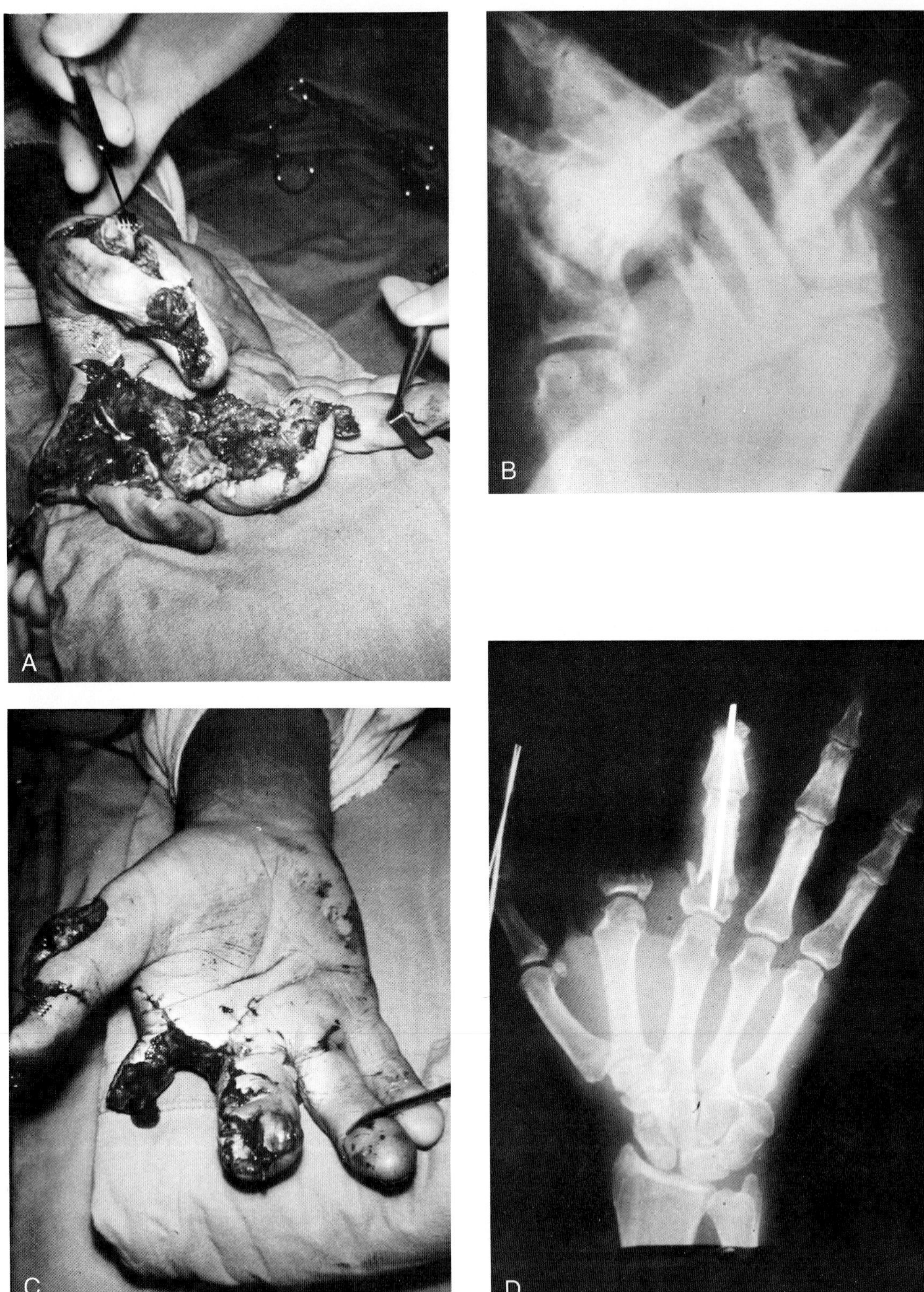

Fig. 27-14. Legend on facing page.

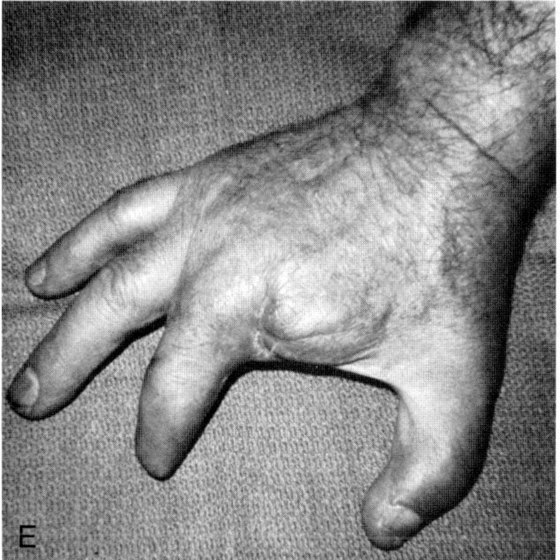

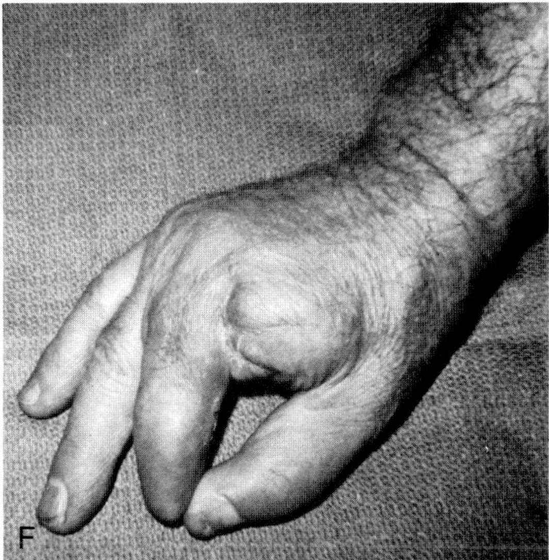

FIG. 27-14. *A*, Massive crush injury to the radial aspect of this 64-year-old man's hand was sustained in an hydraulic press. The thumb was split open from the distal metacarpal area to the tip of the distal phalanx with loss of most of the latter bone. The index and long fingers were virtually filleted from the metacarpus distally. This oblique view was taken after meticulous wound cleansing and irrigation, prior to amputation of the index finger through the PIP joint area. *B*, Corresponding roentgenograph shows complete displacement of long-finger middle phalangeal fracture and diffuse soft-tissue and skeletal injuries. *C*, This palmar view taken 6 days after injury illustrates complete maintenance of the thumb length by insertion of a segment of the deleted index-finger proximal phalanx as an autogenous primary bone graft to stabilize pulp of the distal phalanx. In addition, a viable pedicle of skin on the radial aspect of the index finger was preserved to resurface the proximal phalangeal amputation site. Multiple, interdigitated, jagged, viable skin remnants of the long finger are healing well. Two previous surgical procedures consisting of debridements were carried out 2 days and 4 days after injury. *D*, A corresponding roentgenograph shows longitudinal fixation of the skeletally realigned long finger amputated at the DIP joint area, fixation of the autogenous graft to the thumb distal phalanx, and the amputation site of the index finger at the base of the proximal phalanx. *E*, This photograph taken 6 weeks after injury shows maintenance of viability of the important pulp of the thumb distal phalanx, the severely crushed long finger out to its amputation site at the DIP joint, and the healed amputation of the index finger. *F*, There is strong sensible thumb-long finger pinch and good grasp, even at this early time after injury. This case illustrates the importance of meticulous wound toilet and initial open treatment of a severe crush injury. Conservative initial debridement is followed by staged redebridements to preserve and protect all viable tissue for closure and reconstruction (e.g., proximal phalanx of the deleted index finger as an autogenous primary graft to the thumb distal phalanx, maintenance of full long-finger length out to the DIP joint amputation site by interdigitation of viable ragged skin fragments and delayed primary closure, and delayed primary amputation coverage by pedicled skin to the radial aspect of the index-finger amputation site. (From Sandzén, S. C., Jr.: Atlas of Acute Hand Injuries. New York, PSG Publishing and McGraw-Hill Book Co., 1980.)

tissues. Physiologic immobilization and constant elevation are mandated to reduce edema as soon as and as effectively as possible to minimize chronic edema with its inevitable extensive scarring. At best, the scarring resulting from a severe crush injury hinders the ultimate function of the hand more than does the skeletal trauma.

Emphasis is again directed to early diagnosis and effective treatment of a progressive closed space compression or compartment syndrome of the forearm, metacarpus, and phalanges.

If the crush injury was sustained in hot rollers, the situation is compounded geometrically by the thermal injury insult (Fig. 27-15).

Range of motion exercises must be commenced as soon as symptoms and edema have subsided sufficiently, especially in the treatment of comminuted articular fractures in an attempt to remold the articular surfaces to as acceptable congruency as possible to achieve ultimately functional ranges of joint motion.

Reconstructive attempts at a later date are directed to restoring the underlying skeletal foundation, resurfacing where necessary, and utiliz-

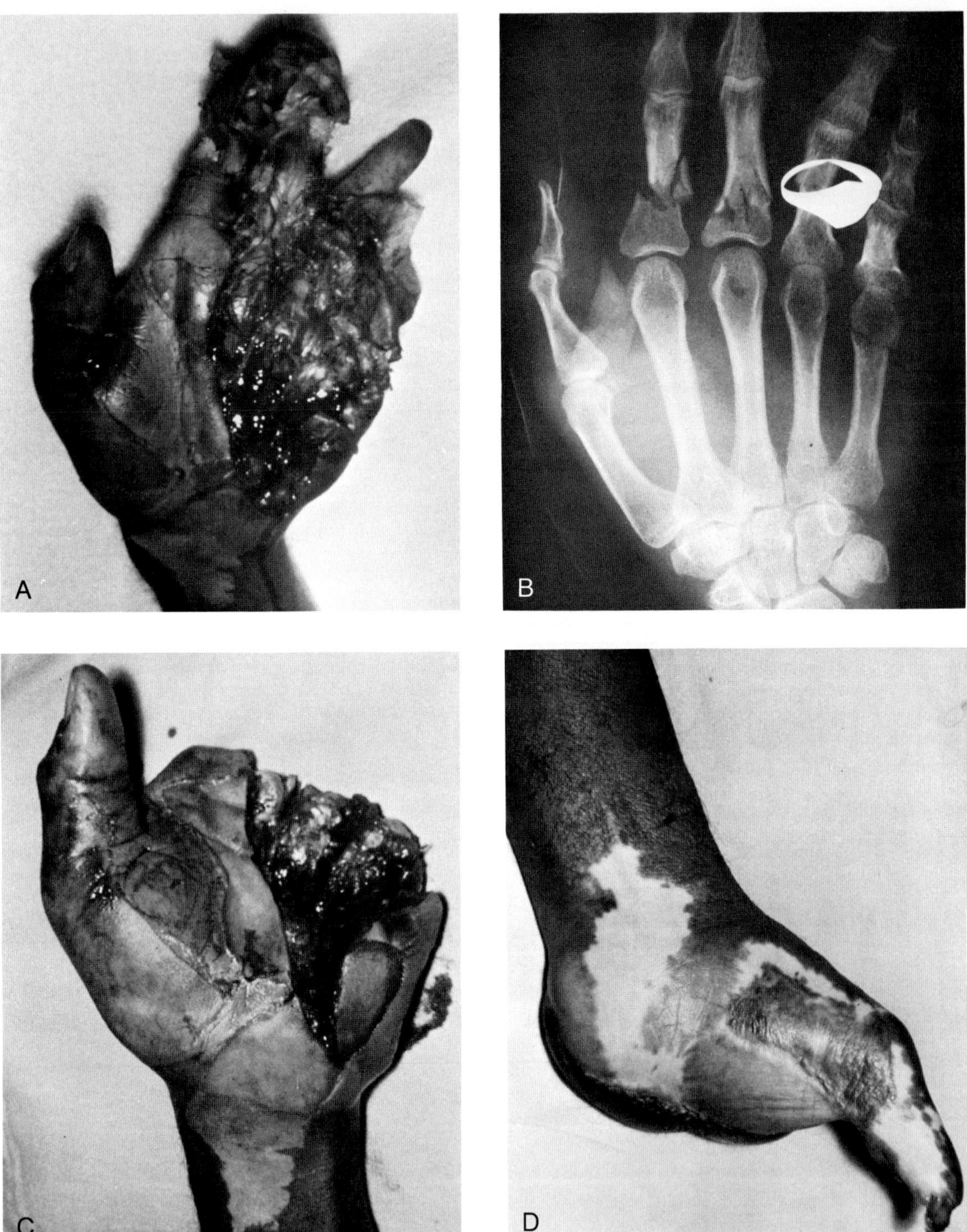

Fig. 27-15. *A*, Severe crush injury compounded by heat sustained in an industrial laundry mangle. *B*, Corresponding roentgenograph shows multiple comminuted proximal phalangeal fractures and distal metacarpal metaphyseal and middle phalangeal fractures of the little finger. *C*, The only viable tissue possible for salvage was the thumb and metacarpus. *D*, Four months after injury the thumb is functional, and oblique amputation through the metacarpus was resurfaced secondarily by a distant abdominal pedicle graft. (From Sandzén, S. C., Jr.: Atlas of Acute Hand Injuries. New York, PSG Publishing and McGraw-Hill Book Co., 1980.)

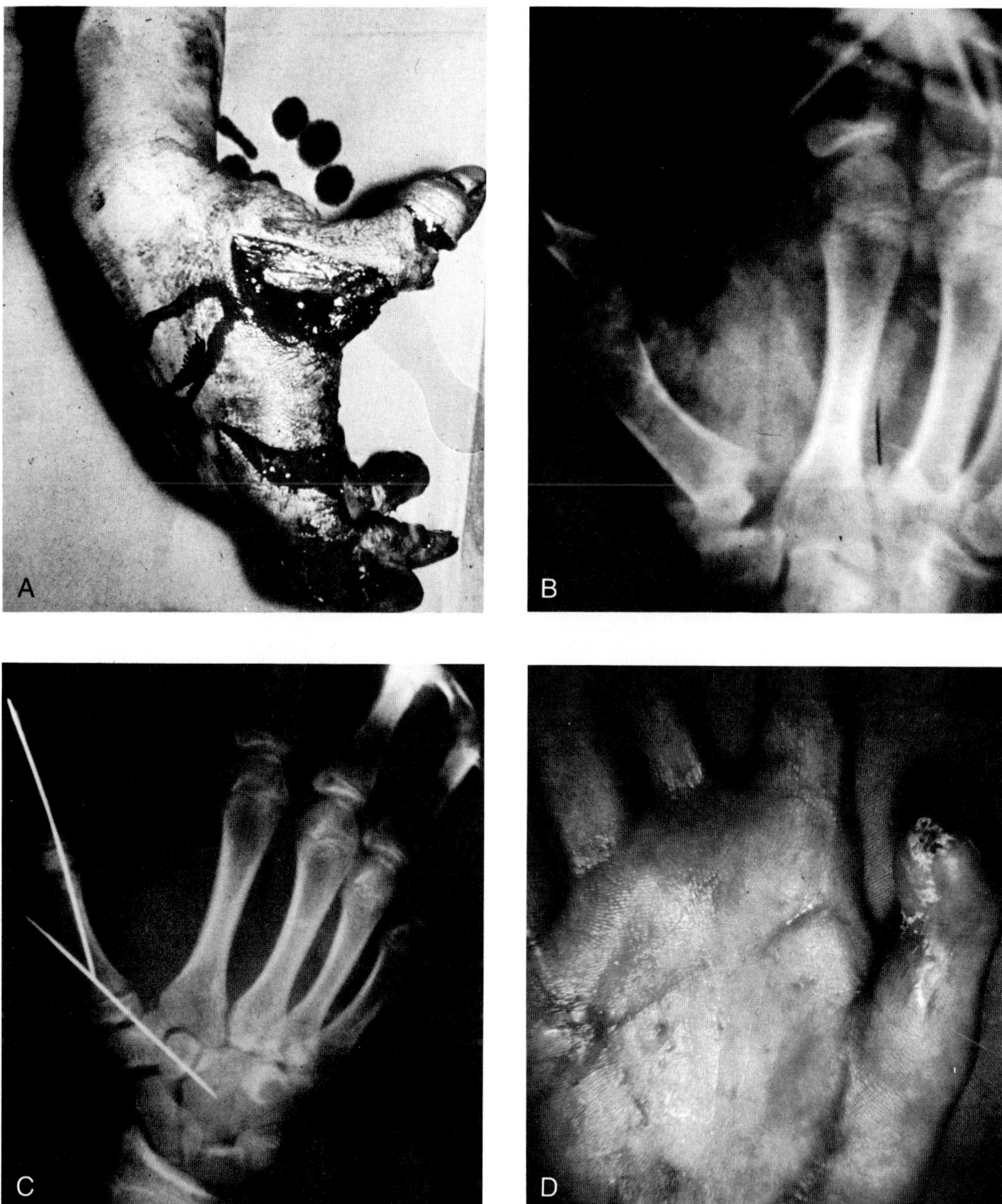

FIG. 27-16. *A*, Blast injury illustrates near avulsion of the radial aspect of the hand, including the thumb and index finger, with completely displaced epiphyseal separation of the index-finger proximal phalanx and partial displacement of those of the thumb metacarpal and proximal phalanx. Both proper neurovascular bundles to the thumb were lost completely, and pulp damage occurred to index-, long-, and ring-finger distal phalanges. The contralateral hand sustained amputation of the index finger through the DIP joint and the long-finger distal phalanx at its midpoint. *B*, Corresponding roentgenograph. *C*, Roentgenograph illustrates the minimal skeletal fixation for maintenance of these epiphyseal growth-plate reductions, necessary only for the thumb metacarpal and proximal phalanx. *D*, Ten weeks after injury, healing is complete with necrosis of a portion of the thumb distal phalangeal pulp, flexion contracture of the thumb IP joint, marked adduction contracture of the thumb-index finger web space, and anesthesia of the thumb, illustrated by dry skin.

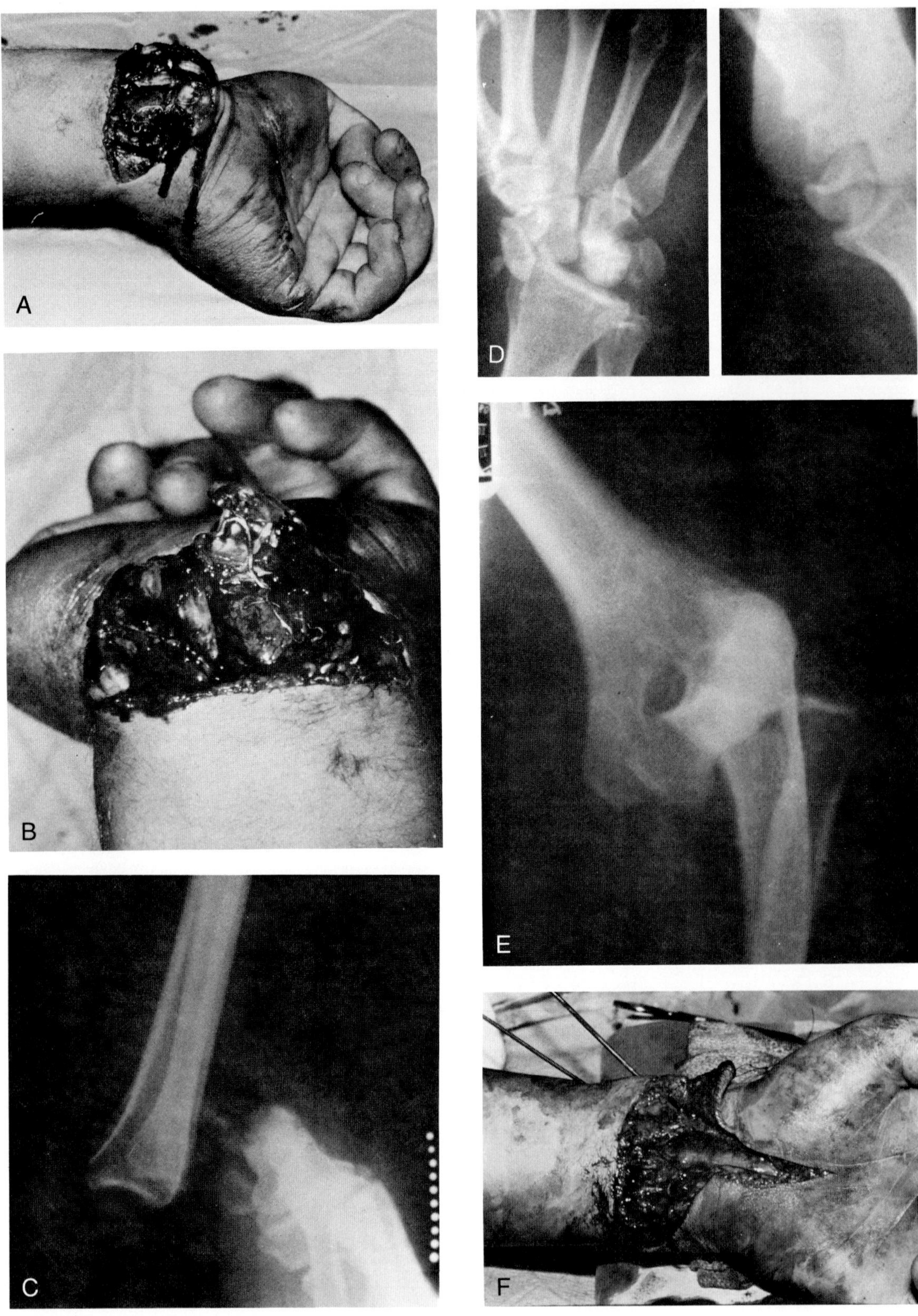

Fig. 27-17. Legend on facing page.

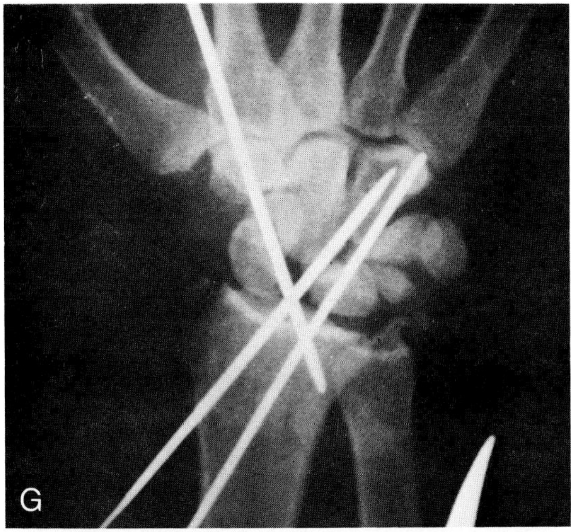

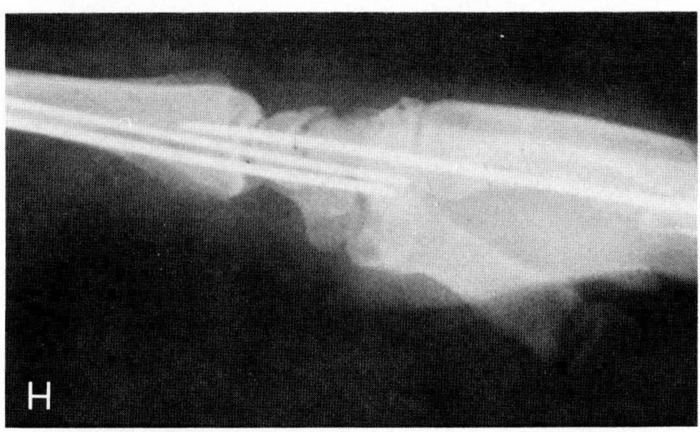

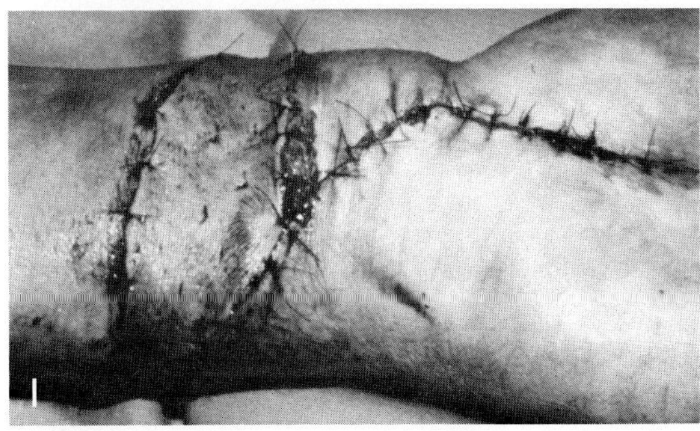

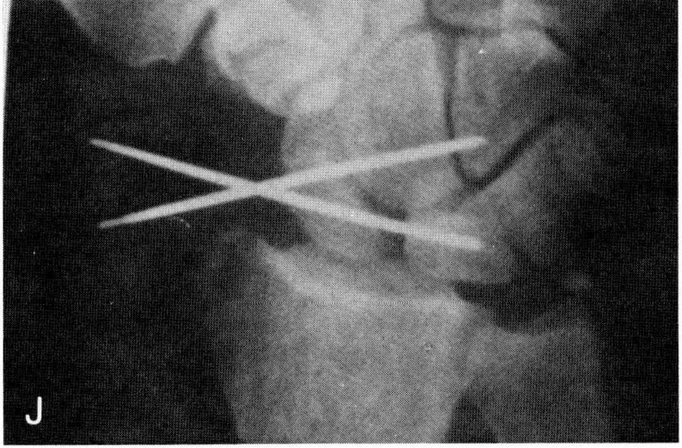

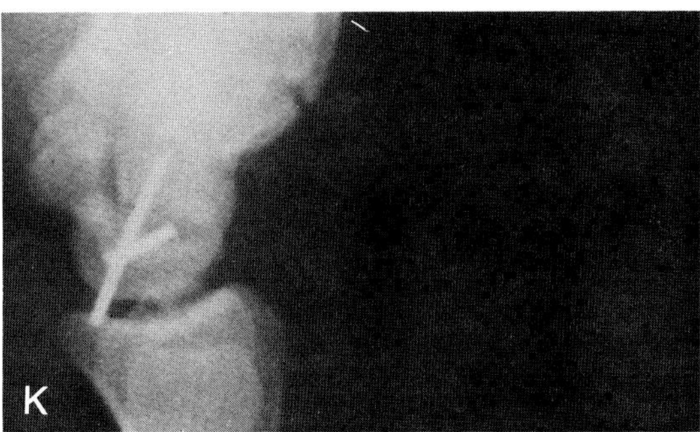

Fig. 27-17. *A*, Severe open impact injury sustained in a motor-vehicle accident. The hyperextension distraction forces avulsed the palmar aspect of the wrist causing avulsive laceration and volar protrusion of the distal radius and lunate. Flexor tendons and the median nerve are radial to the exposed skeletal structures. *B*, This view clearly shows the protruding lunate and the median nerve on its radial aspect. *C*, Lateral roentgenograph illustrates complete dorsal fracture-dislocation of the wrist with the lunate remaining attached to the distal radius. *D*, The posteroanterior view shows complete distortion of wrist anatomy (left). The lateral view shows normal position of the lunate and dorsal fracture dislocation of the remainder of the carpus (right). *E*, Simultaneous open dorsal dislocation of the ipsilateral elbow. *F*, Following wound toilet and open reduction of the elbow dislocation, attention was directed to the wrist. Meticulous wound toilet, fascial release of the distal forearm proximal to the wound, and division of the transverse carpal ligament preceded reduction of the open dorsal perilunate fracture-dislocation with percutaneous Kirschner-wire fixations. *G*, Kirschner wires cross the wrist joint because of apparent gross instability. A minimal Chauffeur's fracture of the radial styloid, as well as persistent diastasis of the scapholunate joint, can be seen. *H*, The lateral roentgenograph shows acceptable restoration of carpal anatomy and wrist joint. *I*, The wound initially was treated open because of massive swelling. Four days later, after removal of Kirschner-wire fixations, reduction of the scapholunate dissociation, and insertion of selected percutaneous Kirschner-wire fixations of the scaphoid, lunate, and capitate (not extending across the wrist joint, which was stable), delayed primary split-thickness skin-graft resurfacing of the wound and closure of the palmar incision were carried out. *J*, Corresponding posteroanterior and lateral roentgenographs show Kirschner-wire fixations and good position of the Chauffeur's fracture. This case illustrates the effects of a severe impact injury with distraction forces centered on the volar aspect of the wrist and compaction focused on the dorsal aspect. Because of massive swelling and extensive soft-tissue injury, open treatment and fascial releases were mandatory to prevent a possible closed-space compression syndrome. In general, the more proximal extremity injuries (in this case the open elbow dislocation) should be treated prior to the more distal injuries (the open displaced dorsal perilunate fracture dislocation). Kirschner wires should extend across the wrist joint only if unstable. If the wrist joint is stable, the unstable components of the carpus should be fixed to one another. (Figures 28-17*A*-17*J* courtesy of John Harmston, M.D.)

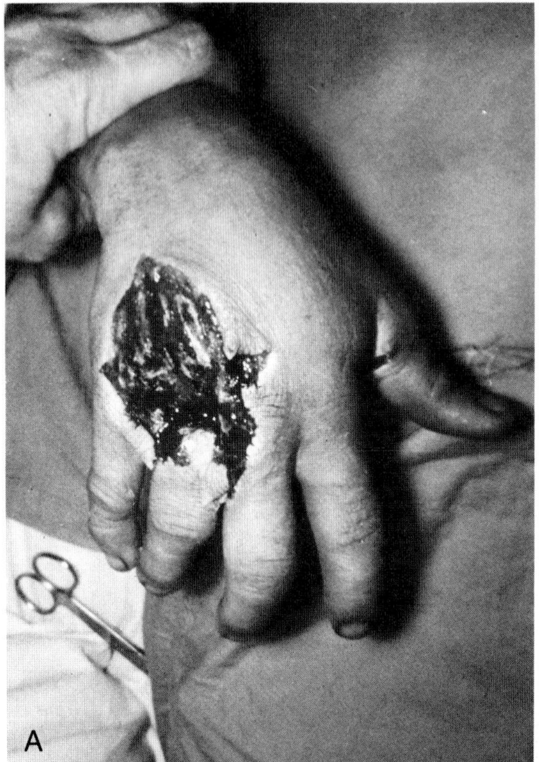

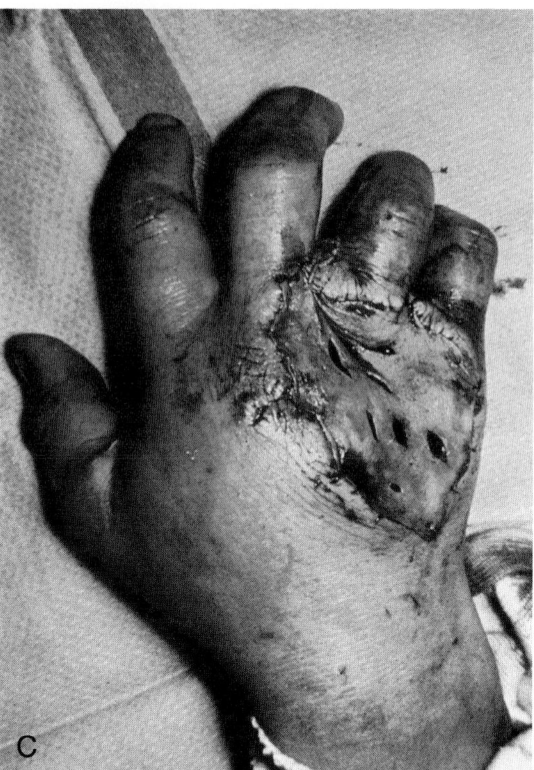

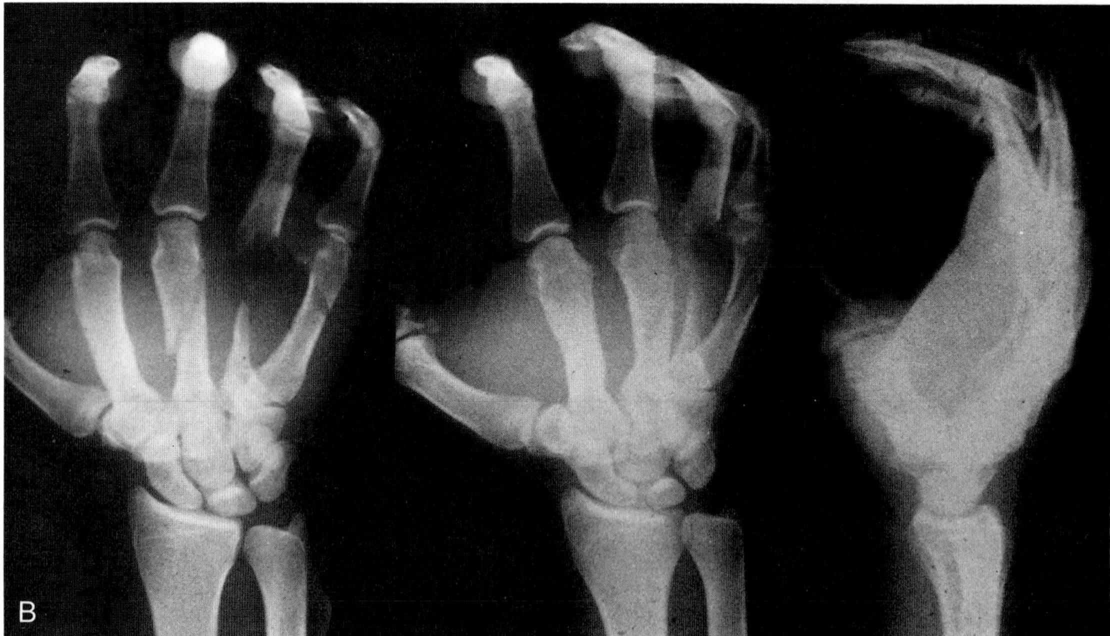

FIG. 27-18. *A*, Through-and-through high-velocity missile injury (AK-47) illustrating small point of entrance in the thumb-index finger web and the much larger exit on the dorsoulnar aspect of the hand. *B*, The corresponding roentgenographs show absence of most of the ring-finger metacarpal and a portion of the proximal phalanx with relatively undisplaced oblique fractures of the long- and little-finger metacarpals. *C*, Initial treatment included wound toilet and application of fenestrated split-thickness skin graft to resurface the dorsal defect.

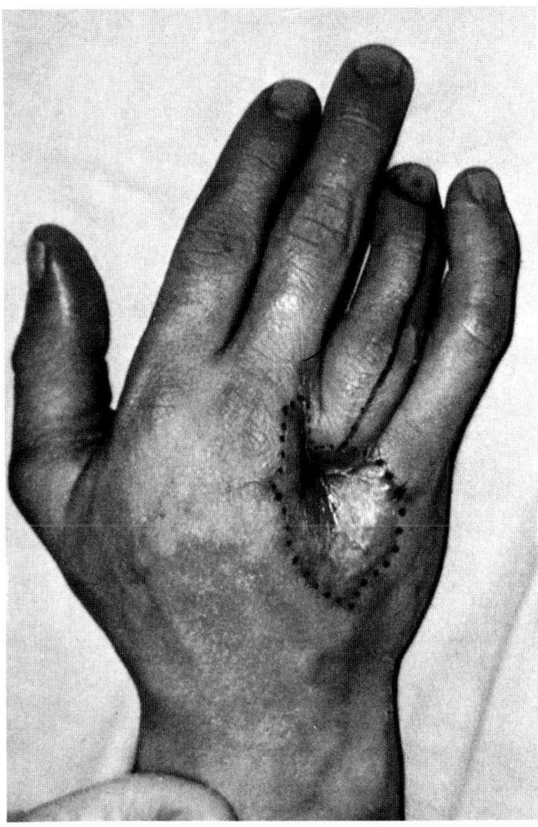

FIG. 27-18 (*continued*). *D*, The appearance of the hand after complete subsidence of edema and healing of the split-thickness skin graft with excellent ranges of motion of all digital joints except the ring finger. (From Sandzén, S. C., Jr.: Atlas of Acute Hand Injuries. New York, PSG Publishing and McGraw-Hill Book Co., 1980.)

ing Z-plasty skin revisions to release scar contractures prior to or simultaneously with applicable tenolyses.

Blast Injuries

Severe blast injuries are discussed separately because of several aspects:

1. The most severe injuries usually involve the radial aspect of the hand, including the thumb and index or thumb, index, and long fingers.
2. Primary split-thickness skin-graft resurfacing may prevent a contracture, particularly if the thumb-index web space is avulsed.
3. Associated trauma usually includes damage to one or both tympanic membranes and/or ocular trauma (Figs. 27-2 and 27-16).

Often one or more digits have precarious viability. The prime responsibility at initial treatment is to debride nonviable tissue and to protect and preserve all viable and marginally viable tissue. Appropriate skeletal fixation and, if possible, primary closure are recommended after meticulous wound toilet. However, initial open treatment is often the procedure of choice with delayed primary or secondary closure or resurfacing effected at a later date. Primary repair of tendon or nerve injuries is rarely indicated.

Reconstruction may include fabrication of a thumb-index web and multiple-system reconstruction of avulsed portions of the hand.

Impact Injuries

A severe impact injury results from striking the hand and wrist against an unyielding object either at high velocity or with extreme force (e.g., a fall on the outstretched arm from a significant height or a motor-vehicle type of injury). Characteristic aspects of this type of injury include:

1. Violent distraction on the side of the hand and wrist hitting the stable object.
2. Comparable compaction of structures on the contralateral side of the hand and wrist.
3. Prevalence of open fractures and open dislocations.

The distraction aspect of the injury causes avulsive lacerations of the skin, ligament avulsions, and open displaced fractures and dislocations (Figs. 27-7 and 27-17).

The compaction of the opposite side of the wrist and hand results in compression fractures and extensive soft-tissue damage caused by the compressive forces.

Meticulous wound toilet is again the most important aspect of initial treatment of the open fractures and dislocations. Primary or delayed primary restoration of skeletal anatomy to as near normal as possible is the second-most important consideration.

Through-and-Through Projectile Injuries

Through-and-through projectile injuries include those incurred by low-, high-, and intermediate-velocity missiles.

Low-velocity missiles travel at less than 1500 ft/sec and include the entire spectrum from 22-caliber through 45-caliber bullets. The amount of permanent functional impairment depends on the course of the projectile and damage caused to tissues in its path; therefore, the large-caliber bullet causes much more extensive local destruction to soft tissues and skeleton.

The .357- and .457-magnum projectiles approach the speed of a high-velocity missile and the mass of a large-caliber low-velocity missile and therefore possess the characteristics of a combination of effects on skeleton and soft tissue.

High-velocity missiles travel 1500 to 2000 ft/sec or faster when fired from hunting rifles and military weapons, such as the M-16 or A-K 47. The high-velocity missile causes a small entry wound and a much larger exit wound and results in tremendous damage, both to tissues directly in the track of the missile and also to tissues circumferentially about the projectile's passage. The latter type of damage is caused by a temporary cavity of circumferentially expanding pressure on adjacent soft tissues and skeleton that follows immediately behind the high-velocity projectile (Figs. 27-18 and 27-19).

The temporary cavity in high-velocity missile injuries is probably the most damaging mechanism of injury. Expansion of that temporary cavity has the effect of an explosion on adjacent soft tissue and skeleton. In addition, the subsequent negative pressure, which contracts the temporary cavity and reapproximates the soft tissue, may suck foreign bodies into the wound from the point of entrance.

Tissue devitalization occurs at varying distances circumferentially about the permanent wound track, depending on the velocity of the missile; most importantly, this irreversible damage is not evident grossly at the initial wound exploration.

Tissues of high specific gravity, primarily cortical bone and muscle, sustain the most serious injuries. Bone fragments may be propelled into the temporary cavity, but usually return either to their site of origin or close to their site of origin. Muscle fibers may swell to four to five times their normal size, accompanied by interstitial extravasation of blood, "clotting" of muscle cytoplasm, and rupture of capillaries. Though larger vessels usually remain intact, thrombosis may occur, often extending far beyond the permanent wound track because of dissipated force along fascial planes. Soft tissues at considerable distances from the obvious wound but adjacent to the fascial planes along which the energy is expended may be damaged.

Treatment must be based on the knowledge that soft-tissue damage is far more extensive than the initial gross wound examination reveals. Therefore, two stages of treatment are recommended:

1. Wide surgical exploration of the wound initially to debride nonviable soft tissue and foreign material; decompression of a markedly edematous area or an area of continuing hemorrhage by fascial lysis; exploration of suspected arterial, nerve, or tendon damage; and meticulous wound toilet and hemostasis.
2. Approximately 3 to 5 days following initial treatment, additional debridement, evacuation of any retained hematoma, and repair of deeper structures (if the wound is clean and uncontaminated) are performed.

Decompression is important at initial treatment to prevent a closed space compression syndrome. Next in importance is repair of any significant arterial damage, conservative debridement with wound excision down to bleeding margins, and copious irrigation with meticulous hemostasis. The wound is loosely packed open initially, and no other attempt is made at primary reconstruction beyond necessary re-establishment of vascular supply.

The second stage, 3 to 5 days later, includes redebridement, evacuation of any hematoma formation, and repair of deeper structures, only if the wound is clean.

The entire rationale of treatment of a high-velocity, through-and-through injury is to prevent retention of nonviable tissue in a closed wound, which would providc an cxccllcnt anacrobic medium for Clostridium welchii growth.

Any extensive reconstruction proceeds after complete subsidence of edema, wound healing, and restoration or maintenance of active and passive joint ranges of motion (Figs. 27-18 and 27-19).

Reconstruction

Basically, reconstruction involves eight distinct considerations:

1. Deletion of the portions of the hand that are functionless, irreparable, or impair overall hand function.
2. Augmentative reconstruction of other damaged areas of the hand with usable portions salvaged from the deleted segment or segments (e.g., skin, bone, tendon and/or nerve).

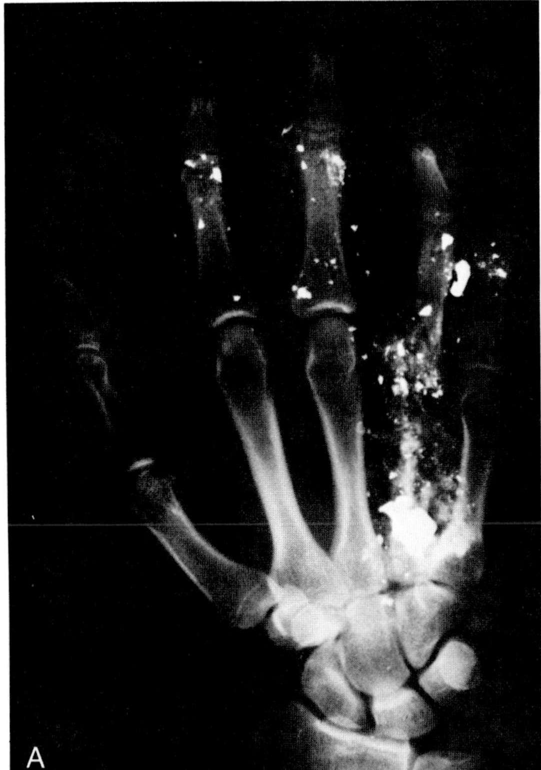

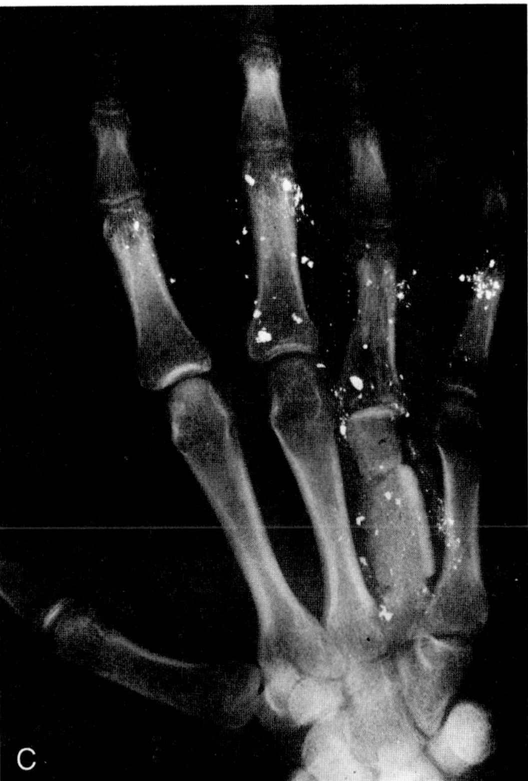

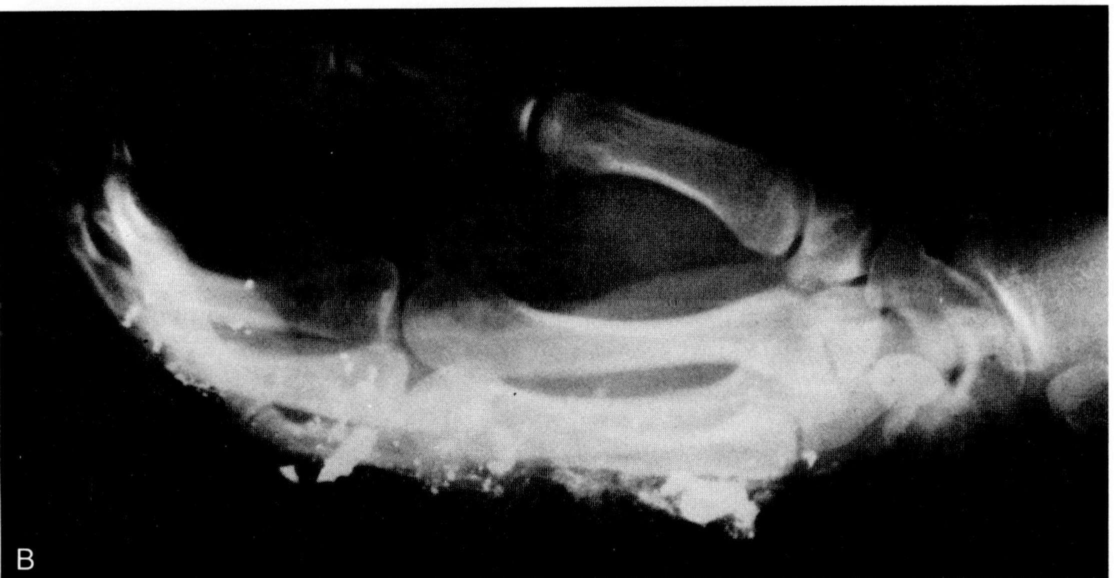

Fig. 27-19. *A*, This posteroanterior roentgenograph shows a similar type of through-and-through high-velocity missile injury (AK-47) with extensive skeletal destruction of the ring-finger metacarpal MP joint and proximal phalanx and multiple retained metallic foreign bodies. *B*, This simultaneous oblique roentgenograph illustrates the numerous metallic foreign bodies dorsally following this high-velocity missile injury. *C*, This posteroanterior roentgenograph illustrates the first procedure of a multiply staged reconstruction of this severely damaged digit—autogenous iliac bone graft for ring-finger metacarpal stability. Additional stages would include MP joint arthroplasty, extensor tendon graft, and extensive therapy. (From Sandzén, S. C., Jr.: Atlas of Acute Hand Injuries, New York, PSG Publishing and McGraw-Hill Book Co., 1980.)

3. Resurfacing, using pedicled skin (local rotational or distant), prior to any extensive deeper reconstruction, and release and revision of scars and contractures by resurfacing or Z-plasty skin revisions.

4. Restoration of the basic skeletal framework as anatomically as possible.

5. Joint arthroplasties (particularly of the wrist) or arthrodeses as indicated.

6. Restoration of sensibility by either nerve graft, neurovascular island pedicle graft, or composite free tissue graft.

7. Restoration of effective muscle-tendon units by tendon graft, tendon transfer, muscle pedicle transfer, or muscle pedicle composite free graft.

8. Establishment of an effective, aggressive program of rehabilitation therapy as soon as possible based on patient understanding and compliance with a specific program that emphasizes self-rehabilitation.

References

1. Committee on Trauma, American College of Surgeons: Early Care of the Injured Patient. 2nd Edition. Philadelphia, W. B. Saunders, 1976.
2. Taleisnik, J.: The ligaments of the wrist. J. Hand Surg., *1*:110, 1976.
3. Dobyns, J. H., et al.: Traumatic instability of the wrist. *In* Instructional Course Lectures: The American Academy of Orthopaedic Surgeons, XXIV. St. Louis, C. V. Mosby, 1975.
4. Linscheid, R. L., et al.: Traumatic instability of the wrist: diagnosis, classification, and pathomechanics. J. Bone Joint Surg., *54-A*:1612, 1972.
5. Flatt, A. E.: *The* Care of Minor Hand Injuries. 3rd Edition. St. Louis, C. V. Mosby, 1972.
6. Eaton, R. G., and Littler, J. W.: Joint Injuries of the Hand. Springfield, IL, Charles C. Thomas, 1971.

Chapter 28 Concomitant Fractures of the Long Bones

SIGVARD T. HANSEN, JR.

All the individual fractures and even some of the combinations covered in this chapter have already been discussed in terms of individual management in earlier chapters. Therefore, this chapter will cover the general philosophy and special considerations that pertain to the patient with injuries of multiple long bones in two or more extremities.

In the Orthopaedic Traumatology Division of the University of Washington's trauma center at Harborview Medical Center, two basic theories have been in force over the past 10 years, and essentially are being tested. Our first working hypothesis is that open fractures, particularly grades II and III, are treated optimally by immediate internal or external fixation. The rationale for this treatment is that it provides the best protection for the soft tissues, assuming that the operative procedure itself will not do enough additional harm to counteract this benefit.[1] This philosophy of treatment extends to all highly unstable fractures, even those in which the skin envelope is closed. In practice, we usually treat closed fractures closed, and open fractures open.

Our second working hypothesis is that either internal or external stabilization of long-bone fractures has a beneficial systemic effect in decreasing the incidence of secondary organ failure, particularly adult respiratory distress syndromes. This effect is greatest when the fractured long bone is the femur, and is present to lesser degrees with a fracture of the tibia and then the humerus.

The summary of our philosophy is that the more severely injured the patient is in terms of the number of fractures sustained and the degree of instability of these fractures, the greater is the need for immediate operative stabilization of the fractures to produce a beneficial effect both regionally and systemically. Several other authors also adhere to this general philosophy.[2–7]

In a simple open fracture, we have found that debridement and careful cleansing, combined with rigid anatomic internal or external stabilization of the skeleton, are more effective in preventing infection than is delaying stabilization of the fracture or leaving it unstabilized. In no case, however, do we perform primary closure of wounds. Rather, we perform delayed primary closures, with further cleansing and debridement if needed, at 5 days or thereafter. In many cases, skin coverage is completed by meshed split-thickness skin grafts at this time.

Several special considerations that may modify or augment our basic treatment concepts must be noted. The surgeon must decide what the goals are to be for the patient with multiple extremity injuries, especially for the common situation in which one or more fractures are open, comminuted, and associated with crushing or soft-tissue injury. This careful assessment and setting of goals may dictate approaches different from those that might be used in a less complex situation.

In especially complex cases, the surgeon must decide whether to give highest priority to saving the patient's life and to preventing early or major complications of secondary organ failure and local infection, or to manage the fracture in the way that would promote the earliest bony union and return to function. The methods for these two options may or may not be the same. For more isolated fractures that do not threaten the patient's life, the management plan usually is related to early functional treatment.

For example, in a patient with an isolated femoral fracture, a closed intramedullary nailing with reaming is geared to provide sufficient stability for early weightbearing and joint motion and is commonly accompanied by rapid union. On the other hand, if a patient has sustained bilateral femoral fractures, one or both of which are open and comminuted, and also has a humeral fracture and a flail chest, the surgeon might not risk closed intramedullary nailing of the femora. Placing the patient in the lateral position, which may compromise pulmonary function, and then reaming the femur, which may cause some additional showering of fat into the blood, might be too risky. Also, intramedullary nailing would ream away more of the internal blood supply of the femur and still might not provide perfect stability at the comminuted open fracture site. The more acceptable course would be to leave the patient supine, so that the chest could be well managed, and, using two or more teams, to address all fractures expeditiously and even simultaneously by plating the femora and the humerus. Plating would quickly make the open unstable femoral fracture anatomic and stable without damaging the internal blood supply; local infection would thus be prevented, or at least the risk of infection would be lowered. The opposite femoral fracture, whether closed or open, could be handled in the same way, at the same time, by the second team; thus, the patient would not need to be moved into different positions.

Closed nailing can be performed with the patient in the supine position. If one of the femoral fractures were closed or were only a grade I fracture with a stable pattern, the second femur might be stabilized in this way. Treatment of one femur by closed nailing would allow the patient to begin bearing weight much earlier, because the intramedullary nail is a weight-sharing device that allows full weightbearing rather early if the fracture pattern is stable. The plate, by contrast, generally requires significant protection.

Plating the humerus would allow the chest to be managed optimally because the arm would not need to be strapped to the chest and the patient would not need to be kept supine in some form of traction. The patient could soon be in an upright position, which would greatly benefit pulmonary management; in addition, the upright position would foster better oral nutrition, which is a distinct advantage because of the high-protein caloric demand of the patient with multiple fractures. Stable internal fixation also markedly decreases the need for pain medication with its accompanying suppression of the body's natural diurnal variation and defense mechanisms in general.

Another special situation is that of an older patient with fractures of two or more limbs, one of which has a significant crushing or soft-tissue injury with vascular damage and loss of skin cover. If the patient's life may be seriously threatened by renal, pulmonary, or liver overload (particularly by renal overload in the presence of crushed tissue), early or possibly immediate ablation or amputation of the most seriously injured lower extremity must be considered. Not only will this ablation or amputation reduce the total load on the organ systems, but it can be of significant benefit in providing a source of vessels, skin, and bone graft material for the other extremity.

An example is the case of an older man with a history of heart disease and alcohol abuse who is changing a tire on his car at night by the side of the road and is struck by a second car. His lower extremities are crushed between the car bumpers. Both limbs have serious distal femoral crush injuries and vascular injuries along with crush injuries to the tibiae, where developing compartmental syndromes will soon be noticed. The function of the patient's visceral organs is already compromised, and he is faced with the probability of long and multiple operations, probably muscle necrosis, and the likely development of sepsis later on. In this case, performing immediate above-the-knee amputation of one limb, being careful to select the most severely injured limb, then giving full attention to the other limb with rigid internal fixation may save the day. The salvaged vessels from the amputated limb, along with skin and bone from the tarsal bones, can be put to excellent use in the reconstruction of the less injured limb. In this instance, one limb is sacrificed to save the patient's life.

In such cases of an older patient already in poor health, sacrifice of one limb may be an acceptable price to pay and frequently prevents a prolonged hospitalization during which the patient may die or end up with severe disability. In other cases, a major problem may be the tremendous financial drain on an estate or on the limited resources of an older couple, where even if the life is saved and disability is not marked, the couple is left penniless.

Amputation performed early may be a necessary consideration, particularly in the older or already compromised patient with multiple-extremity injuries; yet even in these patients, the principles of earliest possible rigid internal fixation of all long bone fractures to prevent both systemic and local complications are valid.

Other special situations may arise in which a less seriously threatened patient may require treatment that allows early function of one limb when multiple long bones have been fractured. An example is the patient who has bilateral open tibial fractures with or without a femoral fracture and/or upper extremity fractures. This patient may be confined to a bed or wheelchair for a rather long time unless at least one extremity is fixed in a way that allows early full weightbearing. In such a case, the use of a prereamed intramedullary nail in a femur or tibia is generally recommended. For open tibial fractures of grade II or III, reaming and intramedullary nailing generally should not be performed in the acute phase of injury. Such treatment threatens the internal blood supply in the tibia when the external blood supply has already been compromised; significant bony necrosis and infection occasionally may result and would be difficult to control. In this special circumstance, however, if one tibia has a good stable fracture pattern in the middle third, one might risk the reaming and nailing to provide a limb that could accept full weightbearing within 2 or 3 weeks. This treatment would allow the patient to move about on crutches and likely would decrease hospital time significantly. One must be sure that marked stripping of the external blood supply from the tibia has not occurred, that the fracture pattern is stable, and that the fracture is in the middle third of the tibia or slightly lower.

The same goal of allowing early function of a limb might occasionally lead to intramedullary nailing of a midshaft humeral fracture that would not normally require any internal fixation. When the patient with lower extremity fractures needs to use crutches or needs both arms for transfers from a bed or wheelchair, intramedullary nailing of the humerus allows early crutch weightbearing and transfers. Moreover, this treatment actually seems to stimulate union of the humerus. Again, nailing can be performed only when the fracture pattern in the humerus is ideal for this treatment, i.e., a fairly transverse pattern in the middle third of the bone.

If one decides that internal fixation should be considered seriously for a given patient, the patient's needs with regard to each of his multiple extremity injuries must be assessed carefully. In a life-threatening situation, one must decide whether a given method of internal fixation will be optimal for preserving tissue and life. When the situation is a little less threatening, one also can consider what method of treatment will be optimal for ultimate union and function. The patient's needs must then be matched carefully with the fixation devices that are available at the hospital and the skills that the individual surgeon has to offer. Furthermore, all decisions must be made with clear knowledge of what each internal or external fixation device offers.

In the lower extremities, intramedullary fixation with prereamed nails is clearly the best treatment if one is concerned primarily with mobilizing the patient to full weightbearing at the earliest possible time. However, this method has a disadvantage in that fractures with comminuted or longitudinal patterns cannot be fixed stably. Interlocking nails can be used for fractures with these patterns, but these nails, like plates, are weightbearing. Thus, full weightbearing cannot be allowed until the locking screw(s) on one end can be removed, usually at 6 or more weeks. A second disadvantage of intramedullary fixation with prereamed nails is its destruction of the intramedullary blood supply; this problem is seldom a major consideration with femoral fractures, but may be a serious consideration with fractures of the tibia. The reaming itself may add somewhat to the shower of fat emboli and may cause slightly more risk to the circulation and system in general. If one is limited to reaming and nailing with the patient in the lateral position, the pulmonary compromise during anesthesia may not be acceptable.

Internal fixation with plates may be performed with the patient in a more standard supine position. Plating does not cause additional harm to the intramedullary blood supply but does cause some additional stripping of the external blood supply to the bone. Also, there is an increased chance of local infection because a larger incision is generally made. In virtually all cases, however, plating results in absolute rigid stabilization of the skeleton, which may provide the best protection from local or regional infection by enhancing the function of the soft tissues. On the other hand, plating does not allow early full weightbearing without protection, and another major operation is required at a later date to remove the hardware. If the hardware is in the diaphysis of a long bone, the bone may require some protection while the plate is in place because of a stress-riser effect at the end of the plate. For the same reason, the stress-protected bone may need protection after plate removal, especially where screws have been removed.

In the early phase of fracture healing, external fixation or stabilization of the skeleton provides some of the advantages of rigid internal stabilization, i.e., protection from regional infection and enough stability to allow the patient to be upright.[8] In general, however, the external fixation device has disadvantages similar to those of the plate in that some protection of weightbearing is needed while the device is affixed to the bone. In addition, pin-tract infections or delayed union may occur occasionally. Again, the stress-relieved bone, especially at the sites of the drill holes, may be susceptible to refracture after removal of the device. Also, external fixation is similar to internal fixation in that if highly developed skills and accuracy in application are lacking, a higher incidence of infection or other complications may result.

Finally, performance of all these fixation procedures requires a high degree of technical skill; any problems are increased almost geometrically in the multiply injured patient. With the extensive soft-tissue damage that is common in these patients, the internal or external fixation device must be applied with great skill so as not to damage the soft tissues further; yet anatomic and rigid stabilization must be gained to allow maximum benefit from the procedure. When multiple fractures must be fixed, either the surgeon must work with great skill and speed or more than one team must be available. Also, if those repairing the fractures must also be concerned with fluids and with abdominal, chest, and other soft-tissue problems at the same time, the level of distraction and confusion will be high. Therefore, it is my strong opinion that these patients must be handled by smoothly integrated teams.

In our trauma center, a specially trained anesthesiologist is familiar with the problems of the multiply injured patient. These problems include head injuries, high levels of alcohol or other drugs, and fluid- and blood-replacement requirements. The anesthesiologist, in conjunction with a specially trained trauma surgeon, must be able to anticipate blood loss, clotting problems, and the need for special nutritional supplements. With pelvic or other fractures that are accompanied by significant blood loss, the early use of platelet replacement may be critical. Post-trauma pulmonary problems are now referred to as adult respiratory distress syndromes (ARDS) and include among their various causes the so-called "fat embolism syndrome," classically associated with major long-bone fractures. Pulmonary failure often becomes the most significant life-threatening problem that must be managed by the anesthesiologist and trauma surgeon.

Ideally, all nonorthopaedic problems should be managed competently by a trauma surgeon, anesthesiologist, and neurosurgeon so that the orthopaedist can turn his attention to and develop his skills in the care of musculoskeletal problems alone. He can then use his time to become skilled in the demanding techniques of adequate debridement and cleansing of soft tissues in open wounds and to develop accuracy and speed in the application of internal or external fixation devices. Even if the orthopaedist is highly skilled, thought must always be given to inviting in a second or even a third orthopaedic team for the patient with multiple long-bone fractures. The team approach not only decreases the total anesthesia and open wound time, but also solves the problems of fatigue and inattention that come from working late at night and performing several complicated procedures in succession.

In our trauma unit, we have worked with these well-integrated teams for almost 10 years, and for approximately 8 years, we have held rigidly to the protocol requiring immediate internal fixation of open or complex fractures (Illustrative case—Figs. 28-1 through 28-18). With extensive experience in this area, we have been gratified to discover that a high percentage of patients with three or more long-bone fractures in three or more extremities come through not only the acute phase but also the rehabilitation phase and go back to work without significant limitation. It has become evident that the immediate use of internal fixation in open fractures does not pose a significant added risk to the patient, especially when closure of wounds is delayed in all cases. In every area except the tibia, the infection rate has been under 5%; with larger numbers of patients, this figure could be under 2%. When an infection does occur, it tends to be managed easily.

As orthopaedic surgeons have found with any method of treatment in grade III open tibial frac-

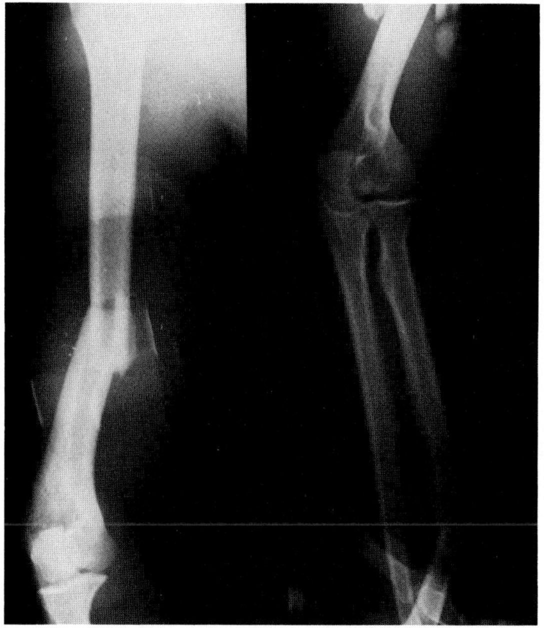

Fig. 28-1. A 19-year-old motorcyclist was brought to the trauma center shortly after he struck a tree at high speed. He had no significant head, chest, or abdominal injuries, but had fractures of almost all major long bones on the right side of his body. These roentgenograms of the upper extremity show a comminuted fracture of the midshaft of the humerus, which fortunately was closed and was not associated with major nerve or vessel damage. Also visible is the distal fracture of the radius, which is seen more easily in Figure 28-2.

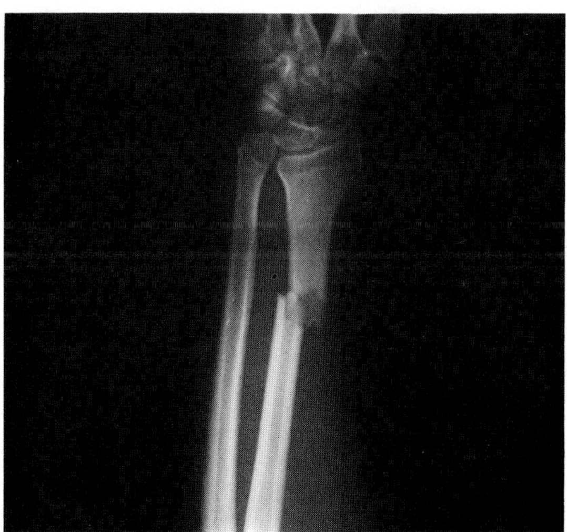

Fig. 28-2. A roentgenogram of the forearm shows a slightly displaced oblique fracture of the radius and shortening of the radius compared with the ulna. Also seen is a Malgaigne-type fracture with at least partial disruption of the radioulnar joint. The radial fracture also was closed and was not associated with major nerve or vessel damage.

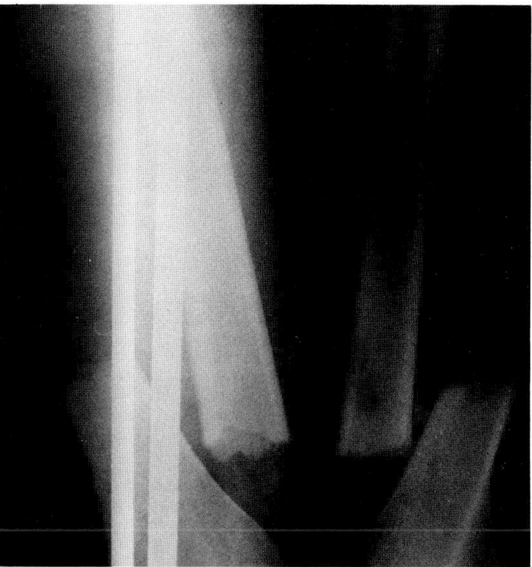

Fig. 28-3. Roentgenograms of the distal femur, also on the motorcyclist's right side. This distal transverse fracture of the shaft had minimal comminution, but was a grade II open fracture; the distal portion of the proximal fragment protruded directly through the quadriceps just above the patella, thus producing a large laceration in the muscle and the skin. Again, no neurologic or vascular damage was apparent.

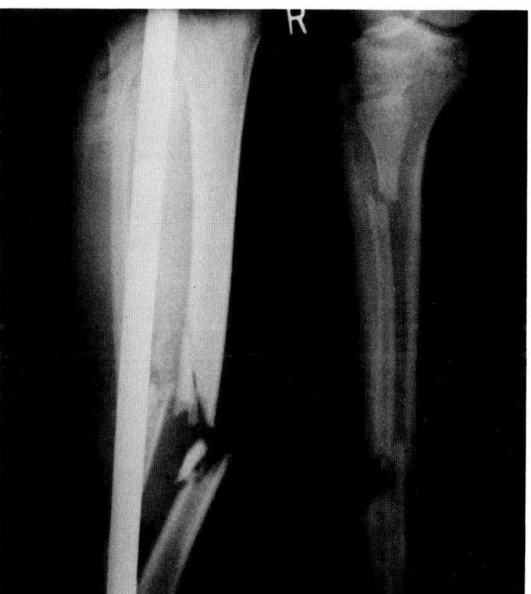

Fig. 28-4. The right lower leg of the same motorcyclist sustained a somewhat severely comminuted fracture of the tibia and fibula as well as a second, higher-level fracture of the fibula. This grade III open fracture caused significant damage to skin and local musculature with gross contamination and contusion of soft tissues. The major nerves and muscles were intact, however, and the foot was in good condition.

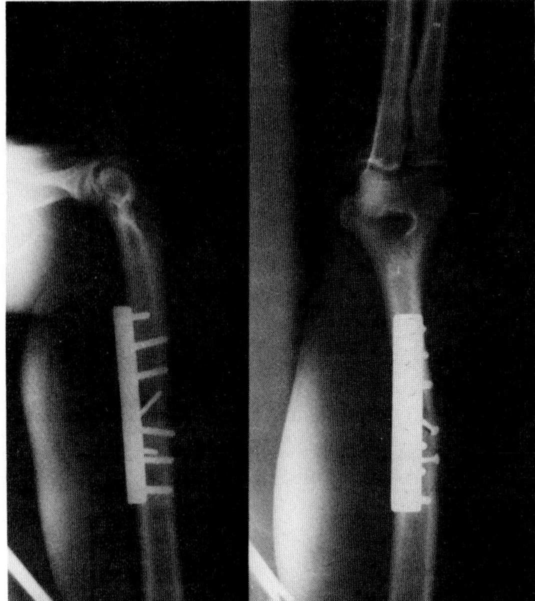

Fig. 28-5. Postoperative films of the upper extremity show fixation of the humerus. A broad plate was applied with intrafragmental screws affixing major comminuted fragments and crossing the oblique fracture. The fracture was plated at a slight angle, and the screws were placed at various angles to avoid splitting the bone. Note that excellent rigid fixation has been achieved. Fixation of the humerus was the last of four operative procedures performed: the tibia was fixed initially, then the femur, followed by the radius and wrist, and finally the humerus.

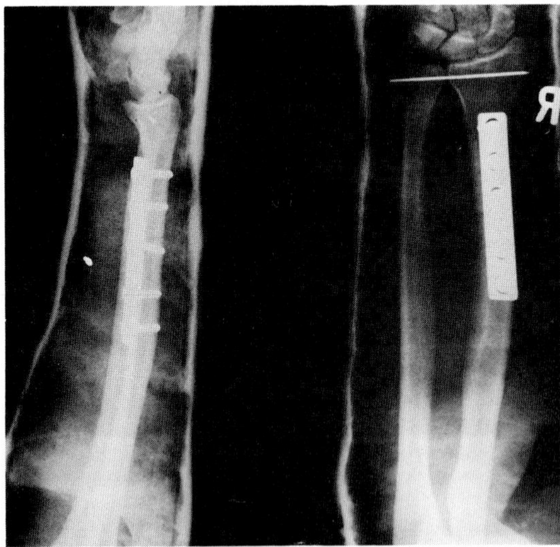

Fig. 28-6. Immediate postoperative films of the Malgaigne fracture show dynamic compression plate fixation of the radius with one screw crossing through the oblique fracture. The unstable radioulnar articulation has been transfixed with a Kirschner wire.

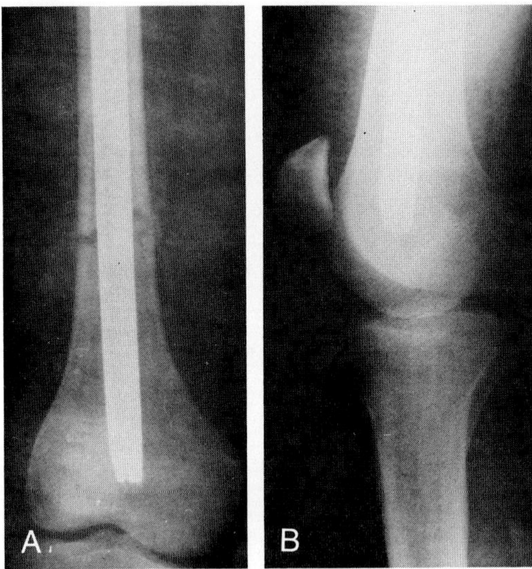

Fig. 28-7. *A* and *B*, Anteroposterior and lateral views of the distal femoral fracture, which is a grade II open fracture. A standard antegrade femoral nailing, the second operation in the sequence, was performed after copious irrigation and limited debridement of the open wound site. The wound was left open after completion of the nailing.

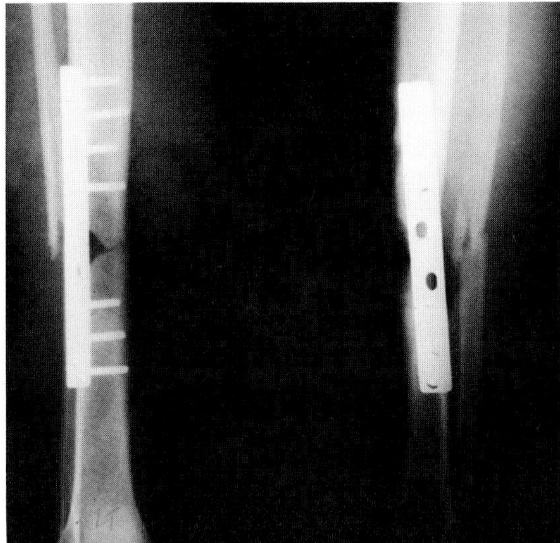

Fig. 28-8. Postoperative films of the grade III comminuted open tibial fracture show stabilization on the lateral side by a broad dynamic compression plate with a slight residual anterior angulation. This fixation was chosen over treatment with an external fixation device to meet the goal of providing rigid anatomic stabilization of the bone to encourage soft-tissue healing. Bone union was a secondary consideration after salvage of the soft tissues. A broad plate was used because of the loss of cortical bone and the need for stronger and more rigid fixation. The plate was placed on the lateral side so it would not be exposed in the open wound; the original wound was left open, although extensions for the plate were closed.

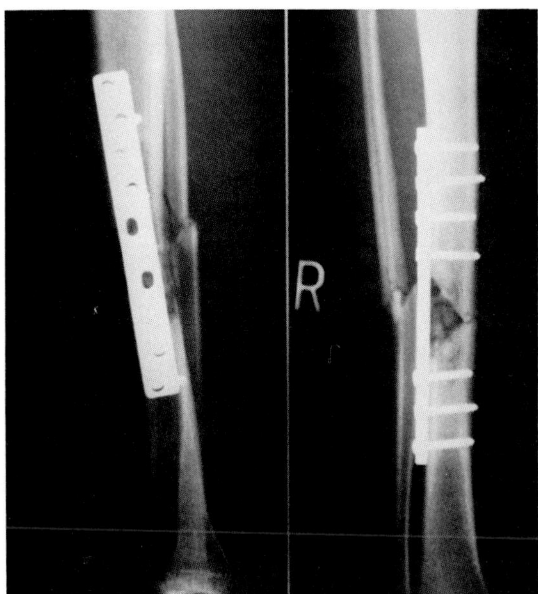

Fig. 28-9. Films of the tibia taken approximately 10 weeks after injury show a bone graft in place and the fracture still relatively stable. At this time, touch-down weightbearing on the lower extremity had been permitted for approximately a month. Although the patient had been confined to a wheelchair for the first 6 weeks of recovery because of the multiple injuries to both upper and lower extremities, he had been free of casts and had been mobilizing the extremities during that time.

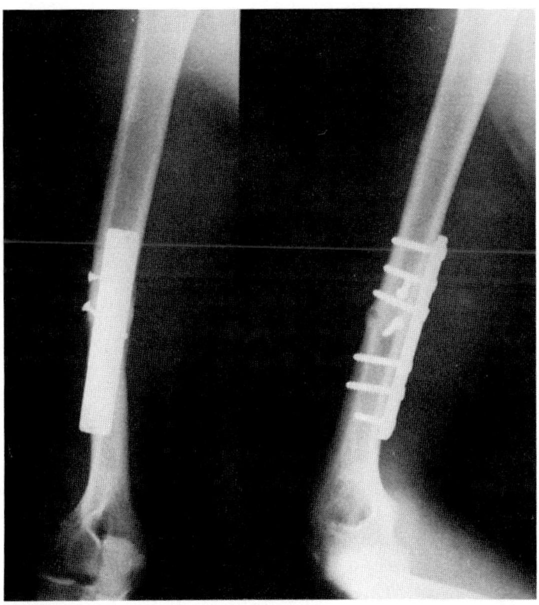

Fig. 28-10. Roentgenograms of the humeral fracture 3 months after injury show a good, sound, early union. The patient returned to his work as a warehouseman at this time and was able to do light lifting.

tures, infection on occasion is a serious problem. The situation is no different with the methods we have described. On the other hand, early rigid stabilization of the tibia does foster improved care of the patient as a whole. Even if infection supervenes in the tibia when it has been rigidly and anatomically fixed, the infection is quite manageable. The ultimate result may still be a functionally normal lower extremity.

In the younger, healthy patient, an increased number of fractures does not seem to affect healing or the patient's resistance to infection locally, provided that increased nutritional requirements of the patient are met. However, in the older patient whose health is already compromised by peripheral vascular disease locally or by heart, lung, liver, or kidney problems generally, we may have to modify our treatment plan significantly. Especially when these older patients have sustained a significant soft-tissue crush injury, they cannot seem to rally the defenses and the pulmonary, liver, or kidney function necessary to survive this insult. As mentioned previously, early amputation of one or more crushed limbs may be an acceptable price for an older patient to pay in such instances.

With regard to other aspects of postoperative care, we tend to cover with a cast all open fractures that have been fixed internally, and we use no special type of dressing except silk or other fine-mesh dressing close to the skin. We have not proved that any special moistening agent provides an advantage. We do not remove the cast and dressing until the patient is returned to the operating room in 5 days, at which time each dressing is removed carefully and inspected, and the wound is cleansed gently. If no further debridement is needed and there is no other major problem at that time, we either close the skin primarily, if this can be done with no tension and with no dead space, or cover the area with a one-to-one meshed split thickness skin graft. This graft always can be excised and some cosmetic or plastic work can be done later if the scar is unsightly, but we take no chances with dead space, dead tissue, hematoma, or tension in the early phase of healing.

On occasion, when wounds are contaminated or soft-tissue damage is too extensive to allow any kind of early closure, we may treat the wounds with wet-to-dry or wet-to-wet dressings for a period of time. Occasionally, split cadaver or pig skin is used to encourage good granulation. When the time is optimal, an autogenous

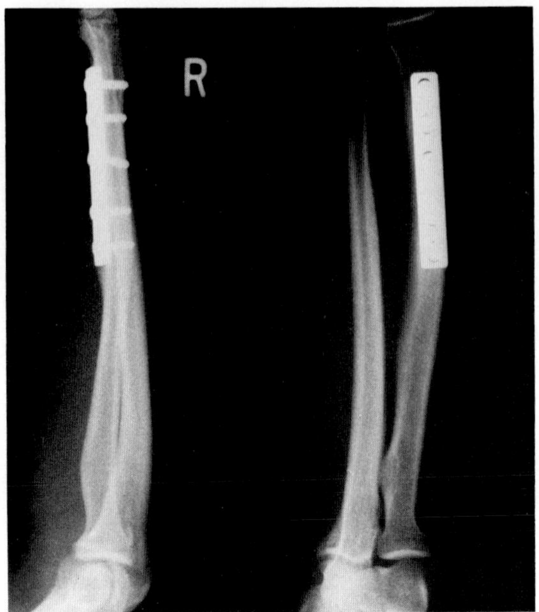

Fig. 28-11. These roentgenograms of the right forearm were taken sometime later, but show solid union; the fracture had united well enough to allow the patient to return to work at 3 months.

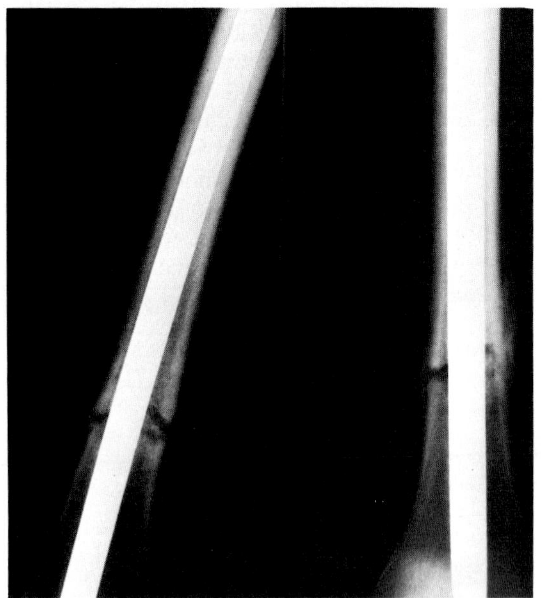

Fig. 28-12. Films taken at 10 weeks show the early union of the femur that had allowed the patient to begin bearing weight on this bone at about 6 weeks and to return to work at 3 months. Note that although the fracture seems rather distal, stable and anatomic fixation was achieved. This result is common in patients of this age group, where the metaphyseal bone in the distal femur provides excellent fixation around a full-length nail.

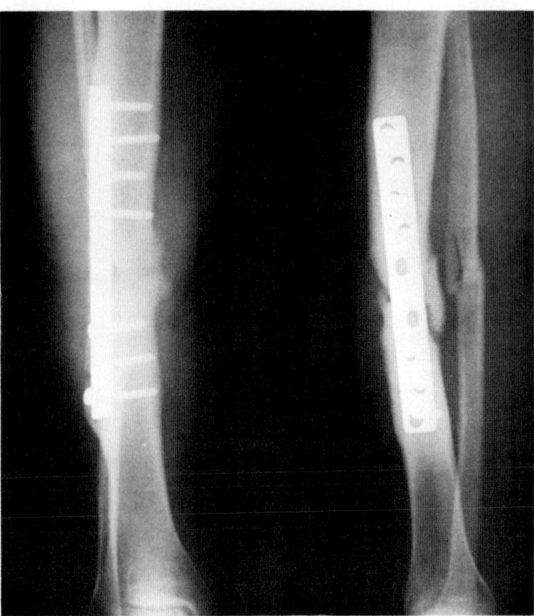

Fig. 28-13. Films of the tibia taken at 1 year show some slight angulation, a broken screw distally, and some hypertrophy, but probable fibrous nonunion. At this time, the patient had been working for approximately 9 months with minimal discomfort in this leg.

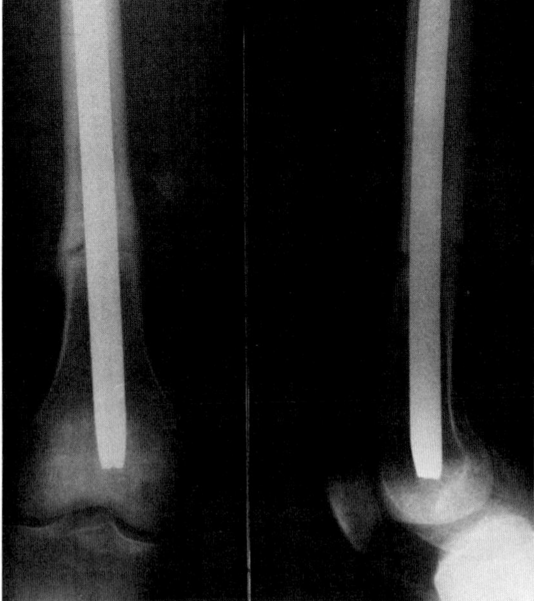

Fig. 28-14. Final roentgenograms of the femur show solid union of the bone in an anatomic position. Despite the damage to the quadriceps caused by the open injury, the patient had regained full motion of the knee by this time; he did have some slightly decreased power in full extension, although he had no lag.

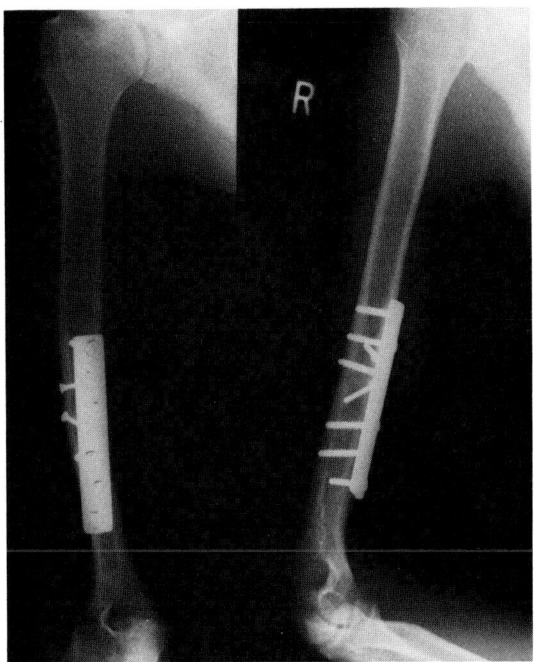

Fig. 28-15. At 18 months the humerus showed solid union and remodeling with no evidence of stress protection.

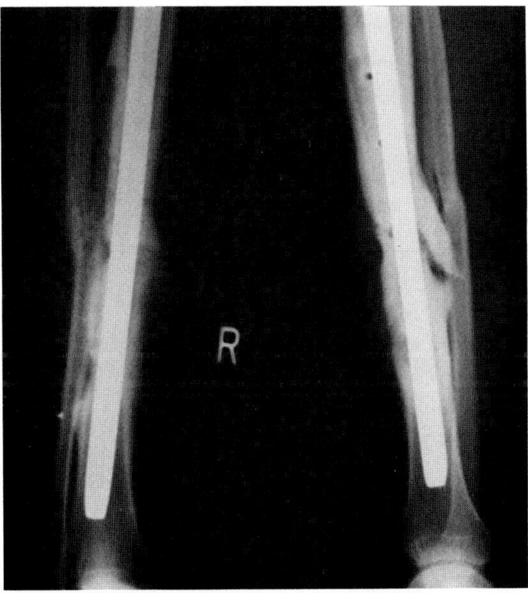

Fig. 28-16. Films show the treatment of fibrous tibial nonunion first noted 6 months earlier (see Fig. 28-13). The plate was removed, and the tibia was treated with closed intramedullary nailing with reaming. This procedure has been proved quite safe after initial plating. However, our experience and that of others[8] has shown that closed intramedullary nailing after initial external fixation can be accompanied by a significant infection rate.

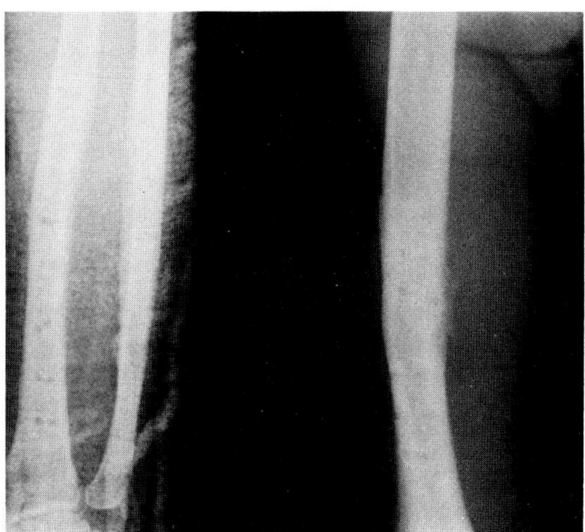

Fig. 28-17. At 18 months the hardware was removed from both the radius and the humerus at the time the tibial fracture was renailed. Hardware removal is not always necessary, but was elected in this case because the man was only about 20 years of age, was active, and was undergoing other surgery.

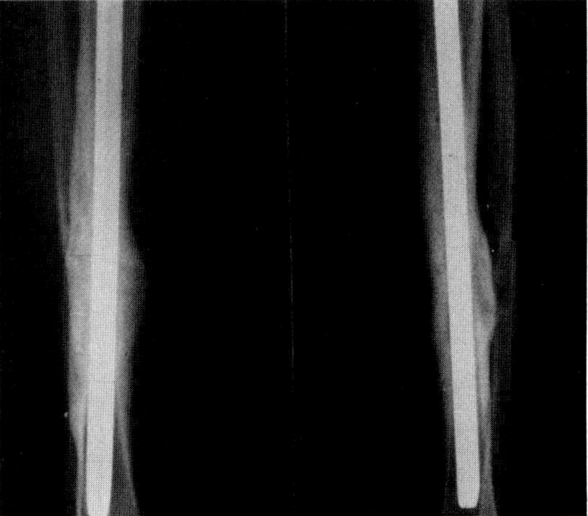

Fig. 28-18. Final roentgenograms of the tibia taken 4 years after injury demonstrate solid union of the tibial fracture 2½ years after the secondary nailing. The patient had been working almost continuously from 3 months after his accident and, on examination, had no functional abnormalities and few, if any, measurable anatomic abnormalities. At the time this film was taken, the patient had returned for tibial nail removal because he felt a slight irritation at the tibial tubercle area when kneeling. The patient's hospitalization time for these multiple injuries totaled approximately 2 weeks: the initial hospitalization of 10 days, an additional 3-day admission for removal of upper extremity hardware and replacement of a tibial plate with a tibial nail, and the final 1-day admission for removal of the tibial nail 4 years after injury. His total time away from gainful employment was approximately 4 months. A residual disability rating was not necessary because he claims no disability.

split-thickness skin graft is then used. With good internal fixation, we also may be able to put the patient into a whirlpool for wound cleansing before we do definitive grafting in a wound that has been contaminated or has a superficial infection.

We also agree with Dr. Border that the earliest possible mobilization of the patient into the upright position through the use of multiple fixation of long-bone fractures is a desirable goal in terms of protecting the patient from chest problems.[9] This treatment is given in association with PEEP (positive end-expiratory pressure) and other special pulmonary support measures that the intensive-care specialists can provide.

Finally, I urge that every multiply injured patient be treated aggressively in the initial phase of treatment. We have seldom found that our operative procedures were too long or too extensive in this phase. On the contrary, we frequently have wished that we had fixed an additional fracture when the only fracture we did not fix became the sole residual problem.

Patients with multiple injuries once had a discouraging and downhill course. By contrast, today's multiply injured patient can be turned about rapidly and put into early rehabilitative programs with expectations of complete functional recovery. Such results require a smoothly functioning and integrated team, each member performing his part of the treatment with a high degree of skill. In the care and recovery of the patient with multiple concomitant long-bone fractures, the orthopaedic traumatologist has a particularly important role to play.

References

1. Allgower, M., and Willenegger, H.: Introduction. *In* The Open Fracture. Assessment, Surgical Treatment, and Results. Edited by P. Matter, and W.-W. Rittmann. Bern, Hans Huber, 1978.
2. Chapman, M. W.: The use of immediate internal fixation in open fractures. Orthop. Clin. North Am., *11*:579, 1980.
3. LaDuca, J. N., Bone, L. L., Seibel, R. W., and Border, J. R.: Primary open reduction and internal fixation of open fractures. J. Trauma, *20*:580, 1980.
4. Matter, P., and Rittmann, W.-W.: The Open Fracture. Assessment, Surgical Treatment and Results. Bern, Hans Huber, 1978.
5. Meek, R. N., Vivoda, E., Crichton, A., and Pirani, S.: Comparison of mortality of patients with multiple injuries according to method of fracture treatment. *In* Proceedings of the Canadian Orthopaedic Association Annual Meeting, June 8–12, 1980, Calgary, Alberta. J. Bone Joint Surg., *63-B*:456, 1981.
6. Rittmann, W. W., Schibli, M., Matter, P., and Allgower, M.: Open fractures—long-term results in 200 consecutive cases. Clin. Orthop., *138*:132, 1979.
7. Tscherne, H., Ostern, H. J., and Sturm, J.: Osteosynthesis of major fractures in polytrauma. World J. Surg., *7*:80, 1983.
8. Karlstrom, G., and Olerud, S.: Percutaneous pin fixation of open tibial fractures. Double-frame anchorage using the Vidal-Adrey method. J. Bone Joint Surg., *57-A*:915, 1975.
9. Border, J.: Cardiopulmonary failure. *In* Basic Surgery. Edited by J. A. McCredie. New York, Macmillan, 1977.

Index

A *t* following a page number indicates a pertinent table on that page; an *f* following a page number indicates a pertinent illustration on that page.

Abdominal injuries, 207–208
Acetabular fractures
  traction for, 138
  treatment of, 201–203, 202*f*, 205*f*
Acid-base disturbances, 105
Acidosis
  metabolic, 20, 105
  respiratory, 105
Acromioclavicular joint, 140
  mechanism of injury to, 342
  treatment of dislocation of, 342–343, 343*f*
Acromion fractures, 342
Adult respiratory distress syndrome (ARDS)
  arterial oxygen content in, 46–47
  chest x-ray of, 45
  classification of, 44*t*
  definition of, 42
  diagnosis of, 43*t*, 44–47
  etiologic factor associated with, 44–45
  fat embolism syndrome vs, 68
  functional residual capacity of lungs in, 45, 46*f*
  incidence of, 42
  morbidity and mortality of, 42–43
  pathology and pathogenesis of, 43–44, 43*f*
  pulmonary compliance in, 45–46
  sepsis associated with, 44
  therapy for, 47–52
    blood replacement in, 52
    cardiovascular, 50–52
    diuretics in, 52
    endotracheal intubation in, 48
    nutrition in, 52
    oxygen, 47–48
    positive end-expiratory pressure in, 49–50
    positive-pressure ventilation in, 48–49
    pulmonary toilet, 47
    weaning patient from ventilation in, 50
  venoarterial shunt in, 46
Aerodigestive tract, 9
Airway
  abnormal upper, 10–17
  anesthetic considerations with obstructions in, 97–98, 107–108
  with breathing obstruction, 13–17
  in central nervous system control loss, 12–13
  in chest injuries, 18–19
  in deglutition, 9–10
  examination of, 14–16
  nasopharyngeal, 12
  normal upper, 9–10
  oropharyngeal, 12
  problems with, following trauma, 13, 13*t*
  in pulmonary insufficiency and toilet, 10–12
  in respiration, 10
Albumin
  in hemorrhagic shock, 37
  in nutritional assessment, 130
Aldolase, 79
Aldosterone in hemorrhagic shock, 33
Alkalosis
  metabolic, 105
  respiratory, 105
Amino acids, 129
Amputation
  digital, 365–366
  indications for, 117
  leg, 402
Analgesics, 99
Anesthesia, 96–111
  acid-base disturbances during, 105
  with airway obstruction, 107–108
  assessment of patient prior to, 97–99, 98*t*
    airway and ventilation difficulties in, 97–98
    gastric contents in, 99
    hemorrhage in, 98–99
    intoxication, 99
    multiple injuries in, 97
    trauma status in, 98*t*
  blood pressure during, 100
  with burns, 109
  with chest and heart trauma, 108–109
  coagulopathies during, 105–106
  electrocardiogram during, 100
  with eye injuries, 109
  fluid balance during, 101
  fluid therapy with, 103–104
  general, 100
  with hand and wrist injury, 369
  with head injury, 106–107, 136–137
  hypotension during, 104–105
  hypothermia during, 104
  induction agents for, 102
  induction and intubation with, 101–102
  inhalation agents in, 103
  with intoxication, 109–110
  maintenance of, 102
  with massive trauma and hemorrhage, 106
  with maxillofacial injuries, 107–108
  mortality rate with use of, 97
  muscle relaxants in, 103
  narcotics in, 103
  with neck and cervical spinal injuries, 107
  patient monitoring during, 100–101
  pharmacologic considerations in, 102–103
  postoperative considerations of, 110–111
  premedication, 99
  regional blocks, 99
  respiratory function during, 100
  spinal, 99
  technique, 99–100
  temperature during, 100–101
  urine output during, 100
Ankle fractures, 154
  classification of, 292–294

Ankle fractures (*Continued*)
complex, 291–311
diagnosis of, 294–297
malleolar, 291
mechanism of injury and incidence of, 292
pilon, 292, 298*f*
postoperative regimen for, 306–310
pronation dorsiflexion type, 292, 293*f*, 294*f*
pronation external rotation type, 292, 295*f*
spiral extension, 292, 299*f*
supination external rotation type, 292, 295*f*
tibial length loss in, 291, 291*f*, 304
treatment of, 297–310
complications of, 310
instruments for, 301–302, 302*f*
with Kirschner wires and Steinmann pins, 297–299
with plaster of Paris, 297
with plates, 300, 301
results of, 310–311
with screws, 296–297*f*, 299–300
type I, 302–303, 303*f*
type II, 299*f*, 300*f*, 303
type III, 303–304, 305–309*f*
from vertical compression forces, 292
Ankylosis, 142
Antacids, 99
Anterior cord syndrome, 164
Antibiotics, 115
Anticholinergic drugs, 99
Antidiuretic hormone in shock, 33
Aortic rupture, 28–30, 108
Aortography
for aortic rupture diagnosis, 29, 30
indications for, 30*t*
Arcuate artery, 326
ARDS. *See* Adult respiratory distress syndrome.
Arm, 158. *See also* Forearm
Arrhythmias, 33–34
Arterial anastomoses, 93, 94*f*
Arterial occlusion
in compartment syndrome pathogenesis, 72, 73*f*
compartment syndrome vs, 79, 79*t*
treatment of, 81
Arterial trauma with fractures
compartment syndromes and, 86, 88*f*
initial evaluation and diagnosis of, 90–91
therapy for, 91–95, 91*f*, 92*f*, 94*f*
Arteriography
for arterial injury diagnosis, 90–91
for fractures with neurovascular or tendinous injury, 117
for renal injuries, 56, 57*f*
Arthrography, 256
Arthroscopic examination, 256
Arthrosis, traumatic, 310
Atlas, 185–186, 186*f*
Atropine, 99
Axillary artery, 326, 339
Axillary nerve, 158, 339
Axis fractures, 187–189, 190*f*
Axonotmesis, 157

Balanced salt solution (BSS), 103–104
Barbiturates, 99, 102
Barton's fracture, 376, 377
Beck's triad, 39
Bennett's fracture, 387
Bladder rupture, 55–56
extraperitoneal, 61–62, 61*f*
intraperitoneal, 60–61, 60*f*
Blalock technique, 373, 373*f*
Blast injuries of hand and wrist, 371*f*, 383*f*, 397
Bleeding disorders
compartment syndromes from, 73
intraoperative considerations of, 105–106
in treatment phase of stabilization, 6
Blood gases
in adult respiratory distress syndrome, 46–47, 47*f*
in fat embolism syndrome, 69
Blood pressure
with hemorrhage, 19
in hypotension, 32
monitoring of, with anesthesia, 100
Blood replacement therapy for ARDS, 52
Blood tests, 79
Bone grafts, 124–125, 126*f*, 127*f*
for distal humeral fractures, 359, 359*f*, 360*f*
for lumbar fracture-dislocation treatment, 177, 177*f*
for segmental femoral fracture, 220, 229
for segmental tibial fractures, 233
Bone reconstruction, 124–125, 126*f*, 127*f*
Brachial plexus injuries, 140, 157
Brachioradialis muscle, 74
Bradykinin, 34
Breathing obstructions, 13–17
Brevital, 102
Brown-Sequard syndrome, 164
Buck's fascia, 63, 64
Bulbocavernous reflex, 164
Burns
anesthetic considerations with, 109
compartment syndromes from, 73
Burst fractures, 193, 193*f*
atlantal, 186
of atlas, 185, 186

Calcaneocuboid joint, 313
Calories, 128, 129
Campbell's surgical approach to distal humerus fractures, 351, 352, 352*f*, 353*f*
Capitate, 377, 380–381
Carbohydrates, 128
Carbon dioxide, 136
Cardiac injuries, 28–30
anesthetic considerations with, 108–109
Cardiac tamponade, 19, 20
anesthetic considerations with, 108
cardiogenic shock from, 39
pericardiocentesis for, 105
Cardiogenic hypotension, 105
Cardiogenic shock, 33–34, 38–39
Cardiotonic drugs, 52
Cardiovascular system
in ARDS, 50–52
blood replacement and, 52
diuretics and, 52
fluid therapy and, 51–52
inotropic support and, 52
monitoring of, 50–51, 51*f*
nutrition and, 52
in chest injuries, 19–20
Carpal bones, 377, 380–381
Cassebaum's transolecranon approach to humeral fractures, 353–355, 353*f*, 354*f*
Cast traction, 138, 138*f*
Casts, 150
for clavicular fractures, 324
for femur fractures, 275
at distal end, 275, 275*f*
segmental, 220–221*f*
for foot fractures, 315
for glenohumeral joint dislocation, 337
for ipsilateral fractures of hip and femur, 213
for segmental tibial fractures, 233
Catecholamines, 33
Cauda equina injury, 164–165
Central cord syndrome, 164
Central nervous system, 12
Central venous pressure
in chest injuries, 19

Central venous pressure (*Continued*)
determination of, 38
as fluid replacement index, 101
technique for obtaining, 101
Cephalosporins, 115
Cervical spinal injuries
airway problem with, 13–14
anesthetic considerations with, 107
delayed recognition of, 135, 135*t*
examination of, 16–17, 16*f*
extension, 192
flexion, 189–190
fracture-dislocations, 179–194
of atlas, 185–186, 186*f*
of axis, bilateral pedicle, 187–189, 190*f*
burst, 193, 193*f*
CT of, 184, 185*f*
diagnostic evaluation of, 181–184
emergency management of, 179–181
myelography of, 184
of odontoid, 186–187, 188*f*, 189*f*
radiographs of, flexion-extension of, 182–184, 184*f*, 185*f*
radiographs of, plain, 181–182, 181*f*
tomography of, 182, 183*f*
locked facet, bilateral, 191–192
locked facet, unilateral, 190–191, 191*f*
from penetrating wounds, 193
in polytrauma patient, 194
Chance fractures, 168–169, 169*f*, 173
Chauffeur's fracture, 376, 377
Chest injuries
airway and ventilation with, 18–19
anesthetic considerations with, 108–109
aortic rupture, 28–30
cardiovascular function with, 19–20
hemothorax, 25–26
initial management and considerations of, 18–20
innominate artery avulsion, 30
myocardial contusion, 28
pneumothorax, 23–25
pulmonary contusion, 20–23
clinical features of, 21–23
radiographic findings of, 20
rib fractures, 26–27
sternal fractures, 27–28
subclavian artery injuries, 30
to wall, 26–28
Chondromalacia, 229
Clavicle, 140, 157
in acromioclavicular joint sprains, 342
fractures of, 323–325
classification of, 323
injuries associated with, 324
mechanism of injury in, 323–324
treatment of, 324–325
Closed space compression syndrome, 370
Coagulopathies, 105–106
Colles' fascia, 63, 64, 65*f*
Colles' fracture, 376
Coma, 135–136
Compartment syndromes
anatomy of, 73–75, 75*f*
arterial injuries in, 86, 87*f*
blood and urine tests in, 79, 79*t*
burns in, 73
causes of, 71–73, 72*f*, 73*f*
in children, 71
clinical findings of, 75–77, 76*f*, 77*f*
complications of, 87–88
definition of, 71
diagnosis of, 71–73
differential diagnosis of, 79–80, 79*t*
drug overdose-limb compression and, 72–73, 74*f*
early evaluation and care of, 80–81
electromyography and nerve conduction in, 77
forearm decompression for, 81
forearm volar and dorsal fasciotomy for, 82
operative technique, 83–84, 83*f*
fractures causing, 71–72, 76
indications/contraindications for decompression in, 80
intramuscular pressure measurements of, 77, 78*f*
laboratory tests of, 77–79
leg decompression for, 81–82
leg double-incision fasciotomy for, 82
anterolateral approach, 84–85
posteromedial approach, 85–86, 85*f*, 86*f*
skin incisions, 84
leg fasciotomy prophylactically for, 86–87
pathogenesis of, 73*f*
peripheral circulation assessment in, 77–79
of plantar region, 314
post-ischemic swelling in, 72
pressure increase with, 76, 76*f*, 77
radius fracture in, 86
soft tissue injury in, 72
tibial fracture in, 86
time of injury vs onset of findings in, 87–88, 88*f*
treatment of, 80–88
ulna fracture in, 86
Volksmann's contracture from, 87–88, 88*f*
Compression rods, 172*f*, 173, 176
Congestive heart failure, 33
Conus medullaris injury, 164–165
Coracoid fractures, 342
Corticosteroids, 40
Cranial nerves
in deglutition, 9
in hypotension, 32
Creatine phosphokinase, 79
Creatinine, 131
Cricoarytenoid muscle, 10
Cricopharyngeus muscle, 10
Cricothyrotomy, 16
Cruciate ligaments of knee, 260–262
in knee dislocation, 268, 269
Crush injuries
of femur, 402
of hand and wrist, 389, 391, 392*f*
of tibia, 402
Crush syndrome
as compartment syndrome complication, 87
drug overdose-limb compression and, 72
laboratory test values in, 79, 79*t*
Cubitus valgus, 158
Cuneiform joints, 313, 315
Cushing reflex, 34
Cystography
of bladder rupture, 60, 60*f*
in trauma workup, 55, 56*f*
of urethral rupture, 63, 63*f*
Cystostomy, 61

Darrach procedure, 142
Deglutition, 9–10
Dextran, 69
Deyerle pins, 213
Digits, 365–366
Disseminated intravascular coagulopathy, 106
Distraction rods, 171, 171*f*
Diuretics, 52
Dopamine, 105
Drug overdose, 72–73, 74*f*

Eating, 9–10
Elbow
anatomy of, 347
dislocation of, 361
fracture of, 347–363

Elbow, fracture of (*Continued*)
distal humerus fracture in, 348–361
with head injury, 140*f*, 141
immobilization of, with plaster cast, 137–138
in Monteggia's fracture-dislocation, 361–362
with nerve injury, 158–159
olecranon fracture in, 363
proximal forearm fracture in, 362
radial head fracture in, 362
treatment of, 347–348
Electrocardiogram, 100
Electromyography, 77
Emphysema, subcutaneous, 23, 25
Ender pins, 213, 214–215, 217
Endotracheal intubation
with laryngeal or cervical tracheal fracture, 19
with pulmonary contusion, 22
topical anesthesia for, 102
tracheostomy vs, 15
tubes for, 11*f*
Energy stores in body, 128–130
Epiglottis in deglutition, 10
Epinephrine, 369
Escharotomy, 73
Ethacrynic acid, 22
Ethrane, 103
Examination, physical
of acromioclavicular joint sprains, 342
of ankle fractures, 295
of foot fractures, 313
of hand and wrist injuries, 366, 367–368
of knee ligament injuries, 253
of lumbar spinal fracture-dislocations, 162
of pelvic fracture, 198*t*
in preanesthetic evaluation, 97
Exsanguination, 106
Extensor carpi radiolis longus and brevis muscles, 74
Eye injuries, 109

Facet
cervical, bilateral locked, 191–192
cervical, unilateral locked, 190–191
lumbar, fracture of, 177
Fasciotomy
in arterial injury treatment with fracture, 93
of forearm, 82–84, 83*f*, 84*f*
for hand and wrist injuries, 366, 370
of leg, 82, 272
prophylactic, 72, 73, 86–87
Fat, 129
Fat embolism syndrome, 67–70
ARDS vs, 68
clinical manifestations of, 68
historical aspects of, 67
incidence of, 67
laboratory findings of, 68–69
pathogenesis of, 68
treatment of, 69–70
Fatty acids, 129
Femur fractures
angular deformities with treatment of, 148*f*, 150
bilateral, 402
of distal end, 275–290
classification of, 277, 277*f*
closed treatment of, 278
complications of, 290
diagnosis of, 276–277
instruments for surgery on, 279–281, 284*f*
internal fixation of, 278–279, 280*f*, 281*f*, 282*f*
lateral surgical approach to, 281, 283, 285*f*
mechanism of injury of, 276
open treatment of, 279–281
operative technique for, 281–288, 285*f*, 286*f*, 287*f*, 288*f*
physical findings for, 276–277
postoperative management of, 288–290, 289*f*
preoperative planning for, 281
radiographic assessment of, 277
treatment of, 277–290
healing of, 139, 139*f*, 149*f*, 150
intramedullary nailing of, 150, 224–226, 225*f*, 226*f*, 227*f*
diagnosis of, 210–211, 211*t*
treatment of, 211–217, 212*f*, 213*f*, 215*f*, 216*f*
with knee ligament injuries, 250
malpositioned healing of, 149*f*, 150
plating of, 402
segmental, 218–230
complications of, 229–230
external fixation of, 220, 222*f*
in floating knee, 239–243, 240–242*f*
intramedullary nailing of, 224–226, 225*f*, 226*f*, 227*f*, 228*f*
nonoperative treatment of, 220, 221*f*
plates for, 220, 224*f*
postoperative management of, 227–229
results of, 229
treatment alternatives for, 220–227
types of, 219–220
stress testing of, 254
traction of, 138, 150
Fentanyl, 103
Fibula
in ankle fractures, 292, 304
in knee dislocations, 273
Flaps
cross-leg, 124, 124*f*
distant, 124, 124*f*
for knee ligament injuries, 258
latissimus dorsi free, 124, 124*f*
muscle, for skin defects about tibia, 118–124
pedicled, 118
rotational, 118
for segmental tibial fractures, 232–233
Flexor carpi radialis, 73
Flexor carpi ulnaris, 73
Flexor digitorum superficialis and profundus, 73–74
Flexor pollicis longus, 74
Fluids
balance of, during anesthesia, 101, 103–104
for hyperalimentation, 131
Foot fractures, 154
closed reduction and casting of, 315
complex, 313–321
complications from treatment of, 321–322
diagnosis of, 313–314
metatarsal shaft, 313, 315, 321
of metatarsophalangeal joints, 313, 315, 321
navicular, 313, 315, 319–321
open reduction and internal fixation of, 315
of os calcis, 313, 315, 318–319
results of treatment of, 322
soft-tissue problems with, 314–315
of talus, 313, 315, 316–318
tarsometatarsal, 313, 315, 321
treatment options with, 315–316, 316*f*, 317*f*, 318*f*, 319*f*, 320*f*
Foot joints, 313
Forearm
anatomy of, 73–74, 75*f*
decompression of, 81
dorsal compartment of, 74
fasciotomy of, 82
dorsal approach, 83, 83*f*
postoperative care with, 83–84
volar approach, 83, 83*f*
fractures of, 141–142, 362

Forearm, fractures of (*Continued*)
with head injury, 141–142
with nerve injury, 158
volar compartment of, 73–74
Fractures
acetabular, 146, 146*f*
traction for, 138
treatment of, 201–203, 202*f*, 204*f*
involving acromioclavicular joint, 140, 342
acromion, 342
of ankle. *See* Ankle fractures
of arm, 158
arterial injuries from, 86
arterial trauma associated with, 90–95
initial evaluation and diagnosis of, 90–91
therapy for, 91–95, 91*f*, 92*f*, 94*f*
of atlas, 185–186, 186*f*
of axis, bilateral pedicle, 187–189, 190*f*
Barton's, 376, 377
Bennett's, 387
burst, 193
carpal bone, 380
of cervical spine, 179–195
burst, 193, 193*f*
CT of, 184
diagnostic evaluation of, 181–184
emergency management of, 179–181
from extension injuries, 192
from flexion injuries, 189–190
from locked facet, bilateral, 191–192
from locked facet, unilateral, 190–191
myelography of, 184
from penetrating wounds, 193
in polytrauma patient, 194
radiography of, 180, 181–184
tomography of, 182
Chauffeur's, 376, 377
clavicular, 140, 323–325
Colles', 376
compartment syndromes from, 71–72, 73*f*
coracoid, 342
definition of, 113
delayed recognition of, 135
of elbow, 137–138, 347–363
with dislocations, 361
with head injury, 140*f*, 141
with nerve injury, 158–159
treatment of, 347–348
extremity, with head injuries, 134–154
anesthesia for treatment of, 136–137
delayed recognition of trauma and, 135
healing of, 139
lower, 142–154
plaster casts for, 137–138
prognosis for, 135–136
traction for, 138–139
upper, 140–142
facet, 177
of femur, 148*f*, 149*f*, 150
bilateral, 402
cast-brace for, 150
complications from, 229–230
external fixation of, 220, 222*f*
in floating knee, 239–243, 240–242*f*
healing of, 139, 139*f*, 149*f*, 150
intramedullary nailing of, 224–226, 225*f*, 226*f*, 227*f*, 228*f*
nonoperative treatment of, 220, 221*f*
plates for, 220, 223*f*
postoperative management of, 227–229
results of, 229
segmental, 219–230
traction for, 138, 150
treatment alternatives for, 220–227
types of, 219–220
of femur, at distal end, 275–290
classification of, 277, 277*f*
closed treatment of, 278
complications of, 290
diagnosis of, 276–277
instruments for surgery on, 279–281, 284*f*
internal fixation of, 278–279, 280*f*, 281*f*, 282*f*, 283*f*
lateral surgical approach to, 281, 283, 285*f*
mechanism of injury for, 276
open treatment of, 279–281
operative technique for, 281–288, 282*f*, 283*f*, 284*f*, 285*f*, 286*f*, 287*f*, 288*f*
physical findings for, 276–277
postoperative management of, 288–290, 289*f*
preoperative planning for, 281
radiographic assessment of, 277
treatment options for, 277–290
of floating knee, 239–246
of foot, 153, 154
complications from treatment of, 322
diagnosis of, 313–314
metatarsal shaft, 315, 321
of metatarsophalangeal joints, 313, 315, 321
navicular, 313, 315, 319–321
of os calcis, 313, 315, 318–319
results of treatment of, 322
soft-tissue problems with, 314–315
of talus, 313, 315, 316–318
tarsometatarsal, 313, 315, 321
treatment options with, 315–316, 316*f*, 317*f*, 318*f*, 319*f*, 320*f*
types of, 313
of forearm, 141
with head injury, 141–142
with nerve injury, 158
proximal, 362
Galeazzi's, 377
with glenohumeral joint dislocation, 338
glenoid, 326
in hand and wrist injuries, 373, 374–375
healing of, 139, 139*f*
heterotopic bone formation with, 141
of hip, 148
with head injury, 147*f*, 148–150
with nerve injury, 159
traction for, 138
treatment of, 203–205, 205*f*, 206*f*
of humerus, 36, 140
bilateral, 402
blood supply in, 326
classification of, 327, 328*f*
diagnosis of, 327–328
distally, 348–361, 349*f*, 352*f*, 353*f*, 354*f*, 355*f*, 356*f*, 357*f*, 358*f*, 359*f*, 360*f*
proximally, 326–333
treatment of, 328–333, 329*f*, 331*f*, 333*f*
immobilization of, 138
of interphalangeal joints, 138
Jefferson, 186, 186*f*
of knee, 150
with dislocation, 273, 273*f*
with head injury, 150–153, 151*f*, 152*f*
with nerve injury, 159
with knee ligament injuries, 249–263
arthrography of, 256
arthroscopic examination of, 256
classification of, 252–253, 252*f*
diagnosis of, 253–256
history and physical examination of, 253

Fractures, with nerve injury (*Continued*)
mechanism of, 250–251, 250*f*, 251*f*, 252*f*
nonoperative management of, 256–257
operative closure in, 262
operative management of, 258–262
postoperative care of, 262
radiographic examination of, 254–255, 254*f*, 255*f*
repair of cruciate ligaments in, 260–262, 261*f*, 262*f*
repair of lateral supporting structures in, 260
repair of medial supporting structures in, 258–260
repair of posterior supporting structures in, 260–262, 261*f*, 262*f*
stress radiographs of, 255, 256*f*, 257*f*
stress testing of, 253–254
treatment options for, 256–262
laryngeal, 19
long bone, concomitant, 401–410, 405*f*, 406*f*, 407*f*, 408*f*, 409*f*
of lumbar spine, 162–178
anterior surgical approach to, 176–177
clinical patterns of paralysis with, 164–166, 165*t*
CT of, 167, 167*f*
diagnosis, priorities, and pitfalls of, 162–163, 168–169
diagnostic tests for, 166–167
initial management of, 169
instrumentation for surgical treatment of, 170–173, 171*f*, 172*f*
lateral tomograms of, 166, 166*f*
myelography of, 167
neurologic evaluation with, 163–164, 164*f*
operative complications of, 177–178
posterior internal fixation and stabilization for, 175–176
postoperative complications of, 178
postoperative management of, 176
roentgenographic evaluation of, 166
from seat belt injury, 168–169, 169*f*
short compression rods for surgery of, 176
spinal stability vs instability with, 167–168, 168*f*
surgical indications/contraindications for, 169–174
surgical stabilization of, 170
surgical techniques for treatment of, 175–177
treatment options and recommendations for, 174–175
unilateral motor weakness and sensory loss with, 166
with major nerve injuries, 156–160
classification of, 156–157
management program for, 160
mandibular, 10
metacarpal, 382–384, 383*f*
of metacarpal phalangeal joints, 138
Monteggia's, 361–362
odontoid, 186–187, 188*f*, 189*f*
olecranon, 363
open vs closed, 113
open, with major skin and bone defects, 113–127
amputation for, indications for, 117
bone reconstruction for, 124–125
classification of, 114, 114*t*
concept of, 114–115
distant flaps for, 124
grade I, 115
grade II, 116
grade III, 116–117
historical background on, 113–114
initial management of, 115–117
muscle flaps for, 118–124
neurovascular or tendinous injury with, 117
pedicled flaps for, 118
soft-tissue reconstruction for, 117–118
pelvic, 36, 145*f*, 146
abdominal and urologic injuries with, 207–208
bed rest for, 199
classification of, 196–198, 197*f*
diagnostic procedures for, 198–199
early mobilization for patient with, 206–207
emergency management of, 198–199, 198–199*t*
hemorrhage with, 205–206
open, 208
pelvic slings for, 199–200
postural reduction and casting for, 199
reduction and external fixation for, 200
reduction and internal fixation for, 200
spinal trauma with, 207
traction for, 138, 199–200
of phalanges, 385
Piedmont, 377
of radius, 376
articular, 376, 376*f*
distal, 141*f*, 142, 143–144*f*
at head, 362
metaphyseal, 376, 376*f*
treatment of, 376–377, 378–379*f*
rib, 26–27
scapular, 140, 325–326
seat belt, 168–169, 169*f*, 173
segmental, of lower extremity, 218–239
femoral, 219–230
with floating knee, 239–246
tibial, 230–239
treatment goals for, 218–219
treatment plan for, 218
of shoulder, 140
clavicle in, 323–325
complicated, 334–335
with head injury, 140
impression defects with, 333–334
with nerve injury, 157–158
neurovascular deficit with, 334–335, 336*f*
proximal humerus in, 325–333
scapula in, 325–326
Smith's, 376, 377
sternal, 27–28
of thumb, 138, 387, 389*f*, 391*f*
tibial, 71, 86, 153, 153*f*, 154*f*
bilateral, 402
casts for, 233
complications of, 237–239
external fixation device for, 233, 234*f*
in floating knee, 243, 244–245*f*
infection from, 237–238
intramedullary nails for, 236, 237*f*
with knee dislocations, 273
malunion of, 238
nonunion of, 238
plates for, 233–236, 235*f*
postoperative management of, 236–237
segmental, 230–239
soft-tissue injury with, 230, 231
stabilization of, 233–263
stiffness from, 238–239
swelling from, 239

Fractures (*Continued*)
wedge compression, of vertebral body, 189
of wrist, 138, 365–382
Frank-Starling curve, 33, 34*f*
Furosemide, 22

Galeazzi's fracture, 377
Gastrocnemius muscle for muscle flaps, 118–121, 119*f*, 120*f*, 121*f*
Genitourinary system
bladder rupture, 60–62
diagnosis of injury to, 55–56
genital injuries, 64–65
renal injuries, 56–59
trauma workup on, 55, 56*f*
ureteral injuries, 59–60
urethral rupture, 62–64
Glasgow coma scale, 135–136, 135*t*
Glenohumeral joint dislocation
anterior, 335–339
complications of, 338–339
diagnosis of, 337
fractures associated with, 338
irreducible, 338
management of, 337–338
mechanism of injury of, 335
nerve injury with, 339
pathology and pathogenesis of, 335–337
roentgenographic interpretation of, 337
rotator cuff injury with, 338–339
unrecognized, 338
vascular injury with, 339
inferior, 339
posterior, 340–342
acute traumatic, 341
chronic unreduced, 341–342
diagnosis of, 341
management of, 341
mechanism of injury of, 340
pathology and pathogenesis of, 340–341
roentgenographic interpretation of, 341
Glenoid fractures, 326
Glossopharyngeal nerve, 10
Glucagon in hemorrhagic shock, 33
Glucose, 129
Glycogen, 128
Glycopyrrolate, 99
Grafts
bone, 124–125, 126*f*, 127*f*
for femoral fractures, 220, 229
for humeral fractures, 359, 359*f*, 360*f*
for lumbar fracture-dislocations, 177, 177*f*
for tibial fractures, 233
skin, 118
for hand and wrist injuries, 370–372
for long bone fractures concomitantly, 407, 410*f*
types of, 372

Hagie pins, 213
Halothane, 103
Hamate, 377
Hand
anatomy of, 365, 382
reconstruction of, 398–400
Hand injuries
closed space compression syndrome from, 370
examination of, physical, 367, 368–369
fractures in, 374–375, 385–387, 386*f*, 388*f*, 390*f*
of ligaments, 385–387, 386*f*
of long bones, 382–385
management of, 365
anesthesia for, 369
with blast injuries, 371*f*, 393*f*, 397
with crush injuries, 389, 392*f*, 397
by fasciotomy, 366
hemorrhage in, 366
immobilization in, 375
with impact injuries, 394–395*f*, 397
indepth wound evaluation in, 372
initial, 366–368
laboratory tests in, 368
with massive injuries, 387–398
mobilization and rehabilitation in, 375
open treatment in, 370
primary wound closure and resurfacing in, 365, 370–372
principles of, 365–366, 367*f*
projectile injuries, 396*f*, 397–398, 397*f*, 399*f*
reconstruction of hand in, 398–400
secondary wound closure and resurfacing in, 372
tetanus prophylaxis in, 368
wound culture and gram stains for, 369
wound toilet in, 369–370, 371*f*
of metacarpals, 382–385, 383*f*, 384*f*, 385*f*
pain of, 366–367
patient history in, 367, 368
of phalanges, 385
roentgenography of, 369
skeletal system in, 374–375, 375*f*
tendons and nerves in, 373–374, 373*f*
of thumb, 387, 389*f*, 390–391*f*
vascular system in, 372
Hangman's fracture, 187
Harrington instruments, 171, 171*f*
Hauser procedure, 71
Head injury
anesthetic considerations with, 106–107
deaths from, 136, 136*t*
extremity fractures with, 134–154
type of trauma and age group resulting in, 134*t*
Heart murmur, 29
Hematomas, 56, 57*f*, 58
Hemodynamics, 5
Hemoperitoneum, 36
Hemopneumothorax, 26
Hemorrhage
anesthetic considerations with, 98–99
with hand and wrist injuries, 366
of hemoperitoneum, 36
in hemothorax, 25–26
hypotension from, 35
with pelvic fractures, 205–206
reduced cardiovascular function with, 19
retroperitoneal, 36
venous return to heart with, 19
Hemorrhagic shock
blood pressure in, 32–33
evaluation of, 35–36
metabolic response to, 33
neural response to, 32
physical signs and symptoms of, 98*t*
treatment of, 36–38
Hemothorax, 25–26
anesthetic considerations with, 109
diagnosis of, 35
signs of, 19
Heparin, 69
Heterotopic bone, 141
Hill-Sachs lesion, 327, 337
Hip
fracture of,
diagnosis of, 210–211, 211*t*
extracapsular, 213
with head injury, 147*f*, 148–150
intracapsular, 213
ipsilateral femur fracture with, 210–217
with knee ligament injuries, 251
with nerve injury, 159
treatment of, 203–205, 211–217

Horner's syndrome, 157
Humeral circumflex artery, posterior, 326
Humeral fracture, 36
Humerus
  dislocation of, 327
  displacement of, 327
  in elbow joint, 347
  fracture of,
    bilateral, 402
    with head injury, 140
    with nerve injury, 156, 158
  fracture of, distal, 348–361
    bone grafts for, 359, 360*f*
    Campbell's surgical approach to, 352, 352*f*
    Cassebaum's transolecranon approach to, 353–358, 353–358*f*
    classification of, 349, 349*f*
    extra-articular, 352–353, 352*f*, 353*f*
    intra-articular, 353–358, 353*f*, 354*f*, 355*f*, 356*f*, 357*f*, 358*f*
    open reduction and internal fixation of, 350–358, 356–357*f*, 358*f*, 359*f*
    operative technique for, 351, 352*f*
    postoperative management of, 361
    preoperative planning for, 351
    surgical approach to, 351
    treatment options for, 349–350
  fracture of, proximal, 327–333
    blood supply in, 326
    classification of, 327
    diagnosis of, 327–328
    treatment of, 328–333, 329*f*, 331*f*, 333*f*
  impression defects of, 333–334
Hyperalimentation, 131–133
  composition of solutions for, 133
  routes for, 131–132
  sepsis from, 132–133
  technique for, 132
Hypercarbia, 136
Hyperextension injuries, 185, 187, 192
Hypertension, 58
Hypoproteinemia, 129
Hypotension
  during anesthesia, 104–105
  bradykinin in, 34
  cardiogenic, 105
  of cardiogenic shock, 38–39
  evaluation and treatment of, 35–40
  of hemorrhagic shock, 35–38
  hypovolemic, 105
  neural response to, 32
  of neurogenic shock, 39
  of septic shock, 39–40
  vasogenic, 105
Hypothermia, 104
Hypovolemia, 19, 33
  anesthetic considerations with, 98–99
  hypotension from, 105
  shock from, 35–38
Hypoxemia, 21
  of fat embolism syndrome, 68–69
  post-anesthetic, 104
Hypoxia, 19

Impact injuries of hand and wrist, 394*f*, 395, 397
Infection
  from ankle fracture treatment, 310
  from arterial injury with fractures, 93–95
  of open fractures, 116
  with segmental femoral fractures, 220, 229
  with segmental tibial fractures, 237–238
  from surgical treatment of lumbar fracture-dislocations, 178
Innominate artery avulsion, 30
Insulin in hemorrhagic shock, 33
Interphalangeal joints, 138
Intoxication, 99, 109–110
Intramedullary nailing
  of bilateral fractures, 402–403
  of femoral fractures, 150, 224–226, 225*f*, 226*f*, 227*f*
  for ipsilateral fractures of hip and femur, 213
  myositis ossificans from, 150
  for tibial fractures, 236, 237*f*, 402
Ischemia
  in compartment syndrome diagnosis, 76, 77*f*
  compartment syndrome from, 72, 73*f*

Jefferson fractures, 186, 186*f*
Jewett nail, 213

Ketamine, 101, 102
Ketone bodies, 129
Kidney
  injury to, 55, 56–59
  operative approach to, 58–59
  in treatment phase of stabilization, 6
Kirschner wires, 297–299, 315
Knee
  dislocation of, traumatic, 265–274, 266*f*, 267*f*
    anterior, 265, 266*f*
    anteromedial parapatellar approach to, 269, 270*f*
    concomitant fractures with, 273
    diagnosis of, 267
    fasciotomy of leg compartments for, 272
    lateral, 265, 266*f*, 268*f*
    lateral approach to, 269, 271*f*
    medial, 265
    medial approach to, 269, 270*f*
    nerve injuries with, 272–273
    posterior, 265, 266*f*
    posterior approach to, 271, 272*f*
    treatment of, 267–271
    types of, 273–274, 273*f*
    vascular complications from, 271–272
  floating, 218, 239–246
    complications of, 246
    femoral fracture of, 239–243, 240–242*f*
    results of treatment of, 243–246
    tibial fracture of, 243, 244–245*f*
  fracture of,
    with head injury, 150–153, 151*f*, 152*f*
    with nerve injury, 159
  stiffness of, 230
    with segmental femoral fracture, 230
    with segmental tibial fractures, 238–239
Knee ligament injuries, 249–263
  arthrography of, 256
  arthroscopic examination of, 256
  cast-brace for, 257
  classification of, 252–253, 252*f*
  fractures associated with, 249, 250–251
    diagnosis of, 253–256
    treatment of, 256–262
  with hip fracture-dislocations, 257–258
  history and physical examination of, 253
  mechanism of, 250–251, 250*f*, 251*f*, 252*f*
  nonoperative management of, 256–257
  operative closure with, 262
  operative management of, 258–262
    for repair of cruciate ligaments, 260–262, 262*f*, 263*f*
    for repair of lateral supporting structures, 260
    for repair of medial supporting structures, 258–259
    for repair of posterior supporting structures, 260–262, 262*f*, 263*f*
  postoperative care of, 262

Knee ligament injuries (*Continued*)
radiographic examination of, 254–255, 254*f*, 255*f*
stress radiographs of, 255, 256*f*, 257*f*
stress testing of, 253–254
traction for, 257, 258*f*
Knodt rods, 172*f*, 173, 176
Knowles pins, 213, 214, 217
Kocher's operation, 58
Kuntscher nail, 213, 214, 217
Kyphosis, 171

Laboratory tests
for compartment syndrome diagnosis, 77–79, 78*f*, 79*t*
for hand and wrist injuries, 368
for nutritional assessment, 130
Lactic acid, 33
Laryngoscopes, 11
Laryngotracheal trauma, 13
management of, 17*t*
signs and symptoms of, 14*t*
Larynx
in deglutition, 9
fracture of, 19
trauma to, 13, 14*t*, 17*t*
Latissimus dorsi free flap, 124, 124*f*
Leg
anatomy of, 74–75, 75*f*
compartments of, 74
decompression of, 81–82
anterolateral approach to, 84–85, 84*f*
posteromedial approach to, 85–86, 85*f*, 86*f*
postoperative care for, 86
skin incisions for, 84
fasciotomy of, double-incision, 82
for knee dislocation, 272
nerves of, 74–75, 76*f*
Ligamentous injuries of knee, 249–263
cast brace for, 257
classification of, 252–253, 252*f*
diagnosis of, 253–256
by arthrography, 256
by arthroscopic examination, 256
by history and physical examination, 253
by radiographic examination, 254–255, 254*f*, 255*f*
by stress radiographs, 255, 256*f*, 257*f*
by stress testing, 253–254
mechanism of, 250–251, 250*f*, 251*f*
nonoperative management of, 256–257
operative closure in repair of, 262
operative management of, 258–262
for repair of cruciate ligaments, 260–262, 261*f*, 262*f*
for repair of lateral supporting structures, 260
for repair of medial supporting structures, 258–260
for repair of posterior supporting structures, 260–262, 261*f*, 262*f*
postoperative care of, 262
treatment options for, 256–262
Lisfranc's joint fractures, 314, 315
Lordosis, 171
Lumbar spinal fracture-dislocations
clinical patterns of paralysis with, 164–166, 165*t*
CT of, 167, 167*f*
diagnosis of, 162–163
pitfalls in, 168–169
initial management of, 169
lateral tomograms of, 166, 166*f*
neurologic evaluation of paraplegic patient with, 163–164, 164*f*
roentgenographic evaluation of, 166
from seat belt injury, 168–169, 169*f*
spinal stability vs instability with, 167–168, 168*f*
surgical treatment of, 169–178
anterior approach to spine for, 176–177
complications after, 178
complications during, 177–178
contraindications to, 173–174
indications for, 169–173
instrumentation for, 170–173, 171*f*, 172*f*
operating techniques for, 175–178
with posterior internal fixation and stabilization, 175–176
postoperative management with, 176
with short compression rods, 176
treatment options for, 174
Lunate, 377, 380
Lungs
in ARDS, 45–46
collapse or compression of, 19
in response to trauma, 44*f*

Malgaigne's hemipelvis fracture-dislocations, 197, 199
Mandibular fractures, 10
Mannitol, 92, 93
MAST garment, 38
Maxillofacial trauma
airway examination with, 14
anesthetic considerations with, 98, 107–108
McIntosh laryngoscope, 11
Median nerve, 74
with distal radius fracture, 142
with elbow fractures, 158
neuropathies involving, 135
Medical antishock trouser, 38
Medical history
of ankle fractures, 294
of hand and wrist injuries, 367
in preanesthetic evaluation, 97
Metacarpal phalangeal joints, 138
Metacarpals, 377, 382–384, 383*f*
Metatarsophalangeal joints, 321
Methohexital sodium, 102
Methylprednisolone, 69
Milk of magnesia, 99
Miller laryngoscope, 11
classification of, 361
diagnosis of, 361–362
operative technique for, 362
Monteggia's fracture-dislocations, 159
Moore pins, 213
Muscle flaps
distant, 124, 124*f*
pedicled, 118
for skin defects about the tibia 118–124, 119*t*, 119*f*, 120–121*f*, 122*f*, 123*f*
Muscles
envelopes of compartments of, 81*f*
of forearm, 73–74
gastrocnemius, 118–121
latissimus dorsi, 124
soleus, 121–124
Myelography
of cervical spinal fracture-dislocation, 184
of lumbar spinal fracture-dislocations, 167
Myocardial contusion, 19, 20, 28
anesthetic considerations with, 108
Myocardial infarction, 39
Myocutaneous flap, 119–121
Myoglobinuria, 79, 79*t*
Myositis ossificans, 139
from intramedullary nailing, 150

Nasopharyngeal airways, 12
Nasotracheal intubation, 11
anesthesia with, 98
Navicular fractures, 313, 315, 319–321
Neck injuries. *See also* Cervical spinal injuries
airway problem with, 13*t*

Neck injuries (*Continued*)
anesthetic considerations with, 107
examination of, 15–17, 15*f*, 16*f*
Nephrography, 56, 57*f*
Nephrostomy, 59, 59*f*
Nerves
axillary, 158, 339
in compartment syndrome diagnosis, 76
cranial, 9, 32
of forearm, 74
in glenohumeral joint dislocation, 339
in hand and wrist injuries, 373–374
injury to
classification of, 157
delayed, 157
with fractures, 117
of arm, 158
classification of, for prognosis, 156–157
of elbow, 158–159
of hip, 159
of knee, 159
of shoulder, 157–158
by interruption, 156
in knee dislocation, 272–273
by manipulation or pressure, 157
median, 74, 135, 142, 158
in neurapraxia, 79, 79*t*, 157
peroneal, 74–75, 135, 159
radial, 140, 158
sciatic, 159
ulnar, 74, 135, 141, 158
Neufeld pin, 213, 214
Neurapraxia
compartment syndrome vs, 79, 79*t*
in nerve injury classification, 157
treatment of, 81
Neurogenic shock, 34, 39
Neuropathies
delayed recognition of, 135, 135*t*
median, 142
sciatic, 159
ulnar, 141
Neurotmesis, 157
Nitrogen balance, 131
Nitrous oxide, 103
Nutrition
for ARDS, 52
assessment of, 130–131
energy stores on body and, 128–130
hyperalimentation and, 131–133
trauma affecting, 130
for wound repair, 114

Obturator nerve injury, 159
Odontoid fractures, 186–187, 188*f*, 189*f*
Olecranon
in distal humeral fractures, 353–355, 353*f*, 354*f*, 355*f*
in elbow joint, 347
fracture of, 363
osteotomy of, 354
reduction of, 358
Operative procedures
delayed, phase of, 6–7
immediate, phase of, 4–5
Oropharyngeal airways, 12
Orotracheal intubation, 11, 11*f*
anesthesia with, 98, 102
Os calcis fractures, 313, 315, 318–319
compartmental syndromes with, 314
internal fixation of, 315
Osteomyelitis, 193
Osteoporosis, disuse, 288
Oxygen
alveolar-arterial difference in, 53
in ARDS therapy, 47–48
arterial content of, in ARDS, 46–47
measurement of consumption of, 53
measurement of delivery of, 53
for post-anesthetic hypoxemia, 104
in shock treatment, 37
in treatment phase of stabilization, 5–6

Pain
of aortic rupture, 29
with compartment syndrome, 75–76
of hand and wrist injuries, 366–367
of myocardial contusion, 28
of rib fractures, 27
of sternal fractures, 27, 28
Palatal valving, 10
Palmaris longus, 73
Pancuronium, 101, 103
Paralysis
clinical patterns of, 164–166, 165*t*
with lumbar injuries, 165
with thoracic injuries, 164
with thoracolumbar junction injuries, 164–165
Paraplegic patient, 163–164, 164*f*
Pelvic fractures, 36
abdominal and urologic injuries with, 207–208
bed rest in treatment of, 199
bladder rupture with, 61, 61*f*
classification of, 196–198, 197*f*
diagnostic procedures for, 198–199
early mobilization of patient with, 206–207
emergency management of, 198–199, 198–199*t*
hemorrhage with, 205–206
open, 208
orthopedic management of, 199–200
pelvic slings for, 199–200
postural reductions and casting for, 199
reduction and external fixation of, 200, 201*f*
reduction and internal fixation of, 200
spinal trauma with, 207
traction for, 138, 199–200
Pelvic slings, 199–200
Pentothal, 102
Pericardicentesis, 20
in knee dislocation, 272–273
Peroneal nerve, 74–75
with femoral traction, 159
with knee injury, 159
neuropathies involving, 135
Phalanges, 385
Piedmont fracture, 377
Plasmanate, 37
Plaster casts
circular, 137
circumferential, 137
for clavicular fractures, 324
for femoral fractures, 375, 375*f*
for foot fractures, 315
for fractures of patients with head injuries, 137–138
for hip fractures, 213
muscle activity with, 137, 137*f*
for tibial fractures, 233
Plaster of Paris, 297
Plates
for ankle fractures, 300–301
for bilateral fractures, 402, 403–404
for segmental femoral fractures, 220, 223*f*, 224*f*
for segmental tibial fractures, 233–236, 235*f*
Pneumothorax
anesthetic considerations with, 109
cardiogenic shock from, 39
closed, 23–25
communicating vs noncommunicating, 23
open, 19, 25
signs of, 19
simple, 23–24
tension, 19, 24–25
Positive end-expiratory pressure, 22

Positive end-expiratory pressure
(*Continued*)
for ARDS, 49–50
side effects of, 49–50
therapeutic effects of, 49
Posterior interosseous nerve, 74
Pressure measurement, intramuscular, 77, 78*f*
Pressure sores, 178
Pressure-regulated ventilator, 48
Projectile injuries of hand and wrist, 396*f*, 397–398, 397*f*, 399*f*
Pronator quadratus, 74
Pronator teres, 73
Proteins, 129
Pulmonary capillary wedge pressure, 51
Pulmonary compliance in ARDS, 45–46
Pulmonary contusion
anesthetic considerations with, 109
clinical features of, 21–23
management of, 22*t*
roentgenographic findings of, 20
Pulmonary vascular resistance, 53

Quadriplegia, 193

Radial artery, 372
Radial nerve
in elbow fracture, 158
in humeral shaft fracture, 140, 158
Radiography. *See* Roentgenography
Radius
in elbow joint, 347
fracture of, 362
articular, 376, 376*f*
distal, 141*f*, 142, 143–144*f*
metaphyseal, 376, 376*f*
treatment of, 376–377, 378*f*, 379*f*
at wrist joint, 377
Reconstruction
bone, 124–125, 126*f*, 127*f*
hand and wrist, 398–400
Recovery phase of treatment, 7
Renal injuries, 55, 56–59
Respiration
mechanics of, 10
monitoring of, with anesthesia, 100
obstruction of, 13–17
Resuscitation, 4
colloid vs crystalloid fluids in, 51–52
Retroperitoneal bleeding, 36
Rib fractures, 26–27
anesthetic considerations with, 109
with clavicular fractures, 324
Ringer's lactate solution, 37
Roentgenography
of acromioclavicular joint sprains, 342
of ankle fractures, 295
of aortic rupture, 29
of ARDS, 45, 45*f*
of burst fractures, 193, 193*f*
of cervical spinal fracture-dislocation, 180, 180*f*
with flexion-extension radiographs, 182–183, 184*f*, 185*f*
with plain radiographs, 181–182, 181*f*
of extremity fractures with head injury, 135
for femur fracture at distal end, 277
of foot fractures, 313–314
of glenohumeral joint dislocation, 337, 341
of hand and wrist injuries, 369
of knee dislocation, 267
of knee ligament injuries, 254–255, 254*f*, 255*f*, 256*f*
of lumbar spinal fracture-dislocations, 162, 162*f*, 166
of pelvic fractures, 198
of pneumothorax, 24
of pulmonary contusion, 20
of scapular fractures, 325
of segmental femoral fractures, 219
Rotator-cuff tear, 338

Sacroiliac joint, 146
Saphenous vein, 93
Scaphoid, 377, 380
Scapula, 323
fractures of, 140, 325–326
diagnosis of, 325
treatment of, 326
Sciatic nerve, 159
Scoliosis, 171
Scopolamine, 99
Screws, 299–300
Scrotum, 65
Seat belt fracture, 168–169, 169*f*, 173
Sellick maneuver, 101
Sepsis
adult respiratory distress syndrome and, 44
from hyperalimentation, 132–133
Septic shock, 34–35, 39–40
Shock
cardiogenic, 33–34, 38–39
grading of, 36*t*
hemorrhagic, 32–33, 35–38
physical signs and symptoms of, 98*t*
hypovolemic, 35–38
neurogenic, 34, 39
septic, 34–35, 39–40
Shotgun wounds, 159–160, 208
Shoulder dislocations
acromioclavicular joint in, 342–343, 343*f*
anterior glenohumeral, 335–339
complications of, 338–339
diagnosis of, 337
fractures associated with, 338
irreducible, 338
management of, 337–338
mechanism of injury of, 335
nerve injury from, 339
pathology and pathogenesis of, 335–337
postoperative complications of, 339
roentgenographic interpretation of, 337
rotator-cuff injury from, 338–339
unrecognized, 338
vascular injury from, 339
inferior glenohumeral, 339
posterior, 340–342
diagnosis of, 341
management of, 341
mechanism of injury of, 340
pathology and pathogenesis of, 340–341
roentgenographic interpretation of, 341
Shoulder fractures
of clavicle, 323–325
complicated, 334–335
with head injury, 140
of humerus, proximal, 325–333
blood supply in, 326
classification of, 327
closed treatment of, 328–330, 329*f*
diagnosis of, 327–328
open treatment of, 330, 331*f*
impression defects with, 333–334
with nerve injury, 157–158
neurovascular deficit of, 334–335, 336*f*
of scapula, 325–326
Skin grafts, 118
in ankle fracture treatment, 304
for hand and wrist injuries, 370–372
homografts, 372
for long bone fractures concomitantly, 407, 410
xenografts-heterografts, 372
Smith's fracture, 376, 377
Snakebites, 73

Sodium bicarbonate, 105
Sodium pentothal, 102
Soft palate, 10
Soft tissue
in foot fractures, 314–315
reconstruction of, 117–118
in tibial fractures, 230, 231
Soleus muscle, 121–124, 122*f*, 123*f*
Spinal cord injury, 164
emergency management of, 179–180
Spinal injuries
cervical
airway problems with, 13–14
anesthetic considerations with, 107
delayed recognition of, 135, 135*t*
examination of, 16–17, 16*f*
fracture-dislocations, 179–194
lumbar, 162–178
anterior operative approach to, 176–177
clinical patterns of paralysis with, 164–166, 165*t*
complications in treatment of, 177–178
diagnosis of, 162–163, 168–169
diagnostic tests for, 166–167, 166*f*, 167*f*
initial management of, 169
neurologic evaluation of paraplegic patient with, 163–164, 164*f*
posterior internal fixation and stabilization of, 175–176
roentgenographic evaluation of, 166
seat belt triad of, 168–169, 169*f*
short compression rods for, 176
stability vs instability with, 167–168, 168*f*
surgical treatment of, 169–174, 175–178
treatment options for, 174
unilateral motor weakness and sensory loss with, 166
neurogenic shock from, 39
with pelvic injuries, 207
Spondylolisthesis, traumatic, 187
Stabilization phase of treatment 5–6
for bleeding disorders, 6
hemodynamics, 5
kidney function in, 6
in oxygenation and organ perfusion, 5–6
Steinmann's pin, 254
for ankle fractures, 297–299
for foot fractures, 315
Sternum, 27–28, 27*t*
Steroids, 69
Straddle fractures, 196, 197
Stridor, 14, 14*f*
Subclavian artery injury, 30
Succinylcholine, 101, 103
Suckling chest wound, 23, 25
Sural nerve, 271
Swallowing, 9–10
Swan-Ganz catheter, 50–51, 51*f*
Symphysis pubis, 146

Talocalcaneal joint, 313
Talonavicular joint, 313
Talus fractures, 313, 315, 316–318
Tarsometatarsal dislocation, 321
Tarsometatarsal joints, 313, 315, 321
Team approach, 3
Temperature, 100–101
Tension pneumothorax, 19, 24–25
cardiogenic shock from, 39
Testis rupture, 64
Tetanus prophylaxis, 115, 368
Thiopental sodium, 102
Thoracic injuries. *See* Chest injuries
Thornton pin, 213
Thrombophlebitis, 178, 310
Thrombus extraction, 91
Thumb fracture, 138, 387, 389*f*, 391*f*
Tibia
in ankle fractures, 292, 304
fractures of, 71, 86
bilateral, 402
casts for, 233
complications of, 237–239
external fixation devices for, 233, 234*f*
in floating knee, 239, 243
infection from, 237–238
intramedullary nails for, 236, 237*f*
with knee dislocations, 273
with knee ligament injuries, 250
malunion of, 238
nonunion of, 238
open, 153, 153*f*, 154*f*
plates for, 234–236, 235*f*
postoperative management of, 236–237
segmental, 230–239
soft-tissue injury with, 230, 231, 243
stabilization of, 233–236
stiffness from, 238–239
stress testing of, 254
swelling from, 239
treatment of, with head injuries, 153
in knee dislocation, 265, 266*f*
muscle flaps for skin defects about, 118–124
gastrocnemius muscle for, 118–121
soleus muscle for, 121–124
Tibial nerve, 271
Tolazine hydrochloride, 93
Tomography
of ankle fractures, 295
of cervical spinal fracture-dislocation, 182, 183*f*
of lumbar spinal injuries, 166, 166*f*
Tongue
in airway obstruction, 12, 12*f*
in deglutition, 10
in sniffing position, 12
Tracheostomy, 11–12, 15, 19, 22
anesthesia with, 98
for ARDS, 48
with maxillofacial trauma, 98
Traction, 138–139, 138*f*
for femur fracture at distal end, 275–276, 276*f*, 278
for ipsilateral fractures of hip and femur, 213
for knee ligament injuries, 257
for pelvic fracture, 199–200
for segmental femoral fractures, 220
Transfusions, blood
for ARDS, 52
bleeding disorders with, 106
Transureteroureterostomy, 59
Trapezium, 377
Trapezoid bone, 377
Trauma center, 404
Triquetrum, 377, 380
Tubocurarine, 101

Ulna
in elbow joint, 347
fracture of, 86
at wrist joint, 377
Ulnar artery, 372
Ulnar nerve, 74
in elbow fracture, 141, 158–159
neuropathies involving, 135
Ureteral injuries, 59–60
Ureteropyelostomy, 59
Ureteroureterostomy, 59
Urethra
reconstruction of, 62
rupture of, 62
classification and diagnosis of, 62–64
confined to Buck's fascia, 63–64, 64*f*
confined to Colles' fascia, 63, 64, 65*f*
inferior to urogenital diaphragm, 63–64

Urethra, rupture of (*Continued*)
superior to urogenital diaphragm, 62–63, 62*f*
Urethrography
in trauma workup, 55
of urethral rupture, 63, 63*f*
Urine tests, 79
Urography, 55
Urologic assessment of injured patient
bladder injuries,
diagnosis of, 55–56
rupture of, 60–62
diagnosis of, 55–56
genital injuries, 64–65
with pelvic fracture, 207–208
renal injuries,
diagnosis of, 55–58
operative approach to, 58–59
trauma workup in, 55
ureteral injuries, 59–60
urethral rupture, 62–64

Vagus nerve, 10
Vasogenic hypotension, 105
Vein graft, 92
Venography, 90–91
Ventilation
anesthetic considerations with obstructions in, 97–98
for ARDS, 48–49
in cervical spinal injuries, 13
in chest injuries, 18–19
determination of status of, 19
for respiratory acidosis, 105
weaning patient from mechanical, 50
Ventilators, 48
Vesicostomy, 63
Volkmann's contracture
from compartment syndromes, 71, 72*f*, 87
incidence of, 87
prevention of, 88, 88*f*
from drug overdose-limb compression, 73
Volume-regulated ventilator, 48

Wainwright splint, 213
Wrist injuries
of carpal bones, 380–381
closed space compression syndrome from, 370
diagnosis of, 377–380
dislocations, 367*f*, 380
examination of, physical, 367, 368–369
fractures, 138, 374–375
of ligaments, 381–382
management of, 365
anesthesia in, 369
with blast injuries, 371*f*, 393*f*, 397
with crush injuries, 389, 392*f*, 397
by fasciotomy, 366, 370
hemorrhage in, 366
immobilization in, 375
indepth wound evaluation in, 372
initial, 366–368
by laboratory tests in, 368
with massive injuries, 387–398
mobilization and rehabilitation in, 375
open treatment of, 370
primary wound closure and resurfacing in, 365, 370–372
principles of, 365–366, 367*f*
with projectile injuries, 396*f*, 397–398, 397*f*, 399*f*
reconstruction of joint in, 398–400
secondary wound closure and resurfacing in, 372
tetanus prophylaxis in, 368
wound culture and gram stains for, 369
wound toilet in, 369–370, 371*f*
pain of, 366–367
patient history of, 367, 368
roentgenography of, 369
skeletal system in, 374–375, 375*f*
tendons and nerves in, 373–374, 373*f*
vascular system with, 372
Wrist joint, 365, 377

Zickel nail, 213, 214